Handbook of Informatics

for Nurses and Healthcare Professionals

Sixth Edition

Toni Hebda, PhD, RN-C, CNE MSIS
Professor MSN Program
Chamberlain College of Nursing, Downers Grove, IL 60515

Kathleen Hunter, PhD, FAAN, RN-BC, CNE
Professor MSN Program
Chamberlain College of Nursing, Downers Grove, IL 60515

Patricia Czar, RN
Information Systems Consultant
Pittsburgh, PA

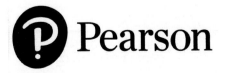 Pearson

330 Hudson Street, NY NY 10013

Publisher: Julie Alexander
Director of Portfolio Management, Nursing: Katrin Beacom
Editorial Assistant: Erin Sullivan
Managing Content Producer: Melissa Bashe
Content Producer: Michael Giacobbe
Design Coordinator: Mary Siener
Vice President of Sales and Marketing: David Gesell
Vice President, Director of Marketing: Brad Parkins
Director, Digital Studio: Amy Peltier
Digital Project Manager: Jeff Henn
Full-Service Project Management and Composition: SPi Global
Full-Service Project Managers: Sreemeenakshi Raghothaman, Anitha Vijayakumar, SPi Global
Editorial Project Manager: Dan Knott, SPi Global
Manufacturing Buyer: Maura Zaldivar-Garcia, LSC Communications, Inc.
Cover Designer: Laurie Entringer

Notice: Care has been taken to confirm the accuracy of information presented in this book. The authors, editors, and the publisher, however, cannot accept any responsibility for errors or omissions or for consequences from application of the information in this book and make no warranty, express or implied, with respect to its contents.

Cataloging in Publication data is available at the Library of Congress

1   18

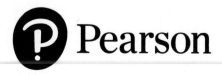

ISBN 10:   0-13-471101-7
ISBN 13: 978-0-13-471101-0

Contents

Preface

The idea for *Handbook of Informatics for Nurses & Healthcare Professionals* first came from the realization that there were few resources that provided practical information about computer applications and information systems in healthcare. From its inception, this book served as a guide for nurses and other healthcare professionals who needed to learn how to adapt and use computer applications and informatics in the workplace. Over time, this text became a reliable resource for students in a variety of healthcare professions who needed to develop informatics competencies. This book serves undergraduates who need a basic understanding, as well as those who require more depth, such as informatics nurse specialists, clinical nurse leaders, doctoral students, and other healthcare professionals.

After a thorough revision in response to reviewers and users of the book, the sixth edition reflects the rapid changes in healthcare information technology (HIT) and informatics. The authors endeavour to provide an understanding of the concepts, skills, and tasks that are needed for healthcare professionals today and to achieve the federal government's national information technology goals to help transform healthcare delivery.

The sixth edition builds upon the expertise provided by contributors currently involved in day-to-day informatics practice, education, and research. Both the primary editors and the contributors share an avid interest and involvement in HIT and informatics, as well as experience in the field, involvement in informatics groups, and a legacy of national and international presentations and scholarly publications.

New to This Edition

- New! All chapters thoroughly revised to reflect the current and evolving practice of health information technology and informatics
- New! Chapter on informatics theory and practice connects theoretical concepts to applications (chapter 2)
- New! Coverage of technology and caring and their symbiotic relationship

- New! Content on ethical use of information encompasses appropriate and inappropriate behaviour and actions, and of right and wrong.
- New! Information on analytics and data science that explains how Big Data applies to healthcare
- New! Cutting-edge content on wearable and mobile technology security, and its impact on nursing and patient care
- New! Academic electronic health record resources and the role they play in educating the next generation of healthcare providers on documentation principles
- New! Hardware and software appendix (appendix A)
- New! Guide to the Internet (appendix B)
- New! An Overview of Tools for the Informatics Nurse (appendix C)

Changes to This Edition

- The sixth edition streamlines content by combining chapters with topics that fit together, and shifting hardware, software, and information on the Internet to new appendices.
- This edition reworks previous content on information systems training and presents it within the context of workforce development. The content still retains the emphasis upon privacy and confidentiality, introduction of information policies, educational methods and resources. New content on evaluation models and training on backup procedures has also been added.
- Former content on integration, interoperability and health information exchange is now presented within the context of information networks and information exchange.
- Moves from defining evidence-based practice to a discussion of levels of evidence and using informatics to support evidence-based practice and research.
- Separate chapters on policy, legislation, regulatory, reimbursement, and accreditation issues were combined to better show the connection among these

areas and the relationship between them and information system design and use.

- Experts from various health disciplines cover the latest on the interprofessional aspects of informatics with more emphasis on interdisciplinary approaches.

- Increases focus on current electronic health record issues while decreasing coverage of the historical evolution of EHRs.

- Highlights strategic planning and project management.

- Underscores the importance of patient engagement and shared decision making.

- Expands content on simulation and virtual learning environments.

Hallmark Features

Learning Objectives—Learning Objectives appear at the beginning of each chapter and identify what readers can expect to learn in the chapter.

Future Directions—As the last section in each chapter, Future Directions forecasts how the topic covered in the chapter might evolve in the upcoming years.

Case Study Exercises—Case studies at the end of each chapter discuss common, real-life applications, which review and reinforce the concepts presented in the chapter.

Summary—The Summary at the end of the chapter highlights the key concepts and information from the chapter to assist in the review.

References—Resources used in the chapter appear at the end.

Glossary—The glossary familiarizes readers with the vocabulary used in this book and in healthcare informatics. We recognize that healthcare professionals have varying degrees of computer and informatics knowledge. This book does not assume that the reader has prior knowledge of computers. All computer terms are defined in the chapter, in the glossary at the end of the book, and on the Online Student Resources Web site.

Organization

The book is divided into three sections: Information and Informatics, Information Systems Development Life Cycle, and Specialty Applications. The major themes of privacy, confidentiality, and information security are woven throughout the book. Likewise, project management is a concept introduced in the strategic planning chapter and carried through other chapters. Chapters include content on the role of the informatics professional, future directions relative to the topic, summary bullet points, and a case study.

Section I: Information and Informatics

This section provides a foundation for why information and informatics are important to healthcare. It details the relationship between policy, legislation, regulation and accreditation and reimbursement and information system use.

- Chapter 1: Provides a definition of informatics and its significance for healthcare, discusses healthcare professionals as knowledge workers, addresses the need for uniform data and the relationship between data, big data, and evidence. This chapter also addresses the increased prevalence of information technology in healthcare, major issues in healthcare that are driving the adoption of information technology, what is necessary to create an informatics culture, and includes a special section on caring and technology.

- Chapter 2: Provides information on informatics theory and practice, and nursing informatics as a discipline.

- Chapter 3: Emphasizes effective and ethical use of data and information, and includes a discussion of big data challenges and issues. Data characteristics, types, integrity, and management are covered. Clinician and informaticist roles pertaining to this area are discussed.

- Chapter 4: Addresses electronic resources for healthcare professionals, basic concepts and applications of the Internet, including criteria for evaluating the quality of online information.

- Chapter 5: Discusses informatics to support evidence-based practice and research. Concepts include levels of evidence, information literacy, managing research data and information, creating and maintaining the infrastructure needed to support research, dissemination of evidence, and effecting practice change.

- Chapter 6: Examines the relationship between policy, legislation, accreditation, reimbursement and HIT design and use.

- Chapter 7: Provides information on electronic health records including definition, components, incentives for adoption, benefits, current status, selection criteria, implications for collection of meaningful data and big data, current issues, and future directions.

- Chapter 8: Provides an overview of types of healthcare information systems, including clinical information systems and administrative information systems, as well as decision support, knowledge representation, and smart data.

Section II: Information Systems Development Life Cycle

This section covers information and issues related to the information systems development life cycle.

- Chapter 9 This chapter discusses the importance of strategic planning for information management, HIT acquisition and use and provides an overview of project management and information system selection considerations. The role of informatics professionals, particularly informatics nurse specialists, in the planning process and project management are addressed, as is the process to introduce change.

- Chapter 10: Addresses the concepts of usability and health informatics applications inclusive of the role that usability plays in the system life cycle and methods of usability assessment.

- Chapter 11: Covers information system implementation, maintenance, and evaluation.

- Chapter 12: Provides a comprehensive look at workforce development in relation to health information technology use.

- Chapter 13: Discusses information security and confidentiality, including practical information on ways to protect information housed in information systems and on mobile devices and addresses security for wearable and implantable information technology.

- Chapter 14: Provides detailed information about health information exchanges.

- Chapter 15: Provides an overview of the role of standardized terminology and language in informatics. Also includes an outline of individual languages and classifications used in healthcare.

- Chapter 16: Discusses the relationship between strategic planning for the organization and the significance of maintaining uninterrupted operations for patient care. Also touches on legal requirements to maintain and restore information. Much of this chapter is geared for the professional working in information services.

Section III: Specialty Applications

This section covers specialty applications of informatics.

- Chapter 17: Details ways that information technology and informatics can support education of healthcare professionals, including sections on simulation and virtual learning environments.

- Chapter 18: Emphasizes the relationship between health and information literacy, patient engagement, shared decision-making, changing healthcare delivery models, patient satisfaction, outcomes, and healthcare reform. Discusses applications of consumer health informatics.

- Chapter 19: Examines telehealth and connected healthcare applications, starting with a historical perspective and including driving forces, applications, and implications for providers as well as informatics professionals.

- Chapter 20: Explores public health informatics and its use to maintain and improve population health.

Three appendices are included. Appendix A provides basic information on hardware and software for the reader who needs a better understanding of this area. Appendix B provides information on the Internet. Appendix C provides an overview of some tools for the informatics nurse.

Instructor Resources

Lecture PowerPoint showcases key points for each chapter.

Test Generator offers question items, making test creation quick and simple.

Student Resources

New! eText offers a rich and engaging experience with interactive exercises. Readers can access online or via the Pearson eText app. Note:
Faculty can opt to package an eText access code
card with the print textbook, or students can
purchase access to the eText online.

Notice Care has been taken to confirm the accuracy of information presented in this book. The authors, editors, and the publisher, however,
cannot accept any responsibility for errors or omissions or for consequences from application of the information in this book and make no
warranty, express or implied, with respect to its contents.

Acknowledgments

Special thanks to Kathy Hunter, who agreed to join me on this 6th edition, lending her knowledge, insights, and support when I most needed it and never said "no" despite her many other commitments.

A special thanks to Patricia Czar, RN, without whom there would be no *Handbook of Informatics for Nurses & Healthcare Professionals* today. Pat actively contributed to the book from the original outline through to the present, providing her knowledge, insights, organizational skills, support, and friendship. Pat was active in informatics for more than 25 years, serving as manager of clinical systems at a major medical center where she was responsible for planning, design, implementation, and ongoing support for all of the clinical information systems. Pat was also active in several informatics groups, presented nationally and internationally, and served as a mentor for many nursing and health informatics students. She is now fully retired and enjoying time with her family.

We acknowledge our gratitude to our loved ones for their support as we wrote and revised this book. We are grateful and excited to have work from our contributors who graciously shared their knowledge and expertise for this edition. We are grateful to our co-workers and professional colleagues who provided encouragement and support throughout the process of conceiving and writing this book. We appreciate the many helpful comments offered by our reviewers. Finally, we thank Lisa Rahn, Michael Giacobbe, Susan Hannahs, Daniel Knott, Taylor Scuglik, and all of the persons who worked on the production of this edition for their encouragement, suggestions, and support.

Thank You

This edition brings in work from multiple contributors for a robust coverage of topics throughout the book. We thank them for their time and expertise. We would also like to thank all of the reviewers who carefully looked at the entire manuscript. You have helped shape this book to become a more useful text for everyone.

Contributors

Diane A. Anderson, DNP, MSN, RN, CNE
Chapter 17: Using Informatics to Educate
*Associate Professor, MSN Specialty Tracks ~ Nurse
Educator, Chamberlain College, Downers Grove, IL*

Ami Bhatt, DNP, MBA, RN, CHPN, CHCI
Chapter 13: Information Security and Confidentiality
*Dr. Bhatt is currently enrolled in the DNP to PhD program
at University of Nevada, Las Vegas, NV*

Sunny Biddle, MSN, RN
Chapter 6: Policy, Legislation, and Regulation Issues
for Informatics Practice
*Circulating Nurse in the Operating Room at Genesis
Healthcare in Zanesville, OH and Clinical Instructor for
Central Ohio Technical College in Newark, OH*

Jane M. Brokel, PhD, RN, FNI
Chapter 8: Healthcare Information Systems
Chapter 14: Information Networks and Information
Exchange
Section Instructor at Simmons College, Boston, MA
Adjunct faculty for the University of Iowa College of
Nursing, Iowa, City, IA

Jennifer A. Brown, MSN, RN, HNB-BC
Chapter 1: An Overview of Informatics in
Healthcare
Faculty, Bronson School of Nursing at Western
Michigan University in Kalamazoo, Michigan in the
undergraduate and RN-BSN programs.

Lisa Eisele, MSN, RN
Chapter 19: Connected Healthcare (Telehealth and
Technology-enabled healthcare)
Chief - Quality, Performance & Risk Management
Manchester VA Medical Center, Manchester VA

Sue Evans, MSN RN-BC
Chapter 11: System Implementation, Maintenance,
and Evaluation
Informatics Nurse II University of Pittsburgh Medical
Center East, Monroeville, PA

Athena Fernandes DNP, MSN, RN-BC
Appendix A: Hardware and Software
Appendix B: A Guide to the Internet and World Wide Web
Senior Physician Systems Analyst, Penn Medicine
Chester County Hospital, West Chester, PA

Carolyn S. Harmon, DNP, RN-BC
Chapter 16: Continuity Planning and Management
Clinical Assistant Professor and Program Director for
the Masters of Nursing Informatics and the Masters
of Nursing Administration at University of South
Carolina, Columbia, SC

Toni Hebda, PhD, RN-BC, MSIS, CNE
Chapter 3: Effective and Ethical Use of Data and
Information
Chapter 18: Consumer Health Informatics
Professor, Chamberlain College of Nursing MSN
Program, Downers Grove, IL

Taryn Hill, PhD, RN
Caring for the Patient Not the Computer in Chapter 1:
An Overview of Informatics in Healthcare
Dean of Academic Affairs for Chamberlain College of
Nursing, Columbus, OH

Diane Humbrecht, DNP, RN
Chapter 12: Workforce Development
Chief Nursing Informatics Officer, Abington Jefferson
Health, Abington, PA

Kathleen Hunter, PhD, RN-BC, CNE
Chapter 3: Effective and Ethical Use of Data and
Information
Chapter 7:   Electronic Health Record Systems
Professor, Chamberlain College of Nursing MSN
Program, Downers Grove, IL

Brenda Kulhanek, PhD, MSN, MS, RN-BC
Chapter 4: Electronic Resources for Healthcare
Professionals
Chapter 12: Workforce Development
AVP of Clinical Education for HCA in Nashville, TN

Susan Matney, PhD, RN-C, FAAN
Chapter 15: The Role of Standardized Terminology
and Language in Informatics
Senior Medical Informaticist, Intermountain
Healthcare, Murray, UT

Julie McAfooes, MS, RN-BC, CNE, ANEF, FAAN
High-fidelity simulation, software, support, and
certification in Chapter 17: Using Informatics to Educate
Web Development Manager for the online
RN-to-BSN Option at the Chamberlain of Nursing,
Downers Grove, IL

Jeri A. Milstead, PhD, RN, NEA-BC, FAAN
Chapter 6: Policy, Legislation, and Regulation Issues
for Informatics Practice
Professor and Dean Emerita, University of
Toledo College of Nursing, Toledo, OH

Patricia Mulberger, MSN, RN-BC
Special Considerations with Mobile Computing in
Chapter 13: Information Security and Confidentiality
Clinical Informatics Quality Supervisor, Kalispell
Regional Healthcare, Kalispell MT

Melody Rose, DNP, RN
Chapter 5: Using Informatics to Support
Evidence-based Practice and Research
Chapter 18: Consumer Health Informatics
Assistant Professor of Nursing. Cumberland University
Jeanette C. Rudy School of Nursing, Lebanon, TN

Carolyn Sipes, PhD, CNS, APN, PMP, RN-BC
Chapter 8: Healthcare Information Systems
Chapter 9: Strategic Planning, Project Management,
and Health Information Technology (IT) Selection
Appendix C: An Overview of Tools for the
Informatics Nurse
Professor, Chamberlain College, Downers Grove, IL

Rebecca J Sisk, PhD, RN, CNE
Virtual Learning Environment in Chapter 17: Using
Informatics to Educate
Professor, Chamberlain College Downers Grove, IL

Rayne Soriano, PhD, RN
Chapter 7: Electronic Health Record Systems
Regional Director for Medicare Operations and Clinical
Effectiveness. Kaiser Permanente, San Francisco, CA

Nancy Staggers, PhD, RN, FAAN
Chapter 10: Improving the Usability of Health
Informatics Applications
President, Summit Health Informatics and adjunct
professor, Biomedical Informatics and College of Nurs-
ing University of Utah College, Salt Lake City, UT

Maxim Topaz PhD, MA, RN
Chapter 2: Informatics Theory and Practice
Harvard Medical School & Brigham Women's Health
Hospital, Boston, MA, USA

Marisa L. Wilson DNSc MHSc RN-BC CPHIMS FAAN
Chapter 20: Public Health Informatics
Associate Professor and Specialty Track coordinator
for the MSN Nursing Informatics program at the University of Alabama at Birmingham School of Nursing.

Reviewers

Janet Baker DNP, APRN, ACNS-BC, CPHQ, CNE
Associate Dean Graduate Nursing Programs
Ursuline College, The Breen School of Nursing
Pepper Pike, Ohio

Theresa L. Calderone, EdD, MEd, MSN, RN-BC
Assistant Professor of Nursing
Indiana University of Pennsylvania
Indiana, PA

Vicki Evans, MSN, RN, CEN, CNE
Assistant Professor of Nursing
University of Mary-Hardin Baylor
Belton, TX

Kathleen Hirthler DNP, CRNP, FNP-BC
Chair, Graduate Nursing; Associate Professor
Wilkes University, Passan School of Nursing
Wilkes Barre, PA

Arpad Kelemen, Ph.D.
Associate Professor of Informatics
University of Maryland School of Nursing
Baltimore, MD

Michelle Rogers, PhD, MS, MA, BS
Associate Professor of Information Science
Drexel University
Philadelphia, PA

Charlotte Seckman, PhD, RN-BC, CNE, FAAN
Associate Professor, Nursing Informatics Program
University of Maryland School of Nursing
Baltimore, MD

Nadia Sultana, DNP, MBA, RN-BC
Program Director and Clinical Assistant Professor, Nursing Informatics
Program
New York University
New York, NY

About the Authors

Toni Hebda, PhD, RN-C, CNE, is a professor with the Chamberlain College of Nursing. MSN Program teaching in the nursing informatics track. She has held several academic and clinical positions over the years and worked as a system analyst. Her interest in informatics provided a focus for her dissertation, subsequently led her to help establish a regional nursing informatics group, obtain a graduate degree in information science, and conduct research related to informatics. She is a reviewer for the *Online Journal of Nursing Informatics.* She is a member of informatics groups and has presented and published in the field.

Kathy Hunter, PhD, FAAN, RN-BC, CNE, is a professor with the Chamberlain College of Nursing MSN Program, teaching in the nursing informatics track. She has more than 40 years of experience in the fields of nursing informatics, healthcare informatics, and nursing education. After conducting clinical practice in critical care and trauma nursing for several years, she began practicing nursing informatics (NI), working with end users and with information systems design, development, testing, implementation and evaluation. She has presented nursing-informatics research in national and international meetings as well as publishing numerous articles in peer-reviewed journals. Collaborating in a community of practice with nursing-informatics faculty at Chamberlain, Dr. Hunter led the work resulting in the development of the TIGER-based Assessment of Nursing Informatics Competencies (TANIC) tool.

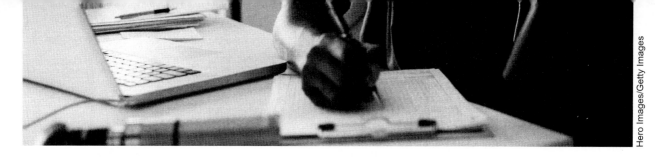

Chapter 1
An Overview of Informatics in Healthcare

Jennifer A. Brown, MSN, RN, HNB-BC
Taryn Hill, PhD, RN
Toni Hebda, PhD, RN-C

 ## Learning Objectives

After completing this chapter, you should be able to:

- Provide an overview of the current state of healthcare delivery.

- Discuss the role that technology plays in healthcare.

- Provide a definition for informatics.

- Discuss the significance of informatics for healthcare.

- Describe the process required to create an informatics culture.

- Examine the relationship between technology, informatics, and caring.

The healthcare delivery system today is a complex system faced with multiple, competing demands. Among these demands are: calls for increased quality, safety, and transparency; evolving roles for practitioners; a shift in consumer-provider relationships; eliminating disparities in care; adopting new models of care; the development of a learning health system (LHS); advanced technology as a means to support healthcare processes and treatment options; and providing a workforce with the skills needed to work in a highly technology-laden environment that is reliant upon data and information to function.

Technology is a pervasive part of every aspect of society including healthcare delivery. Many suggest that health information technology (HIT) provides the tools to enable the delivery of safe, quality care in an effective, efficient manner while improving communication and decreasing costs (Institute of Medicine, 2012). HIT was named as one of nine levers that stakeholders could use to align their efforts with the National Strategy for Quality Improvement in Health Care, a collaborative effort also known as the National Quality Strategy, a mandate of the 2010 Affordable Care Act (ACA). The National Quality Strategy, published in 2011, represented input from more than 300 groups and organizations from various sectors of healthcare industry and the public (Agency for Healthcare Research and Quality, 2017). Yet, the healthcare sector has been slow to adopt and use technology to its full potential. Lucero (2017) noted that the failure for technology in healthcare to live up to its full promise to the present is not surprising given the complexity of healthcare delivery. So, what is information technology? Information technology (IT) is a broad term referring to the process of searching, organizing, and managing data supported by the use of computers. It has also come to include electronic communication. IT represents only a portion of the technology found in healthcare today, but is significant because data leads to information, which in turn provides knowledge. This chapter and the book as a whole will discuss the role that informatics plays to help address the multiple challenges facing healthcare today.

Informatics

Before we can discuss the role of informatics in healthcare, infomatics must first be defined. The American Medical Informatics Association (AMIA) (2017, Para. 1) states that informatics is an interdisciplinary field that draws from, as well as contributes to, "computer science, decision science, information science, management science, cognitive science, and organizational theory." Informatics drives innovation in how information and knowledge management are approached. Its broad scope encompasses natural language processing, data mining, research, decision support, and genomics. Health informatics encompasses several fields that include:

- *Translational bioinformatics.* This area deals with the storage, analysis, and interpretation of large volumes of data. It includes research into ways to integrate findings into the work of scientists, clinicians, and healthcare consumers.

- *Clinical research informatics.* This area concentrates on discovery and management of new knowledge pertinent to health and disease from clinical trials and via secondary data use.

- *Clinical informatics.* The concentration here is on the delivery of timely, safe, efficient, effective, evidence-based and patient-centered care (Levy, 2015). Examples include nursing informatics and medical informatics. Nursing informatics has its own scope and standards for practice as set forth by the American Nurses Association (ANA) as well as certification established by the American Nurses Credentialing Center (ANCC) (American Nurses Association, 2015a). AMIA began the process, in 2007, of defining clinical informatics and its competencies, to lay the foundation for a credentialing process to recognize competence of clinical informaticists (Shortliffe, 2011). There is also discussion at a global level on specialty-board certification for physicians in clinical informatics (Gundlapall et al., 2015).

- *Consumer health informatics.* The focus here is the consumer, or patient, view and the structures and processes that enable consumers to manager their own health.

- *Public health informatics.* Efforts here include surveillance, prevention, health promotion, and preparedness.

As might be surmised from a review of the above list, there are areas of overlap among the fields.

Informatics and its subspecialties—including nursing informatics—continue to evolve as has the terminology used to discuss this field. For example, medical informatics was previously used as the umbrella term under which the subspecialties of health informatics fell.

The Relevance of Informatics for Healthcare

Informatics is an essential component of healthcare today. The Institute of Medicine (2013a) noted its vision for the development of a continuously learning health system in which science, informatics, incentives, and culture are aligned for continuous improvement and innovation, and new knowledge is captured as a by-product of care processes. Together, HIT and informatics have been hailed as tools that can streamline processes, improve the quality of care delivered, reduce mortality, cut costs, and collect data to support learning (Institute of Medicine, 2012, 2015; Kohli & Tan, 2016; Lucero, 2017; Luo, Min, Gopukumar, & Yiqing, 2016; McCullough, Parente, & Town, 2016; Pinsonneault, Addas, Qian, Dakshinamoorthy, & Tamblyn, 2017). In fact, the Institute of Medicine (2013b, p. 1) stated that "digital health data are the lifeblood of a continuous learning health system." Achieving this learning health system will require the work of many individuals and organizations.

There are several factors to consider on the journey to a learning healthcare system. These include:

- Healthcare professionals are knowledge workers.
- Structures must be in place to support the collection, interpretation, and reuse of data in a meaningful way.
- Evidence-based practices are a pre-requisite to achieving optimal outcomes.
- Big data and data analytics are quickly becoming a major source of evidence, augmenting, and even replacing, other traditional forms of evidence such as clinical trials.
- HIT and all forms of technology are present but best use is inconsistent.
- Healthcare reform and a learning healthcare system are intricately linked.
- Patient safety and the need to improve quality of care are drivers for healthcare reform.

Each of these will be discussed briefly.

Knowledge Work

Nurses and other healthcare professionals have a long tradition of gathering data, which is then used to create information and knowledge. When previous knowledge and experience are applied appropriately to take action or intervene in some fashion, it is known as wisdom. These processes constitute a major part of the clinician's day and, when done well, yield good outcomes. As an example, a piece of data without context has no meaning. The number 68 in isolation conveys nothing. It could be an age, a pulse rate, or even a room number, but in and of itself, there is no way to know what it means. However, if 68 is determined to be a pulse rate, the nurse can make the determination that this falls within the normal range, indicating that the patient is in no distress and requires no intervention. On the other hand, if that same number represents the rate of respirations per minute, the patient is in respiratory distress and immediate intervention is required.

Gaberson and Langston (2017) noted that changes in the healthcare system, inclusive of demands for safe, accessible, quality care, have increased both the awareness of and demand for well-prepared knowledge workers. Gaberson and Langston also cited the assertion of the landmark 2010 Institute of Medicine report, *The Future of Nursing: Leading Change, Advancing Health*, that nursing is an appropriate profession to play a major role in transforming the healthcare system; yet, nursing education has not adequately prepared its graduates for this role. As a consequence, there is a need to better prepare nurses—and other healthcare professionals—during their basic education for this role and to provide better options to aid the new professional to assume the knowledge-worker role and to maintain essential competencies in this area.

Structures to Support Meaningful Use of Data

To be useful, data and information must be available when needed, to whom it is needed, and in a form that can be analyzed or used. Historically, the healthcare delivery system has collected huge amounts of data and information from different sources and in different formats, creating data silos within departments and facilities. Without organization, this data and information has limited value, even at its collection site, and is not amenable to sharing for learning purposes. The use of electronic health records (EHRs) moved data and information to a digital format, which is conducive to organization, analysis, and sharing, but differences in format still make analysis difficult. Data exists in raw and processed states and unstructured and structured forms. Examples of unstructured data include documents, email, and multimedia. Structured data fits into predetermined classifications such as that seen with a list of selectable options that can easily be quantified. Even before the widespread adoption of EHRs, there was a growing recognition that improved communication among professionals required the adoption of standardized languages and terminologies to ensure that a concept had the same meaning in all settings; this also makes generalization of research findings possible. One example of a standardized language that is familiar to most nurses is NANDA, which was created by the North American Nursing Diagnosis Association to provide standardized terms for nursing diagnoses. Standardized languages and terminologies can be integrated into EHRs. A lack of data standardization jeopardizes opportunities for learning because important data may not be available for analysis (Auffray et al., 2016). Standardization of data and its collection in a digital format in databases facilitate collecting, sorting, retrieval, selection, and aggregation of data to a degree never before possible. Aggregate data can be analyzed to discover trends and, subsequently, to inform and educate.

Researchers use both qualitative and quantitative methods to analyze data. Qualitative methods focus on numbers and frequencies, with the goal of finding relationships or variables specific to an outcome. Qualitative methods are variable and not focused on counting. These methods can include any data captured. This data can be in the form of questionnaires, surveys including web surveys, interviews, list serves, and email. Electronic data collection tools include personal digital assistants or laptop computers.

Another important facet of information access is related to the electronic literature databases for the health sciences, business, history, government, law, and ethics that healthcare professionals and administrators use to keep up-to-date and inform their practices. Libraries purchase electronic literature databases that users can easily search using keywords, Boolean search operators, title, author, or date to find relevant information. Literature databases use key terms to index collections. Medical subject headings (MeSH) are used by the controlled vocabulary thesaurus of the National Library of Medicine (NLM) to index articles in PubMed, a free search engine maintained by the NLM. PubMed is used to access the MEDLINE bibliographic database. Some other examples of literature databases relevant for healthcare include EBSCO, Ovid, ProQuest, CINAHL, and Cochrane Library. Becoming familiar with the databases most relevant to one's purpose or focus is important. Adept use requires time and practice. When searching a database, one should define the subject and the question; then, search for the evidence in multiple components of the literature: for example, use evidence from multiple studies (not just one random study), incorporate what was learned into practice, and evaluate the impact of what was implemented.

Evidence-Based Practice

Evidence-based practice (EBP) entails using the current best evidence for patient-care decisions in order to improve the consistency and quality of patient outcomes (Mackey & Bassendowski, 2017). It requires critical thought processes. EBP provides the foundation for clinical-practice guidelines and clinical decision-support tools that are widely found in healthcare organizations today. EBP in nursing evolved from Florence Nightingale's idea that she could improve patient outcomes through systematic observations and application of subsequent learning. EBP has been further defined by the International Council of Nurses (2012) as an approach that incorporates a search for the best available, current evidence with clinical expertise and patient preferences.

Big Data and Big Data Analytics

According to the National Academies of Sciences, Engineering, and Medicine (2017), a learning health system is one that uses real-time evidence for continuous improvement and innovation. The implications of real-time evidence are that traditional research and publication cycles where months, or even years, transpire from the time of research until dissemination of results no longer satisfy the criteria for best evidence because data may no longer be current or timely. Real-time data for analysis requires different methods, tools, and dissemination methods. Enter big data and big data analytics.

Big data are very large data sets that are beyond human capability to manage, let alone analyze, without the aid of information technology. Big data has been collected for years by retail-shopping organizations. As an example, consider the shopper's card that nearly everyone has for their favorite grocery store. In exchange for special store discounts on select merchandise or points earned for discounts, the store collects information on shopper preferences every time the card is used. The aggregate data that healthcare providers collect via their EHRs is a type of big data. Another example of big data is seen when healthcare providers submit data collected for meaningful use core data (with one exemplar being smoking status) to the US Centers for Medicare and Medicaid Services (CMS) (2010), CMS analyzes the data for trends, with the intent to better allocate funds and services to improve care coordination and population health.

Big data, and the technologies used to reveal the knowledge within it, provide new opportunities for healthcare to discover new insights and create new methods to improve healthcare quality (Luo, Min, Gopukumar, & Yiqing, 2016). Furthermore, the computing speed associated with big data (Kaggal et al., 2016) provides a promising development to make the LHS possible. A new science, known as data science, has emerged to deal with all aspects of big data including data format, cleaning, mining, management, and analysis.

Analysis of big data, or analytics, looks for patterns in data, then uses models to recommend actions (Wills, 2014). Analytics can be used to forecast the likelihood of an event. Real-time analytics use current data from multiple sources to support decisions; this may result in powerful tools useful at the bedside as well as to support executive-level thought processes. Business intelligence is another term that is used when discussing best use of data, although business intelligence is a broader term that encompasses a plan, strategy, and tool sets to support decisions.

Increased Prevalence of Technology in Care Settings

According to recent projections, US hospital adoption of EHRs is expected to surpass 98% by the end of 2017, with adoption by physicians running slightly below that figure (Bulletin Board, 2016; Orion Market Research, 2017). EHRs are also found in long-term care settings, although adoption rates there lag behind hospital and physician-office settings (EHR Adoption, 2017) . There are also many different types of technology found at the bedside, or point of care. These range from point of care computer terminals to access patient records or literature databases to monitoring biometric measures such as pulse, heart rate and rhythm, blood pressure, oxygen saturation, and many tests that were formally only done in laboratory settings. There are also medication-dispensing cabinets, smart-technology that includes medication-administration infusion pumps that link with provider order entry, pharmacy, and medication-administration systems for greater safety. A growing number of implantable devices such as insulin pumps, pacemakers, and defibrillators, and various telehealth applications such as telestroke consultations that allow the neurologist at another site to evaluate and communicate with the stroke victim and attending family and care givers. There are also telesitter applications that allow an individual at a central location to monitor several patients at one time, observing them for attempts to get out of bed without assistance, and having the capability to verbally reorient them or call for further assistance. Many of these technologies already have the capability to communicate and input data into EHRs. There are also voice-activated, hands-free communication devices for staff use. Technology is supplementing work once done by ancillary staff. There are robots that deliver supplies while other robots use ultraviolet light to disinfect patient rooms and operating rooms.

The range of technology available in the home includes telemonitoring and care devices to track congestive heart patients, the mentally ill, and many more conditions. The number and range of mobile applications available to track wellness and manage chronic healthcare conditions is growing at an exponential rate. Patients have implantable devices to monitor their cardiac function, control seizures, control pain, and control the function of prosthetics. Robots to assist with care are expected to become commonplace in the near future.

The move to a technology-laden environment has implications for informatics. Informatics specialists are prepared to design, implement, and evaluate technologies that support healthcare providers and consumers.

Healthcare Reform

Health reform has many drivers. The United States spends more per capital on healthcare than any other nation in the world, without commensurate results (Robert Wood Johnson Foundation, 2017). In one effort to enact change, value-based payment models reward providers for quality of care provided and efficient resource use rather than volume of services. In another effort, the enactment of the American Recovery and Reinvestment Act (ARRA) in 2009, along with its component Health Information Technology for Economic and Clinical Health (HITECH) Act, provided economic stimuli and incentives for the adoption of EHRs, in alignment with the goal that each person in the United States would have a certified digital health record by 2014. As of 2016, this goal was achieved by more than 98% of nonfederal acute care hospitals. These digital records meet the technical capabilities, functionality, and security criteria promulgated by the Center for Medicaid and Medicare Services (Office of the National Coordinator for Health Information Technology, 2017a). The push for EHRs was consistent with the thinking that a longitudinal health record would improve access to information and consequently improve care. HITECH also ensured the collection of aggregate data that could be used to improve policy decisions relative to allocation of services and population health. Digital data also facilitates collection of data needed to measure quality of healthcare delivery, as well as improving data dissemination, as digitation allows easier data sharing.

Other drivers for healthcare reform include calls for improved safety and quality, transparency, the rise of consumerism with greater patient participation in planning care, and changing provider-patient relationships.

The Push for Patient Safety and Quality

Despite life or death consequences of decisions, healthcare is not as safe as it might be. Ineffective collaboration and poor communication have led to fragmented care and potentially dangerous errors and poor patient outcomes (Titzer, Swenty, & Mustata Wilson, 2015). The World Health Organization (WHO) (2017, Para. 1) refers to patient safety as a "fundamental principle of health care," calling for policy, leadership, data to drive improvements, patient engagement, and a skilled workforce to make healthcare safer. The Joint Commission International publishes patient safety goals that are integrated into the national accreditation process (The Joint Commission, 2017). Joint Commission International (2017) lists six patient safety goals that focus upon correct identification, effective communication, improved safety of high-alert medications, procedures that do not introduce harm, decreased risk of healthcare-acquired infections, and reduced risks of harm secondary to falls. HIT can improve safety and quality through alerts and decision support that help to improve the hand-off process—a point where many errors occur—and through the use of checklists. Zikhani (2016) noted that there are active and latent errors. Active errors include mistakes, slips, and lapses made by clinicians, while latent errors occur with imperfect organization design such as those seen with incomplete procedures, poor training, and poor labeling. Zikhani outlined steps to prevent errors in healthcare that include:

- Checklists that can prevent slips and lapses.
- Tools that improve communication such as hand-off tools.
- Automation when possible.
- Simplification, organization, and standardization.
- Not allowing errors to happen. An example of the latter might be the bar-code administration system that tells the nurse that it is not the correct medication during the medication administration process

Clearly, these processes lend themselves well to automation, or technology.

Technology can also be used to simulate clinical scenarios to educate the members of an interprofessional team (Titzer, Swenty, & Mustata Wilson, 2015). Nurse leaders have recognized the importance of integrating nursing informatics into undergraduate curricula by adding an informatics-competency category to the quality and safety curriculum developed by the Quality and Safety Education for Nurses (QSEN) project (QSEN Institute, 2017a). Many hospitals have elearning systems or use their intranets to provide ongoing education for personnel (Chuo, Liu, & Tsai, 2015).

Another effort to improve the coordination of care has led to new care models such as accountable care organizations (ACOs) and patient medical homes (PMHs). ACOs bring together primary care providers, specialists, and hospitals to share information and coordinate care and payment plans with the aims of greater efficiency and quality at a lower cost and, ideally, with less aggravation for the patient (Dewey, 2016). PMHs also bring together an interdisciplinary team that networks with other practices and networks to deliver or improve access to services (Hefford, 2017). Hefford (2017) noted that PMHs represent a move towards an integrated system of care. Team-based healthcare delivery models require great levels of collaboration (Rajamani et al., 2015). All models are dependent upon data, particularly shared data, for success.

Another model of care is seen with the changing dynamics of the provider-patient relationship. In the past, patients relied upon the judgment of their provider, often without question. However, with the rise in consumerism and widespread recognition that healthcare reform requires input from everyone, including consumers, patients are encouraged to be involved in their healthcare decisions. The transition from passive recipient to active participant requires several skills that include language literacy, health literacy, digital literacy, and transparency. The latter—transparency—requires access to information. The digitization process—making information available in electronic format—makes it easier to post and share information needed to make health decisions.

Provider roles are also changing and evolving. In addition to traditional roles, providers serve as gatekeeper to services, coach, navigator, and, sometimes, informatician (Johnson, 2015). And at a time where not every local practitioner has privileges at local hospitals, or patients are transported to other facilities, the hospitalist fills that void—a role that is still new to many healthcare consumers.

Creating an Informatics Culture

While informatics is much more than data management, knowledge that is derived from data and information is a central tenet. Creating a knowledge strategy and the infrastructure, expertise, and tools required to discover new learning and knowledge in data, particularly big data, fits well within the scope of informatics (Dulin, Lovin, & Wright, 2016; Kabir & Carayannis, 2013) . An informatics culture requires a vision to develop the policies, funding, infrastructure, and education to instill the knowledge and skills needed by all healthcare executives, clinicians, and informaticists, and the tools to gather and analyze amassed data. The process to do this takes time.

The first step in the process is assessing the current state to determine gaps (How Informatics can reshape healthcare, 2016). A highly innovative culture provides a solid foundation with the EHR playing a key role, because it provides a view of what is going on within an organization and beyond as data from healthcare exchanges and national data sets are examined.

Foundational Skills

There are foundational skills that are required for an information-driven culture. These include computer literacy, information literacy, and (for the consumer), health literacy.

Computer literacy is a term used to refer to the basic understanding and use of computers, software tools, spreadsheets, databases, presentation graphics, social media, and communication via email. The fundamentals of basic literacy—the ability to read, write, and comprehend—are prerequisite. Without a basic understanding of literacy, barriers to other forms of literacy cannot be addressed (Nelson & Staggers, 2018). Health informatics is built on overlapping layers of literacies.

Information literacy is the ability to read and understand the written word and numbers as well as the ability to recognize when information is needed. One of the biggest challenges today is making health information accessible to all without regard to background, education, or level of literacy.

Health literacy is the ability to understand and act upon basic healthcare information. A simple example would be how a person acts upon a change in diet in relation to a new medical diagnosis. Clearly each type of literacy is important for both healthcare consumer and healthcare worker.

Creating a Policy, Legal, and Reimbursement Framework

Professional organizations and informaticists have been working to create an informatics culture for some time through their involvement in national and organizational policy-setting. As an example, the American Nurses Association (2014) position statement *Standardization and Interoperability of Health Information Technology: Supporting Nursing and the National Quality*

Strategy for Better Patient Outcomes called for standard representation and interoperability of data collected in EHRs and other HIT. The National Association of Clinical Nurse Specialists (2017) set two goals relative to HIT for their 2016–2018 public policy agenda that included representing the role of the clinical nurse specialist in relevant legislative, policy, and advocacy efforts for increased access to healthcare via the use of technology. The US Office of the National Coordinator for Health Information Technology (ONCHIT), the federal entity charged with coordinating national efforts to implement and use HIT and electronic exchange of health information, invites input from healthcare professionals and consumers (HealthIT.gov, 2016). ONCHIT also has many committees with healthcare professions representation. Informatics groups, inclusive of the American Medical Informatics Association, American Nursing Informatics Association, Health Information Management Systems Society (HIMSS), and the Alliance for Nursing Informatics (ANI), include public policy related to HIT-enabled care among their goals (Collins, Sensmeier, Weaver, & Murphy, 2016; Health Information Systems Society, 2017a).

Ethical Framework

Ethics is the formal study of values, character, and/or conduct of individuals or collections of individuals from a variety of perspectives or viewpoints (American Nurses Association, 2015b). The field of health informatics focuses on using computers to enhance the way health information is processed. Today, the Internet opens up multiple avenues for obtaining information. Most links on the information highway do not have an overseer or monitor screening for good ethical decision making. This process is individual and personal, based on standards and the ability to differentiate right from wrong. Ethical decision making is the basis for this process. There are also issues related to how information collected for one purpose may be used for another. In a work that remains relevant today Beauchamp and Childress (1994) proposed four simple guiding principles for moral action. First is autonomy. Autonomy is the individual's freedom to control interferences by others, retaining a personal capacity for intentional action. Second is nonmaleficence: the obligation for doing no intentional harm, Third is beneficence, which refers to actions that result in positive outcomes in which benefits and utility are balanced. Finally, fourth is justice, which refers to the standards practiced by healthcare professionals. Professional associations for informatics also have codes of ethics that provide guidance for ethical use of data and information.

Workforce Preparation

Fox, Flynn, Clauson, Seaton, & Breeden, (2017, p. 1) noted that "informatics education for clinicians is a national priority," particularly since there is a lack of consistency in teaching informatics competencies. Informatics competencies are needed to help healthcare professionals manage and use technology effectively. The Institute of Medicine (2012) recognized the need for a workforce prepared to work with technology. The Technology Informatics Guiding Education Reform (TIGER) Initiative is another effort that grew out of the need to develop informatics skills among an interprofessional workforce (Healthcare Information and Management Systems Society, 2017). Informatics competencies are delineated for nursing graduates by the American Association of Colleges of Nursing, National League for Nursing, and the QSEN Institute, among others.

QSEN Institute identified quality and safety competencies for nurses that fit well with an informatics culture. These competencies include: patient-centered care, teamwork, evidence-based practice, quality improvement, safety, and informatics. Educators can use the QSEN framework as a guide. Teaching strategies can start with incorporating the QSEN competencies into curricula via classroom, simulation lab, and clinical strategies. The goal of the competencies is to use information and technology to communicate, manage knowledge, mitigate error, and support decision making (QSEN Institute, 2017b). The institute recommends incorporating the competencies beginning in the first semester of education and continuing throughout the nursing program. The competencies are formatted into three categories: knowledge, skill, and attitude. An example of *knowledge* would be the ability to contrast benefits and limitations, understand the value of databases for patient care monitoring, and establish a good understanding of terminology and interoperability of systems. An example of *skills* is for the nurse to play an active role in the design, promotion and modeling of standard practice. Nurses are an important member of the healthcare informatics team that can bring a clinical lens to the development table. *Attitude* incorporates nursing values whether it is in the realm of reporting or preventing errors, improving patient safety in a no-blame environment, and acting as a sentry for self, patients, and family. QSEN (2017c) also lists competencies for nurses prepared at the graduate level.

Hersh et al. (2014) spoke to the need for physicians needing informatics competencies because of their interaction with EHRs, clinical decision support, quality measures and improvement, personalized medicine, personal health records, and telehealth. Obviously, physicians are not the only healthcare professionals who use EHRs, decision support, telehealth, personal health records, or have concerns related to quality measurement and improvement, so all clinicians are impacted.

The Office of the National Coordinator for Health Information Technology (2017b) funded curriculum development centers to develop curricula and education in response to the mandate by the HITECH Act of 2009 to aid institutions of higher learning to establish or expand medical-informatics education programs. Twenty topics were developed originally, and more recently, five additional topics were developed in population health, care coordination and interoperability, value-based care, analytics, and patient-centered care. Materials developed through this effort are available for use at no cost.

Workforce preparation is under review in other areas of the world as well. One exemplar is the collaborative effort between the United States and European Union, which yielded an extensive list of competencies, including an informatics category. The workforce published the list of competencies as a tool for self-assessment. The Health Information Technology Competencies (HITCOMP) tool may be accessed without charge at http://hitcomp.org/

Technical Infrastructure

The technical infrastructure for healthcare informatics and exchange of information is the result of policy, legislation, funding, a multitude of agencies that are working to advance HIT for the benefit of healthcare, and technical standards. Policy and legislation and the relationship with funding will be discussed later in the book. One of the most important US agencies to advance HIT is the Agency for Healthcare Research and Quality (AHRQ). AHRQ is a division of the US Health and Human Services committed to research and evidence to improve the safety and quality of healthcare and to providing education for healthcare professionals that will enable them to improve care (Agency for Healthcare Research and Quality, n.d.).

Another agency that is a division of the US Health and Human Services is the National Institutes of Health (NIH). While NIH does not focus on technology to the same extent as AHRQ, it does provide funding for research to improve health (NIH, n.d.).

The third notable US government agency is the Office of the National Coordinator for Health Information Technology (ONCHIT). This office was funded with money granted by the Public Health Service Act (PHSA) as defined by the Health Information Technology for Economic and Clinical Health Act (HITECH). ONCHIT provides EHR certification, and its structure includes multiple offices that are relevant for HIT as may be seen in Figure 1-1 (HealthIT.gov, 2017).

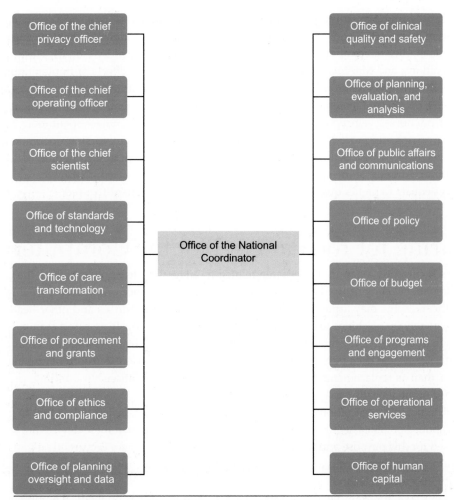

Figure 1-1 • ONC Organization.

SOURCE: From Office of the National Coordinator for Health Information Technology (ONC), Published by U.S. Department of Health and Human Services.

Technical standards provide specific directions to ensure that data and information can be exchanged in a fashion so that uniform meaning is maintained on both sides of the exchange. Health-information data standards may be grouped into the following four categories: content, transport, vocabulary, and privacy/security standards (Health Information Management Systems Society, 2017b). Content standards establish the structure and organization of the content. Transport standards set forth the format for exchange. Terminology standards improve communication through the use of structured terms and facilitate organization of data. (More will be said on terminology standards later). Privacy standards protect personal health information, while security standards provide administrative, physical, and technical actions that provide patient confidentiality as well as the availability and integrity of health information.

It is important to dispel the idea that computers are taking nurses away from the bedside. As nursing practice evolves, technology evolves in tandem. Technology supports all aspects of nursing practice, which include direct care, administration, education, and research (McGonigle, Hunter, Sipes, & Hebda, 2014). In order to create an informatics culture, there must be harmonious interaction between people and technology. While technology changes rapidly, so do the needs of the user. Informaticists play a key role in both system design and nurturing the user's abilities.

EHRs bring a meaningful medium to enhance continuity of care, care coordination, access to information, and satisfaction for both patient and provider, while decreasing costs. Various studies have reported mixed reviews. A study published by Gomes, Hash, Orsolini, Watkins, and Mazzoccoli (2016) intended to determine the effects of implementing an EHR and the direct relationship to patient-centered activities, attitudes, and beliefs. A well-known EHR was implemented, with the study taking place six months post implementation. Data from nurses' self-reports showed that post-implementation, nurses spent more time in patient rooms and more time engaged in purposeful interaction. Nursing documentation time decreased by 4%, which may be related to increased skill in doing documentation via computer. Although time spent in the patients' rooms had increased, that increase did not always equate to higher quality care if interactions were not patient-focused.

Caring for the Patient Not the Computer

There is currently a gap in the research related to integrating technology within the caring nurse-patient relationship. In our current digital world, reliance on technology is high. In healthcare, some may argue that this reliance is even higher. Nurses and other healthcare workers rely on machines to obtain vital signs that were previously assessed manually. The change from manual to automated blood pressures has the ability to change the focus of the healthcare system from person to machine. Using the machines as extensions of nursing care, rather than as replacements for it, can allow for continued relationship building, progress toward optimal health, and reduction in medical errors.

The notable expectation regarding the use of technology is using it as a tool to gather data about a patient's health status. We must always remember that these devices are tools to be used for this purpose and not to replace assessment skills. There is currently a gap in the literature regarding effective ways to integrate the concept of caring with the use of today's health information technology.

Let's take, for example, the concept of alarm fatigue. Alarms on medical equipment are designed to alert the healthcare team of an existing or impending change in the patient's healthcare status. However, it is estimated that "While defects of devices threatened patient safety in the past, alarms indiscriminately generated by the explosive increase in the number of medical devices now threaten their safety. Reports on safety accidents related to the diversity of medical device alarms have raised awareness of the clinical alarm hazard" (Cho, Hwasoon, Lee, & Insook, 2016, p. 46). This alarm fatigue is compounded by the number of potential false alarms during a nurses' work shift. It is important that we visit the reason for the alarm fatigue and the importance of using technology as a means to improve patient outcomes. Cho et al. (2016) noted that when The Joint Commission introduced the latest patient safety goals in 2013, hospitals were asked to identify ways to manage alarms. This included a deep dive into the most important alarms and what type of signals could be identified to improve alarm safety. Hospitals began the task to create policies and procedures to address this issue. As the primary caregiver at the bedside, nurses are empowered to identify ways to improve the safety of patient care through the management of alarm fatigue. Nurse informaticists are especially equipped to identify ways to highlight important alarms and reduce the number of non-actionable alarms. Nurses need to be equipped with the resources needed to make this happen. Part of this process includes the realization that the alarm-generating technology is paramount in providing data to nurses that allows them to make critical decisions about the care of their patients.

The electronic health record provides the nurse with the opportunity to use technology in a caring way that provides direct one-on-one interactions with the patient, using the computer as a tool to gather and store data that is important to patient care. Nurse informaticists can be on the cutting edge in devising technology that focuses on decreasing the frequency of monitor alarms so that the alarms become more actionable to the nurse. Through a systematic review of research articles on physiologic-monitor alarms and alarm fatigue, Paine et al. (2016) identified that the proportion of actionable alarms ranged from less than 1% to 36% across hospital settings. Some studies showed that the amount of alarm exposure affected nurse response time to the alarm. Longer response times may lead to poorer patient outcomes. The findings of this systematic review are further support that nurses need to be well versed in the reasons they use technology as a support. When nurses do not utilize technology to support the care of the patient, but, instead, use it as a substitute for assessing the patient, part of the nurse-patient relationship is lost.

Nursing education is at a pivotal time to be able to educate current and future nurses on the importance of utilizing information technology as a tool for safe patient care. Nursing faculty and nursing staff need to be able to minimize barriers to both training and implementation of tools within a technology-rich environment. Understanding how to use technology for patient intake and assessment, while still creating a trusting nurse-patient relationship, can provide an environment that enhances both quality and safety in nursing.

An important way to assist in creating this type of environment is to ensure that all patients are aware of the type of technology that is used for data collection and communication. It is important that they have the perception that the nurse cares about them. Instilling this value in the relationship is difficult when nurses are so heavily reliant on technology such as computers, specialized communication devices, and telephones that they carry with them during the course of patient care. Limitations to building a trusting, caring relationship come when patients perceive the nurse does not care, or is distracted during interactions—as can be the case when nurses stop to answer the phone or other communication devices during the course of a nurse-patient interaction. Patients need to be able to see the relevance of technology to the quality and safety of the care they receive. A collaborative approach to the use of technology between the patient and the nurse may assist in increasing caring relationships and decreasing patient events related to alarm fatigue.

Future Directions

Over the last few years, the focus has been on health information exchange for care delivery and quality. Over the next ten years, the infrastructure to support interoperability of systems and data exchange must be completed. The Office of Health and Human Services is responsible for increasing the amount of electronic health information and interoperability of HIT. This coincides with the ONC mission to protect the health of all Americans and provide essential human services, especially for those least able to help themselves (Office of the National Coordinator for Health Information Technology, 2015). The ONC roadmap for interoperability is written for both public and private stakeholders who will advance health IT interoperability for the betterment of patient care, smarter spending, and a healthier people. The document is intended to be dynamic as goals are met and new ones created. In order to achieve interoperability and ensure electronic health information security, the ONC proposed the following pathways:

- Improved technical standards and implementation guidance. In short, this means use of commonly known standards and consistency in application of standards.
- A shift in alignment of federal, state, and commercial payment policies away from fee-for-service to a value-based model.
- Coordination among stakeholders to promote and align policies and business practices.

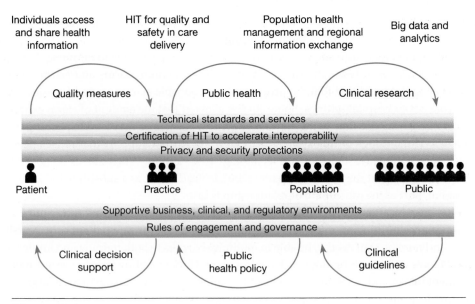

Figure 1-2 • Health IT Ecosystem.

SOURCE: From Office of the National Coordinator for Health Information Technology (ONC), Published by U.S. Department of Health and Human Services.

The IT ecosystem is important as new technology enters the market. At the core of the ecosystem are the patient, practice, population, and public. Surrounding the core of stakeholders are the products and services that allow interoperability to happen. Figure 1-2 depicts the health IT ecosystem.

Nursing informatics will continue to evolve as a specialty, particularly as its visibility increases and the need for all healthcare professionals to develop their own informatics competencies becomes increasingly apparent. Nursing informatics will continue its journey by staying current with technology trends, building strong collaborative teams, promoting standardization, and being proactive. As clients demand more health information and quicker access to it, information research using the tools of technology is a basic must-have skill for the nurse. Just as nurses face the challenges of patient care through competencies, the same approach should be incorporated into practice while facing the future of technology.

New technologies afford the opportunity to create new tools or to use them in new ways. As one example consider the growing use of virtual reality for education. Virtual worlds are found in computerized settings that simulate environments without typical boundaries. Second Life (http://secondlife.com) is one example of a virtual application that allows for creativity although it can be time-intensive, costly, and unable to provide feedback from a sense of smell and touch.

Summary

- The healthcare delivery system faces many demands that include calls for increased quality, safety, and transparency; evolving roles for practitioners; a shift in consumer-provider relationships; eliminating disparities in care; adopting new models of care; the need to develop a learning health system; increased technology; and workforce preparation.

- HIT has the potential to facilitate delivery of safe, quality care in an effective, efficient manner while improving communication and decreasing costs.
- Informatics in healthcare provides the knowledge and skills to harness the potential of HIT.
- Healthcare professionals are knowledge workers, and their work is supported via well-used HIT; but educational preparation for knowledge work has been inconsistent.
- Structures are needed to support meaningful use of data. These include digital formats using standardized languages and terminologies to ensure consistent meanings across all settings.
- Large data sets, known as big data, increasingly provide evidence to support learning and new practices—often supplementing or replacing traditional research findings.
- Healthcare delivery needs to become a learning health system, which is defined as one that uses real-time evidence for continuous improvement and innovation. This real-time evidence can be supplied through big data and analytics or business intelligence.
- Technology is pervasive throughout healthcare delivery inclusive of point of care devices, wearable, implantable, monitoring, as well as information systems and EHRs. Informatics professionals play a role in the design, implementation, and evaluation of that same technology.
- Economic incentives for the adoption of EHRs provides means to measure quality of care and provided learning that can be used for improved allocation of resources.
- Patient safety is a global initiative. HIT can provide or enhance safety through the provision of checklists, improved communication, and prevention of errors, as well as simplification and standardization.
- New care models are reliant upon data to better coordinate patient care.
- The move to consumerism, with care as a partnership, drives the need for available quality data for consumers to facilitate informed decision-making.
- An informatics culture recognizes the value of data, establishes a knowledge strategy, and the infrastructure, expertise, and tools required to discover new learning and knowledge in data.
- An infrastructure conducive to an informatics culture fosters legislative, policy, and advocacy efforts to increase access to information and quality care. Professional groups and government agencies, including the US Office of the National Coordinator for Health Information Technology, have demonstrated efforts to foster an informatics culture.
- Informatics and healthcare professionals have ethical codes to guide the use of data and information.
- All healthcare professionals need informatics knowledge and skills to ensure appropriate use of technology and data, information, and knowledge. Informatics professionals need to provide leadership and informatics to ensure that all healthcare professionals receive these competencies.
- Technology provides a tool to augment, not replace, the care. Informaticists must consider the needs of healthcare professionals and consumers when technology is deployed.
- HIT is not deployed in isolation; instead, it is part of the health IT ecosystem that brings together patients, provider practices, populations, and the public in a system designed to support each through research, policy, guidelines, and decision support, while measuring quality and outcomes.
- The development of new technologies and informatics competencies is a given over time.

Case Study

The community member on your hospital's advisory body has asked you to provide an overview of the relationship between informatics, technology in healthcare, and the status of healthcare delivery today. In your efforts to provide a short answer what would be four points that you would make?

About the Authors

Jennifer A. Brown has been a nurse educator for over eighteen years and has spent the last five years teaching Health Informatics to students in nursing, health information management, interdisciplinary health sciences, and computer science. Board Certified in Holistic Nursing, her passion for holism is threaded throughout each course that Professor Brown teaches. She is a tenured full-time faculty and teaches in the Bronson School of Nursing at Western Michigan University in Kalamazoo, Michigan in the undergraduate and RN-BSN programs.

Taryn Hill serves as Dean of Academic Affairs for Chamberlain College of Nursing. She contributed the content *Caring for the Patient Not the Computer*. She has authored and presented on nursing informatics topics.

Toni Hebda teaches graduate-level informatics courses at Chamberlain College of Nursing.

References

Agency for Healthcare Research and Quality. (2017). About the national quality strategy. Retrieved from www.ahrq.gov/workingforquality/about/index.html

Agency for Healthcare Research and Quality. (n.d). What we do. Retrieved from www.ahrq.gov/

American Medical Informatics Association (AMIA). (2017). The science of informatics. Retrieved from www.amia.org/about-amia/science-informatics

American Nurses Association. (2014). Standardization and interoperability of health information technology: Supporting nursing and the national quality strategy for better patient outcomes. Retrieved from http://nursingworld.org/MainMenuCategories/Policy-Advocacy/Positions-and-Resolutions/ANAPositionStatements/Position-Statements-Alphabetically/Standardization-and-Interoperability-of-Health-Info-Technology.html

American Nurses Association. (2015a). *Nursing informatics: Scope and standards of practice* (2nd ed.). Silver Spring, MD: Author.

American Nurses Association. (2015b). *Code of ethics for nurses with interpretive statements.* Silver Spring, MD: Author.

Beauchamp, T., & Childress, J.F. (1994). *Principles of Biomedical Ethics.* Oxford, United Kingdom: Oxford University Press.

Bulletin Board. (2016). Physician EHR adoption growing, but not physician information exchange. *Journal of AHIMA, 87*(4), 9.

Centers for Medicare and Medicaid Services. (2010). Medicare & Medicaid EHR incentive program: Meaningful use stage 1 requirements overview. Retrieved from www.cms.gov/Regulations-and-Guidance/Legislation/EHRIncentivePrograms/downloads/MU_Stage1_ReqOverview.pdf

Cho, O. M., Hwasoon, K., Lee, Y. W., & Insook, C. (2016). Clinical alarms in intensive care units: Perceived obstacles of alarm management and alarm fatigue in nurses. *Health Informatics Research, 22*(1), 46–53. Published by The Korean Society of Medical Informatics © 2016.

Chuo, Y., Liu, C., & Tsai, C. (2015). Effectiveness of elearning in hospitals. *Technology & Health Care, 23,* S157–S160.

Collins, S., Sensmeier, J., Weaver, C., & Murphy, J. (2016). Speaking with one voice: Alliance for Nursing Informtics policy responses. 2016 update. *CIN: Computers, Informatics, Nursing, 34(11),* 490–492.

Dewey, J. P. (2016). Accountable care organizations (ACOs). *Salem Press Encyclopedia of Health* https://salempress.com/

Dulin, M. F., Lovin, C. A., & Wright, J. A. (2016). Bringing big data to the forefront of healthcare delivery: The experience of Carolina's healthcare system. *Frontiers of Health Services Management, 32(4),* 3–14.

EHR adoption continues to lag for long-term care providers. (2017). *Journal of AHIMA, 88(3),* 10.

Fox, B. I., Flynn, A., Clauson, K. A., Seaton, T. L., & Breeden, E. (2017). An approach for all in pharmacy informatics education. *American Journal of Pharmaceutical Education, 81(2),* 1–13.

Gaberson, K., & Langston, N. F. (2017). Nursing as knowledge work: The imperative for lifelong learning. *AORN Journal, 106(2),* 96–98.

Gomes, M., Hash, P., Orsoline, L., Watkins, A., & Mazzoccoli, A. (2016). Connecting professional practice and technology at the bedside: Nurses' beliefs about using an electronic health record and their ability to incorporate professional and patient-centered nursing activities in patient care. *CIN: Computers, Informatics, Nursing, 34(12),* 578–586.

Gundlapalli, A. V., Gundlapalli, A. V., Greaves, W. W., Kesler, D., Murray, P., Safran, C., & Lehmann, C. U. (2015). Clinical informatics board specialty certification for physicians: A global view. *Studies in Health Technology and Informatics, 216,* 501–505.

Healthcare Information and Management Systems Society (HIMSS). (2017a). What is TIGER? Retrieved from www.himss.org/professionaldevelopment/tiger-initiative.

Health Information Management Systems Society (HIMSS). (2017b). About HIMSS. Retrieved from www.himss.org/about-himss

HealthIT.gov. (2016). About ONC. Retrieved from www.healthit.gov/newsroom/about-onc

HealthIT.gov. (2017). ONC HealthIT certification program. Retrieved from www .healthit.gov/policy-researchers-implementers/about-onc-health-it-certification-program

Hefford, B. (2017). The patient medical home: Working together to create an integrated system of care. *British Columbia Medical Journal, 59(1),* 15–17.

Hersh, W., Gorman, P., Biagioli, F., Mohan, V., Gold, J., & Mejicano, G. (2014). Beyond information retrieval and electronic health record use: Competencies in clinical informatics for medical education. *Advances in Medical Education and Practice,* 2014 (5), 205–212. doi:10.2147/AMEP.S63903.

How informatics can reshape healthcare. (2015). *Health Leaders Magazine, 19(4),* 40–44.

Institute of Medicine. (IOM). (2012). *Health IT and Patient Safety: Building Safer Systems for Better Care.* Washington, DC: The National Academies Press.

Institute of Medicine. (IOM). (2013a). *Core measurement needs for better care, better health, and lower costs: Counting what counts: Workshop summary* by Claudia Grossman, Brian Powers, Julia Sanders. Washington, DC: The National Academies Press © 2013.

Institute of Medicine. (IOM). (2013b). *Digital data improvement priorities for continuous learning in health and health care: Workshop summary.* Washington, DC: The National Academies Press © 2013.

Institute of Medicine. (IOM). (2015). *Genomics-enabled learning health care systems: Gathering and using genomic information to improve patient care and research: Workshop summary.* Washington, DC: The National Academies Press.

International Council of Nurses. (2012). *Closing the gap: From evidence to action.* Geneva: International Council of Nurses.

Johnson, J. D. (2015). Physician's emerging roles relating to trends in health information technology. *Informatics for Health & Social Care, 40*(4), 362–375. doi:10.3109/17538157.2014.948172

Kabir, N., & Carayannis, E. (2013). Big data, tacit knowledge and organizational competitiveness. *Proceedings of the International Conference on Intellectual Capital, Knowledge Management & Organizational Learning*, 220–227.

Kaggal, V. C., Komandur Elayavilli, R., Mehrabi, S., Pankratz, J. J., Sunghwan, S., Yanshan, W., . . . Hongfang, L. (2016). Toward a learning health-care system—knowledge delivery at the point of care empowered by big data and NLP. *Biomedical Informatics Insights*, (8), 13–22. doi:10.4137/Bii.s37977

Kohli, R., & Tan, S. S. (2016). Electronic health records: how can researchers contribute to transforming healthcare? *MIS Quarterly, 40*(3), 553–574.

Lucero, R. J. (2017). Information technology for health promotion & care delivery. Improving health promotion and delivery systems through information technology. *Nursing Economics, 35*(3), 145–146.

Luo, J., Min, W., Gopukumar, D., & Yiqing, Z. (2016). Big data application in biomedical research and health care: A literature review. *Biomedical Informatics Insights*, (8), 1–10. doi:10.4137/BII.s31559

Mackey, A., & Bassendowski, S. (2017). The history of evidence-based practice in nursing education and practice. *Journal of Professional Nursing, 33,* 51–55. doi:10.1016/j.profnurs.2016.05.009

McCullough, J. S., Parente, S. T., & Town, R. (2016). Health information technology and patient outcomes: The role of information and labor coordination. *RAND Journal of Economics (Wiley-Blackwell), 47*(1), 207–236.

McGonigle, D., Hunter, K., Sipes, C., & Hebda, T. Everyday informatics: Why nurses need to understand nursing informatics. *AORN Journal, 100*(3), 324–327. http://dx.doi.org/10.1016/j.aorn.2014.06.012

National Academies of Sciences, Engineering, and Medicine. (2017). *Real-world evidence generation and evaluation of therapeutics: Proceedings of a workshop*. Washington, DC: The National Academies Press. doi: https://doi.org/10.17226/24685.

National Association of Clinical Nurse Specialists. (2017). 2016–2018 Public Policy Agenda. Retrieved from http://nacns.org/advocacy-policy/public-policy-agenda/

National Institutes of Health (NIH). (n.d.). What we do. Retrieved from www.nih.gov/about-nih/what-we-do

Nelson, R., & Staggers, N. (2018). Theoretical foundations of health informatics In Ramona Nelson & Nancy Staggers (Eds), *Health informatics: An interprofessional approach* (pp. 10–37). St. Louis, MO: Elsevier.

Office of the National Coordinator for Health Information Technology. (2015). Connecting health and care for the nation: A shared nationwide interoperability roadmap—version 1.0. Retrieved from www.healthit.gov/sites/default/files/hie-interoperability/nationwide-interoperability-roadmap-final-version-1.0.pdf

Office of the National Coordinator for Health Information Technology. (2017a). Health IT dashboard: Quick stats. Retrieved from https://dashboard.healthit.gov/quickstats/quickstats.php

Office of the National Coordinator for Health Information Technology. (2017b). Health IT education opportunities. Retrieved from www.healthit.gov/providers-professionals/health-it-education-opportunities

Orion Market Research. (2017). Global healthcare information systems market research and analysis 2015–2022. Retrieved from www.omrglobal.com/industry-reports/healthcare-information-systems-market/

Paine, C. W., Goel, V. V., Ely, E., Stave, C. D., Stemler, S., Zander, M., & Bonafide, C. P. (2016). Systematic review of physiologic monitor alarm characteristics and pragmatic interventions to reduce alarm frequency. *Journal of Hospital Medicine*, *11*(2), 136–144.

Pinsonneault, A., Addas, S., Qian, C., Dakshinamoorthy, V., & Tamblyn, R. (2017). Integrated health information technology and the quality of patient care: A natural experiment. *Journal of Management Information Systems*, *34*(2), 457–486.

QSEN Institute. (2017b). QSEN. Retrieved from http://qsen.org/about-qsen/

Quality and Safety Education for Nurses (QSEN). (2017a). Competencies. Retrieved from http://qsen.org/competencies/

Quality and Safety Education for Nurses (QSEN). (2017c). Graduate QSEN competencies. Retrieved from http://qsen.org/competencies/graduate-ksas/#informatics

Rajamani, S., Westra, B. L., A. Monsen, K., LaVenture, M., & Gatewood, L. C. (2015). Partnership to promote interprofessional education and practice for population and public health informatics: A case study. *Journal of Interprofessional Care*, *29*(6), 555–561.

Robert Wood Johnson Foundation. (2017). What is the national quality strategy? Retrieved from www.rwjf.org/en/library/research/2012/01/what-is-the-national-quality-strategy-.html

Shortliffe, E. H. (2011). President's column: Subspecialty certification in clinical informatics. *Journal of the American Medical Informatics Association*, *18*(6), 890–891. doi:10.1136/amiajnl-2011-000582.

The Joint Commission. (2017). 2017 National patient safety goals. Retrieved from www.jointcommission.org/assets/1/6/2017_NPSG_HAP_ER.pdf

Titzer, J. L., Swenty, C. F., & Mustata Wilson, G. (2015). Interprofessional education: Lessons learned from conducting an electronic health record assignment. Journal Of Interprofessional Care, 29(6), 536–540. doi:10.3109/13561820.2015.1021000

Wills, M. J. (2014). Decisions through data: Analytics in healthcare. *Journal of Healthcare Management*, *59*(4), 254–262.

World Health Organization. (WHO). (2017). Health topics: Patient safety. Retrieved from www.who.int/topics/patient_safety/en/

Zikhani, R. (2016). Seven-step pathway for preventing errors in healthcare. *Journal of Healthcare Management*, *61*(4), 271–281.

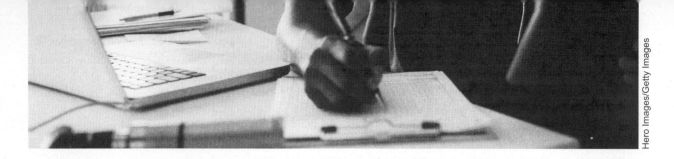

Chapter 2

Informatics Theory and Practice

Maxim Topaz, PhD, MA, RN

 ## Learning Objectives

After completing this chapter, you should be able to:

- Discuss the relevance of theory for informatics research and practice.
- Apply the DIKW framework to a situation in your lived experience.
- Examine ways that informatics may use the wisdom-in-action framework to support clinical care.
- Compare and contrast the different informatics subdisciplines found within healthcare.
- Weigh how the scope of informatics practice determines the types and levels of competencies needed.
- Discuss future needs and directions for nursing informatics.

Overview of Theory

Theory Definition

In general, theory is defined as a scientifically acceptable general principle—or constellation of principles—offered to explain phenomena (Meleis, 2015). Scientific disciplines are often based on some central theories that define the general school of thought accepted within a discipline. For example, a theory of evolution formalized by Darwin (1859) states that through a process called natural selection, live organisms are changing over time while passing their new traits to the next generations. This process results in evolution of simple creatures to complex organisms. Eventually, the changes accumulate and produce an entirely different organism. This theory is fundamental to several fields, for example, biology, where a common assumption states that all life on Earth has evolved from a common ancestor. Similarly, health sciences are based on several core theories, and each health discipline provides its own unique lens into ways of achieving optimal health and well-being.

As stated in the theory definition, all theories explain specific phenomena, large or small. The word phenomenon is often defined as an aspect of reality that can be consciously sensed or experienced otherwise (Meleis, 2015). Within a particular discipline, phenomena reflect the domain or the boundaries of the discipline. Phenomena are often used to describe an idea about an event, a situation, a process, or a group of events. A phenomenon may be geographically or time bound. Phenomena can be things that can be seen, heard, smelled, or felt (e.g., patient's pulse or blood-pressure measures). A phenomenon can also take a more abstract form and be based on evidence that is grouped together through presumed connections (e.g., the observation that individuals with surgical incisions that live alone and have multiple medications are more likely to be readmitted to a hospital after cardiac-surgery hospitalization). In the example of Darwin's theory, the studied phenomenon is that of natural selection and the theory describes the phenomenon's characteristics in detail.

Theories have two major purposes: to guide research and practice (Meleis, 2015). In research, theory is used to formulate a minimum set of generalizable statements to explain a maximum number of observable relationships among the research variables. Theory informs research and vice versa; research results can be used to verify, alter, or defy theories. In practice, theories help healthcare professionals in general, and nurses in particular, to construct a framework needed to set the goals of assessment, diagnosis, and intervention. For example, a theory can be used to set a general goal of nursing care to promote a patient's self-care through patient-focused decision-support tools and reminders for symptom management and a healthy diet, sent to a patient's smartphone.

Nursing Theory

One of the most comprehensive definitions of nursing theories is suggested by Afaf I. Meleis: "Nursing theory is conceptualization of some aspect of nursing reality communicated for the purpose of describing phenomena, explaining relationships between phenomena, predicting consequences, or prescribing nursing care" (Meleis, 2015, p. 29). In nursing, theories are often labeled as conceptual frameworks, models, paradigms, etc., but in essence, they all share the same properties and aim to achieve the same results.

Some scholars identify three levels of abstraction into which nursing theories can be categorized: grand theories, middle-range theories, and situation-specific theories. Grand theories aim to describe the broadest scope of nursing phenomena and relationships between them and do not lend themselves to empirical testing. Grand theories mostly emerged in 1950–1960s and helped differentiate between nursing practice and the practice of medicine.

For example, Orem's theory of self-care, first published around 1950, emphasized the person's need to care for oneself (Orem, 1985). The self-care theory identified three types of nursing systems: wholly compensatory, in which the nurse cares for all the patient needs; partly compensatory, in which the nurse assists the patient to care for himself or herself; and supportive-educative, when the nurse assists the patient to learn how to care for himself or herself. According to Orem, nursing is needed when a person is limited or incapable in the provision of effective and continuous self-care. The theory identifies several types of needed actions: guiding, supporting, or teaching others; acting for and doing for others; and creating an environment promoting personal development in an effort to meet future demands.

Middle-range theories are more limited in scope, focus on a specific phenomenon, and reflect practice (teaching, clinical, or administrative). These theories cross different nursing fields and reflect a wide variety of nursing-care situations. Middle-range theories are a good fit for empirical testing, because they are more specific and can be readily operationalized.

For example, Riegel, Jaarsma, and Strömberg (2012) have recently developed a middle-range theory of self-care among individuals with chronic illness. Based on the observation that not everyone is capable of performing self-care, Riegel and colleagues identified key concepts playing a role in individual decision making. For example, the theory makes the assumption that in order to make the right decisions, patients with chronic illness need focused attention and sufficient working-memory capacity. On the other hand, people with limited memory and attention (e.g., individuals with dementia) have little ability to interpret their symptoms and thus, may not be able to perform self-care. Situational influences on attention and memory (e.g., emotional stress or sleep deprivation) also affect decision making and interfere with effective self-care. According to Riegel, shared care, dependent care, or community support might be needed to help individuals experiencing these situations (Riegel et al., 2012). Middle-range theories were also applied to describe concepts like incontinence, uncertainty, social support, and quality of life, among others.

Situation-specific theories focus on a specific nursing phenomenon. They are often bound to a specific type of clinical practice and focus on a specific population. These theories are not meant to transcend time or go beyond a particular social structure, but rather they fit well within a certain social context (Meleis, 2015).

The previously described middle-range theory of self care among patients with chronic illness (Riegel et al, 2012) has been applied to patients with heart failure. This work has led to a situation-specific theory of heart failure self-care (Riegel, Dickson, & Faulkner, 2016; Riegel, Dickson, & Topaz, 2013; Riegel & Dickson, 2008.) This resulted in a situation-specific theory of heart failure self-care. Riegel and Dickson (2008) described self-care as a naturalistic decision-making process involving the choice of behaviors to maintain physiologic stability and the response to symptoms when they occur. In the theory, four propositions are used to specify the key assumptions: (a) symptom recognition is the key to successful self-care management; (b) self-care is better in patients with more knowledge, skill, experience, and compatible values; (c) confidence moderates the relationship between self-care and outcomes; and (d) confidence mediates the relationship between self-care and outcomes. Other examples of situation–specific theories are menopausal experiences of Korean immigrants, lived experiences of Asian American women caring for their elderly relatives, and preventive models for HIV among adolescents (Meleis, 2015).

Critical Theories Supporting Informatics

Health informatics is formed by a merger of several disciplines, including information science, computer science, and a specific health discipline; for example, nursing or medicine. Thus, the study of health informatics is informed by several theories from the related fields. In this review, I will describe one central theory, called the data, information, knowledge, and wisdom theory (DIKW), and provide a general approach that can be applied to connect the different disciplines and create a shared theoretical framework to guide nursing-informatics practice and research (Ronquillo, Currie, & Rodney, 2016; Topaz, 2013). Following this extensive review, a summary of other supporting theories is provided.

The Data, Information, Knowledge, and Wisdom Theory

HISTORICAL DEVELOPMENT The origins of the DIKW theory can be tracked to the early 17th century, when ideas about taxonomies emerged (Ronquillo, Currie, & Rodney, 2016). However, it wasn't until the late 1980s that the framework was adapted to health informatics by Blum (1986). In this classic work, he identified three types of systems used in health informatics, including:

1. Data-oriented systems. For example, systems designed for patient monitoring, clinical laboratory data, diagnostic systems, and imaging (e.g., computed tomographic scan);

2. Information-oriented systems. For example, clinical information systems that can provide administrative support (e.g., reduce errors) and healthcare decision support (e.g., alerts and reminders to support clinical decision making);

3. Knowledge-oriented systems. Examples include large knowledge databases (e.g., medical-articles collections) and artificial-intelligence systems (i.e., smart systems capable of applying advanced clinical reasoning).

Blum's work was widely adopted and created a foundation for theorizing in health informatics. The concept of wisdom is sometimes attributed to Ackoff's 1989 address to the Society for General Systems (Ackoff, 1989). Ackoff suggested that data is leads to information, information to knowledge and finally, knowledge leads to wisdom that guides the application of knowledge in clinical practice.

THE DATA, INFORMATION, KNOWLEDGE, AND WISDOM THEORY IN NURSING

The theory was first adapted to nursing in Graves and Corcoran's (1989) seminal paper, "The Study of Nursing Informatics" that established nursing informatics as a field of scholarly inquiry. This work was well accepted and implemented by the international nursing community. For example, the American Nurses Association (ANA) has adopted DIKW to guide the development of the scope and standards of practice in nursing informatics, suggesting that "Nursing informatics is a specialty that . . . communicates data, information, knowledge and wisdom in nursing practice" (American Nurses Association, 2008, p. 2). Nelson (2002) and most recently, Matney et al. (2011), studied and further adapted the theory to guide nursing informatics.

THE DATA, INFORMATION, KNOWLEDGE, AND WISDOM THEORY: CENTRAL CONCEPTS

- Data are the most discrete components of the DIKW framework. They are mostly presented as discrete observations with little interpretation. These are the smallest factors describing the patient, disease state, health environment, and so forth. Examples include a patient's principal medical diagnosis (e.g., International Statistical Classification of Diseases (ICD-10) diagnosis # N18.1: Chronic kidney disease, stage 1) (World Health Organization, 2014) or marital status (e.g., married, divorced, single, etc.). A discrete data-point observation (datum) is not meaningful when presented in isolation from other observations.

- Information might be described as data plus meaning. A meaningful clinical picture is constructed when different data points are put together and presented in a specific context. Information is a continuum of progressively developing and clustered data; it answers questions such as who, what, where, and when. For example, a combination of a patient's ICD-10 diagnosis # N18.1: Chronic kidney disease, stage 1 and marital status of 'Divorced' has a certain meaning in a context of an older, homebound individual.

- Knowledge is information that has been processed and organized so that relations and interactions are identified. Knowledge is constructed of meaningful information built of discrete data points. Knowledge is derived by discovering patterns of relationships between different clusters of information and affected by assumptions and central theories of a scientific discipline with which it is concerned. Knowledge answers questions of why and/or how.

  For nurses, the combination of different information clusters, such as the ICD-10 diagnosis #N18.1: Chronic kidney disease, stage 1, coupled with the fact the patient is divorced, and additional information that an older man (78-years old) was just discharged from hospital to home with a complicated surgical-incision treatment, prescription could indicate that this person is at a high risk for hospital readmission.

- Wisdom is an appropriate use of knowledge to manage and solve human problems (Matney et al., 2011). Wisdom includes ethics or knowing why certain things or procedures should or should not be implemented in specific cases. Wisdom guides the nurse in recognizing the situation at hand, based on the nurse's expertise, patient's and patient's family's values, and patient's healthcare knowledge. Using wisdom and a combination of all these components, the nurse decides on a nursing intervention or action. Benner (2000) presents wisdom as a clinical judgment integrating senses, emotions, and intuition. Using the previous examples, wisdom will be displayed when the homecare nurse considers prioritizing the elderly kidney-disease patient with complex surgical-incision care for an immediate intervention, such as a first nursing visit within the first hours of discharge from hospital to assure appropriate wound care and prevent complications.

The elements of the DIKW framework have certain hierarchical structure: data constructs information; information grows into knowledge informed by a particular setting or a problem; and knowledge progresses to wisdom to be applied in practice. However, the hierarchy is not strictly linear but rather, circular, and DIKW elements are interrelated. In a still relevant work, Nelson defined this phenomenon as a "constant flux" between the framework parts (Nelson, 2002, p. 27). See Figure 2-1 for a depiction of this flux. Simply put, new knowledge derived from specific data coupled with wisdom might warrant assessment of new data elements (Matney et al., 2011). In clinical practice, for example, a nurse administering inpatient medications can discover that a patient refuses to take the prescribed lipid medication as scheduled (data and knowledge and medication nonadherence). This, in turn, will trigger the nurse to explore the reasons for patient nonadherence (new data), and then, a nurse might discover that the patient uses a different medication for lipid management at home. Using clinical wisdom, the nurse will discuss the situation with the attending physician who can reconcile the discrepancies in the patient's medication list. In this scenario, information about

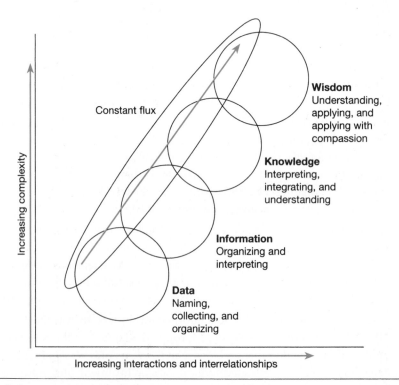

Figure 2-1 • Nelson's depiction of the data-information-knowledge-wisdom (DIKW) continuum.

SOURCE: Based on Nelson, R. (2002). Major theories supporting health care informatics. In S. Englebardt & R. Nelson (Eds.), Health Care Informatics: An Interdisciplinary Approach (pp. 3–27). St Louis, MO: Mosby.

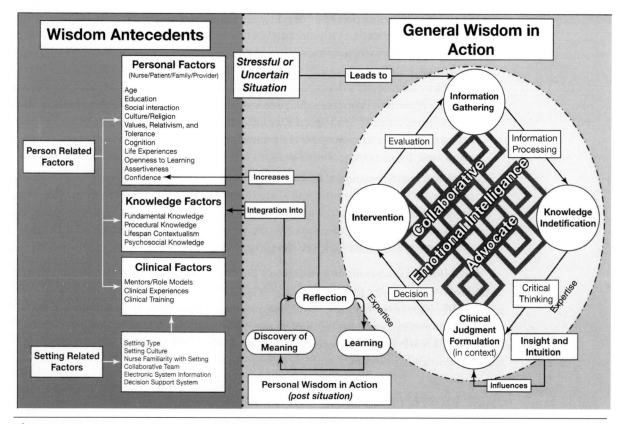

Figure 2-2 • The theory of wisdom in action for clinical nursing©.

SOURCE: The Theory of Wisdom in Action for Clinical Nursing from Development of a Theory of Wisdom in Action for Clinical Nursing. Copyright © 2015 by Susan A. Matney.

a patient's nonadherence triggered further data assessment, which, in turn, resulted in new information that was used to resolve the problem using wisdom.

EXPLORING WISDOM While data, information, and knowledge are often described as fairly straightforward constructs, the concept of wisdom may be quite confusing. Nelson and Joos are cited as the first to expand on the concept of wisdom in nursing; they described wisdom as "knowing when and how to use knowledge to manage a patient need or problem." (Nelson & Joos, 1989, p. 6). Later on, the ANA defined wisdom as nurses' ability to evaluate the knowledge and information within the context of caring and then use judgment to make care decisions (ANA, 1994).

Most recently, Matney (2015) developed a middle-range theory called the theory of wisdom in action for clinical nursing, using derivation and synthesis based on models from other disciplines and nursing literature. The theory comprised of four interrelated dimensions that are described here and depicted in Figure 2-2.

1. Person-related factors affecting wisdom include personal and clinical factors. Personal factors would include simple concepts, such as nurse and/or patient age, education, marital status, and more complex concepts (e.g., values, beliefs, or life experiences). Clinical factors include clinical training and experience and mentors and role models.

2. Environment-related factors affecting wisdom include setting-related and information-system factors. In term of settings, setting type and culture are important because they define, to some extent, how nurses act. Information-systems factors include the use of computerized data, which leads to clinical information in a certain context.

3. Knowledge is constructed of three different knowledge types, increasing in complexity: rich factual knowledge, rich procedural knowledge, and lifespan contextualism. Factual knowledge refers to the knowledge of nursing process and patient care. This kind of knowledge is often presented in nursing textbooks and then refined and further bolstered by continuous professional development. Procedural knowledge is comprised of clinical procedures, processes, and interventions required for care. Procedural knowledge is often acquired in a specific type of setting based on the accepted norms and rules of behavior. Lifespan refers to the understanding of others as well as understanding oneself. It can change over a person's lifespan, based on the acquired experiences.

4. Wisdom in action requires "knowledge mastery when dealing with uncertain or stressful situations. Knowledge impacts and insight and intuition influence the clinical judgment in context of the situation. The judgment leads to a care decision. After a care decision is applied, reflection, and discovery of meaning occur, which results in learning. Gained knowledge is integrated back into the knowledge dimension" (Matney, 2015, p. 135).

According to the wisdom-in-action theory, nurses make decisions in stressful or uncertain situations in an iterative process that includes applying knowledge based on skilled clinical judgment. Implemented decisions produce consequences, which, in turn, initiate reflection, discovery of meaning, and learning. Finally, new information is integrated back into changing and refining knowledge and judgment, when necessary. This theory provides a framework for translating wisdom into clinical nursing practice and learning about wisdom development.

Applying DIWK to Guide Nursing Research

As an example, the DIKW framework provides a generic structure describing how data is used to produce wisdom. However, to apply the DIKW in practice to guide nursing or other research, one needs to identify the theory describing the data and information in a specific research domain. Thus, the DIKW, ideally, needs to be used in combination with a specific theory. For example, in his dissertation, Topaz (2014) combined a mid-range nursing-transitions theory (Meleis, 2010) with DIKW to guide his research.

Transitions theory emerged in the late 1970s, and since then, it was constantly developed and refined by Meleis and others (Meleis, Sawyer, Im, Hilfinger Messias, & Schumacher, 2000; Meleis, 2010). In general, a transition can be defined as a passage from one state to another, a process triggered by change. Transitions theory has been applied to various types of transitions, for example, immigration transition, health-illness transition, and administrative transition, among others (Meleis, 2010). The transitions theory includes six central components: types and patterns of transitions; properties of transition experiences; transition conditions: facilitators and inhibitors; process indicators; outcome indicators; and nursing therapeutics (see Figure 2-1).

Topaz's study focused on a particular type of transition: transition from hospital to homecare. In his preliminary work, the author found that nurses' decisions on whom to prioritize for the first homecare visit vary among different homecare agencies, which results in delays of care and high risk for hospital readmissions. The goal of the study was to create a clinical-decision support tool that will help homecare nurses to identify a patient's priority for a first homecare nursing visit. The study used the transitions theory to conceptualize the different data points for further inclusion in the study.

The transitions theory suggests that the nature of the transition is affected by several elements; for example, transition type. One type of transition is health-illness transition. For the majority of patients, admission to a hospital is a major health-illness transition. This type of transition includes sudden or gradual role change resulting from moving from wellness to acute or chronic illness or vice versa. For instance, the most common reasons for hospitalization in the US are newly diagnosed illness conditions (such as heart failure) or exacerbation of a chronic disease (such as chronic obstructive pulmonary disease). Thus, the timing of the diagnosis and comorbid conditions played an important role in the data collection and analysis of Topaz's study.

According to transitions theory, it is necessary to uncover the personal, community, and societal conditions that facilitate or hinder progress toward achieving a healthy transition, also called transition facilitators and inhibitors (Meleis, 2010). Personal conditions include meanings that patients attribute to the transitions; these meanings might facilitate or hinder healthy transition. Transitions affect and are affected by cultural beliefs and attitudes. Socioeconomic status might serve as an inhibitor or facilitator of an optimal transition. In practice, it meant that the study needed to incorporate a patient's sociodemographic variables (e.g., age, gender, education level) and information about community supports available (e.g., caregiver's availability and willingness to help). The goal of the study was to create and validate a decision support tool (nursing therapeutics according to transitions theory) to assist clinicians to identify a patient's priority for the first nursing visit. See Figure 2-3 for more details on the transitions-theory domains and factors.

For his dissertation, Topaz merged two theories to create a cohesive guiding theoretical framework using the discipline-specific transitions theory to examine the individual's transition from hospital to home-health settings. The transitions theory guided the analysis of factors (disease characteristics, medications, patient needs, and social-support characteristics).

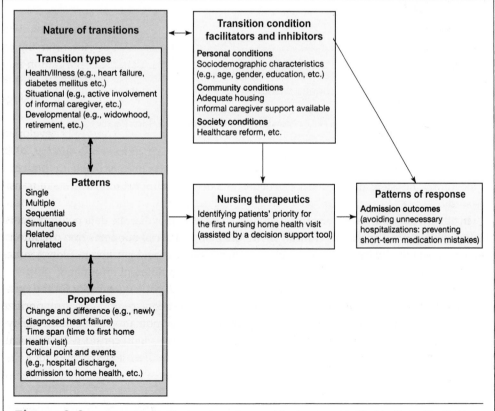

Figure 2-3 • Transitions-theory domains and factors as applied in Topaz's study.

SOURCE: From Developing a Tool to Support Decisions on Patient Prioritization at Admission to Home Health Care by Maxim Topaz. Copyright © 2014 by University of Pennsylvania. Used by permission.

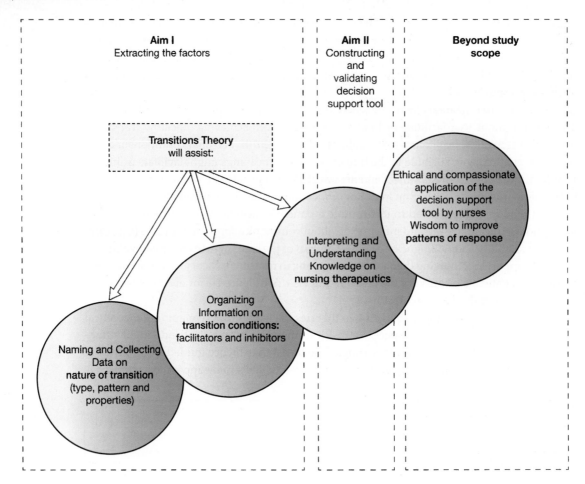

Figure 2-4 • The data information knowledge wisdom theory coupled with the transitions theory as applied in Topaz's dissertation study.

SOURCE: From Developing a Tool to Support Decisions on Patient Prioritization at Admission to Home Health Care by Maxim Topaz. Copyright © 2014 by University of Pennsylvania.

The DIKW framework (American Nurses Association, 2008) was used to explicitly present all the informatics steps during the construction of a decision-support tool, the final goal of this study.

In other words, the transitions theory guided the selection of discrete data points during the transition process (patient's clinical, environmental, and social-support characteristics); creation of meaningful information about the patient's medical-and-social conditions (organized into case studies); and analysis of the linkages between different information clusters to create a hierarchy of factors representing the knowledge of patient's priority for the first home-health nursing visit. This knowledge was used to create a tool to support patient prioritization at admission to home health. Figure 2-4 presents the combination of the frameworks to address study goals. Other researchers in nursing informatics might consider this merged approach to generate useful theoretical frameworks for their studies.

Additional Supporting Theories and Sciences

These additional theories and sciences include communication theory, information sciences, computer science, group dynamics, change theories, organizational behavior, learning theories, management science, and systems theory.

Theory/Science	Key Ideas
Information Communication Model	"The fundamental problem of communication is that of reproducing at one point, either exactly or approximately, a message selected at another point" (Shannon, 1948, p. 379). Sender → Medium (Noise and Distortion) → Receiver Encoder and Decoder Focus—Analyze information transfer and communication effectiveness and efficiency
Information Sciences	Exploitation of scientific and technical information of all kinds and by all means. Application of science and technology to general information handling. Branches: • Information retrieval • Human-computer interaction • Information handling within a system
Computer Science	Engineering and technology of hardware, software, and communications. Includes aspects of information and cognitive science.
Group Dynamics	Focuses on the nature of groups. Influence of a group may rapidly become strong, influencing or overwhelming individual proclivities and actions. Within every organization, there are formal and informal group pressures.

Change Theories	Change in people or social systems, such as healthcare organizations.
	Informatics specialists are change agents.
	Seek to manage impact of IS to yield positive results.
	Two perspectives:
	• Planned Change—Kurt Lewin
	  • Unfreezing
	  • Moving
	  • Freezing
	• Diffusion of innovations—E. Rogers
	  • Process for communicating an innovation throughout a social system.
	    • Innovators
	    • Early adopters
	    • Early majority
	    • Late majority
	    • Laggards
	  • Rogers identified five perceived characteristics of an innovation that affect the rate of adoption:
	    • Relative advantage
	    • Compatibility
	    • Complexity
	    • Trialability
	    • Observability
	  • Adoption of an innovation by an individual is dependent on the perceptions the individual has of that innovation.

Theory/Science	Key Ideas
Organizational Behavior	Focuses on small groups and individuals within organizations. Organizational health requires a balance, among participants, of: • Autonomy • Control • Cooperation Guides plans for system implementation.
Learning Theories	Changes in knowledge, skills, attitudes and values. More than 50 major theories of learning. Types of theories: • Behavioral • Cognitive • Adult learning • Learning styles
Management Science	Use mathematics and other analytical methods to help make better decisions of all kinds, including clinical decision-support applications. Methods: • Forecasting • Decision analysis • Inventory models • Linear programming • Graph theory and network problems • Queuing theory and waiting line problems • Simulation
Systems Theory	Studies the properties of systems as a whole. Focuses on the organization and interdependence of relationships. Boundaries: • Open • Closed Systems are constantly changing. • Dynamic homeostasis • Entropy • Negentropy • Specialization • Reverberation • Equifinality

Informatics Specialties within Healthcare

In general, informatics, as it applies to healthcare, is comprised of several specialties based on areas of application and inquiry. Historically, two terms were interchangeably used to refer to the field: medical informatics and bioinformatics. These terms reflected either a medical orientation of the profession (e.g., the use of information-technology tools and approaches by medical doctors) or a biological orientation focused on issues around basic biology (e.g., the human genome project that determined the sequence of human DNA and mapped all of the genes). Over time, with emergence of new health-informatics disciplines, such as nursing informatics or imaging informatics, both of the terms were used to refer to the new subfields. These traditional terms were also incorporated into the names of the major health informatics organizations, for example, International Medical Informatics Association (IMIA).

More recently, however, with a growing understating of the expanding body of work within the field, many organizations have revised their agendas and visions to incorporate a broader scope of informatics specialties. For the purposes of a more detailed description of specialties, the general view of informatics suggested by the American Medical Informatics Association (AMIA) will be used (Kulikowski et al., 2012). AMIA now refers to the discipline as *biomedical informatics*, defined as "the interdisciplinary field that studies and pursues the effective uses of biomedical data, information, and knowledge for scientific inquiry, problem solving, and decision making, driven by efforts to improve human health" (Kulikowski et al., 2012, p. 933).

As depicted in Figure 2-5, this definition suggests that biomedical informatics is a core discipline that provides methods, techniques, and theories to its subdisciplines including (1) bioinformatics and structural (imaging) informatics; (2) health informatics, including clinical informatics (with subfields of nursing, medical, and dental informatics) and public-health informatics (also referred to as population informatics to incorporate global health informatics); (3) and informatics in translational science with subfields of translational bioinformatics and clinical-research informatics. AMIA's definition also suggests that biomedical informatics lends its approaches to solve problems across the spectrum, ranging from molecular and cellular levels to the patient and population levels. The following descriptions define each of the subdisciplines:

- Bioinformatics is often defined as studying biology (e.g., physical and/or chemical structures of macromolecules) by applying informatics skills to understand and organize the information associated with these molecules on a large-scale. Bioinformatics is primarily concerned with three types of data from molecular biology: macromolecular structures, genome sequences, and the results of functional genomics experimentation (e.g., gene expression data). Additional types of data that are often used in bioinformatics might include the scientific literature (e.g., large collection of articles from Pubmed on genomic associations), taxonomies and standard terminologies (e.g., gene taxonomies),

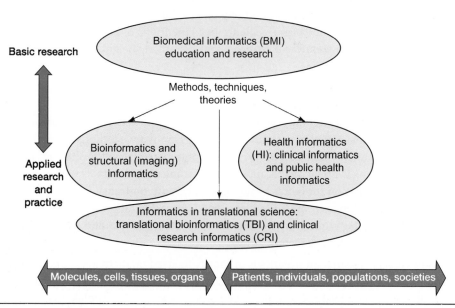

Figure 2-5 • Biomedical informatics and its areas of application and practice, spanning the range from molecules to populations and society.

SOURCE: From AMIA Board White Paper: Definition Of Biomedical Informatics And Specification Of Core Competencies For Graduate Education In The Discipline by Casimir A Kulikowski, Edward H Shortliffe, Leanne M Currie et.al. in Journal of American Medical Informatics Association. Used by permission of Oxford University Press/ on behalf of the sponsoring society if the journal is a society journal.

and protein-protein interaction data. Informatics techniques are applied on these data to achieve clinically meaningful tasks, such as designing new drugs.

- Structural (imaging) information refers to research and practical applications concerned with representing, managing, and using information about the physical organization of the body (Brinkley, 1991). The notion of structural in the subdiscipline name often refers to the structure of objects in space. Informatics methods are used to store, study, and use data from studies about human-body structure. For example, a chest computerized-tomography (CT) image can be classified via image recognition with machine learning to identify or rule out a presence of lung cancer (van Rikxoort & van Ginneken, 2013).

- Nursing informatics is a subdiscipline of clinical informatics included in the general domain of health informatics. Nursing informatics uses nursing knowledge, along with information and communication technology to promote the health of individuals, families, and entire populations. For more information, see chapter 1 of this book.

- Medical informatics is another subdiscipline of clinical informatics included in the general domain of health informatics. Medical informatics refers to research and practice in clinical informatics that focuses on disease and predominantly involves the role of physicians. This term was used interchangeably with other terms in the past to refer to the discipline of biomedical informatics as a whole (Kulikowski et al., 2012).

- Dental informatics is yet another subdiscipline of clinical informatics included in the general domain of health informatics. It is defined as a multidisciplinary field that seeks to improve health care through the application of health-information technology and information science to dental-health delivery, information management, healthcare administration, research, and knowledge sharing.

- Public-health informatics, included in the general domain of health informatics, is the science of applying information technology in areas of public health, including prevention, preparedness, health promotion, and surveillance. Public-health informatics takes a perspective of groups of individuals and focuses on work, neighborhoods, and environment of work and living places, among others. Some of the common areas in public-health informatics include biosurveillance (e.g., mentions of new spreading viruses on social media), epidemic-outbreak management, or ranking neighborhoods in one county in terms of health problems.

- Translational bioinformatics, included within the domain of informatics in translational science, combines applications of health informatics, bioinformatics, and structural informatics to identify genomic and cellular mechanisms to explain and predict clinical phenomena. Translational bioinformatics develops innovative techniques for the integration of biological and clinical data to create a more personalized healthcare. The recent emergence of precision medicine, aimed at providing all individuals with access to personalized information for better health, builds heavily on translational-bioinformatics methods to develop accurate and personalized characterization of patient populations based on molecular, clinical, environmental exposures, lifestyle, and other patient information (Frey, Bernstam, & Denny, 2016).

- Lastly, clinical-research informatics is primarily focused on methods supporting clinical and translational research. Its goals are discovery and management of new knowledge about diseases and health. Clinical-research informatics is often applied to identify ways for secondary research use of clinical data or to manage information related to clinical trials (Kulikowski et al., 2012).

All the subdisciplines of biomedical informatics interact among each other to provide a comprehensive suite of informatics tools for better healthcare practice and research. Nursing informatics draws on informatics disciplines, such as medical or public-health informatics to advance its goals of promoting health worldwide. On the other hand, other informatics sub-disciplines need nursing informatics to achieve their goals; for example, medical-informatics problems will often depend on nursing data to identify appropriate solutions. For instance, physicians prescribing medications need to understand a patient's adherence status to be able to match complex medication regimes for a specific patient.

Informatics Competencies for Healthcare Practitioners

To achieve its goals, biomedical informatics needs to define a set of competencies for its practitioners and academics. However, before diving into competencies, several interesting professional challenges should be addressed. First, biomedical informatics is an inherently interdisciplinary field that draws on theories and problem-solving approaches from healthcare, computer science, statistics, decision science, and other relevant fields. To achieve a common goal, representatives of all the different disciplines need to share a set of common terms and understandings. This set is sometimes referred to as the biomedical-informatics core competencies (Kulikowski et al., 2012). Second, some competencies are more geared towards biomedical-informatics practitioners (for example, a nursing informatics specialist working in a hospital system needs to understand specifics of standards for health-information exchange) while other competencies are critical for informatics researchers in academia (e.g., researchers need skills in situation-specific theory development while analyzing data from interviews with nurses who use electronic-health-records systems). These complexities shape the nature of the biomedical-informatics competency recommendations. The next few paragraphs will describe some early and recent work on biomedical-and-nursing-informatics competencies.

Work of Staggers, Gassert, and Curran

In the early 2000s, Staggers, Gassert, and Curran (2002), conducted an influential Delphi study that was one of the first to produce a research-based list of informatics competencies for nurses. The study also differentiated the competencies by levels of nursing practice. Nursing informatics experts ($n = 72$) surveyed in this study agreed on a list of 281 competencies for nurse informaticians.

The study stratified nurses into four categories by which the list of expected competencies was organized:

Level 1—Beginning nurse: expected to have fundamental information-management and computer-technology skills and use existing information systems and established information-management practices. Forty-three skills-and-knowledge competencies were identified in the domains of administration (e.g., using applications for structured data entry), system (e.g., using computer technology safely), and impact (e.g., recognizing that health computing will become more common), among others.

Level 2—Experienced nurse: expected to have a specific area of expertise (e.g., public health, education, administration); be skilled in using information management and computer technology; have strong analytic skills to learn from relationships between different data elements; and be able to collaborate with the informatics nurse specialist to suggest improvement to systems. The 35 identified skills and knowledge competencies included domains of desktop software (e.g., using desktop publishing), evaluation (e.g., evaluating the accuracy of health information on the Internet), and systems maintenance (e.g., performing basic trouble-shooting in applications), etc.

Level 3—Informatics specialist: defined as a nurse with advanced skills specific to health-information management and computer technology. Nurse specialist was expected to focus on information needs for the practice of nursing, which included education, administration, research, and clinical practice and use critical thinking, process skills, data-management skills (including identifying, acquiring, preserving, retrieving, aggregating, analyzing, and transmitting data), expertise in the systems development life cycle, and computer skills. One-hundred-eighty-six skills and knowledge competencies were in the domains of data (e.g., constructing data structures and maintaining data sets), design and development (e.g., developing screen layouts, report formats, and custom views of clinical data through working directly with clinical departments and individual users), and training (e.g., producing short-term and long-term training plans), etc.

Level 4—Informatics innovator: expected to be educationally prepared to conduct informatics research and generate informatics theory and have advanced understanding and skills in information management and computer technology. Forty skills and knowledge competencies were identified in the domains of research (e.g., developing innovative and analytic techniques for scientific inquiry in nursing informatics), practice (e.g., applying advanced analysis and design concepts to the system life cycle process), and fiscal management (e.g., obtaining research funding), among others (Staggers et al., 2002).

The work of Staggers, Curran, and Gassert was used as the basis for many further competency initiatives and full list of competencies can be found at http://himssni.pbworks.com/f/Delphi+Study+Article.pdf

AMERICAN NURSES ASSOCIATION COMPETENCIES IN NURSING INFORMATICS SCOPE OF PRACTICE In the US, the ANA is one of the largest nursing professional organizations, representing more than 3.4 million nurses. Since the early 1990s, ANA dedicated a significant amount of effort towards development of the specialty of nursing informatics. To accomplish this goal, ANA engaged nursing-informatics leaders from academia and practice to develop a scope of practice. Formal recognition of nursing informatics as one of the specialty practice areas for nursing occurred in 1992 (American Nurses Association, 1994).

In its first edition of the nursing-informatics scope of practice, the ANA defined nursing informatics as "Nursing informatics is the specialty that integrates nursing science, computer science, and information science in identifying, collecting, processing, and managing data and information to support nursing practice, administration, education, research, and the expansion of nursing knowledge" (American Nurses Association, 1994, p. 4). A nursing-informatics practitioner, referred to as an informatics nurse, was defined as a nurse with bachelor's degree in nursing and additional experience and knowledge in informatics. ANA defined 18 competencies for the informatics nurse, including systems design and analysis, use of software, and application of computer-programming tools. At the next level of practice, the informatics nurse specialist was defined as a nurse with a masters' degree in nursing and graduate-level courses in bioinformatics. These nurses were expected to master an additional seven competencies, such as nursing-informatics theory development, consulting skills, and the ability to develop procedures and policies for evaluating and improving nursing-information technology applied in clinical practice.

Following this initial seminal document, the ANA revised and enhanced the scope of nursing practice throughout the years. Some of the major consecutive changes reflected the growth and maturation of nursing informatics as a discipline. For example, the 2001 revised edition of *Scope and Standards of Informatics Practice* (American Nurses Association, 2001), placed more focus on management and communication of data, information, and knowledge (based on the DIKW framework) in nursing practice compared to the original focus on activities related to identification, collection, processing, and management of information. This was reflected in the renewed definition of nursing informatics as a "specialty that facilitates the integration of data, information, and knowledge to support patients, nurses, and other providers in their decision-making in all roles and settings." (American Nurses Association, 2001, p. 122).

In 2008, ANA's approach was revised, which resulted in a new document—that was better aligned with other nursing specialties—titled *Nursing Informatics: Scope and Standards of Practice* (American Nurses Association, 2008). In this document, the concept of wisdom (the last part of the DIKW theory) was added to the definition of nursing informatics. Also, the document included a matrix of skills addressing the competencies identified by Staggers et al. (2002).

The 2015 revision of the scope and standards of practice in nursing informatics followed its predecessors with more content about competencies for all nurse informaticians and additional competencies for the informatics nurse specialist. Competencies now are structured to fall under each of the 16 nursing informatics practice standards, presented below:

- Standard 1. Assessment
- Standard 2. Diagnosis, Problems, and Issues Identification
- Standard 3. Outcomes Identification
- Standard 4. Planning
- Standard 5. Implementation
- Standard 5A. Coordination of Activities
- Standard 5B. Health Teaching and Health Promotion
- Standard 5C. Consultation
- Standard 6. Evaluation and Standards of Professional Performance for Nursing Informatics.
- Standard 7. Ethics
- Standard 8. Education
- Standard 9. Evidence-Based Practice and Research
- Standard 10. Quality of Practice
- Standard 11. Communication
- Standard 12. Leadership
- Standard 13. Collaboration
- Standard 14. Professional Practice Evaluation
- Standard 15. Resource Utilization
- Standard 16. Environmental Health

THE AMERICAN ASSOCIATION OF COLLEGES OF NURSING ESSENTIALS The American Association of Colleges of Nursing (AACN) is a US-based organization that establishes quality standards for nursing education, assists schools of nursing in implementing those standards, and provides accreditation for baccalaureate and graduate nursing education. AACN's accreditation process evaluates the curricula of each particular educational organization and ensures that an essential set of professional competencies are addressed. In 2008, AACN published the set of baccalaureate educational-program requirements titled *The Essentials of Baccalaureate Education for Professional Nursing Practice* where one of the nine essentials is focused explicitly on health-information technology (American Association of Colleges of Nursing, 2008).

AACN identifies several aspects of information management and application of patient-care technology that every baccalaureate graduate should master. For example, graduates are supposed to be able to "use standardized terminology in a care environment that reflects nursing's unique contribution to patient outcomes" (American Association of Colleges of Nursing, 2008, p. 29). Some other competencies are more general and relate to ethical and high-quality application of health-information technology, ability to evaluate the existing systems, etc. See page 18 of the *Essentials* report for full list of graduate competencies required (American Association of Colleges of Nursing, 2008). Similarly, the AACN required in 2011 that master's-prepared nurses are able to use patient-care technologies to deliver and enhance care and use communication technologies to integrate and coordinate care (American Association of Colleges of Nursing, 2011). For the doctoral level of education (AACN regulates the Doctor of Nursing Practice—DNP—education), AACN requires that DNP graduates must be proficient in the use of information-technology resources to implement quality-improvement initiatives and support practice-and-administrative decision-making. Graduates also need to learn and be proficient in selecting and evaluating information systems and patient-care technology, and related ethical, regulatory, and legal issues (American Association of Colleges of Nursing, 2006).

TIGER

In 2004, an initiative called Initiative for Technology Informatics Guiding Education Reform—or TIGER—was formed to advance nurses' competencies related to informatics. TIGER's primary objective was to develop a US nursing workforce capable of using electronic health records to improve the delivery of health care. The TIGER initiative brought together nursing stakeholders to develop a shared vision, strategies, and specific actions for improving nursing education, practice, and the delivery of patient care through the use of health-information technology (Health Information Management Systems Society, 2013). In 2006, the TIGER initiative published a summary report titled *Evidence and Informatics Transforming Nursing: 3-Year Action Steps toward a 10-Year Vision* (Skiba et al., 2006).

TIGER's participants reviewed the existing literature and outlined a minimum set of competencies to focus on for all nurses. TIGER generated three categories of competencies, and each of the three categories had several subcategories.

> Basic Computer Competencies: includes areas such as hardware, software, security, Internet, and email use, among others. For each area, several subcategories with specific competencies are offered; for example, users are supposed to understand that some devices are both input and output devices, such as touch screens (hardware domain) or be able to forward an email (email domain).

> Information Literacy: a set of abilities allowing individuals to recognize when information is needed and to locate, evaluate, and use that information appropriately, according to the Association of College and Research Libraries (2000). Information literacy builds on computer literacy and refers to a user's ability to identify information needed for a specific purpose, locate pertinent information, evaluate the information, and apply it correctly.

> Information Management: consists of (a) collecting data, (b) processing the data, and (c) presenting and communicating the processed data as information or knowledge. DIKW theory served as the basis for this set of competencies.

In recent years, TIGER's work was adopted and now is managed by HIMSS (Healthcare Information and Management Systems Society), a professional association of health-information-technology stakeholders and venders (Healthcare Information and Management Systems Society, 2013).

TANIC and NICA

Several instruments exist to assess nurses' competencies in informatics. For example, Hunter, McGonigle, and Hebda (2013) have developed a set of tools to assess informatics competencies at all levels. First, they used the competency recommendations from the TIGER initiative to identify and validate a comprehensive list of competencies in the domains of: Basic Computer Skills (e.g., ability to sort files or rename files and folders); Clinical Information Management (e.g., ability to print standardized reports or knowledge of procedures to maintain security of organizational information); and Information Literacy (e.g., ability to synthesize conclusions based upon information gathered or understanding of free versus fee-based access to information). The developed instrument is called TIGER-based Assessment of Nursing Informatics Competencies (TANIC)©.

In later work Hill, McGonigle, Hunter, Sipes, and Hebda (2014) also developed an instrument for assessing advanced nursing informatics competencies called the Nursing Informatics Competency Assessment L3/L4 (NICA - L3/L4)©. The tool is using three domains to assess competencies: Computer Skills (e.g., determine the impact of computerized information management on manager and executive roles through program evaluation); Informatics Knowledge (e.g., use cognitive-science principles and artificial-intelligence theories to participate in the design of technology appropriate to the cognitive abilities of the user); and Informatics Skills (consult with clinical, managerial, educational, and or research entities about informatics).

Future Directions

So what is the future of nursing informatics competencies? One possible direction can be found in a recent survey conducted by a group of nursing informatics students with the International Medical Informatics Association–Nursing Informatics Working Group (IMIA-NI) (Peltonen et al., 2016; Topaz et al., 2015). The survey was focused on the current and future trends in nursing informatics with more than 500 nurse-informatician participants from more than 40 countries. When responding to the question "What should be done (at a country or organizational level) to advance nursing informatics in the next 5–10 years?". Survey participants' responses identified five key themes: (a) Education and training; (b) Research; (c) Practice; (d) Visibility; and (e) Collaboration and integration (Topaz et al., 2016).

Several existing nursing-informatics-competency recommendations (e.g., TIGER) can be used to help make progress in the five key areas. However, there are also gaps in existing competencies; for instance, in-service education for practicing nurses and their competencies remain largely unaddressed. Also, there are only a few separate initiatives aimed at identifying competencies necessary to promote nursing informatics visibility or ability to collaborate and integrate with other professions. These gaps can help set agendas for future competency development (Ronquillo, Topaz, Pruinelli, Peltonen, & Nibber, 2017; Topaz et al., 2016).

In addition, several new areas for future nurse informaticians have recently emerged and are becoming more prevalent. For example, big data is a recent term referring to large, unstructured datasets that are becoming increasingly available in health-related domains. Examples include millions of social-media postings (e.g., Twitter or Facebook) about new side effects to an established or new medication (e.g., Topaz, Lai, et al., 2016) or patients' opinions about a certain hospital. All these data can help nurses better understand their clients while, on the other hand, presenting multiple challenges, e.g., noise reduction, signal detection, free-text analytics etc. Thus, big-data science will require a variety of techniques for analyzing inputs, from traditional statistics to visualization techniques, data mining, and natural-language processing (Topaz & Pruinelli, 2017). With the increasingly growing role of big data in health analytics, nurses are starting to develop new tools and approaches to turn this data into information and wisdom to guide clinical practice.

Summary

- Theories serve to guide research and practice.
- Nursing theory serves to describe phenomena, explain relationships, predict consequences, and prescribe care.
- Nursing theory can be categorized as grand, middle-range, or situation-specific theory.
- Grand theories are broad and not amenable to empirical testing.
- Middle-range theories focus on specific phenomena, reflect practice, and lend themselves to empirical testing.
- Situation-specific theory focus on a specific nursing phenomenon and are often bound to a specific type of clinical practice and population.
- Several theories inform and support informatics including, but not limited to, the data, information, knowledge, and wisdom (DIKW) theory, the theory of wisdom in action, and transitions theory.
- Communication theory, information sciences, computer science, group dynamics, change theories, organizational behavior, learning theories, management science, and systems theory also contribute to the underpinnings of informatics.
- Several informatics specialties exist within healthcare. These include biomedical informatics, bioinformatics, structural (imaging) informatics, and nursing informatics.
- Competencies must be defined to accomplish informatics goals.
- Development and evolution of nursing informatics competencies draw from the work of diverse contributors.
- Informatics competencies have been identified for nurses and other healthcare professionals by several groups including, but not limited to, the American Nurses Association, the American Association of Colleges of Nursing, the Technology Informatics Guiding Education Reform (TIGER) Initiative, and the Health Information and Management Systems Society.
- Several instruments exist to assess informatics competencies both at basic and advanced levels. The TIGER-based Assessment of Nursing Informatics Competencies (TANIC)© and Informatics Competency Assessment L3/L4 (NICA - L3/L4)© represent tools developed to test competencies at four levels of practice—beginner and experienced nurses, informatics nurse specialist, and innovator, respectively.

About the Author

Maxim Topaz is a postdoctoral research fellow at the Harvard Medical School and Brigham Women's Health. His passion is applying new technologies to improve people's health. Maxim's expertise includes nursing and health informatics theory, clinical decision support, and data and text mining (including natural language processing).

References

Ackoff, R. (1989). From data to wisdom. *Journal of Applied Systems Analysis, 16*(1), 3–9.

American Association of Colleges of Nursing. (2006). *The essentials of doctoral education for advanced nursing practice.* Retrieved from www.aacn.nche.edu/dnp/Essentials.pdf

American Association of Colleges of Nursing. (2008). *The essentials of baccalaureate education for professional nursing practice* © 2008. Retrieved from www.aacn.nche.edu/publications/order-form/baccalaureate-essentials

American Association of Colleges of Nursing. (2011). *The essentials of master's education in nursing.* Retrieved from www.aacn.nche.edu/education-resources/MastersEssentials11.pdf

American Nurses Association. (1994). *Scope of practice for nursing informatics* © 1994. Washington, DC: Author.

American Nurses Association. (2001). *Scope and standards of nursing informatics practice* © 2001. Silver Spring, MD: Author.

American Nurses Association. (2008). *Nursing informatics: Scope and standards of practice* © 2008. Washington, DC: Author.

American Nurses Association. (2015). *Nursing informatics: Scope and standards of practice* (2nd ed.). Washington, DC: Author.

Association of College and Research Libraries. (2000). *Information literacy competency standards for higher education.* Retrieved from www.ala.org/acrl/ilcomstan.html.

Benner, P. (2000). The wisdom of our practice. *The American Journal of Nursing, 100*(10), 99–105.

Blum, B. (1986). *Clinical information systems.* New York: Springer-Verlag.

Brinkley, J. F. (1991). Structural informatics and its applications in medicine and biology. *Academic Medicine: Journal of the Association of American Medical Colleges, 66*(10), 589–591.

Darwin, C. (1859). *On the origin of species by means of natural selection, or, the preservation of favoured races in the struggle for life.* London, UK: Murray.

Frey, L. J., Bernstam, E. V., & Denny, J. C. (2016). Precision medicine informatics. *Journal of the American Medical Informatics Association: Journal of the American Medical Informatics Association, 23*(4), 668–670. doi:10.1093/jamia/ocw053

Graves, J., & Corcoran, S. (1989). The study of nursing informatics. *Journal of Nursing Scholarship, 21*(4), 227–231.

Hill, T., McGonigle, D., Hunter, K. M., Sipes, C., & Hebda, T. L. (2014). An instrument for assessing advanced nursing informatics competencies. *Journal of Nursing Education and Practice, 4*(7), 104. doi:10.5430/jnep.v4n7p104

Health Information Management Systems Society. (2013). The TIGER Initiative. Retrieved from www.himss.org/professionaldevelopment/tiger-initiative

Hunter, K. M., Mcgonigle, D. M., & Hebda, T. L. (2013). TIGER-based measurement of nursing informatics competencies: The development and implementation of an online tool for self-assessment. *Journal of Nursing Education and Practice, 3*(12), 70–80. doi:10.5430/jnep.v3n12p70

Kulikowski, C. A., Shortliffe, E. H., Currie, L. M., Elkin, P. L., Hunter, L. E., Johnson, T. R., & Williamson, J. J. (2012). AMIA Board white paper: Definition of biomedical informatics and specification of core competencies for graduate education in the discipline. *Journal of the American Medical Informatics Association, 19*(6), 931–938. doi:10.1136/amiajnl-2012-001053

Matney, S. (2015). *Development of a theory of wisdom in action for clinical nursing.* (Unpublished doctoral dissertation). Salt Lake City, UT: The University of Utah. Published by Susan A. Matney, © 2015.

Matney, S., Brewster, P. J., Sward, K. A., Cloyes, K. G., & Staggers, N. (2011). Philosophical approaches to the nursing informatics data-information-knowledge-wisdom framework. *ANS. Advances in Nursing Science, 34*(1), 6–18. doi:10.1097/ANS.0b013e3182071813

Meleis, A. I. (2010). *Transitions theory: Middle range and situation specific theories in nursing research and practice.* New York: Springer Publishing Company.

Meleis, A. I. (2015). *Theoretical nursing: Development and progress* (5th ed.). Philadelphia: Wolters Kluwer Health © 2011.

Meleis, A. I., Sawyer, L. M., Im, E. O., Hilfinger Messias, D. K., & Schumacher, K. (2000). Experiencing transitions: An emerging middle-range theory. *ANS. Advances in Nursing Science, 23*(1), 12–28.

Nelson, R. (2002). Major theories supporting health care informatics. In S. Englebardt & R. Nelson (Eds.), *Health Care Informatics: An Interdisciplinary Approach* (pp. 3–27). St. Louis, MO: Mosby.

Nelson, R., & Joos, I. (1989). On language in nursing: from data to wisdom. *PLN Visions,* Fall, 6–7. Published by Elsevier, © 1989.

Orem, D. E. (1985). A concept of self-care for the rehabilitation client. *Rehabilitation Nursing: The Official Journal of the Association of Rehabilitation Nurses, 10*(3), 33–36.

Peltonen, L.-M., Topaz, M., Ronquillo, C., Pruinelli, L., Sarmiento, R. F., Badger, M. K., & Alhuwail, D. (2016). Nursing informatics research priorities for the future: Recommendations from an international survey. *Studies in Health Technology and Informatics, 225*, 222–226. Published by IMIA and IOS Press, © 2016.

Riegel, B., & Dickson, V. V. (2008). A situation-specific theory of heart failure self-care. *The Journal of Cardiovascular Nursing, 23*(3), 190–196. doi:10.1097/01.JCN.0000305091.35259.85

Riegel, B., Dickson, V. V., & Faulkner, K. M. (2016). The situation-specific theory of heart failure self-care: Revised and updated. *The Journal of Cardiovascular Nursing, 31*(3), 226–235. doi:10.1097/JCN.0000000000000244

Riegel, B., Dickson, V. V., & Topaz, M. (2013). Qualitative analysis of naturalistic decision making in adults with chronic heart failure. *Nursing Research, 62*(2), 91–98.

Riegel, B., Jaarsma, T., & Strömberg, A. (2012). A middle-range theory of self-care of chronic illness. *ANS. Advances in Nursing Science, 35*(3), 194–204. doi:10.1097/ANS.0b013e318261b1ba

Ronquillo, C., Currie, L. M., & Rodney, P. (2016). The evolution of data-information-knowledge-wisdom in nursing informatics. *ANS. Advances in Nursing Science, 39*(1), E1–18. doi:10.1097/ANS.0000000000000107

Ronquillo, C., Topaz, M., Pruinelli, L., Peltonen, L., & Nibber, R. (2017). Competency recommendations for advancing nursing informatics in the next decade: International survey results. *Studies in Health Technology and Informatics, 232*, 119–129.

Skiba, D., Delaney, C., Dulong, D., Walker, P., Mcbride, A., Sensmeier, J., & Weaver, C. (2006). The TIGER initiative evidence and informatics transforming nursing: 3-Year action steps toward a 10-year vision. Retrieved from www.tigersummit.com

Shannon, C. E. (1948). A mathematical theory of communication. *The Bell System Technical Journal, 27*, 3, 379–423; 27, 4, 623–656. © 1948.

Staggers, N., Gassert, C. A., & Curran, C. (2002). A Delphi study to determine informatics competencies for nurses at four levels of practice. *Nursing Research, 51*(6), 383–390.

Topaz, M. (2013). The hitchhiker's guide to nursing informatics theory: Using the data-knowledge-information-wisdom framework to guide informatics research. *Online Journal of Nursing Informatics, 17*(3). Available at http://ojni.org/issues/?p=2852

Topaz, M. (2014). Developing a tool to support decisions on patient prioritization at admission to home health care (Doctoral dissertation). Retrieved from *Publicly Accessible Penn Dissertations*. 1473.https://repository.upenn.edu/dissertations/1473

Topaz, M., Lai, K., Dhopeshwarkar, N., Seger, D. L., Sa'adon, R., Goss, F., & Zhou, L. (2016). Clinicians' reports in electronic health records versus patients' concerns in social media: A pilot study of adverse drug reactions of aspirin and atorvastatin. *Drug Safety, 39*(3), 241–250. doi:10.1007/s40264-015-0381-x

Topaz, M., & Pruinelli, L. (2017). Big data and nursing: Implications for the future. *Studies in Health Technology and Informatics, 232,* 165–171.

Topaz, M., Ronquillo, C., Peltonen, L.-M., Pruinelli, L., Sarmiento, R. F., Badger, M. K., . . . Alhuwail, D. (2016). Advancing nursing informatics in the next decade: Recommendations from an international survey. *Studies in Health Technology and Informatics, 225,* 123–127. Published by IMIA and IOS Press, © 2016.

Topaz, M., Ronquillo, C., Pruinelli, L., Ramos, R., Peltonen, L.-M., Siirala, E., & Badger, M. K. (2015). Central trends in nursing informatics: Students' reflections from International Congress on Nursing Informatics 2014 (Taipei, Taiwan). *CIN: Computers, Informatics, Nursing, 33*(3), 85–89. doi:10.1097/CIN.0000000000000139

van Rikxoort, E. M., & van Ginneken, B. (2013). Automated segmentation of pulmonary structures in thoracic computed tomography scans: a review. *Physics in Medicine and Biology, 58*(17), R187–220. doi:10.1088/0031-9155/58/17/R187

World Health Organization (WHO). (2014). International classification of diseases (ICD). Retrieved from www.who.int/classifications/icd/en/

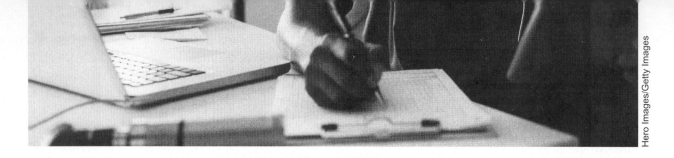

Chapter 3
Effective and Ethical Use of Data and Information

Toni Hebda, PhD, RN-C
Kathleen Hunter, PhD, RN-BC, CNE

 ## Learning Objectives

After completing this chapter, you should be able to:

- Distinguish between the metastructures of data, information, knowledge, and wisdom.

- Detail prerequisite conditions for effective and ethical use of data and information.

- Provide exemplars of effective and ethical use of data and information within healthcare.

- Relate issues and concerns for effective and ethical use of healthcare data and information.

- Discriminate between the terms big data, data science, data analytics, and data modeling.

- Summarize the current state of big data use within healthcare.

- Differentiate between clinician and informatics roles with big data and analytics.

Overview of Data and Information

Before one can discuss effective and ethical use of data and information, it is necessary to define data and information. *Nursing informatics: Scope and standards of practice* used the classic work of Graves and Corcoran to define **data** as "discrete entities that are described objectively without interpretation" and **information** as "data that have been interpreted, organized, or structured" (American Nurses Association, 2015a, p. 2). The scope-of-practice section also referenced the same work to define **knowledge** as synthesized information that showed formally recognized relationships. Knowledge is important to the ability to effectively use data. But it is the fourth metastructure of nursing informatics, wisdom, which is critical to effective and ethical use of data, information, and knowledge. **Wisdom** is the ability to appropriately use knowledge to recognize and handle complex problems.

Ethical Use of Data and Information

Effective and ethical use of data and information is consistent with professional standards of practice and essential to safe, efficient healthcare delivery, a learning healthcare delivery system, attainment of optimal individual and population health outcomes, and the transformation of the current, inefficient healthcare delivery system to one that provides quality, personalized care, at lower costs. As an example, the American Nurses Association's (ANA) (2015b) code of ethics calls for the nurse to respect the client whether that is one person, a family, a group, or a population. As patient advocate, the nurse is charged with protecting the health, safety, and rights of the patients. This protection extends to information and the use of systems that house patient information. The code of ethics also calls for nurses to actively participate in shaping social and health policy for the benefit of all. The code of ethics for nurses provides a foundation for nursing informatics practice. The specialty of nursing informatics then builds upon this foundation with a practice standard for ethics, Standard 7 (American Nurses Association, 2015a). Standard 7 delineates competencies for two levels of informatics practice—informatics nurse and informatics nurse specialist. Informatics nurses are called upon to:

- Evaluate factors related to handling data, information, and knowledge
- Help resolve ethical issues involving consumers, other healthcare providers (HCPs), and stakeholders
- Report or take action when illegal, unethical, or inappropriate behaviors are noted that could harm individuals or organizations
- Question practices as necessary for the purpose of maintaining or promoting safety and quality improvement
- Promote effective workflows
- Advocate for consumer access to their records and work to reduce disparities in access and related issues such as eliteracy.

In addition to the above competencies, Standard 7 calls for the informatics nurse specialist to:

- Actively participate in interprofessional teams that address ethical concerns, consumer benefits, and outcomes
- Apprise administrators of ethical concerns, consumer benefits, and outcomes
- Foster engagement of all stakeholders in the oversight and management of data, information, and knowledge.

The International Medical Informatics Association (IMIA) approved its updated code of ethics for health information professionals in 2016 (International Medical Informatics Association, 2016). The preamble to the IMIA code calls for flexibility to accommodate an ever-changing environment without sacrificing the application of basic principles. IMIA also notes that health informatics professions interact with, and need to weigh, the needs and sometimes conflicting demands of consumers, HCPs, administrators, healthcare delivery organizations, payers, researchers, governments, and society while adhering to the IMIA code of ethics. The principles and rules of ethical conduct outlined by IMIA, like the ANA *Code of Ethics*, provide guidance for informatics practice that includes directions for effective and ethical use of data and information. Clearly informatics professionals have major responsibilities related to shaping how data and information are used.

Data Sharing versus Data Silos

Today's healthcare system has many databases maintained by different groups—often designed to meet the needs of a specific population. Within a single healthcare delivery system, each entity maintains its own records—the hospital, specialty areas, and the physician. There are also local urgent-care clinics, public health departments, subacute and long-term care facilities, and pharmacies, which may or may not share information with other providers. This situation leads to different versions of data, missing data, redundant data collection, and contributes to potentially dangerous errors and wasted resources. As an example, Jane Doe's primary healthcare record lists the antibiotic Keflex and latex for her allergies, but when Jane is taken to the trauma center unconscious, unaccompanied, and without a medical-alert bracelet, the only allergy listed at the trauma center is antibiotic Keflex. This example of incomplete information could expose Jane to an allergen with potentially deadly results because information was not shared.

Sharing health information, otherwise known as health information exchange (HIE), provides a means to reduce redundant tests, improve quality of care, and improve public confidence (Bailey et al., 2013; Kuehn, 2014). In one example, Bailey et al. (2013) examined longitudinal HIE data for a region that connected 15 hospitals and two clinic systems to find decreased diagnostic testing and improved adherence to evidence-based guidelines for the care of patients evaluated for headaches in the emergency department. But HIE alone is not enough. A 2016 report that interviewed more than 500 clinical EHR users noted that meaningful exchange of data requires data to be available when needed, easy to find, within the workflow, and delivered in an effective way—yet participants reported the presence of all four criteria only 6% of the time (Leventhal & Hagland, 2017). In 2016, several major healthcare information-system vendors committed to a framework for interoperability and data-sharing principles set forth by Carequality, a public-private collaborative and an initiative of the Sequoia Project, which released its interoperability framework in 2015. The Sequoia framework established legal, policy, and technical specifications for sharing data as well as processes for governance. This initiative reflected a major change among vendors which historically had not previously cooperated. The next anticipated breakthrough is to ensure that shared elements remain the same across vendor platforms.

The issue of sharing data goes beyond HIE to include study findings. Not all research is published (Kuehn, 2014). Some findings are submitted to clinical-trial registries, to regulators as a requirement for marketing approval, or alternately, may never be seen by anyone but the researchers. This uneven access fosters inappropriate assumptions and violates the ethical obligation that researchers have to their subjects. In other developments, recent years have witnessed the creation of international collaboratives for research and biobanks, both of which entail extensive sharing (Dove, 2015). Biobanks collect human biological material and related data that are stored for research purposes, which may not even be defined at the time that materials are stored.

Sharing data is an ethical and scientific imperative that can expedite health gains, create new public health value, and fulfill patient expectations that data will be used in the best ways (Bauchner, Golub, & Fontanarosa, 2016; Davidson, 2015; Haug, 2017), but no common ethical and legal framework yet exists to connect healthcare providers with regulators, funders, and research projects that will link genomic and clinical data, limiting potential benefits (Knoppers, Harris, Budin-ljosne, & Dove, 2014).

Using Data for Quality Improvement

Increasingly, data is viewed as a strategic resource (Otto, 2015). One of the most pressing concerns is the ability to generate and use sufficient data related to quality. Organizations use data to meet regulatory requirements, to facilitate the move from fee-for-service to a value-based model of care, to measure quality of care, outcomes, and services, and day-to-day operations, in order to remain solvent (Using data, 2016; Smith, 2013). The ability to meaningfully measure quality requires the presence of several data attributes. In addition to a full or complete set of data from all necessary sources (as was mentioned under data sharing), data must be clear, accurate, available when needed, precise, verifiable by other means, without bias, current, appropriate to the needs of the user, and in a convenient form for interpretation, classification, storage, retrieval, and updates. High quality data are essential for better information, better decision-making, and better outcomes (Chen, Hailey, Wang, & Yu, 2014; Otto, 2015).

Data Quality

Data integrity is a comprehensive term that encompasses the notion of wholeness when data is collected, stored, and retrieved by the user. For data to be complete and orderly, a systematic approach must be used to ensure preservation of data integrity. Data integrity is crucial in the healthcare environment because data serves as a driving force in determining treatments. Information technology (IT) must ensure that healthcare decisions are based on authentic data. If the quality of data is flawed or incorrect, so are subsequent decisions. If data is faulty or incomplete, the quality of derived information will be poor, resulting in inappropriate and possibly harmful decisions. For example, if the nurse interviewing a client collects data related to allergies but fails to document all reported allergies, the client could be given drugs that cause an allergic reaction. In this case, the data were collected but not stored. Computer systems can be designed to facilitate data collection (although entry of incorrect data through input errors is still possible). Input errors can include hitting the wrong key on a computer keyboard or selecting the wrong item from a list. Input errors may be decreased through staff education, periodic system checks, and providing opportunities to verify data prior to entry.

Although the initial data collection and entry process provides an excellent opportunity to verify data accuracy and completeness, it should not be the only time that this is done. Healthcare consumers should be able to review their records at any time and furnish additional information that they believe is important to their care or to dispute portions of their record with which they do not agree. A **system check** is a mechanism provided by the computer system to assist users by prompting them to complete a task, verify information, or prevent entry of inappropriate information. After data has been collected, its quality may be improved via the process of **data cleansing** or **data scrubbing** so that it will be accurate enough to support analysis. These terms are used interchangeably to refer to removing incorrect, incomplete, duplicate, or improperly formatted items using special software designated for this purpose.

Quality Improvement

Quality improvement is a scientific approach to the analysis of performance and ways to improve it (Wilson, 2016). Quality improvement is built upon the following principles:

- Commitment to quality and collaborative efforts. The organization must demonstrate clear and consistent dedication to quality from its mission statement all the way through its policies and actions.
- Quality must be measurable, and measurability allows one to determine if change resulted in improvement.
- Systems thinking, which focuses on processes and the improvement of processes.
- Quality is ongoing and results from rigorously repeated efforts.

The following items, while far from inclusive, provide some specific examples of data that are tracked for the purpose of improved quality:

- *The Consumer Assessment of Healthcare Providers and Systems (CAHPS®).* This survey instrument collects data on patients' perceptions of their care, permitting comparison across settings, providers, and financial incentives in the form of increased or decreased Medicare reimbursement for hospitals to improve the quality of care provided (Centers for Medicare and Medicaid Services [CMS], 2017). Results are public.

- *Patient falls.* Hospitals voluntarily submit patient fall data to the national database of nursing quality indicators (NDNQI), a database created by the American Nurses Association. Hospitals can then compare their fall rates against other hospitals of similar type and size (Mennella & Holle, 2016).

- *30-day readmission rates.* The hospital readmissions reduction program provides financial incentives to hospitals to reduce patient readmissions within 30 days for Medicare beneficiaries (Mennella & Key, 2016). This is the reason why organizations collect information on their patients with acute myocardial infarction, heart failure, pneumonia, chronic obstructive pulmonary disease, and elective hip and/or total knee replacement to determine ways that they can improve both patients' outcomes and the organization's subsequent reimbursement.

It should be noted that the concept of quality management is not realized until data collected is used to support decisions for the purpose of improvement (Rivenbark, Roenigk, & Fasiello, 2017). The Patient Protection and Affordable Care Act mandates the creation of a national strategy for quality, and more efforts in this area can be expected (Smith, 2013).

Data Management

Data management is the process of controlling the collection, storage, retrieval, and use of data to optimize accuracy and utility while safeguarding integrity. Efficient and effective data management optimizes the value of the data for informed decision-making (Shankaranarayanan, Even, & Berger, 2015). Good data management requires thorough planning (Wills, 2014). On the organizational level, it is critical to consider what information is needed as well as the tools and resources required to manage it and realize its value. This planning should start with the organization's strategic plan. It should be noted. However, that it may not be possible to anticipate every future need.

Several levels of personnel are involved in data management. Personnel at the point of data entry include employees and, in some cases, clients. System analysts help the users to specify the data that are to be collected and how data collection will be accomplished. Programmers create the computer instructions, or program, that will collect the required data. They also build **databases**, the file structure that supports the storage of data in an organized fashion and allows data retrieval as meaningful information. Some facilities also employ **database administrators**, who are responsible for overseeing all activities related to maintaining the database and optimizing its use. Another common strategy used within organizations is the data warehouse. A **data warehouse** is a repository for storing data from several different databases so that it can be combined and manipulated as needed and to provide answers to various queries (Shankaranarayanan, Even, & Berger, 2015).

Costs and benefits are considerations in the management of data. Organizations must invest in storage systems, software, and personnel to derive the optimal benefit from analyzing data that they manage. Data management is cost- and labor-intensive but must be viewed as an investment needed to yield high-quality data.

Data Types and Formats

Data management is complicated by the fact that data comes in different forms. Data may be raw or processed or come in unstructured or structured formats. Unstructured data include documents such as consults, emails, and multimedia resources. Structured data are typically organized into a repository or database for effective processing. An example of structured data can be seen with a pick list on a nursing documentation screen where the user is forced to select an option. Structured data can be used to generate reports while unstructured data do not lend themselves to such quick analysis. While the healthcare industry still has some paper documents that it maintains, this situation is becoming uncommon. The widespread conversion of data and information to electronic format so that it can be accessed, processed, stored, or transmitted via the use of computer technology is known as **digitization**. Digitization increases the amount of information available electronically.

Data Governance

Data Governance is the term used to refer to the collection of policies, standards, processes, and controls applied to an organization's data to ensure that it is available to appropriate persons when and where it is needed, in the format that is needed, and is otherwise properly secured (Dutta, 2016). Data governance is an extremely important part of data management. Data governance may seem fairly straightforward—when one organization or healthcare delivery system is involved—but becomes more complicated in the presence of HIE and other, larger efforts to share data for big data purposes. At the local level, data governance establishes the screens and data that each user class is able to access, configures the view for each user class, has oversight for the creation, dispersal, and revocation of individual user names and passwords to log on to the system, and drafts and enforces access policies. With HIE, traditional governance issues include privacy and security of data, liability for inappropriate disclosure, and possible unfair market advantages (Allen et al., 2014). Data-sharing agreements (DSAs) among exchange partners spell out responsibilities and meet legal requirements.

Big Data, Data Analytics, and Data Modeling

The term **big data** refers to very large data sets that are beyond human capability to analyze or manage without the aid of technology. These large data sets are then used to reveal patterns and discover new learning. The availability of large data sets, decreased storage costs, and increased computing power support the big data phenomenon (Tattersall & Grant, 2016). Although the arrival of big data in healthcare lags behind its use in other industries, it is nonetheless of vital importance due to the increasing complexity of healthcare and its need for informed decision-making (Tharmalingam, Hagens, & Zelmer, 2016; Wills, 2014). Big data includes data of different types, levels of complexity, and formats (structured, unstructured, and semi-structured), as well as processed and unprocessed items from several sources that is then analyzed for patterns (Jukić, Sharma, Nestorov, & Jukić, 2015; Manerikar, 2016).

The process of examining big data for patterns is known as **data mining**, and sometimes the term **analytics** is used interchangeably. Data mining is a process that uses software to uncover relationships within large data sets via the use of artificial intelligence, statistical computation, and computer technology (Brown & White, 2017). Data mining has been used in marketing and politics to determine buying and voting trends within society. It has even been used to discover financial fraud (Albashrawi, 2016) and has only recently been added to the repertoire of healthcare industry tools to determine a variety of outcomes. Analytics actually goes beyond the discovery of patterns in data as it systematically uses data and insights from models that it incorporates to offer solutions and drive decisions (Wills, 2014).

Analytics is seen in three forms: small data, predictive modeling, and real-time analytics (Wills, 2014). Small data refers to limited data sets such as that seen with EHR information for a select patient population at a single hospital or healthcare delivery system. A specific example might include using EHRs to determine the patients admitted with congestive heart failure for a specific timeframe. Small data is ideal to report benchmarks and can be used very effectively for case-management purposes. Costs and expertise needed to run and use small data are nominal; needed resources are already in place at most facilities (Wills, 2014). Analysis of small data most typically requires the presence of a data repository, staff training, and possibly some changes to existing workflows.

Predictive modeling, also known as **predictive analytics**, uses past and current data to forecast the likelihood of an event (Kakad, Rozenblum, & Bates, 2017; Wills, 2014). In healthcare, predictive analytics can use medical information derived from EHRs to evaluate health risks for patients, the likelihood that they will utilize services in the future, or predict who is at risk for complications. In one specific example, Vesely (2017) detailed the use of this type of tool to identify which patients were at high-risk for central-line infections, so that that active measures could be employed to prevent infections before they occurred. In addition to improving outcomes, predictive analytics can help eliminate waste (Kakad, Rozenblum, & Bates, 2017). Despite the potential to improve the efficiency and effectiveness of healthcare delivery, adoption of predictive analytics by healthcare organizations has been slow.

Real-time analytics (RTA) examines current data in real-time. RTA is unfettered by the time lag associated with the use of historical data, which may no longer apply and can negatively impact decisions (Dobrev & Hart, 2015). RTA allows a move from a reactive to proactive stance and can foster both learning and predictions in administrative and clinical areas. RTA at the point of care use data available through device integration comparing it against data from the EHR, registries, and other information systems and databases, to present immediate, actionable information to clinicians. Examples of actionable information would include alerts of possible drug interactions or complications, and suggested interventions. RTA requires integration of systems, a data repository, a master data management environment, architecture that supports data creation, integration, interception for analysis, a mature business intelligence (historical data helps to provide context and meaning) and data warehouse, the ability to configure and re-engineer processes, information-technology expertise with subject matter/business knowledge, rule definition, established goals and requirements, and decisions upon whether to build or contract for RTA services.

Business intelligence (BI) is another term used when discussions of best use of data arise. BI is the integration of data from different sources for the purpose of optimizing its use and understanding (Pinto & Fox, 2016). BI refers to a strategy, processes, and a tool set (Obeidat, North, Richardson, Rattanak, & North, 2015). That is to say that analytics can be, and frequently are, a part of business intelligence. BI is a very important part of healthcare delivery today but is not the primary focus of this chapter.

The knowledge gleaned from large data sets and big data is sometimes referred to as **knowledge discovery in databases (KDD)**. KDD can be defined as a process of an iterative sequence that entails the following steps: understanding the domain; understanding the data used in the domain; data preparation that handles missing values or removes redundant or irrelevant data; applying methods to extract data (namely data mining); and finally, data presentation (Afshar, Ahmadi, Roudbari, & Sadoughi, 2015). Clinical databases hold huge amounts of information about patients and their medical conditions. The potential to discern patterns and relationships within those databases that would contribute to new knowledge was recognized some time ago, but until recently, discovery of useful information was hampered by a lack of tools to reveal it. Clinical repositories are now available for research and utilization purposes.

A foundational concept to useful data and information is **data modeling**. Data modeling is a process to define and analyze data requirements to support processes required within an organization. Data modeling is an important step in the design of a database such as an EHR, because it establishes what information must be collected and in what format. On a larger scale, data modeling provides a platform for BI and data analysis and can help to address the gap between data that are available and information that is required (LaMacchia & Egan, 2017). Data modeling also supports exchange and re-use of data (Goossen & Goossen-Baremans, 2013).

Challenges in Finding and Using Big Data in Healthcare

The challenges to finding and using big data in healthcare are many. Among the most notable are:

- *Incentives to share data.* Without data sharing, the amount of big data is limited, which minimizes its value. When addressing the Zika outbreak, Littler et al. (2017) noted that there were limited incentives for researchers and responders to share data. Reluctance to share may stem from concerns over intellectual property rights or attribution issues.

- *Proprietary issues.* In the United States, the rivalry among healthcare vendors historically made it difficult to readily share data resident on competing products. And competing healthcare systems have been loathe to share patient information for fear that it would afford their rivals an unfair advantage. These types of issues limit the amount of data shared and, consequently, the amount of big data. Data has value and can be sold for other uses. HIEs sell secondary data. The American Medical Association and US Centers for Medicare and Medicare also sell provider data (Kaplan, 2015).

- *Lack of appropriate infrastructure.* Creating the infrastructure to share data and support big data is quite involved. First, a governance structure must be created that provides a balance between privacy and access while complying with state, national, and international ethical and legal requirements (Littler et al., 2017; Moorthy, Roth, Olliaro, Dye, & Kieny, 2016). Terms for data use must be clear. It is only after governance issues are addressed that the data repository, special software, and experts can follow.

- *Data quality.* Wills (2014) noted that much healthcare data is available but not enough has sufficient applicable information accompanying it. Presumably that statement refers to metadata. **Metadata** is defined as the data that provides information about how, when, and by whom data are collected, formatted, and stored. Without metadata and data dictionaries, the correct or meaningful re-use of information cannot occur. More work is needed to develop data-sharing platforms that can standardize, clean, and curate data into usable forms (Merson, Gaye, & Guerin, 2016).

- *Culture.* Organizations and their leaders need to adopt new processes.

- *Costs.* Investment in technology, including the infrastructure and technology required for the aggregation and analysis of big data by healthcare, has been limited with some notable exceptions (Wills, 2014). Not all healthcare systems have the same resources, and costs can be difficult to justify when balanced against many competing needs (Dobrev & Hart, 2015).

- *Complexity of healthcare.* The nature of healthcare has limited the ability to incorporate the same level of sophistication in analytic tools found in other industries (Wills, 2014).

- *Insufficient expertise.* Big data presents a steep learning curve for administrators and clinicians, and the data scientists needed to help them understand big data are highly sought-after, making them scarce commodities in the healthcare sector (Gelinas, 2016).

- *A lack of nursing visibility.* Gelinas (2016) noted there is a danger that decisions will be made without nursing representation, because there are no posted big data positions for nurses and nurse informaticists. Nurses and nurse informaticists are needed to communicate clinician needs to data scientists, and nurses must work with data scientists to advance both nursing knowledge and practice using big data. Another visibility issue for nursing relates to the low levels of adoption of standardized nursing language in EHRs, leaving nursing with limited measures of its clinical accomplishments.

- *Big promises but limited progress.* The potential of big data in healthcare has barely been tapped. There are inequities in the ability to support big data, and gaps in pre-requisite knowledge and skill-sets among administrators and clinicians, that currently hinder the best use of big data.

Information and Knowledge Management

Good information management ensures access to the right information at the right time to the people who need it. Vast amounts of information are produced daily. This information may or may not be readily available when it is needed. Its volume exceeds the processing capacity of any single human being. Part of good information management ensures that care providers have the resources that they need to provide safe, efficient, quality care. Some examples of these resources include clinical guidelines, standards of practice, policy and procedure manuals, research findings, drug databases, and information on community resources. IT can help to ensure access to the most recent versions of these types of resources via tools such as intranets and electronic communities. This type of version control within an organization eliminates the uncertainties of what may or may not be available in various locations, and whether or not it is the most recent version. Good information management also eliminates redundant data collection, which wastes resources. In the era of big data, good information management is more important than ever before.

Although the terms information management and knowledge management are sometimes used interchangeably, the concepts are different. **Knowledge management (KM)** refers to the process of selectively applying knowledge gained from previous experiences and decision-making to current and future situations for the express purpose of improved effectiveness (Karlinsky-Shichor & Zviran, 2016). **Knowledge management systems** are sets of information systems that enable organizations to tap into the knowledge, experiences, and creativity of their staff to improve performance (Karlinsky-Shichor & Zviran, 2016). KM is a structured process for the generation, storage, distribution, and application of both tacit knowledge (personal experience) and explicit knowledge (evidence) in organizations. Knowledge is a valued commodity and one that can provide a competitive edge. While many organizations collect and store vast amounts of data, not all are equally successful in discovering hidden knowledge in that data (Dastyar, Kazemnejad, Sereshgi, & Jabalameli, 2017). Data mining can provide a valuable asset to knowledge management.

Effective KM in an organization requires the presence of the following infrastructure elements: human, process, and IT (Dastyar et al., 2017). As to the human infrastructure, there must be an understanding of foundational concepts such as data and information, and a process to support individual knowledge becoming group knowledge. Process infrastructure includes practices, regulations and laws. And lastly, IT infrastructure would include a network, a data warehouse, individual databases, and data mining tools.

Using Analytics to Support Healthcare Delivery

Analytics can support healthcare delivery day-to-day operations and clinical care of healthcare delivery systems. As one example at the organizational level, predictive analytics can help determine what services the facility should offer, helping to maintain the bottom line while meeting healthcare-consumer needs (Drell & Davis, 2014). Real-time analytic tools can offer significant and measurable improvements, help organizations remain competitive, and, in the long run, drive strategic business objectives from a grass roots level (Dobrev & Hart, 2015). Many of the larger healthcare delivery systems have been using analytics to improve operations and improve patient care (Wills, 2014).

On the clinical side of operations, big data and analytics provide tools to help deliver care more effectively, efficiently, and at lower cost (Bates, Saria, Ohno-Machado, Shah, & Escobar, 2014). Furthermore, big data findings are a form of evidence used to supplement traditional research findings, or as a source of evidence on their own (de Lusignan, Crawford, & Munro, 2015; Kennedy, 2016).

On a larger scale, big data and analytics can also uncover new learning and evidence to improve patient outcomes and population health. If that sounds familiar, it should be, as that intent precipitated the American Recovery and Reinvestment Act of 2009 that provided financial incentives to providers to adopt electronic health records so that data could be collected and shared electronically for analysis and subsequent learning to improve healthcare. This legislation arose from a health policy that helped to establish a framework for big data. Big data and the resulting evidence can then be used to inform policy makers, who in turn make decisions that impact funding and delivery of services.

Clinician Roles in Using Big Data and Analytics

Clinicians need to understand the relationship between big data and evidence-informed practice (Brennan & Bakken, 2015). They also need to have a voice in the selection and use of tools, such as real-time analytics at the bedside, and predictive analytics, to ensure that the tools provide value for clinicians and patients. Both activities require the acquisition of new knowledge and skills, although nurses start with a good foundation given their theoretical background, patient-centered focus, basic understanding of standards, standardized languages, and research as a source for evidence-based decisions. Even as many nurses struggle to grasp the concepts of nursing informatics, now in addition they must learn about big data. **Data science** is the systematic study of digital data (National Consortium for Data Science, 2017, Para. 2)—analytics, business intelligence, knowledge management, and discovery informatics so that they have context for the time and place in which they practice. **Discovery informatics** uses scientific models and theories to create computer-based discovery of new learning in big data, replacing human cognition with the idea that discovery and learning can be accelerated (Honavar, 2014).

Ethical Concerns with Data and Information Use

Rapid developments with data sharing, new models for research, secondary use, and big data enable opportunities to improve health and healthcare, yet exacerbate some concerns (Kaplan, 2016), and give rise to new ones, which are briefly addressed here:

Ownership of Patient Data. Ownership of patient data is not clearly addressed from a legal perspective either in the US or abroad (Kaplan, 2016).

Data sharing. There are numerous questions here that include control and implications of when data is shared. Participants in a summit on aligning incentives for data sharing wanted their data quickly so that others could benefit (Haug, 2017). Study participants also wanted results shared directly with them along with explanation of what results meant, a change from current practices. Also, in treatment trials, early sharing may bias results.

The meaning of informed consent. This has several aspects. One is that some patients believe it to mean that they will receive the best treatment in a research trial. There are also differences across the US and Europe in what consent conveys (Haug, 2017). And yet another issue occurs with data mining and biobanking, because consent implies awareness and choice—neither of which are true in this instance (Al-Saggaf, 2015; Meir, Cohen, Mee, & Gaffney, 2014). And finally, big data creates a shift with research so that the informed consent relationship is no longer with a person or research institution.

Secondary use of data. De-identified, aggregate data is commonly sold for purposes other than the original reason for collection. This can pose problems because ownership is not well-defined (Kaplan, 2016). Secondary data has been used to target persons for marketing purposes even though it should be de-identified.

Privacy versus confidentiality. Research findings, biobanks, and big data are typically de-identified, or kept confidential, but there are occasions when personal information can be identified and information released, causing harms that include discrimination in obtaining credit, insurance, housing, or employment, social stigma, and even reuse of DNA collected for research for criminal profiling (Dove 2015; Kaplan, 2016).

Future Directions

The amount of data and information produced within healthcare will continue to grow, particularly as new data sources and models of sharing such as biobanks evolve, and data streams from wearable and consumer devices are incorporated. As the amount of data and information increases we look forward to a commensurate increase in knowledge and wisdom created with the use of big data, data science, and the tools supporting big science. Along with that knowledge and wisdom, there will be major changes in the way we diagnose and treat patients.

Informatics professionals, and informatics nurses in particular, must be active participants in advocating for consumers and infusing their knowledge, skills, and experience into the analysis of big data (Booth, 2016). The transformation of healthcare requires evidence, plus the infrastructure provided by informatics, to support knowledge discovery and dissemination gained through effective use of data and information (Delaney, Kuziemsky, & Brandt, 2015). At the same time, the INS must never lose sight of the need to collaborate interprofessionally to achieve this transformation, while working to decrease errors and promote safety.

Summary

- A discussion of effective and ethical use of data and information requires definition of the concepts of data, information, knowledge, and wisdom, as well as a discussion of responsibilities delineated in professional codes of ethics and practice standards for informatics nursing.
- Healthcare data has long resided in a series of separate silos with limited sharing and benefits to the larger community.
- Sharing data is an ethical and scientific imperative because it can bring great good to the many, yet no common ethical and legal framework exists that will connect healthcare providers and data in EHRs with research findings, regulators, collaboratives, and various other databases.
- Data is a strategic resource that can be used to track day-to-day operations, patient outcomes and services, and more.
- Quality improvement and quality management, requires data that is complete, reliable, without error, and reliable (data quality).
- Data quality can be fostered through the use of computer-system checks that remind users to complete a task, verify information, or that prohibit entry of inappropriate information.
- Data scrubbing, or cleansing, is a process that improves data quality to improve analysis.
- Healthcare follows multiple metrics to determine if improvements have occurred. Some examples include patient satisfaction, patient outcomes, and readmissions.
- Data management is the process of controlling the collection, storage, retrieval, and use of data to optimize accuracy and utility, while safeguarding integrity in the process of controlling the collection, storage, retrieval, and use of data to optimize accuracy and utility.
- Data management is complicated by the various formats that data come in.
- Digitization is the widespread conversion of data and information to electronic format so that it can be accessed, processed, stored, or transmitted via the use of computer technology.
- Data governance is the collection of policies, standards, processes and controls applied to an organization's data to ensure that it is available when, where, and by who it is needed, in the format that is needed, and is properly secured.
- Big data is the term used to refer to very large data sets (that are beyond human capability to analyze or manage without the aid of technology) that are now being examined for patterns that can be used to drive decisions.
- Data mining is the process that uses software to uncover relationships within large data sets via the use of artificial intelligence, statistical computation, and computer technology.
- Analytics uses data and insights from models that it incorporates to offer solutions and drive decisions.
- Predictive modeling, or predictive analytics, use past and current data to forecast the likelihood of an event.
- Real-time analytics (RTA) examines current data in real-time.
- Business intelligence (BI) refers to the strategy, processes, and tool set that integrate data from different sources for the purpose of optimizing its use and understanding.

- The knowledge gleaned from large data sets and big data is sometimes referred to as knowledge discovery in databases.
- Data modeling is a process to define and analyze data requirements to support processes required within an organization.
- Challenges to big data use include: limited incentives to share data; proprietary issues; lack of infrastructure; uneven data quality; organizational culture; costs; the complexity of healthcare; limited available expertise; limited nursing visibility; and limited progress toward creation and support.
- Knowledge management is the process of applying knowledge gained from experience to current and future situations for the express purpose of improved effectiveness.
- Analytics can bring value to healthcare delivery.
- Clinicians need to acquire knowledge and skills to use big data.
- Unresolved ethical issues related to data and information use include unanswered questions of ownership of patient data and secondary use, control with data sharing, clarifying "informed consent," and patient harms related to disclosure of information.
- The amount and types of data will continue to grow, providing new opportunities for learning as well as new challenges.
- Nurses, and informatics nurses in particular, must take an active role with all things related to effective and ethical use of data and information.

Case Study

You have been asked to speak to senior nursing students enrolled in a nursing informatics class at the local university on the implications of big data for healthcare delivery and nursing. You are trying to condense your presentation to ten key points—what would they be and what is your rationale for their selection?

About the Authors

Toni Hebda teaches graduate-level informatics courses at Chamberlain College of Nursing. She graduated from Washington Hospital, earned her BSN from Duquesne University, and her MNEd, PhD, and MSIS from the University of Pittsburgh. She has taught in formal nursing programs, staff development, and instructed hospital staff in the use of information systems. Kathleen (Kathy) Hunter graduated from Church Home & Hospital and served with the Army Nurse Corps. She earned her BSN, MS in nursing, and PHD at the University of Maryland. Nursing informatics is her area of practice. Dr. Hunter has taught online for several years. Her contributions to nursing informatics include starting the MSN informatics track at Chamberlain College, leadership roles, and research on nursing informatics competencies. Dr. Hunter is a Professor with the Chamberlain MSN Program and has been recognized as an American Academy of Nursing Fellow.

References

Afshar, H. L., Ahmadi, M., Roudbari, M., & Sadoughi, F. (2015). Prediction of breast cancer survival through knowledge discovery in databases. *Global Journal of Health Science*, 7(4), 392–398. doi:10.5539/gjhs.v7n4p392

Albashrawi, M. (2016). Detecting financial fraud using data mining techniques: A decade review from 2004 to 2015. *Journal of Data Science, 14*(3), 553–569.

Allen, C., Des Jardins, T. R., Heider, A., Lyman, K. A., McWilliams, L., Rein, A. L., . . . Turske, S. A. (2014). Data governance and data sharing agreements for community-wide health information exchange: Lessons from the Beacon communities. EGEMS. (*Generating Evidence & Methods to Improve Patient Outcomes, 2*(1), 1–9. doi:10.13063/2327-9214.1057

Al-Saggaf, Y. (2015). The use of data mining by private health insurance companies and customers' privacy. *Cambridge Quarterly of Healthcare Ethics, 24*, 281–292.

American Nurses Association. (2015a). *Nursing informatics: Scope and standards of practice* (2nd ed.). Silver Spring, MD: Author.

American Nurses Association. (2015b). Code of ethics for nurses with interpretative statements. Retrieved from nursingworld.org

Bailey, J., Wan, J., Mabry, L., Landy, S., Pope, R., Waters, T., & Frisse, M. (2013). Does health information exchange reduce unnecessary neuroimaging and improve quality of headache care in the emergency department? *Journal of General Internal Medicine, 28*(2), 176–183. doi:10.1007/s11606-012-2092-7

Bates, D. W., Saria, S., Ohno-Machado, L., Shah, A., & Escobar, G. (2014). Big data in health care: Using analytics to identify and manage high-risk and high-cost patients. *Health Affairs, 33*(7), 1123–1131.

Bauchner, H., Golub, R. M., & Fontanarosa, P. B. (2016). Data sharing: An ethical and scientific imperative. *The Journal of the American Medical Association, 315*(12), 1237–1239.

Booth, R. G. (2016). Informatics and nursing in a post-nursing informatics world: Future directions for nurses in an automated, artificially intelligent, social-networked healthcare environment. *Nursing Leadership (Toronto, Ont.), 28*(4), 61–69.

Brennan, P. F., & Bakken, S. (2015). Nursing needs big data and big data needs nursing. *Journal of Nursing Scholarship, 47*(5), 477–484.

Brown, G. E., & White, E. D. (2017). An investigation of nonparametric data mining techniques for acquisition cost estimating. *Defense Acquisition Research Journal: A Publication of The Defense Acquisition University, 24*(2), 302–332. doi:10.22594/dau.16756.24.02

Centers for Medicare & Medicaid Services. (Revised 06/20/2017). Consumer Assessment of Healthcare Providers & Systems (CAHPS). Retrieved from www.cms.gov/Research-Statistics-Data-and-Systems/Research/CAHPS/

Chen, H., Hailey, D., Wang, N., & Yu, P. (2014). A review of data quality assessment methods for public health information systems. *International Journal of Environmental Research & Public Health, 11*(5), 5170–5207. doi:10.3390/ijerph110505170

Davidson, A. J. (2015). Creating value: Unifying silos into public health business intelligence. *Frontiers in Public Health Services & Systems Research, 4*(2), 1–13. doi:10.13063/2327-9214.1172

Dastyar, B., Kazemnejad, H., Sereshgi, A. A., & Jabalameli, M. A. (2017). Using data mining techniques to develop knowledge management in organizations: A review. *Journal of Engineering, Project, and Production Management, 7*(2), 80–89.

Delaney, C. W., Kuziemsky, C., & Brandt, B. F. (2015). Integrating informatics and interprofessional education and practice to drive healthcare transformation. *Journal of Interprofessional Care, 29*(6), 527–529.

de Lusignan, S., Crawford, L., & Munro, N. (2015). Creating and using real-world evidence to answer questions about clinical effectiveness. *Journal of Innovation in Health Informatics, 22*(3), 368–373.

Dobrev, K., & Hart, M. (2015). Benefits, justification and implementation planning of real-time business intelligence systems. *Electronic Journal of Information Systems Evaluation, 18*(2), 105–119.

Dove, E. S. (2015). Biobanks, data sharing, and the drive for a global privacy governance framework. *The Journal of Law, Medicine & Ethics: A Journal of The American Society of Law, Medicine & Ethics, 43*(4), 675-689. doi:10.1111/jlme.12311

Drell, L., & Davis, J. (2014). Getting started with predictive analytics. *Marketing Health Services, 34*(3), 22–27.

Dutta, A. (2016). Ensuring the quality of data in motion: The missing link in data governance. *Computer Weekly*, 1–4.

Gelinas, L. (2016). Big data: Big roles in big demand for nurses. *American Nurse Today, 11*(2), 1–1.

Goossen, W., & Goossen-Baremans, A. (2013). Clinical professional governance for detailed clinical models. *Studies in Health Technology & Informatics, 193*, 231–260. doi:10.3233/978-1-61499-291-2-231

Haug, C. J. (2017). Whose data are they anyway? Can a patient perspective advance the data-sharing debate? *The New England Journal of Medicine, 376*(23), 2203–2205. doi:10.1056/NEJMp1704485

Honavar, V. G. (2014). The promise and potential of big data: A case for discovery informatics. *Review of Policy Research, 31*(4), 326–330.

International Medical Informatics Association (IMIA). (2016). The IMIA code of ethics for health information professionals. Retrieved from http://imia-medinfo.org/wp/wp-content/uploads/2015/07/IMIA-Code-of-Ethics-2016.pdf

Jukić, N., Sharma, A., Nestorov, S., & Jukić, B. (2015). Augmenting data warehouses with big data. *Information Systems Management, 32*(3), 200–209.

Kakad, M., Rozenblum, R., & Bates, D. W. (2017). Getting buy-in for predictive analytics in health care. *Harvard Business Review Digital Articles*, 2–5.

Kaplan, B. (2015). Selling health data: de-identification, privacy, and speech. *Cambridge Quarterly of Healthcare Ethics, 24*(3), 256–271.

Kaplan, B. (2016). How should health data be used? *Cambridge Quarterly of Healthcare Ethics, 25*(2), 312–329.

Karlinsky-Shichor, Y., & Zviran, M. (2016). Factors influencing perceived benefits and user satisfaction in knowledge management systems. *Information Systems Management, 33*(1), 55–73.

Kennedy, M. A. (2016). Adaptive practice: Next generation evidence-based practice in digital environments. *Studies in Health Technology and Informatics, 225*, 417–421.

Knoppers, B. M., Harris, J. R., Budin-ljøsne, I., & Dove, E. S. (2014). A human rights approach to an international code of conduct for genomic and clinical data sharing. *Human Genetics, 133*(7), 895–903.

Kuehn, B. M. (2014). IOM outlines framework for clinical data sharing, solicits input. *The Journal of the American Medical Association, 30*(7), 665.

LaMacchia, C., & Egan, W. (2017). Smart data modeling. *Proceedings for the Northeast Region Decision Sciences Institute (NEDSI)*, 466.

Leventhal, R., & Hagland, M. (2017). Healthcare's latest interoperability push. Healthcare Informatics, 34(1), 35–37.

Littler, K., Wee-Ming, B., Carson, G., Depoortere, E., Mathewson, S., Mietchen, D., . . . Segovia, C. (2017). Progress in promoting data sharing in public health emergencies. *Bulletin of the World Health Organization, 95*(4), 243–244. doi:10.2471/BLT.17.192096

Manerikar, S. (2016). Big data. *Aweshkar Research Journal, 21*(2), 95.

Mennella, H. A., & Holle, M. O. (2016). Falls, accidental: Incident reports—risk management. CINAHL Nursing Guide. Glendale, CA: EBSCO.

Mennella, H. A., & Key, M. C. (2016). Case management: Readmissions. CINAHL Nursing Guide. Glendale, CA: EBSCO.

Meir, K., Cohen, Y., Mee, B., & Gaffney, E. F. (2014). Biobank networking for dissemination of data and resources: An overview. *Journal of Biorepository Science for Applied Medicine*, 229–242. doi:10.2147/BSAM.S46577.

Merson, L., Gaye, O., & Guerin, P. J. (2016). Avoiding data dumpsters—Toward equitable and useful data sharing, *The New England Journal of Medicine, 374*(25), 2414–2415.

Moorthy, V. S., Roth, C., Olliaro, P., Dye, C., & Kieny, M. P. (2016). Best practices for sharing information through data platforms: Establishing the principles. *Bulletin of the World Health Organization, 94*(4), 234, 234A.

National Consortium for Data Science. (2017). About the National Consortium for Data Science. Retrieved from http://datascienceconsortium.org/about/

Obeidat, M., North, M., Richardson, R., Rattanak, V., & North, S. (2015). Business intelligence technology, applications, and trends. *International Management Review, 11*(2), 47–56.

Otto, B. (2015). Quality and value of the data resource in large enterprises. *Information Systems Management, 32*(3), 234–251. doi:10.1080/10580530.2015.1044344

Pinto, B., & Fox, B. I. (2016). Clinical and Business Intelligence: Why it's important to your pharmacy. *Hospital Pharmacy, 51*(7), 604. doi:10.1310/hpj5107-604

Rivenbark, W. C., Roenigk, D. J., & Fasiello, R. (2017). Twenty years of benchmarking in North Carolina: Lessons learned from comparison of performance statistics as benchmarks. *Public Administration Quarterly, 41*(1), 130–148.

Shankaranarayanan, G., Even, A., & Berger, P. D. (2015). Optimizing data management with disparities in data value. *Journal of International Technology & Information Management, 24*(3), 1–24.

Smith, H. L. (2013). Public reporting of Medicare quality data. *PT in Motion, 5*(10), 44–47.

Tattersall, A., & Grant, M. J. (2016). Big Data—What is it and why it matters. *Health Information and Libraries Journal, 33*(2), 89–91. doi:10.1111/hir.12147

Tharmalingam, S., Hagens, S., & Zelmer, J. (2016). The value of connected health information: perceptions of electronic health record users in Canada. *BMC Medical Informatics & Decision Making*, 161–169. doi:10.1186/s12911-016-0330-3

Using data for quality management and care collaboration: PART 1. (2016). *Long-Term Living: For the Continuing Care Professional, 65*(4), 54–55.

Vesely, R. (2017). Predictive analytics: IU health knows the patient in room 103 is at high-risk for CLABSI. Would you? *H & HN: Hospitals & Health Networks, 91*(2), 20–25.

Wills, M. J. (2014). Decisions through data: Analytics in healthcare. *Journal of Healthcare Management, 59*(4), 254–262.

Wilson, D. M. (2016). Quality model for improvement: Plan-do-study-act. CINAHL Nursing Guide, Nursing Reference Center Plus. Accessed Februaury 4, 2017

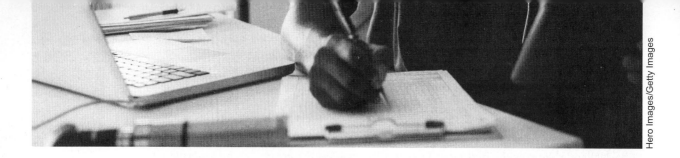

Chapter 4
Electronic Resources for Healthcare Professionals

Brenda Kulhanek, PhD, MSN, MS, RN-BC

 ## Learning Objectives

After completing this chapter, you should be able to:

- Choose methods to locate reliable information online.

- Propose ways to determine the veracity of online information.

- Demonstrate responsible use of social media for healthcare professionals.

- Identify reliable resources for health information and services.

- Discuss the benefits of online services for healthcare professionals.

- Name specific professional organizations and watchdog groups focused on electronic resources.

- Discuss the benefits and drawbacks to eLearning.

- Describe technology used to organize and use electronic information.

This chapter provides a brief overview of electronic resources available for healthcare professionals, including online resources for information and learning. Also included is information about how to determine the veracity of information, services available for healthcare providers, organizing information, and future directions of electronic resources for healthcare professionals.

Information Literacy

The Internet contains many sources of information, some credible and some not credible. Effective use of the Internet requires information literacy. Information literacy involves both the ability to locate information and to interpret information in a manner that is relevant to the user.

Historically, database and literature searches involved a trip to a library and hours of time to comb through paper-based literature. Databases are now easily accessible and available through the Internet as public libraries, colleges and universities, subscriptions, and open access database engines—such as Google Scholar—allow the user to access journals, publications, and periodicals quickly and easily from any device with an Internet connection. Databases that contain information that can be used for research—such as de-identified patient records or self-reported patient databases—allow for the ability to study specific patient populations.

Although some databases are open to any user, most databases containing scholarly publications require a subscription or access through a school or organization. There are sites that provide pay-per-article access to literature; however, these sites may not have the full spectrum of literature found in a scholarly database.

Internet Searches

The average computer user can quickly and easily access large amounts of information on the Internet. However, the ability for consumers to identify and utilize health information for positive change remains uncertain (Diviani, van den Putte, Giani, & van Weert, 2015; Medlock et al., 2015), although accurate use of online health information by health professionals appears to be related to improve patient knowledge and outcomes (Laugesen, Hassanein, & Yuan, 2015). More concerning is the ability of both the consumer and healthcare professional to identify and recommend valid and reliable health-information websites (Buultiens, Robinson, & Milgrom, 2012).

Critical Assessment of Online Information

The number of websites and resources on the Internet is ever increasing. Healthcare professionals must possess the skills to critically evaluate information and guide healthcare consumers to accurate information sources. The National Library of Medicine provides tutorials that can be used to assist in determining the validity of health information found on the Internet, in magazines, and on television. Table 4-1 provides some tips that can be used for evaluating health information. In addition to the general guide for evaluating information, another good rule of thumb is that larger organizations—such as hospitals, the government,

Table 4-1   Evaluating Online Health Information

Evaluation Criteria	Questions to Ask
Provider	Who is in charge of the website? Why are they providing the site? Can you contact them?
Funding	Where does the money to support the site come from? Does the site have advertisements? Are they labeled?
Quality	Where does the information come from? How is the content selected? Do experts review the information that goes on the site? Does the site avoid unbelievable or emotional claims? Is it up-to-date?
Privacy	Does the site ask for your personal information? Do they tell you how it will be used? Are you comfortable with how it will be used?

SOURCE: *Based on Evaluating Internet Health Information: A Tutorial from the National Library of Medicine.* Retrieved from www.nlm.nih.gov/medlineplus/webeval/webeval_start.html#

universities and other health organizations—will have the most reliable sites. The owner of the website can often be verified by clicking on the "about us" link, or the publisher information at the bottom of the web page.

It is important to assume that information is not accurate until it has been verified as coming from a reputable source that accurately cites information and research contained on the site. Research studies cited in a magazine or on a website should contain all of the details of the research study, rather than a general statement that information is clinically proven or from a recent research study. Information should be thorough, without any noticeable gaps or omissions.

Information should contain a date, although this rule is not always followed. General information published on websites by the government does not always contain dates written or published; yet, these are reputable sites. The quality of the writing and the look of the website should be professional and well-organized. A website with misspelled words, poor organization, or a confusing design may contain information that is not reliable, especially if the website is also selling a product or service.

The Health on the Net Foundation (www.healthonnet.org) was formed in 1995 as a nonprofit, private organization dedicated to ensuring quality health information on the Internet through a code of ethics that guides websites to develop objective and high-quality information that is carefully designed to meet the unique needs of the identified audience. The HONcode principles as identified on the HON website are shown in Table 4-2.

When a website has been certified, it receives the HONcode designation (www.healthonnet.org). Any website that applies for HONcode certification undergoes an initial expert review process, as well as annual expert reviews. The HONcode certification does not appear on the web page unless the HONcode toolbar has been installed on the end user's web browser. Once the toolbar has been installed, the HONcode seal will appear in color if the website has been certified.

The type of certification granted by HON for quality content differs from a certificate that indicates the security of the data passing between the end user's browser and the website's server, as exemplified with URL addresses that begin with HTTPS rather than HTTP typically seen to submit financial information. HTTPS refers to the hypertext transfer protocol over secure socket layer used to transfer and display content securely. An organization must go through a validation process in order to obtain a certificate that commences with verification that the domain is owned by the purchaser of the certificate. At this level, there is no guarantee of the legitimacy of the business. The highest level of certification—extended validation—provides proof of legitimacy of the business and may be designated by a lock icon on the URL toolbar (Figure 4-1).

Table 4-2 HONcode Principles

Principle	Evidence of Support
Principle 1—**Authority**	Give qualifications of authors
Principle 2—**Complementarity**	Information to support, not replace
Principle 3—**Confidentiality**	Respect the privacy of site users
Principle 4—**Attribution**	Cite the sources and dates of medical information
Principle 5—**Justifiability**	Justification of claims/balanced and objective claims
Principle 6—**Transparency**	Accessibility, provide valid contact details
Principle 7—**Financial disclosure**	Provide details of funding
Principle 8—**Advertising**	Clearly distinguish advertising from editorial content

SOURCE: "Health on the Net Foundation (HON), (2014). The HONcode: Principles. Retrieved from www.healthonnet.org/HONcode/Patients/Visitor/visitor.html. Used by permission. Copyright © 2014 by Health On the Net Foundation."

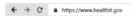

Figure 4-1 • Extended Validation

Health information abounds on the Internet, on television, and in magazines. Information may be presented in order to sell a product or service, information may be incorrect, or the website may exist to capture personal information for other uses. It is important to validate the accuracy of health and medical information by using certified or secured websites and through careful evaluation of key characteristics of the website.

Social Media—Responsibilities and Ethical Considerations

The first social-media site was created in the late 1990s, with minimal use or notice. The next iteration of social media to emerge was Myspace (www.myspace.com), which captured the attention of young people in 2003. However, it wasn't until Facebook and Twitter were implemented in 2004 and 2006 that the potential of social media captured the attention of the business and healthcare community. Since that time, new approaches to social media emerged on a regular basis, some based on sharing photos and some based on common interests. While use of social media has become second nature for many healthcare providers, and this use provides some valuable support of healthcare information, there are also many legal and ethical considerations to understand and apply.

One of the most widely used social-media sites is Facebook (www.facebook.com), which can be accessed on smartphones, tablets, and web browsers. Launched in 2004 for Harvard students, the rapid growth in popularity of the application resulted in a world-wide launch shortly after the original launch. Facebook allows users to connect with family, friends, and colleagues and provides the ability to share photos, thoughts, videos, web links, blogs, and other information. Facebook supports private user groups, public groups, and semi-private groups with common interests or relationships. Because Facebook is such an accepted part of the social structure for many people, it becomes a risk for HIPAA violations as healthcare-worker behavior has ranged from posting patient pictures, to describing patient situations, to discussing the interesting patient that they worked with that day. Despite the potential for oversharing of private and protected patient information, Facebook has become a powerful tool used for promoting businesses and healthcare organizations, for sharing healthcare information, and for advertising health products, both valid and not valid. An important consideration for users of social media is to assume that anyone may be able to access any information that is posted; therefore, best practice is to not share any professional information on this site. In addition, posting questionable pictures of one's own social life may backfire when seeking employment or even when a patient may choose to look up a caregiver on a site.

Based on a post of 140 or fewer characters, Twitter (www.twitter.com) is a widespread social-media tool that allows users to share small bits of information, web links, photos, and videos. Accessible through smart phones, tablets, and web browsers, Twitter is frequently used by businesses and healthcare organizations to share health information, provide remote live access to conferences or events, links to blogs, and to quickly share the latest news or information. Although Twitter users have experienced fewer issues with HIPAA violations, care should be taken to share only information that is not private or protected or that could be traced back to a patient.

LinkedIn (www.linkin.com) is another social-networking application that was designed to facilitate communication among business professionals. LinkedIn allows for posting and sharing of resumes, job opportunities, work experience, educational background, and other professional and social activities. LinkedIn is also used to enhance business awareness and advertising through sharing of white-paper-type articles, blogs, educational events, and advertisement of products.

Blogs (a derivation from "web log") provide an Internet-based forum for lectures, journaling, or discussions about specific topics or personal thoughts. These web logs may or may not be interactive, depending on the topic, format, and audience. Blogs may be found in text or video format or a combination of the two. The blogger or audience is often able to share comments, images, files, and videos on the blog site. News articles may also include the ability to comment and respond to the article content. Blogs may also be linked to Facebook, Twitter, LinkedIn, or other social-media formats, in order to broaden the reader base.

A wiki is another web application that allows users to write, collaborate, and edit information and documents on a shared site. Wikipedia.org is the most widely known example of a wiki site. Because wiki collaborators are typically providing experience and opinion rather than scholarly information based on literature, a wiki may not be a highly reliable source of information. Wikis can be used in a private capacity where a higher degree of trust and confidence in the contributors can provide the format for an evolving body of information. Typically, wikis can support audio, video, images, text, and other types of files to be shared. Wikis may be used for the ongoing work of committees as the software provides a means for tracking history and changes.

RSS, which stands for "really simple syndication" is a code that provides for a streamlined delivery of web content to subscribers to the information feed. When a user subscribes to an RSS feed, the content is often viewed through an RSS aggregator, an application designed to post all feeds in one location. Some web browsers, such as yahoo.com, contain feeds from many different sites; however, an RSS aggregator allows the user to determine the sites and content for the feed rather than relying on the information that Yahoo has chosen to share with its readers.

In contrast to the term social media, social networking refers to the process of using online technologies, such as Twitter, Facebook, LinkedIn, and other sites, to expand the number of contacts for either business or social purposes (Merriam Webster, www.merriam-webster.com/dictionary/social%20networking). Both social-media tools and the process of social networking are being increasingly used in the healthcare community to help patients connect with each other, to allow healthcare providers to connect with each other, to allow the government and other regulatory bodies to remain connected with their healthcare constituents, for recruiting, and for students to connect with each other and with instructors. In addition, information and education are distributed to a broader audience through the use of blogs, wikis, podcasts, Twitter, and other social-media tools.

Healthcare Information and Services

Navigating and locating data on the web can be difficult without the use of web-based tools designed to help locate desired information and sort search results. The use of information technology to obtain health information, generate and identify evidence for practice, or to interact with patients varies by discipline (Ventola, 2014). Tools used to search for information may range from commonly used search engines to academic databases. As the number-one-ranked search engine, Google experiences more than 40,000 searches per second (www.Internetlivestats.com/google-search-statistics/). Despite the popularity of search engines such as Google or

Yahoo, the user may not be aware that many search engines will rank search results based on either relevance to the keywords used or weight results according to the popularity of the sites containing matching information. Ranked or weighted search results may result in placing the articles of interest towards the end of the search results, providing top search results that have less relevance to the search topic because of their use as marketing tools (Glick, Richards, Sapozhnikov, & Seabright, 2014).

In contrast with popular and commonly used web-search engines, browsers designed to search for healthcare-related information can help narrow search results and decrease the time spent sorting through search results. Healthcare-specific browsers include such sites as Springer Publishing's biomedcentral.com, the metasearch engine Omni Medical Search (www.omnimedicalsearch.com), and the Consumer and Patient Health Section (CAPHIS) of the Medical Library Association. CAPHIS provides a ranking of the best websites for topic-specific health information searches that is available to members for a nominal fee. Often, peer-reviewed health research is only accessible through academic or publisher resources such as EBSCO, CINAHL, Ovid, and other sites. Some search engines, such as Medline, will provide the abstracts and locations for articles of interest, but full-text access is only obtained through a paid subscription site.

One of the most important parts of a data search on the Internet is the effective use of keywords to narrow and direct the search. A keyword search utilizes the most important words for the topic of interest; for example, if the information of interest was related to the average age of the nursing workforce, the keywords used might include nurse, age, and workforce. Changing the search terms can provide additional results, such as nurse, average age, and United States. To eliminate extraneous terms that the search engine may assume are valid, the search terms can be limited to only keywords with the use of quotation marks before and after the words.

For convenience and search speed, many publisher search engines index common search terms; these can often be seen as suggested searches that display as keywords are entered into the search-criteria fields. In order to increase the visibility of articles and publications, authors often identify keywords that are most closely related to the article topic; these keywords enhance or speed the search.

To locate the most relevant information for a web-based data search, it is usually necessary to use several different search tools to locate all relevant information. When subsequent Internet searches begin to produce the same information as prior searches, it can be assumed that most of the available information has been located. Additional challenges for web-based data searches include security filters that may block valid information.

Metasearch engines are search engines that utilize existing search engines to locate information, bypassing the indexing that is normally present. Search engines, such as Unabot, utilize other metasearch engines to conduct an Internet search. Some other metasearch engines include mamma (mamma.com), iBoogie (www.iboogie.com), Vroosh (www.vroosh.com), Turbo Scout (www.turboscout.com), Dogpile (www.dogpile.com), and more. The same concepts can be found in publisher search engines such as EBSCO's Academic Search Complete (www.ebscohost.com/academic/academic-search-complete), which searches through multiple databases for literature that would otherwise only be found within database-specific searches. OmniMedicalSearch (www.omnimedicalsearch.com) was developed to aggregate multiple sources of medical and patient information together into one searchable location. The site focuses on information that is regarded as reliable for users of the site. Medical World Search (www.mwsearch.com) is a search tool for selected medical sites that requires a subscription fee. It uses indexing and a thesaurus of uniform healthcare terms, which users can view before conducting a search.

Additional sites include PubMed (www.pubmed.com), a free database of medical and healthcare-related journal articles managed by the National Library of Medicine, a part of the National Institutes of Health. Medline (www.medline.com) contains over 22-million biomedical articles. The Cochrane Database of Systematic Reviews (www.cochranelibrary.com/cochrane-database-of-systematic-reviews/) provides access to meta-analyses and systematic reviews of research studies. Google Scholar (https://scholar.google.com/) is a free search engine able to retrieve medical and healthcare-related journal articles from multiple databases (HealthWriterHub, www.healthwriterhub.com/medical-journal-search-engines/).

Online Services for Healthcare Professionals

There are many online services and educational websites available for healthcare professionals. A rich source of health-information-technology (HIT) information for healthcare providers and consumer is www.healthit.gov. The site contains HIT information ranging from foundations of HIT to implementations and effective use of information technology for providers to consumer information about reliable health information and the role of information technology in improving personal health. The site also provides information for those working with health policy and the latest changes in the HIT landscape. The government's Health Resources and Services Administration (www.HRSA.gov) provides information about healthcare initiatives throughout the United States, along with funding opportunities and strategic plans for this organization.

The American Nurses Association (www.nursingworld.org) provides links to continuing education, certification, and nursing information. Much of the information on this site is available free to non-members; however, some resources are for members only.

There are many commercial sites on the Internet that advertise free CE-credit courses for nurses. Care should be taken to ensure that the education provided by any of these sites is approved by the appropriate credentialing body for the particular licensure or certification requirements.

Most professional organizations offer links to further information on licensure and certification applications and renewals. State boards of nursing maintain websites providing information on practice regulations, licensure requirements, and necessary application and renewal forms. Nursys (www.nursys.com) is a website that provides licensure information for all members of the National Council of State Boards of Nursing as a single source for verification of licensure. Nursys may also be used by individuals to verify the nursing license of any nurse. Nurses can opt to use the Nursys renewal reminder service to alert them when licenses are due to expire, a convenience when nurses are tracking licenses in multiple states.

Online services have added a level of transparency, efficiency, and convenience to information and credentialing access that was previously not possible when records were kept on paper.

Online Publication and Journals

Online journals provide the ability to cost-effectively publish literature that is available to a broad audience without the costs of printing and postage. A fully online journal may be printed by the reader but is not offered in a paper-based format. Some journals may be offered in a print format at a different cost than the identical online version. Some of the benefits of online publication include:

- *Efficient peer-review process.* Distribution of content for peer review can be conducted quickly via email or other computer technology, and responses from peers are received instantly.

- *Decreased cost.* While costs for editing and review may remain the same, costs for printing and mailing are eliminated.

- *Technology facilitates collaboration.* Electronic tools, such as email, wiki sites, and document-sharing sites, allow for near-synchronous collaboration.

- *Enhanced graphics.* Expensive color printing and static images can be replaced with full color images, moving images, or interactive diagrams.

- *Instant availability.* The most recent journal edition is available immediately to any subscriber with an Internet connection.

- *Enhanced information sharing.* Journal articles may be available in PDF format for printing and sharing, and many online journals contain links that provide easy email sharing of selected articles.

- *Enhanced searching.* Journal readers can search electronically within or across issues for specific words or phrases and may be able to link to references and other related materials.

- *Eliminated storage space.* Electronic journals do not require space to store printed materials.

Informatics journals available in an online format include the *Online Journal of Nursing Informatics* (www.ajni), the *Journal of Informatics Nursing* (www.ania.org/publications/journal), *CIN: Computers, Informatics, Nursing* (journals.lww.com/cinjournal/Pages/default.aspx), and *Journal of the American Medical Informatics Association* (www.amia.org/news-publications/jamia) are some examples of fully or partially online informatics-related journals. A web search using the terms online+journal+nursing will produce a list of many additional online journals. It is important to remember that some journals identified through this type of search may require a subscription to view the contents.

Professional Organizations and Watchdog Groups

In response to the immense amount of information to be found on the Internet, both reliable and unreliable, numerous organizations and watchdog groups have arisen to monitor and promote the quality of healthcare information posted on the Internet. Despite the issues presented by false and misleading information to be found on the Internet, none of these watchdog organizations possess any authority to control content. Rather, watchdog groups function by review and validation of information and education of the public to increase awareness. The Health on the Net Foundation (HON) places a symbol on health content that it deems valid and reliable (www.healthonnet.org/). URAC (www.urac.org) was founded in 1990 to provide standards for healthcare quality, including accreditation services for healthcare websites. Websites that have been accredited by URAC will display a seal on the web page. The federal Department of Health and Human Services (DHHS) provides information for consumers about how to assess the accuracy and validity of online health information through the healthit.gov website (www.healthit.gov/patients-families/find-quality-resources).

The eHealth Code of Ethics was developed in 2000 (Rippen & Risk, 2000), and the eight points in this document have been used by many other organizations for accreditation and educational purposes. The presence of a seal on a website can promote trust in the content; however, the proliferation of eHealth information on the Internet far outstrips the ability of any number of organizations to monitor or accredit. One of the best ways to determine the veracity of online health information remains vigilance and education, for both consumers and healthcare providers.

Healthcare Websites of Interest for Healthcare Providers

Nurses and other healthcare providers rely heavily on the Internet for information on health and healthcare related topics. The following websites noted in Table 4-3 were designed to service nurses and other healthcare providers by placing related information into easily

Table 4-3   Healthcare Websites of Interest for Healthcare Providers

Organization	Web Link	Mission and Purpose
Agency for Healthcare Research and Quality (AHRQ)	www.ahrq.gov	The mission of AHRQ is to produce evidence that will make healthcare safer and improve quality, accessibility, and affordability.
American Nurses Credentialing Center (ANCC)	www.nursecredentialing.org	The mission of ANCC is to promote excellence in nursing and healthcare throughout the world through credentialing programs and educational materials for nursing specialty-practice areas. In addition, ANCC recognizes healthcare organizations that meet standards of nursing excellence, quality patient outcomes, and safe, positive work environments. Healthcare organizations that provide and approve ANCC continuing nursing-education programs are accredited through this organization.
Centers for Disease Control (CDC)	www.cdc.gov	The CDC's focus is to protect America from health, safety, and security threats, both foreign and in the United States, through critical science and health information that responds to, and protects our nation against, expensive and dangerous health threats.
Centers for Medicare and Medicaid Services (CMS)	www.cms.gov	CMS is part of the Department of Health and Human Services (DHHS) and is focused on health insurance and improving the quality of healthcare and the healthcare system.
Food and Drug Administration (FDA)	www.fda.gov	As a part of DHHS, the FDA is responsible for protecting public health by assuring the safety, efficacy, and security of human and veterinary drugs, biological products, medical devices, our nation's food supply, cosmetics, and products that emit radiation. In addition, the FDA advances public health through innovations that make medicines more effective, safer, and more affordable and by helping the public get the accurate, science-based information it needs to use medicines and foods to maintain and improve health. The FDA ensures the security of the food supply and fosters the development of medical products designed to respond to deliberate and naturally emerging public health threats.
HealthIT.gov	www.healthit.gov	Managed through the Office of the National Coordinator for Health Information (ONC), healthit.gov assists healthcare providers to better manage patient care through secure use and sharing of health information, including the use of electronic health records (EHRs) to manage people's health information.

Organization	Web Link	Mission and Purpose
Health Resources and Services Administration (HRSA)	www.hrsa.gov	HRSA's mission is to improve health and health equity through development of a skilled health workforce, innovative programs, and access to quality services.
National Institutes of Health (NIH)	www.nih.gov	The mission of the NIH is to seek fundamental knowledge about living systems and to apply that knowledge to enhance health, lengthen life, and reduce illness and disability.
National Library of Medicine-National Institutes of Health (NLM-NIH)	www.nlm.nih.gov	NLM manages the world's largest biomedical library and produces electronic information resources on a wide range of topics. It also supports and conducts research, development, and training in biomedical informatics and health-information technology.
Quality and Safety Education for Nurses (QSEN) Institute	www.qsen.org	The Quality and Safety Education for Nurses Institute was founded to build the capacity for nursing to continuously improve the quality and safety of healthcare.
The National Academies of Sciences, Engineering, Medicine; Health and Medicine Division (HMD)	www .nationalacademies .org	Formerly known as the Institute of Medicine, the HMD helps those in government and the private sector to make informed health decisions through evidence. Each year, more than 3,000 individuals volunteer their time, knowledge, and expertise to advance the nation's health through the work of the HMD.
Department of Health and Human Services (DHHS)	DHHS.gov	The mission of the DIs to enhance and protect the health and well-being of all Americans through quality health and human services and through promoting advances in medicine, public health, and social services.

searchable locations. Although the following list is not comprehensive, the websites are widely used and accepted as primary resources for health-information-technology topics. Information about each of these resources is based on the mission or purpose statements on their websites.

ELearning

The Internet is increasingly used as a resource for lifelong learning, either as a course-delivery method for degree programs, for healthcare-facility-delivered training, for work-related knowledge delivery, and for continuing-education opportunities. Learning obtained through the use of computer technology is referred to as eLearning, web-based learning, computer-based learning, or, when combined with classroom learning elements, technology-assisted learning is referred to as blended learning or distance learning.

Studies have shown that blended learning can be just as effective as a full classroom-learning program, with reports of cost savings ranging from nothing (Cook, 2014) to a reported 24% decrease in training costs (Maloney et al., 2015). eLearning presents benefits unrelated to cost savings such as the ability to deliver education asynchronously in order to reach learners at the times they are available to learn, increased convenience in the learning process by eliminating a commute to the classroom, flexibility to allow the learner to manage learning time around family time and other commitments (Neal, 2013), and consistency of the educational content (content that does not vary based on instructor style and preferences). Studies have shown little difference between classroom and eLearning outcomes for the learner (Delf, 2013).

Successful eLearning is dependent on the ability of the learner to be motivated and self-directed. Because the learner is not relating to fellow learners or instructors in real time, the learner can experience feeling of isolation or disconnectedness when first experiencing online learning. In addition, the eLearning participant must have a degree of technical skills and ability to be able to navigate and manage the various elements within the course environment.

Similar to classroom-based learning, eLearning typically utilizes a course schedule that students must follow in order to remain in synchronization with the rest of the class, with the course topics, and with their assignments. A certain number of communication entries in the course room by certain times each week is the expectation for most academic eLearning programs, and grades are based on both participation and the quality of the course work presented.

Online learning environments are designed to provide learning opportunities that reflect best practices for adult learning and maximize interactivity in an asynchronous environment. Typically, learners interact through electronic discussion boards where responses to specific questions are posted and discussed among the learners and instructors. Many learning platforms are designed so that there are additional online spaces where learners can hold conversations not related to the course topics; these are created so the learner does not become distracted by other discussion. Online learning platforms also provide the opportunity for links to electronic materials that can be shared and downloaded. In addition, colleges and universities are increasingly utilizing electronic textbooks, which eliminates the need for learners to obtain and access printed materials and books and provides for easy updates to the most recent textbook version.

Virtual Learning Environments

Virtual online worlds provide the opportunity for students to practice and demonstrate skills, knowledge, communication abilities, and critical thinking. Virtual environments can be designed to reflect real-world environments or any variation in the spectrum from realistic to fantasy. Virtual worlds provide the opportunity for many users in different locations to interact synchronously or to interact asynchronously with elements of the virtual world. Virtual worlds have been used for playing games for many years, and most recently, virtual worlds are being used for training and educational purposes. An example of a virtual world designed for nursing informatics is the TIGER Virtual Learning Environment (VLE) sponsored by HIMSS (Healthcare Information and Management Systems Society, 2016). Another popular virtual world is Second Life, which hosts multiple sites devoted to healthcare.

Using Information Technology to Organize and Use Information Effectively

Advances in information technology provide the ability to add efficiency to daily work through communication and organization tools such as email. The average employee in the United States spends one quarter of his or her day sorting through emails (Smith & Giang, 2014). Although email presents a potentially efficient way to communicate, the volume of email can produce a loss of productivity, and the quality of email communication can either enhance or degrade a professional image. Email's functional structure can provide efficiency through the use of folders and rules for incoming messages.

Rules are a function within many email programs that allow the system to automatically perform functions that would otherwise be done manually, taking up valuable work time. A rule can be configured to enable incoming messages conforming to the created rule to undergo automatic action, based on the rule specifications. Examples of this might be emails from a certain sender that would be automatically placed into a subject-specific folder or into the delete-mail folder.

Folders provide a way to sort emails by sender or by topic. Folders are easily set up in an email program and provide the ability for quick search and storage of key information. Examples of folders might be a folder set up for informatics topics, a folder set up for messages from co-workers, or folders set up by tasks that need to be completed.

An additional function found in some email programs is the ability to link an email to a task or action that can be scheduled for a certain date. This process becomes handy when an action is required from an email but the date for action is in the future. If the email is left in the common inbox, it will soon move towards the bottom of the list, out of sight and out of mind. Linking the email to a task will produce a reminder and keep the original email attached to the reminder until the task is satisfied.

Effective use of email can also enhance or decrease a professional image, based on how email is used. An article in *Business Insider* (Smith & Giang, 2014) provides recommendations for professional use of email.

- *Include a clear, direct subject line.* This allows the recipient to quickly identify important emails for timely review.
- *Use a professional email address.* Emails received from nonprofessional email addresses such as "sexynurse.com" will not convey a professional message to the recipient and may be deleted before being read.
- *Do not use "reply all."* Using the reply-all function can clutter inboxes with information not relevant to a major of the people on the original email thread.
- *Use professional salutations.* Do not use nicknames, colloquial expressions, or slang when addressing emails in a professional environment.
- *Minimize use of exclamation points.* Overuse of exclamation points can add emotional drama or immaturity to an email message.
- *Use humor cautiously.* Much of humor is conveyed through body language. Unless the sender is certain of how the recipient will receive and understand humor, it should be left out of emails.
- *Be culturally sensitive.* Email use may differ by culture; be aware of social norms for other cultures when formatting an email message.
- *Reply to emails.* Good email etiquette dictates that emails should get a response, even when sent to the wrong person. A short acknowledgement is appropriate and polite.
- *Proofread your email message.* Mistakes in spelling and grammar can discredit the sender's reputation, in addition, spellcheck can sometimes substitute very inappropriate words into a professional email.
- *Double check the recipient.* Many organizations have employees with similar names; it is important to ensure the correct recipient is identified.

Spreadsheets

Spreadsheets are electronic tools that can be used to organize data such as lists of related data. The row and column format support calculations, but spreadsheet software can also be used to create staff schedules, track information, and make simple reports. A spreadsheet can perform some simple functions of a database but cannot provide the complex relationship linking and reporting that is found in a true database.

Databases

A database is an electronic format for storing, organizing, and retrieving data in an organized manner. Databases provide the backbone for any organizations that need to store, retrieve, and organize data—including EHR systems—and other uses for data in healthcare. Some commonly seen types of databases include relational databases, distributed databases, operational databases, and hierarchical databases. The most common type of database is the relational database, which provides the ability to sort and retrieve data through its relationship with other data fields such as linking a name with an address or a gender with a diagnosis. At the simplest end of the spectrum, a spreadsheet can store, organize, and retrieve data in a limited fashion. On the other end of the spectrum, a data warehouse can store and associate data from multiple systems in one location so that information from a billing system, a pharmacy system, patient-care documentation, data from physician records, and even state immunization records can all be linked together. The more complex the database, the more work is involved in designing the database and ensuring that the data is valid, reliable, and internally consistent.

Future Directions

The rise of information technology has changed healthcare in many ways, by providing quick and easy access to reliable health information, by enhancing the speed of dissemination of new information, by providing availability of information to anyone with an Internet connection, by facilitating communication and networking through social-media tools, and by increasing access to learning and information. Some challenges associated with the explosion of information accessed through technology include the need to validate information found on the Internet, enforcement of responsible use of the Internet and social media by healthcare workers, development and promotion of reliable information sources for healthcare workers and consumers, and protection of consumers from unethical uses of information technology and information.

Glimpses into the future of information technology produce visions of improvements in the usability and information-sharing abilities of electronic health records, development and use of standards for the efficient use of health-information technology, and increased sharing and use of health data to improve patient care and population health (DeSalvo, Dinkler, & Stevens, 2015; Department of Health and Human Services, 2015). Although health-information technology has advanced tremendously in the past decade, further enhancement and sharing of information will be needed to fully realize the benefits that have been promised.

Summary

- Information literacy, the ability to locate and interpret information in a manner that is relevant to the user, is key to effective use of the Internet.
- Online information can increase access to information and decrease search time.
- The US National Library of Medicine provides tutorials that can be used to help determine the validity of health information.
- In general, large organizations, such as hospitals, the government, universities, and other large health organizations, have the most reliable online information.
- When evaluating information quality, look for qualified, credible sources, and specific details and dates that enable independent verification of information.

- Health on the Net Foundation is a nonprofit, private organization dedicated to ensuring quality health information on the Internet through an accreditation process; once accreditation is achieved, the HONcode seal appears on the website and may be verified by browser searches.
- Social media can provide valuable information for healthcare professionals but must be used with caution to avoid compromising patient information or organization policies.
- Key search terms and healthcare-specific browsers can yield more relevant results.
- Metasearch engines send out simultaneous queries to other search tools, bypassing indexing structures for faster results than independent searches of the individual tools yield.
- HealthIT.gov is a rich source of HIT information.
- Professional organizations and government agencies provide valuable links to continuing education, relevant legislation, certification and licensure information, and practice updates.
- Professional online publications shorten traditional timelines to disseminate information, help to hold down costs, support search capability, and save space.
- elearning, inclusive of virtual learning environments, provides additional flexibility for both traditional and continuing education.
- Technology opens us to an overwhelming amount of information but also provides tools to manage information that include, but are not limited to:
  - Email rules
  - Email folders
  - Linking email to a task or conversation stream
  - Clear, concise professional use of electronic communication limiting copies to individuals with a need to know
  - Really simple syndication (RSS)
  - Spreadsheets
  - Databases.

About the Author

Brenda Kulhanek is the AVP of Clinical Education for HCA in Nashville, Tennessee. She has served on the board of the American Nursing Informatics Association since 2012 and currently fills the role of president elect. Dr. Kulhanek is an adjunct and visiting professor for graduate and postgraduate nursing informatics programs at Walden University and Chamberlain College of Nursing.

References

Buultiens, M., Robinson, P., & Milgrom, J. (2012). Online resources for new mothers: Opportunities and challenges for perinatal health professionals. *Journal of Perinatal Education, 21*(2), 99–111. doi:10.1891/1058-1243.21.2.99

Cook, D. A. (2014). The value of online learning and MRI: Finding a niche for expensive technologies. *Medical Teacher, 36*(11), 965–972. doi:10.3109/0142159X.2014.917284

Delf, P. (2013). Designing effective eLearning for healthcare professionals. *Radiography, 19*(4), 315–320. doi:http://dx.doi.org/10.1016/j.radi.2013.06.002

DeSalvo, K. B., Dinkler, A. N., & Stevens, L. (2015). The US Office of the National Coordinator for Health Information Technology: Progress and promise for the future at the 10-year mark. *Annals of Emergency Medicine, 66*(5), 507–510. doi:http://dx.doi.org/10.1016/j.annemergmed.2015.03.032

Department of Health and Human Services. (2015). ONC releases interoperability roadmap. *Journal of AHIMA, 86*(4), 10.

Diviani, N., van den Putte, B., Giani, S., & van Weert, J. C. (2015). Low health literacy and evaluation of online health information: A systematic review of the literature. *Journal of Medical Internet Research, 17*(5), e112-e112. doi:10.2196/jmir.4018

Glick, M., Richards, G., Sapozhnikov, M., & Seabright, P. (2014). How does ranking affect user choice in online search? *Review of Industrial Organization, 45*(2), 99–119. doi:10.1007/s11151-014-9435-y

Healthcare Information and Management Systems Society (HIMSS). (2016). TIGER Virtual learning environment. Retrieved from www.himss.org/professional-development/tiger-initiative/virtual-learning-environment

Laugesen, J., Hassanein, K., & Yuan, Y. (2015). The impact of Internet health information on patient compliance: A research model and an empirical study. *Journal of Medical Internet Research, 17*(6), e143–e143. doi:10.2196/jmir.4333

Maloney, S., Nicklen, P., Rivers, G., Foo, J., Ooi, Y. Y., Reeves, S., . . . Ilic, D. (2015). A cost-effectiveness analysis of blended versus face-to-face delivery of evidence-based medicine to medical students. *Journal of Medical Internet Research, 17*(7), e182–e182. doi:10.2196/jmir.4346

Medlock, S., Eslami, S., Askari, M., Arts, D. L., Sent, D., de Rooij, S. E., & Abu-Hanna, A. (2015). Health information-seeking behavior of seniors who use the Internet: A survey. *Journal of Medical Internet Research, 17*(1), e10–e10. doi:10.2196/jmir.3749

Neal, J. (2013). Innovation in education: Using elearning to improve the quality of education for practice nurses. *Practice Nurse, 43*(6), 40–43.

Rippen, H., & Risk, A. (2000). eHealth code of ethics. *Journal of Medical Internet Research, 2*(2). doi:http://doi.org/10.2196/jmir.2.2.e9

Smith, J., & Giang, V. (2014). 11 email etiquette rules every professional should know. *Careers.* Retrieved from www.businessinsider.com/email-etiquette-rules-everyone-should-know-2014-9

Ventola, C. L. (2014). Social media and health care professionals: Benefits, risks, and best practices. *Pharmacy and Therapeutics, 39*(7), 491–520.

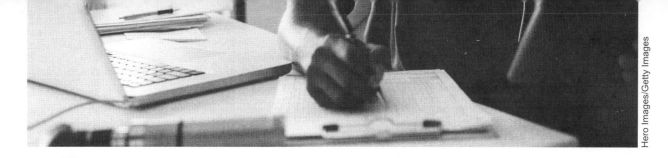

Chapter 5
Using Informatics to Support Evidence-Based Practice and Research

Melody Rose, DNP, RN

 ## Learning Objectives

After completing this chapter, you should be able to:

- Identify the role of outcomes research and transformational research in modern healthcare.

- Explain the need for defining levels of evidence in healthcare research.

- Identify existing models of integration for evidence-based practice into clinical practice.

- Define the need for research databases and data repositories related to research.

- Identify ethical and legal principles of research related to patient privacy and security.

- Identify and discuss methods of research dissemination based on current government funding practices.

- Identify key government agencies that influence healthcare research through management and funding.

- Discuss the role of nursing in the future of healthcare research.

Evidence-based practice comes from the culmination of many years of research and research styles that have been modeled into empirical databases feeding best clinical practices. Historically, quantitative and qualitative models of research have been followed and utilized. Studies suggest an average qualitative/quantitative research project takes 17 years to disseminate results (Munro & Savel, 2016). The need for a quicker, more healthcare-specific model of research was met in the last half of the 20th century when outcomes research (OCR) became the standout model that strove to measure outcomes through quality indicators

(In & Rosen, 2014). The ultimate goal of OCR is to improve quality of care through examination of outcomes (In & Rosen, 2014).

The main concepts of OCR are to minimize variations in practice by developing quality guidelines, providing ways to systematically measure the functioning and well-being of patients, linking treatments and outcomes data through databases, and analyzing databases so results can be quickly and easily disseminated (In & Rosen, 2014). Measurable outcomes are defined as biological endpoints, survival, quality-of-life, functional status, costs, cost-effectiveness, and patient satisfaction (In & Rosen, 2014).

History

In the last half of the 20th century, the terms comparative effectiveness research (CER), health services research (HSR), and outcomes research (OCR) were all types of research used in healthcare. Within the decade of the 1990s, the importance of OCR was realized through participation from several major organizations. Of those, the Agency for Health Care Policy and Research (AHCPR) (National Archives, 2016), which later became the Agency for Healthcare Research and Quality (AHRQ), established OCR programs to sponsor trial research programs and develop research networks (Agency for Healthcare Research and Quality, 2002; In & Rosen, 2014).

In 2001, the Institute of Medicine's (IOM) report *Crossing the Quality Chasm: A New Health System for the 21st Century* indicated that information technology (IT) was integral to achieving substantial quality improvement for the delivery of high-quality healthcare (Institute of Medicine, 2001). As a result of this recommendation, the AHRQ supported multiple projects that explored the potentials of IT.

Integrated Delivery System Network

The AHRQ operated the Integrated Delivery System Research Network (IDSRN) from 1999–2005. This project used a model of field-based research and joined with top researchers from some of the nation's largest healthcare systems (Agency for Healthcare Quality and Research, 2002). The uniqueness of this program was the strategy of establishing partnerships between researchers and consumers of the research (Gold & Taylor, 2007). This approach put relevant research into the hands of users that had typically been outside of the research community (Gold & Taylor, 2007). As a result of the IDSRN project, many clinical databases have been developed such as the National Comprehensive Cancer Network (NCCN) and Oncology Outcomes Database. National registries have also been developed. Examples of cancer registries include American College of Surgeons (ACS), Commission on Cancer (CoC), and Centers for Disease Control and Prevention's (CDC) National Program of Cancer Registries (NPCR) (Centers for Disease Control and Prevention, 2016).

Accelerating Change and Transformation in Organizations

The IDSRN project was followed by the Accelerating Change and Transformation in Organizations and Networks (ACTION) program. The overall goal of the ACTION project was accelerating the diffusion of research into practice (AHRQ, 2015a). The ACTION project continued to use the field-based collaborative relationship model established within the IDSRN project. ACTION focused on finding results, both successful and unsuccessful, to improve healthcare outcomes and disseminating results (AHRQ, 2006). Topics of study for the ACTION project were suggested by participating members and approved by AHRQ. Topic research timeframe was an average completion of 15 months (AHRQ, 2006). ACTION was a five-year initiative that began in 2005. Since its initiation, ACTION II and ACTION III have been launched as continuations of this initiative. All ACTION III projects are scheduled to be complete by 2018 (AHRQ, 2016).

Practice-Based Research Networks

In the 1970s, primary care physicians in the United States followed the lead provided by European counterparts and began developing research networks. Through the AHRQ, federal grant funding has been available for practice-based research networks (PBRN) since the early 21st century (AHQR, 2012a). Information aggregated from PBRN improves practice for the primary care provider and patient. Through this network, information becomes relevant to the clinician and can be introduced quickly into practice (AHQR, 2012a).

Translating Research into Practice

Translating research into practice (TRIP) and, later, TRIP II were studies funded by AHRQ beginning in 1999 and designed to look at the way primary-care teams were using health-information technology (HIT) (AHRQ, 2013b). The TRIP and TRIP II studies looked at Practice Partner Research Network (PPRNet) participants for project-specific electronic health data and the effect on practice in improving quality that came from this translated information (AHRQ, 2013b). A total of 27 projects were funded through TRIP and TRIP II (AHRQ, 2015).

Levels of Evidence

Finding the best quality of research to follow and implement has been a problem for healthcare. In a still-relevant article, Ebell et al. (2004) discussed this problem. Sorting out what is credible and what is not can be time-consuming and resource-intensive. Discovery of level-of-evidence has been the topic of discussion and a point of deliberation for many nurses and nurse administrators. By the early 2000s, many evidence-grading scales had been developed by a variety of organizations. Adding confusion to the mix, various scales that were in use were inconsistent in what was scored, used no standardized criteria for comparison, and sometimes offered opinion of reviewer rather than scientific review (Ebell et al., 2004). Early scales were reported in many different formats, A through E, one through five, or V through I. Many of the grading scales were so complex that the clinical user would not or could not take time to review the results in depth for application value (Ebell et al., 2004). Research that is not translatable is not viable research. This lack of consistency left the clinical healthcare and research communities looking for a better way to evaluate and translate the level of evidence in healthcare research.

Grading of Recommendations Assessment Development and Evaluation

In 2000, a collaboration of people formed the Grading of Recommendations Assessment, Development, and Evaluation (GRADE) work group with a goal to address levels of evidence (Grade Working Group, 2016). The GRADE approach was to get input from many contributors including representatives of other grading systems. The thought behind this strategy was to bring forward previous work and ideas and promote the development of a transparent approach for grading research evidence. Among the international organizations represented in the initial work group were the World Health Organization, Centers for Disease Control and Prevention, and Oxford Center for Evidence-Based Medicine. Upon conclusion of the original product from this workgroup, groups that actively supported the use of the result of GRADE workgroup included the Cochrane Collaboration, the World Health Organization, and Up To Date. The most recent update to GRADE was made in April of 2016 (GRADE Working Group, 2016).

The GRADE approach provides four levels of rating of evidence—high, moderate, low, and very low. An algorithm of concrete rules was developed that can be applied to evidence, guiding research into the appropriate rating. Four areas of criteria were constructed for the algorithm: (1) number of participants, (2) risk of bias of trials, (3) heterogeneity, and (4) methodological quality of the review. As the algorithm is applied, the reviewer determines if downgrades to the level of evidence should be applied. The total number of downgrades applied determines the level rating the evidence receives.

Agency for Healthcare Research and Quality Methods Guide

The Agency for Healthcare Research and Quality (AHRQ) recognized that healthcare decision-making should be done through systematic reviews. The Evidence-Based Practice Council (EPC), initiated in 1997, has worked with a variety of organizations and agencies to establish a comprehensive method of comparative effectiveness reviews. The Effective Health Care (EHC) Program, initiated in 2005, was challenged to improve healthcare delivery in the United States by improving quality, efficiency, and effectiveness (AHRQ, 2014). Both groups are sponsored by the AHRQ.

There are 14 EPCs throughout the country. In 2004 to 2005, the councils developed methodologies to assess the level of evidence within research. From this preliminary work, a *Methods Guide* was developed. The initial *Methods Guide* was based on the approach developed by the GRADE working group (AHRQ, 2014). Differences include terminology: EPC refers to strength of evidence, GRADE refers to quality of evidence. EPC identifies three domains as directness, consistency, and precision while GRADE identifies three domains as indirectness, inconsistency, and imprecision. EPC design is intended more for individual studies that are not necessarily compared to other studies. This methodology is intended for a more diverse type of user than the researcher. EPC also does not make or grade clinical recommendations (AHRQ, 2013a).

American Association of Critical-Care Nurses Levels of Evidence

The American Association of Critical-Care Nurses (AACN) taskforce developed an evidence-rating scale in 1995. The original rating scale used Roman numerals and rated evidence with lower numbers representing lower levels of evidence (Armola et al., 2009; Peterson et al., 2014). This system was considered confusing as other rating systems used a reverse order. The AACN established a volunteer workgroup in 2007 to focus on developing resources for the bedside clinician. This group was called the Evidence-Based Practice Resources Workgroup (EBPRWG) and developed many valuable tools for clinicians. In 2008, the EBPRWG was challenged to review and make recommendations for improving the AACN rating tool (Armola et al., 2009; Peterson et al., 2014). The end product was an alphabetical rating scale using A for the highest level of evidence and moving down through the alphabet to letter E as reliability decreased. The letter M was reserved for evidence that was recommended only by the industry or manufacturer. In 2011 to 2012, the EBPRWG revised the rating tool to discriminate between randomized control trials and reviews of other studies (Armola et al., 2009; Peterson et al., 2014).

Strength of Recommendation Taxonomy

Through encouragement and directives from the Federal government, primary-care physicians and providers have been collecting and storing patient data in practice-based research networks (AHRQ, 2012a). Physicians and providers collected data but did not have a reliable way to qualify evidence-based outcomes from outside sources. Several journals and the Family Practice Inquiries Network (FPIN) developed a taxonomy for this purpose (Ebell et al., 2004). The Strength of Recommendation Taxonomy (SORT) provides a strength of recommendation based on a body of evidence. The strength of recommendation is based on an A, B, C scale with A indicating consistent, good-quality patient-oriented evidence; B indicating inconsistent or limited-quality patient-oriented evidence; and C indicating consensus, disease-oriented evidence, usual practice, expert opinion, or case series for studies of diagnosis, treatment, prevention, or screening (Essential Evidence Plus, 2016). The body of evidence is evaluated by four elements: (1) study quality, (2) diagnosis, (3) treatment/prevention/screening, and (4) prognosis.

Applying Information Literacy to Find the Highest Levels of Evidence

Searching and researching for evidence has changed exponentially since the 1990s with the introduction of the Internet and the personal computer. The Internet has made millions of data bits available to researchers, and the development of the computer and the personal computer has brought accessibility to the level of the individual in their home. For the curious, if you have a question and resources to access the Internet, you can probably find some form of an answer.

Meta-analysis of multiple controlled studies, systematic reviews, and randomized controlled trials (RCT) are considered potentially high-level evidence resources (Peterson et al., 2014; AHRQ, 2014; AHRQ, 2012b; Facchiano & Snyder, 2012). Searching for this level of resources can be accomplished in several ways. If using a search engine from the Internet, please use a scholarly search engine. Electronic libraries provide access to databases that specifically house scholarly medical resources. Many of the electronic databases have restricted access and can only be used by members. Entities that house electronic libraries include colleges/universities, healthcare institutions, service organizations, and professional organizations. Databases specific to health and healthcare provide methods to help narrow searches. Primary searches can be done from a word or phrase. Advanced searches allow the user to expand or restrict a search in many different areas. Examples of expanding search criteria are searches through Boolean phrases (connectors such as "and," "or," "not"), searches for partial match of phrase, or related words. Examples of restricting search criteria are limiting publish date ranges and specifying full text, peer-reviewed articles. Clinical practice guidelines can be searched for by using the key term "clinical practice guideline" in search criteria and naming the specific topic desired.

Filtered resources are resources that have been preappraised for quality and content. Filtered resources will often make practice recommendations (Facchiano & Snyder, 2012; Walden University, 2016). Unfiltered resources are typically primary or original research studies that have not been appraised as a filtered resource has (Facchiano & Snyder, 2012; Walden University, 2016).

When searching for a specific topic using a keyword or term, add additional defining terms through an advanced search as necessary to narrow the search in the desired direction. If a specific type of research is desired, this can be included in the search criteria. Examples are qualitative, quantitative, peer-reviewed, randomized-controlled study, and population-intervention-comparison-outcome (PICO) (Facchiano & Snyder, 2012).

The following databases are specific to systematic research reviews:

- Cochrane Library.
- Joanna Briggs Institute EBP Database.
- Database of Abstracts of Reviews of Effects (DARE).

The following databases are commonly used when searching for original research articles:

- CINAHL.
- MEDLINE.
- Proquest Nursing & Allied Health.
- PsychINFO.
- PubMed.

Integration of EBP into Clinical Systems and Documentation

Knowledge translation (KT) from the point of valid research to implementation at the bedside can take place through many well documented models. Most strategies agree there has to be an existing culture that is willing to accept a change of practice, appropriate facilitation of implementation methods, key stakeholders that include bedside clinicians with administration involvement, and some form of evaluation post implementation conducted (Roe & Whyte-Marshall, 2012; Schaffer, Sandau, & Diedrick, 2013; Hubbel & Greenbaum, 2014; Kitson & Harvey, 2016). Multiple models exist for the purpose of integrating evidence-based practice (EBP) into use. While many of these models were developed several years ago, they remain relevant. Top models include the Stetler model, the Iowa model of evidence-based practice to promote quality care, the ACE star model of knowledge transformation, and the PARIHS framework (Schaffer et al., 2013). Other viable models exist and are well documented in scholarly literature.

Promoting a culture of change is necessary for successful implementation of evidence-based practice (Hubbell & Greenbaum, 2014). Change cannot be successfully implemented unless there is agreement—from the very top levels of administration through the clinical caregivers—that change in practice is necessary and will happen. The same message has to be delivered throughout the project to all facility members affected by the coming change. Transparency and consistency are paramount when implementing change.

Regardless of the implementation strategy (method) chosen, several key points of representation have been identified in documented methods. Identified stakeholders need to include those being impacted most significantly by the change (Roe & Whyte-Marshall, 2012; Schaffer et al., 2013; Hubbel & Greenbaum, 2014; Kitson & Harvey, 2016). Senior administration needs to be present as a stakeholder to encourage ownership and commitment throughout the project and also to be aware of any long-term risks that arise as the project continues (Dogherty, Harrison, Graham, Vandyk, & Keeping-Burke, 2013). Potentially, multiple or additional projects can present a risk to a long-running project through impacts on resources and commitment. Having senior administration as a stakeholder provides a clear focus of priorities for project resources and commitment.

Evaluation is the process used to determine if the evidence-based intervention(s) implemented are/have been successful. Evaluation should be planned based on the model of implementation. Immediate evaluation at the time of implementation should be done to determine if patient safety issues or major financial issues exist. Barring these, no changes should be made to the newly implemented system for approximately 30 days, allowing the end user learning curve to level off. At 30 days—or in many cases prior to this mark—the true value of the new system can start to be realized. At this point, an evaluation process can begin.

Stetler Model

The original Stetler model was developed in 1976 and was revised specifically to the needs of EBP in 1994 and again in 2001 (Gray, Grove, & Sutherland, 2017). The model is divided into five phases: (1) preparation, (2) validation, (3) comparative evaluation/decision-making, (4) translation and application, and (5) evaluation. The Stetler model can be oriented toward the individual or team approach (Schaffer et al., 2013).

Iowa Model of Evidence-Based Practice to Promote Quality Care

The Iowa model of evidence-based practice (EBP) was originally developed in 1994 and revised in 2001 by Titler and colleagues (Gray et al., 2017). The Iowa model stresses the importance of prioritizing triggers based on the need for change and the needs of the clinical agency. Once supporting evidence of change is found, the change is introduced in a pilot environment. Evaluation of the pilot leads the facility to the decision of adopting the change or not (Gray et al., 2017; Schaffer et al., 2013). If the change is implemented facility-wide, ongoing evaluation with dissemination of results will be continuing components of the model (Schaffer et al., 2013).

ACE Star Model of Knowledge Transformation

The Academic Center for Evidence-Based Practice (ACE) developed the ACE star model to address translation and implementation aspects of the evidence-based practice process. The model applies evidence to clinical nursing by considering factors that determine the likelihood of adoption of practice. There are five steps in the ACE star model: (1) discovery of new knowledge; (2) rigorous review process of evidence followed by summary; (3) translation of evidence for clinical practice; (4) integration of intervention into practice; and (5) evaluation of the practice change (Schaffer et al., 2013).

PARIHS Framework

The PARIHS (Promoting Action on Research Implementation in Health Services) framework is considered less structured than a true model of practice, providing a theory of practical application (Schaffer et al., 2013). PARIHS framework defines three key elements that, when used together, will mutually influence each other for a successful EBP implementation (Schaffer et al., 2013). The three elements are: (1) evidence—sources of knowledge from multiple stakeholders, (2) context—quality of the environment EBP is to be implemented, and (3) facilitation—how change will be supported (Kitson & Harvey, 2016; Schaffer et al., 2013). The PARIHS framework had been redefined to i-PARIHS utilizing F-facilitation, I-innovation, R-recipients, and C-context (Kitson & Harvey, 2016).

Managing Research Data and Information

Organizing captured data and making it accessible has become a topic of great interest with the increase of health information technology (HIT). Part of the success of outcomes research is combining researchers with consumers of research (clinicians) so results can become more transparent. A bigger picture arises when determining what to do with all of the data that is being collected. How can this data be saved, archived, and made available to researchers and consumers as needed?

A newer approach, through translational science, attempts to understand the scientific and operational principles that support each step of generalizing research from one environment to the next. The aim of translational science is to move data gained from the translational research process to the level of the clinician and patient, quickly (NCATS, 2015). The National Center for Advancement of Translational Science (NCATS), part of the National Institutes of Health (NIH), was established in 2012 to improve strategies of developing and disseminating research for translations science (NCATS, 2015).

Data collected for research and subsequently stored is subject to the Office of Human Research Protections policy providing guidance to institutional review boards (IRB) regarding anonymity. The IRB review also validates protection of the rights and welfare of human subjects within the research project (Food and Drug Administration, 2106). Patient information that has not been de-identified is also protected by Health Insurance Portability and Accountability Act (HIPAA) rules and cannot be shared without patient consent (Bardyn, Resnick, & Camina, 2012).

Databases

The National Library of Medicine (NLM) sponsors the National Network of Libraries of Medicine (NN/LM) program with a goal to improve access of biomedical information to US health professionals and the public's access to information (National Institutes of Health, 2016). Eight regional medical libraries and five national centers provide outreach efforts to researchers, health professionals, the public workforce, and the public, providing access to quality health information through research databases. Access to NN/LM information is by membership, which can include libraries, information centers, or other types of organizations.

The White House Office of Science and Technology Policy (OSTP) required that federal agencies make results of federally funded scientific research available to the public, industry, and scientific communities. The AHRQ established guidelines for this compliance to be complete by October 2015. The guidelines apply to all scientific publications and data in a digital format (AHRQ, 2015). The intent of these guidelines is to provide public access to scientific research results, including field data, lab data, quality-control samples, sample ID data, and instrument-calibration data, in a digital format. Final result formats can be viewed or down-loaded without charge (AHRQ, 2015). Data that has personal identifiers is out of scope for this reporting. AHRQ stores data through a commercially contracted data repository. AHRQ research submitted for storage will be cross-referenced using the AHRQ-funded identifications number (PubMed Central Identification—PMCID) providing linkage into PubMed records (AHRQ, 2015).

Data Mining

Scientific research that involves searching and researching large networks and databases of information for collaborative purposes can be defined as escience (Bardyn, Resnick, & Camina, 2012). Escience can span many types of digital data sources including (but not limited to) academic, institutional, private, public, government, and research databases/repositories. Digital curation maintains data long-term for retention of value and risk of digital obsolescence (Bardyn et al., 2012). Data sets of clinical research can be stored in many different formats and are/will be used for retrospective analysis. The ability to recall these formats must be maintained as part of the curation process.

Long-Term Management

Preservation and sustainability balanced with cost-effective data management brings the project plan of contracting to a commercial repository and periodic reviews to identify coverage gaps and needs (AHRQ, 2015). The Office of Extramural Research, Education and Priority Populations (OEREP) has been tasked with this responsibility. A data management plan must now be submitted with any grant application for project funding through the AHRQ process (AHRQ, 2015).

Creating and Maintaining the Infrastructure to Support Research

Creating and maintaining an environment to house research is multifaceted in nature. Organizations that maintain a sustainable health-services-research infrastructure have considerations in some, if not all, of the following areas: research staff with expertise and experience; financial considerations that include contracts and grants; research facilities and equipment; and partnerships for dissemination of information (AHRQ, 2011).

Research Staff

Although the researcher is typically thought of as the only necessary person for research, this statement is not true. A competent research office requires a team of multiple people, dependent on the size of the facility. The facility director and/or manager will help select research projects, organize the daily running of the office, validate credentialing of researchers, organize validation of project time lines, and generally keep the office running. Researchers, research students, and staff may be permanently assigned to the facility or work on conditional/contractual projects. All people involved with research projects have to be documented to the project. Daily, weekly, and ongoing reporting is necessary for projects. This work may be designated by the director/manger to researchers or other staff.

Financial contracts and grant applications are an essential part of research. Writing and reviewing these documents are roles of the research staff. Both researchers and grant writers can author contracts and grant applications. In some organizations, these documents will be diverted through a legal department for review before submission to an intended recipient. This can be done by a designated contract/grant role or be left to the individual researcher, but follow-through on this process has to be complete.

Every research project has to follow predetermined rules of ethics and compliance. Research proposals have to be approved by an Food to validate protection of the rights and welfare of human subjects within the research project (Food and Drug Administration, 2016). If the research facility is associated with an IRB, this may provide an easier portal of entry for this process. If not, an IRB site will need to be established for review of research projects. All elements of the HIPAA have to be observed for privacy and confidentiality.

Appropriate policies and procedures (P&Ps) must be in place for a research facility. These P&Ps will range from mission statements to personnel statements and include all facets of the functioning of the facility. It is the responsibility of the research staff to make sure appropriate P&Ps are in place and reviewed on a routine schedule.

Financial Considerations

Research is an expensive proposition. Many research projects are funded by government grants, nonprofit agencies, and academic institutions (Mick, 2015; AHRQ, 2015). Another method of supporting research is encouraging corporate entrepreneurship strategies, creating an environment that supports competitive yet collegial research that will return profit for the corporation (Holmes, Zahra, Hoskisson, DeGhetto, & Sutton, 2016).

Budgeting and project management are ways to monitor cost, check expense, and project status of the project at hand. Outside of the actual research, reporting on total amount spent, amount spent by category, total labor hours, labor hours by category, indirect costs incurred, percentage of total budget remaining, and percentage of time remaining on grant or contract are reportable items (AHRQ, 2011).

Research Facility

The actual research facility is a consideration. The research office (physical location of researchers, managers, directors, grant writers, etc.) may or may not be located where the information technology (IT) servers are located. In the situation of academic health services databases, the physical location of the research office may be on the same campus but logistically distant from the IT servers. In a professional or corporate environment, these entities may be united in the same location. IT server storage space can also be commercially contracted and located remotely in comparison to the actual research office.

Technology infrastructure is a consideration. The only guaranteed factor in technology is that it will change. The known facts are that data must be stored, data must be retrieved, and data must be aggregable. The physical technology has evolved and is capable of processing collected data. Within the data collection process, it is important to define data parameters for extracting data (Cole, Stephens, Keppel, Hossein, & Baldwin, 2016). Data is more easily collected and aggregated from discrete data fields rather than narrative fields. Rigorous documentation of parameters and processes should be stored with research data.

Partnerships

Multiple facets of research exist. Researchers may need a relationship with an organization to do research. Organizations may have an identified need and resources for research. Government agencies may have grant monies available for research projects. Independent data warehouses may have servers that can store, aggregate, and report data. Forming a partnership between any of these entities could be mutually beneficial. Partnerships can be formed with academic institutions, individuals, businesses, foundations, think tanks, nonprofit organizations, different levels of government—the list is endless. Partnerships can also be formed nationally and internationally. Partnerships should have well-defined roles, be mutually beneficial, and promote the culture of research.

Ethical and Legal Principles for Handling Data and Information in Research

Evidence-based practice is driven by research. The way research data is completed and processed must be done ethically and with legal precision. Accessibility through Internet and research networks has made research materials much more available and accessible. Elements that must be considered in the ethical and legal handling of data for research are the use of informed consent, respect of privacy and confidentiality for the patient and protective laws, the respectful and appropriate use of intellectual property, and the potential for multiple or conflicting roles of the researchers and/or writers.

Informed Consent

Informed consent is the modern basis for medical treatment. Patients expect transparency in care and treatment. This begins with conversation and education from the first point of contact and can include signing legal documents that give permission (consent) for treatments, surgeries, blood transfusions, and so on. This process of transparency in care and treatment transfers from caregiver to caregiver as the level of care changes. If the patient, procedure, or any part of the procedure is specifically used in a research project, the patient must be made aware and consent must be obtained.

Privacy and Confidentiality

The **Health Insurance Portability and Accountability Act (HIPAA)** became public law in 1996 (DHHS, 2016). The purpose of HIPAA was multi-focused but has generally become known for its effect on patient privacy and confidentiality within the electronic health record (EHR). The American Psychological Association (APA) indicates that maintaining confidentiality within the research environment is a priority (APA, 2010). Any breach of confidentially within the healthcare environment is subject to the penalties of HIPAA. This can lead to fines for the facility involved and fine and jail sentences for individual violators. The Office of Civil Rights (OCR) enforces HIPAA (DHHS, 2016).

Intellectual Property

Transformational science exists because of the research communities' ability to network and share information. Digital information transferred electronically through networks and Internet capabilities has made national and international sharing a reality. With this capability comes the need to define and protect intellectual property. Intellectual property (IP) can be defined in many contexts and somewhat unclearly for writing research. National and international copyright laws govern this area. The APA indicates authorship credit is determined by substantial contribution to a published work (APA, 2010). Primary source references are reports written by the original researcher(s) regarding their work, while secondary source references summarize or quote primary sources (Grove, Gray, & Burns, 2015). Acknowledgment of IP can be done through appropriate citations and references.

Ghostwriting, the practice of a professional writer paid to write books, articles, stories, etc. that are credited to someone else, has been identified as an issue (Wnukiewicz-Kozlowska, 2011; Stretton, 2014). Ghostwriters are not acknowledged in writing credits but medical writers are acknowledged. The ghostwriter (a person with no medical education) does not operate as a contributor to content but rather an interpreter of literature, opening the opportunity for misrepresentation of results. Attention to this topic has gained attention. Suggestions of using peer reviewers with expertise, closely monitoring the internal and external validity of study data, and noting if data is appropriately interpreted in context to current practices will help isolate a true author from a ghostwriter.

Conflicting Roles

Researchers must be aware of and clearly state any economic or commercial interests in a product or service used in a research project. Providing full disclosure of activities, interests, relationships, or conflicts that might have an influence or present a bias should be defined within the research definitions (APA, 2010). This will not always be defined a conflict of interest, but without doing this, transparency of the research may never be achieved (APA, 2010).

The commercial contribution to research by industry, corporations, and business cannot be denied. Ethical standards require full disclosure of financial interests. Research and development is an expensive business and sometimes takes years of work to meet federal safety regulations before a product can be delivered safely to the public. The commercial element of research and development has to be allowed to be profitable but not at the expense of monopoly or safety (Moses, Matheson, Cairns-Smith, Palisch, George, & Dorsey, 2015). Government regulations have been put in place and carefully maintained through checks and balances to provide safety for the public, fair compensation for the commercial industries, and a somewhat speedy process of development (Holmes et al., 2016). This is an ongoing and ever-developing system.

Practices for Collecting and Protecting Research Data

The Office of Research Integrity (ORI), part of the DHHS, identifies eight key components in the practice of responsible data collection, management, and protections. These are data ownership, data collection, data storage, data protection, data retention, data analysis, data sharing, and data reporting (DHHS, 2016).

Data Ownership

Although many contributors may work on a research project, the legal rights of ownership for the data resulting from the project may not belong to the researchers. Ownership should be established at the time the project is initiated and can be based on employment and/or funding status. If researchers work for the sponsor of the research, unless otherwise stated, the sponsor will be the owner of the data. If the research project is funded by outside organizations, the outside organizations can also expect ownership of research data. The principal investigator (PI) can also be granted stewardship of project data, providing some level of ownership. In some projects, research subjects may be considered partial owners of project data (DHHS, 2016). Ownership of the research data should be established at the beginning of the project and included in the description of the project that is sent before the IRB. This will provide transparency in the project and identify any potential conflicts of interests (Food and Drug Administration (FDA), 2016).

Data Collection

Data collection, in this reference, is the documented process of the project. Providing a framework, map, or model of the project design along with the processes used for data collection will help reviewers validate rigor of the project and help future researchers recreate the study (Grove et al., 2015).

Data Storage

Data storage has been addressed throughout this chapter. AHRQ now requires a data storage plan as part of project grant applications (AHRQ, 2015). Data storage considerations include the amount of data to be stored/retained and the method of storage (electronic or paper). When considering the data to be stored, the means to recreate the project, notes, relevant observations from the researchers, and relevant statistics should be stored. It may not be necessary to store raw data (DHHS, 2016).

Electronic storage can be accomplished several ways. Funded research projects may have a stipulation that project results become accessible through some form of public or membership access (AHRQ, 2015). This has to be considered when storage is determined. Backup storage can also be done with static storage through CDs and removable drives.

Data Protection

Protecting stored data can be approached from multiple directions. Data stored in a physical form (paper or on a physical server) should be kept safe from elements and local damage and secured from theft or loss (DHHS, 2016). A backup of this type of stored data is also recommended. Data stored in an electronic format that is open to outside access should also be protected from outside attacks such as virus, worms, and hackers (DHHS, 2016). An offline backup of this type of stored data is recommended.

Data Retention

Retention of data can have several dependencies. If a project has been funded or contracted, the terms of the funding/contract may define the period of retention (DHHS, 2016). If there are no dictated time parameters, cost of retention may be the determining factor. Continued storage of confidential information has security risks and can also be a factor in discontinuing storage. If data is determined to be no longer needed for retention, it should be completely destroyed through proven and documented methods (DHHS, 2016).

Data Analysis

Methods for data collection are defined in the framework of the research project. Methods for data analysis are not as clearly defined until raw data has been collected and evaluated. Data analysis can include the researcher but also often includes the services of statisticians and biostatistical services. The project investigator, researchers, and statisticians need to work together to make sure data is analyzed in the context and scope of the project (DHHS, 2016).

Data Sharing

The fields of OCR and TR have developed because of the delay in sharing data. Both OCR and TR expedite the timeline of sharing data by including research at the clinical level. Research that has been funded by outside organizations may have reporting and sharing parameters written into the funding agreements creating an obligation to report (AHRQ, 2015; DHHS, 2016). Commercial and industrial research may be completed under proprietary domain, however, the results will typically be translated into commercial products for consumers.

Data Reporting

A vital part of the scientific process is data reporting. Reporting establishes an institution/ organization/researcher's contribution to a field of study. A published report allows a project's outcome to be reviewed for accountability. Published reports also promote discussion and ideas that may lead to additional research (DHHS, 2016).

Supporting Dissemination of Research Findings

Dissemination is simply a term that indicates communication of information, in this case research knowledge, from a source (Primary Health Care Research and Information Service, 2016). A facet of the Affordable Care Act (ACA) mandated that research findings would become more accessible to the public, when it was enacted in 2010 (PCORI, 2016). The rationale for this was to allow for better decisions based on available evidence at the levels of patients, providers, caregivers, insurers, and others involved as stakeholders in healthcare.

Patient and public involvement (PPI) in dissemination of research knowledge improves communications between the patient and caregivers, including the risks of different treatments (PCORI, 2015). McNichol and Grimshaw (2014) suggested the relationship between research and PPI be encouraged to expand the continuum of scope of dissemination. Publicly funded research that fits the ACA mandate is required to submit peer-reviewed preliminary findings to the Patient Centered Outcomes Research Institute (PCORI) (Merino & Loder, 2014). A potential downfall of this is that—as this material continues to be analyzed and reported—journal reviewed versions of these results may provide different or expanded results (Merino & Loder, 2014).

Dissemination at the level of the caregiver continues to translate knowledge into practice (Kelly, Wicker, & Martin, 2016). Because translational research has been taken to the clinical level, changes in practice can be quicker. By making research results available publicly, stakeholders at the clinical level can identify research activities that would be appropriate for their institutions. This practice can encourage contribution and participation by having broader access to research outcomes (Kelly et al., 2016). Dissemination of research findings through mandated public access supports this concept of broader access. Hospitals that have achieved Magnet Recognition demonstrate quality improvement through research, evidence-based practice, and innovation (American Nurses Credentialing Center, 2016). Research should lead clinical areas in a direction that promotes meaningful change for the patient, caregivers, and organization.

Patient Centered Outcomes Research network (PCORnet) is a public database of clinical effectiveness research (CER) data from publically funded projects. This information is available to the public and to healthcare workers (PCORI, 2015). The goal of this network is to make researching specific topics easier (one location instead of many). PCORnet aggregates research information from hospitals, health plans, and practice-based networks for funded projects. This project has been divided into phase I and II. As phase II nears completion, funding is expected to be shifted to agencies such as the National institutes of Health, the Food and Drug Administration, and potentially private industry (PCORI, 2015).

Selected Software

The quest for a single software application that will search and compile all research has gone unanswered. What has developed or become more specific is the importance of advanced search techniques of current search engines used, such as MEDLINE, CINAHL, PubMed, PsychINFO, and so on. As research projects are designed, submitted, enacted, completed, and published, authors should create keywords for easy search and submit to known databases that are included in medical search engines.

Effecting Practice Change

Health information technology (HIT) has been an increasingly active part of healthcare for many years. Until the ACA in 2010, there were few measurable designs to standardize the type of HIT used by healthcare (Murphy, 2010). Since we are a country of private industry, the federal government has made no mandates on specific software systems to purchase and put in place. What have been dictated are the capabilities of electronic health record systems (EHRSs), by setting system standards, capabilities, and accountability (Appari, Johnson, & Anthony, 2013). Through a series of financial incentives that turn into financial penalties as time passes without compliance, eligible providers are requested to meet minimum EHRS compliance. As EHRS compliance achieves a higher level of reportable documentation, reportability occurs, promoting evidence-based data capture.

Prior to the ACA, HIT systems were not always enterprise-wide systems that communicated with each other. Free-standing systems in the emergency department, operating room, laboratory, radiology, inventory control, and other areas were not uncommon, making communication between these systems unlikely (Lyon et al., 2016). As HIT systems evolved and regulations were written, the push for enterprise-wide systems was felt. An enterprise-wide system is an information system by one vendor that houses modules for all (or most) areas of the facility with the ability to share information between modules. This element is key for promoting patient safety and better patient care.

The Centers for Medicare and Medicaid Services (CMS) developed the meaningful use (MU) criteria that EHRSs must meet to be identified as certifiably capable EHR systems (CMS, 2016). The Office of the National Coordinator for Health Information Technology (ONCHIT) has created a voluntary program for testing and certifying health IT systems. Certified HIT systems, including EHRSs meet the criteria for meaningful use (ONCHIT, 2016). As healthcare facilities come into MU standards, even though they may not be using the same software, the software being used should have the same capabilities.

As eligible providers and facilities (those that take payments from CMS) come on line with MU criteria, the groundwork for standardized, reportable, and evidence-based practice becomes available. From this comes the standardized ability to document, collect, and report clinical quality measures (CQMs) (Wilson & Newhouse, 2012). HIT also offers the ability to place clinical decision support (CDS) mechanisms in place based on the patient's current condition. The ability to exchange electronic health information also becomes available, which aides in the transfer and communication of information (Thurston, 2014).

The ability to effectively change practice at the level of the facility can be supported by several different models of change, which have been previously discussed. The need for change can be identified through multiple mechanisms. Burns and Grove (2011) identified the clinical nurse and nurse researcher as key stakeholders in identifying needs for evidence-based changes in practice. Additional identifiers include financial indicators and quality indicators. The necessary elements of change that need to be respected include a culture that is ready and willing to accept change, appropriate stakeholder representation and buy-in, adequate resources and planning, and a comprehensive evaluation-of-change tool.

Future Directions

Evidence-based practice is the direct result of research and has a documented effect on the way clinical care is provided. Research can be chronicled through many styles and methods leading to the more efficient outcomes research and translational research used to promote evidence-based practice. The evolution of health information technology has enabled the capabilities of data collection, data aggregation, data reporting, data storage, and data linkage to become more efficient.

Nursing, as a profession, has the ability to change practice, promote education, and influence health policy. This has to be done credibly through steps of evidence-based research. Through nursing research, value has already been demonstrated. Addressed through national patient safety goals, clinical quality measures, and meaningful use criteria, the impact of nursing research has helped identify patient-centered issues with positive outcomes (Appari et al., 2013; The Joint Commission, 2016; CMS, 2016).

Nursing research can influence the impact of cost containment. Although this topic is bigger than nursing alone, nursing research an have impact by providing solid analytical data that supports patient care issues such as re hospitalization within 30 days. Lundmark (2015) indicates cost-benefit questions are an area that helps drive healthcare systems. Nursing research can be an interdisciplinary effort and often includes nurse clinicians, nurse researchers, nurse informaticists, and nurse leaders (Sousa, Weiss, Welton, Reeder, & Ozkaynak, 2015). The level of credentialing for nursing research has been evaluated by multiple credentialing organizations with a focus on the value of individual nurse certification related to improving patient outcomes (Lundmark, 2015).

Storage of research data has been previously described as public, private, academic, commercial, and in some cases international. There is no one spectacular data repository that houses all data. Retrieval of data is done through search engines and the typical search methods allowed by search engines. The researcher finds catalogued information based on methods of search and the way information is stored. There does not seem to be an alternative for this methodology at this time.

Several methods of quantifying the level of evidence have been identified. Each method has value and solid support in its approach. Researchers are provided guidance on methods of critique to establish validity for research materials if these levels of evidence methods have not been applied.

Multiple models of integration for evidence-based practice have been identified in an overview fashion. Evidence-based practice is the goal of evidence-based research with a continuing quest of improved outcomes for the patient and caregivers. As EBR is implemented, careful documentation of changes should be noted for evaluation, based on the chosen models criteria. The collected data from an EBR implementation can be the beginning of the next EBR project. Changes put in place from EBR can be transmitted to users through presentations, poster projects, and potential journal articles, resulting in an effective dissemination of knowledge. Holsti, et al. (2013) suggested the role of nursing researchers should be developed and encouraged in patient-outcomes research by increasing nursing research programs.

Summary

- The time lag between research findings and integration into practice may average 17 years.
- Comparative effectiveness research (CER), health services research (HSR), and outcomes research (OCR) are types of research used in healthcare.
- The potential of information technology (IT) to support research and improve healthcare has been recognized and has given rise to multiple projects resulting in:
  - The establishment of clinical databases and national registries
  - Research and dissemination of findings related to improved healthcare outcomes
  - The establishment of practice-based research networks
  - Research on how primary-care teams use health information technology
  - A decrease in the length of time from research completion to dissemination of results
- A key factor in the integration of research into practice is the ability to determine the strength or level of evidence and to critique the quality of the study.
- Levels of evidence refer to the strength of evidence or confidence placed in the findings related to the approach used. Confidence in findings is critical to the process of translating findings into practice. Meta-analysis of multiple controlled studies, systematic reviews, and randomized controlled trials (RCTs) are considered to be high-level evidence resources.
- Evaluation of levels of evidence has been complicated by inconsistencies in scales and factors to evaluate the strength of evidence.
- Information literacy is critical to find the highest levels of evidence.
- Knowledge translation (KT) from the point of valid research findings to implementation at the bedside can take place through many well-documented models. KT requires a culture that is willing to accept a change of practice, facilitation of implementation methods, key stakeholders that include bedside clinicians and administrators, and post implementation evaluation.
- Some models for change include the Stetler model, Iowa model of evidence-based practice, ACE star model, and PARIHS framework.
- HIT provides the potential to improve the management of research data inclusive of data management and curation.
- Translational science is an approach that seeks to expedite the move of data gained from the translational research process to the clinician and patient.
- The White House Office of Science and Technology Policy (OSTP) requires that federal agencies make results of *federally funded scientific research* available to the public, industry, and scientific communities.
- Infrastructure to support research includes staff, budgets and funding, institutional review board approval, project management, appropriate policies and procedures,

physical space and accommodations to house staff, information technology and data, and partnerships with organizations that have an identified need.

- Handling research data and information must conform to ethical and legal principles that include informed consent, protection of privacy, confidentiality, and intellectual property, and full disclosure of activities, interests, relationships, or conflicts that might influence or bias study results.
- Practices for collecting and protecting research data need to consider the following components: data ownership, data collection, data storage, data protection, data retention, data analysis, data sharing, and data reporting.
- The Affordable Care Act mandated that research findings would become more accessible to the public as a means to facilitate better decisions based upon evidence.
- HIT has enabled the capabilities of data collection, data aggregation, data reporting, data storage, and data linkage to become more efficient.

Case Study

As the informatics nurse specialist at your facility, you are responsible for implementing the infrastructure to collect and protect research data. How would you go about implementing the eight key components identified by the Office of Research Integrity at your facility? Where would you start?

About the Author

Melody Rose, DNP, RN is a 2014 graduate of Duke University School of Nursing DNP program, 2011 graduate of Walden University School of Nursing MSN—Informatics Specialty, 1986 graduate of Illinois Central College, Associate Degree of Nursing program. Dr. Rose lives in Murfreesboro, Tennessee, and is an Assistant Professor of Nursing at Cumberland University Jeanette C. Rudy School of Nursing, a Visiting Professor of Nursing at Chamberlain College of Nursing, and works PRN as a Nursing Supervisor at Southern Hills Medical Center in Nashville, Tennessee.

References

Agency for Healthcare Research and Quality (AHRQ). (2002). *Integrated delivery system research network (IDSRN)*. Retrieved from http://archive.ahrq.gov/research/idsrn .htm#mission

Agency for Healthcare Research and Quality (AHRQ). (2006). *Accelerating change and transformation in organizations and networks (ACTION)*. Retrieved from www.ahrq .gov/sites/default/files/publications/files/action_0.pdf

Agency for Healthcare Research and Quality (AHRQ). (2011). *An organizational guide to building health services research capacity*. Retrieved from www.ahrq.gov/sites/default/ files/wysiwyg/funding/training-grants/hsrguide/hsrguide.pdf

Agency for Healthcare Research and Quality (AHRQ). (2012a). *AHRQ centers for primary care practice-based research and learning*. Retrieved from www.ahrq.gov/professionals/ systems/primary-care/rescenters/index.html

Agency for Healthcare Research and Quality (AHRQ). (2012b). *Primary care practice-based research networks (PBRN)*. Retrieved from www.ahrq.gov/research/findings/factsheets/ primary/pbrn/index.html

Agency for Healthcare Research and Quality (AHRQ). (2013a). *Grading the strength of a body of evidence when assessing health care*. Retrieved from www.effectivehealthcare .ahrq.gov/ehc/products/457/1752/methods-guidance-grading-evidence-131118.pdf

Agency for Healthcare Research and Quality (AHRQ). (2013). *Synthesizing lessons learned using health information technology*. Retrieved from healthit.ahrq.gov/ ahrq-funded-projects/synthesizing-lessons-learned-using-health-information-technology

Agency for Healthcare Research and Quality (AHRQ). (2014). Effective health care program. Retrieved from www.effectivehealthcare.ahrq.gov

Agency for Healthcare Research and Quality (AHRQ). (2015a). *Accelerating change and transformation in organizations and networks (ACTION) III*. Retrieved from www.ahrq .gov/research/findings/factsheets/translating/action3/index.html

Agency for Healthcare Research and Quality (AHRQ), (2015b). *Public Access to Federally Funded Research*. Retrieved from www.ahrq.gov/funding/policies/publicaccess/index.html

Agency for Healthcare Research and Quality (AHRQ). (2016). *Translating Research Into Practice*. *Retrieved* from www.ahrq.gov/research/findings/factsheets/translating/index.html

American Nurse Credentialing Center (ANCC). (2016). *Magnet recognition program overview*. Retrieved from www.nursecredentialing.org/Magnet/International/ MagnetProgOverview

American Psychological Association (APA). (2010). *Publication manual of the American psychological association* (6th ed). Washington, DC: Author.

Appari, A., Johnson, M. E., & Anthony, D. L. (2013). Meaningful use of electronic health record systems and process quality of care: Evidence from a panel data analysis of US acute-care hospitals. *Health Services Research, 48*(2), 354–375.

Armola, R. R., et al., (2009). AACN levels of evidence: What's new? *Critical Care Nurse, 29*(4), 70–73.

Bardyn, T. P., Resnick, T., & Camina, S. K., (2012). Translational researchers' perceptions of data management practices and data curation needs: Findings from a focus group in an academic health sciences library. *Journal of Web Librarianship, 6,* 274–287.

Burns, N., & Grove, S. (2011). *Understanding nursing research. Building an evidence-based practice.* (5th ed.). Maryland Heights, MO: Elsevier Saunders.

Centers for Disease Control and Prevention (CDC). (2016). *National program of cancer registries*. Retrieved from www.cdc.gov/cancer/npcr/about.htm

Centers for Medicare and Medicaid Services (CMS). (2016). Certified electronic health record technology (CEHRT). Retrieved from www.cms.gov/regulations-and-guidance/ legislation/ehrincentiveprograms/certification.html

Cole, A. M., Stephens, K. A., Keppel, G. A., Estiri, H., & Baldwin, L.-M. (2016). Extracting electronic health record data in a practice-based research network: Processes to support translational research across diverse practice organizations. *eGEMs, 4*(2) 1206. http:// doi.org/10.13063/2327-9214.1206.

Department of Health and Human Services (DHHS). (2016). *Guidelines for responsible data management in scientific research*. Retrieved from http://ori.hhs.gov/images/ddblock/ data.pdf

Dogherty, E.J., Harrison, M.B., Graham, I.D., Vandyk, A.D. & Keeping-Burke, J. (2013). Turning knowledge into action at the: The collective experience of nurses facilitating the implementation of evidence-based practice. *Worldviews on Evidence-Based Nursing, 10*(3), 129–139.

Ebell, M. H., Siwek, J., Weiss, B. D., Woolf, S. H., Susman, J., Ewigman, B., & Bowman, M. (2004). Strength of recommendation taxonomy (SORT): A patient-centered approach to grading evidence in the medical literature. *American Family Physician, 69*(3), 548.

Essential Evidence Plus. (2016). Levels of evidence. Retrieved from www .essentialevidenceplus.com/product/ebm_loe.cfm?show=sort

Facchiano, L., & Snyder, C. H. (2012). Evidence-based practice for the busy nurse practitioner: Part one: Relevance to clinical practice and clinical inquiry process. *Journal of American Academy of Nurse Practitioners, October 24* (10), 579–86. doi: 10.1111/j.1745-7599.2012.00748.x

Food and Drug Administration (FDA). (2016). *Institutional review boards information.* Retrieved from www.fda.gov/RegulatoryInformation/Guidances/ucm126420.htm

GRADE Working Group. (2016). Criteria for applying or using GRADE. Retrieved from www.gradeworkinggroup.org/publications/index.htm

Gray, J., Grove, S., & Sutherland, S. (2017). *Burns and Grove's The Practice of Nursing Research, 8th Edition. Maryland Heights,* MO : Elsevier/Saunders

Grove, S. K., Gray, J. R., & Burns, N. (2015). *Understanding nursing research building and evidence-based practice.* St. Louis, MO: Elsevier.

Gold, M., & Taylor, E. F. (2007). Moving research into practice: Lessons from the US Agency for healthcare research and quality's IDSRN program. *Implementation Science,* (2)9. doi: 10.1 186/1748-5908-2-9

Holmes, R. M., Zahra, S. A., Hoskisson, R. E., DeGhetto, K., & Sutton, T. (2016). Two-way streets: The role of institutions and technology policy in firms; corporate entrepreneurship and political strategies. *Academy of Management Perspectives, 20*(3), 247–272.

Holsti, M., Adelgais, K. M., Willis, L., Jacobsen, K. Clark, E. B., & Byington, C. L. (2013). Developing future clinician scientists while supporting a research infrastructure. *Clinical & Translational Science Journal, 6*(2), 94–97.

Hubbell, B., & Greenbaum, D. (2014). Counterpoint: Moving from potential-outcomes thinking to doing—changing research planning to enable successful health outcomes research. *American Journal of Epidemiology, 180*(12), 1141–1144.

In, H., & Rosen, J. E. (2014). Primer on outcomes research. *Journal of Surgical Oncology, 110,* 489–493.

Institute of Medicine (IOM). (2001). *Crossing the quality chasm: A new health system for the 21st century.* Washington, DC: National Academy Press.

Kelly, L. A., Wicker, T. L., & Martin, D. M. (2016). Utilizing research findings: Nurse leaders and researchers working together. *Nurse Leader, 14(5),* 350–353.

Kitson, A. L., & Harvey, G. (2016). Methods to succeed in effective knowledge translation in clinical practice. *Journal of Nursing Scholarship, 38*(3), 294–302.

Lundmark, V. (2015). Starting a national conversation the institute of medicine workshop on the future directions of credentialing research in nursing. *Journal of Nursing Administration, 45*(1), 1–3.

Lyon, A. R., Lewis, C. C., Melvin, A., Boyd, M., Nicodimos, S., Liu, F. F., & Jungbluth, N. (2016). Health information technologies—academic and commercial evaluation (HIT_ACE) methodology: Description and application to clinical feedback systems. *Implementation Science, 11*(128). doi: 10.1186/s13012-0160495-2

McNichol, E., & Grimshaw, P. (2014). An innovative toolkit: Increasing the role and value of patient and public involvement in the dissemination of research findings. *International Practice Development Journal, 4*(1). Retrieved from www.fons.org/library/journal.aspx

Merino, J., & Loder, E. (2014). PCORI's ambitious efforts to promote transparency and dissemination of research findings. *The BMJ.* doi: 10.1136/bmj.g6261

Mick, J., (2015). Addition of a decision point in evidence-based practice process steps to distinguish EBP, research and quality improvement methodologies. *Worldviews on Evidence-Based Nursing, 12*(3), 179–181.

Moses, H. I., Matheson, D. M., Cairns-Smith, S., Palisch, C., George, B. P., & Dorsey, E. R. (2015). The anatomy of medical research: US and international comparisons. *JAMA-Journal of the American Medical Association, 313*(2), 174–189.

Munro, C. L., & Savel, R. H. (2016). Narrowing the 17-year research to practice gap. *American Journal of Critical Care, 25*(3), 194–196.

Murphy, J. (2010). The journey to meaningful use of electronic health records. *Nursing Economic$, 28*(4), 283–286.

National Archives. (2016). Records of the Agency for Health Care Policy and Research 1964-87. Retrieved from www.archives.gov/research/guide-fed-records/groups/510.html

National Center for Advancing Translational Sciences (NCATS). (2015). Transforming translational research. Retrieved from ncats.nih.gov/files/NCATS-factsheet.pdf

National Institutes of Health (NIH). (2016). National network of libraries of medicine fact sheet. Retrieved from www.nlm.nih.gov/pubs/factsheets/nnlm.html

Office of the National Coordinator for Health Information Technology (ONCHIT). (2016). Health IT Certification Program Overview, v1. 2 January 30, 2016. Retrieved from www.healthit.gov/sites/default/files/PUBLICHealthITCertificationProgramOverview_v1.1.pdf

Patient Centered Outcomes Research Institute (PCORI). (2015). PCORnet: The national patient centered clinical research network.. Retrieved from www.pcori.org/research-results/pcornet-national-patient-centered-clinical-research-network

Patient Centered Outcomes Research Institute (PCORI). (2016). Research dissemination and implementation. Retrieved from www.pcori.org/research-results/research-dissemination-and-implementation

Peterson, M., Barnason, S., Donnelly, B., Hill, K., Miley, H., Riggs, L., & Whiteman, K. Choosing the best evidence to guide clinical practice: Application of AACN levels of evidence. *Critical Care Nurse, 34*(2), 58–68.

Primary Health Care Research & Information Service (PHCRIS). (2016). PHCRIS getting started guides: Introduction to . . . research dissemination. Retrieved from www.phcris.org.au/guides/dissemination.php

Roe, E. A., & Whyte-Marshall, M. (2012). Mentoring for evidence-based practice. *Journal for Nurses in Staff Development, 28*(4), 177–181.

Schaffer, M. A., Sandau, K. E., & Diedrick, L. (2013). Evidence-based practice models for organizational change: Overview and practical applications. *Journal of Advanced Nursing, 69*(5), 1197–1209.

Sousa, K. H., Weiss, J., Welton, J., Reeder, B., & Ozkaynak, M. (2015). The Colorado collaborative for nursing research: Nurses shaping nursing's future. *Nursing Outlook, 63*(2), 204-210. doi:10.1016/j.outlook.2014.08.013

Stretton, S. (2014). Systematic review on the primary and secondary reporting of the prevalence of ghostwriting in the medical literature. *BMJ Open, 4*(7).

The Joint Commission (TJC). (2016). National patient safety goals. Retrieved from www.jointcommission.org/standards_information/npsgs.aspx

Thurston, J. (2014). Brief report: Meaningful use of electronic health records. *The Journal for Nurse Practitioners, 10*, 510–513. doi:10.1016/j.nurpra.2014.05.012

Walden University. (2016). Academic answers-quick answer. Retrieved from http://academicanswers.waldenu.edu/faq/73299

Wilson, M. L., & Newhouse, R. P. (2012). Meaningful use intersections with evidence-based practice and outcomes. *Journal of Nursing Administration, 42*(9), 395–298.

Wnukiewicz-Kozlowska, A. (2011). Legal and ethical aspects of ghostwriting in medicine. *Archivum Immunologia et Therapia Experimentalis, 59*, 1–9.

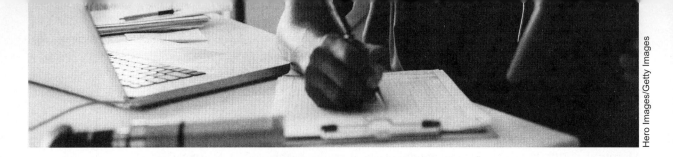

Chapter 6

Policy, Legislation, and Regulation Issues for Informatics Practice

Sunny Biddle, MSN, RN

Jeri A. Milstead, PhD, RN, NEA-BC, FAAN

 Learning Objectives

After completing this chapter, you should be able to:

- Differentiate policy, legislation, and regulation through components, processes, outcomes, and relationship to informatics.

- Contrast how value-based reimbursement differs from pay-for-performance or volume-based delivery models.

- Analyze the implications of health information technology (HIT) and informatics on diagnostic and billing codes.

- Determine points of access for making decisions in the federal rule-making process related to informatics issues.

- Identify the impact of informatics on at least three specific federal regulations.

- Identify the relationship among accreditation decisions, reimbursement, quality of care, and informatics.

- Discuss the pros and cons of working in interprofessional teams related to informatics and public policy-making.

- Discuss ethical issues that impact healthcare providers and organizations in the electronic age.

Policy, legislation, and regulation are related but separate processes that convey values, ideals, and significance to our lives. Students in the healthcare professions must understand the process of policy making and, especially, their obligation to participate in the process. Governmental laws and rules direct the practice of healthcare workers in every aspect of their scopes of practice. This chapter helps the reader differentiate law from rule and policy from procedure. The reader begins to understand how informatics impacts and influences these processes. Presentation of specific legislation and regulations provides examples that directly affect electronic processes that are fundamental in healthcare delivery.

Although central concepts in this chapter are related to governmental processes, policies that have been developed in the private sector also are presented. Policies from private accreditation organizations such as The Joint Commission (TJC) have enormous impact on reimbursement and continued operation of a healthcare agency. Finally, this chapter examines the recent impact of informatics and policy-making on interprofessional learning and teams, evidence-based care, and ethics.

The Policy Process

What Are Policies?

Policies are written documents that reflect the values of administrators of organizations. They should and ought to express what the chief executive officers (CEOs) and their inner circles and confidantes believe. Policies cover a variety of components of an organization. For example, policies at the federal level of the United States reflect the scope of the cabinet-level departments such as commerce, defense, health, transportation, etc. Policies indicate the direction that an organization will take and, very importantly, signal where funding will be directed. For example, after the United States was attacked on September 11, 2001, the policies of President George W. Bush and his cabinet were focused on defense, and funding was concentrated on the military. When Barack Obama was running for president, he campaigned on the promise of healthcare for all Americans, and that is where funding appeared.

Policies can be found in mission statements, organizational objectives, strategic plans, and other documents. The process of developing policies is fairly straightforward but is fluid and does not always follow a straight course. That is, since policies mirror leaders' values, policies will change whenever there is a change in administration. Throughout the processes and components addressed in this chapter, the reader should consider how informatics and the use of data can provide information for decisions that will affect healthcare professionals in their work.

Components

Generally, policy-making is simple: take problems to government and obtain a response. We all know that there is much more to it than that. Policy-making is not a sequential, linear process—it is messy and often takes a zig-zag course. There are several components that can be identified for the purpose of analysis: agenda setting, government response (often law and regulation [rule]), program design and implementation, and evaluation. A model developed by Cohen, March, and Olsen (1972) in their early work on organizational choice depicted the policy-making process as resembling a garbage can into which problems are floated, solutions are proposed, and politics sway choices. This classic model holds up well today. Getting a problem to the attention of government may not be easy, and an idea can be catapulted onto the policy agenda by a catastrophe (e.g., the attack on the Twin Towers and the Pentagon in 2001) or a change in an indicator (e.g., the emergence of the Zika virus in 2016). The federal agenda is always on the mind of the president and his/her confidantes, so having a relationship with a senior congressperson or senator who has the president's ear can help bring about a change. In Kingdon's (1995, 2001) classic research on agenda-setting, he noted that a **policy entrepreneur** is a person who commits interest, time, and money to moving a proposal forward. This person often keeps a proposal from fading on the agenda.

Government response usually occurs in two ways: legislation and regulation. How a bill becomes a law is a standard discussion in every junior-high or senior-high school in this country. A member (Member) of the House or Senate (remember: the president is CEO of the executive branch, and only members of the legislative branch can attend to legislation) introduces a bill. The bill is given a number and sent to a committee or sub-committee for discussion. This group is significant because they actually determine the extent of interest in the problem. Committees determine whether a bill moves forward or dies. Opponents and proponents are given voice through a series of hearings, proposed language is altered or amended, or ideas from bills may be consolidated into a substitute bill. Remember: legislative staff receive and analyze ideas, talk with staff from other offices and federal agencies, and update the Member on the scope and implications of a problem. Informatics experts, including nurses, physicians, pharmacists, and so on, have a tremendous opportunity to provide relevant research, statistical data, results of surveys, and other facts that staff can share with the Member.

If a senator or representative introduces a bill, the healthcare professionals must monitor the progress, suggest amendments if needed, and continuously inform the Member of new information or changes. Bills can authorize (create) a new program; other bills appropriate money to implement a program. One must watch for unfunded mandates; this is a program that has been authorized, but funds have not been appropriated. Bills have a two-year life span. That is, a legislative session is two years; if a bill has not been voted by both the House and Senate and sent to the president within the legislative session, the bill dies; the process must be repeated in the next legislative session.

Often, a bill designates a program that will address a national problem. Bardach's (1977) book remains a classic about games played by officials during policy implementation. Many of the games had to do with how funds would be applied. A program may specify eligibility requirements, that is who can participate. For example, if a free school-lunch program is proposed, who can take part? Children in all grades? All children or just those in public schools? Those whose parents are below the poverty level? Only those with a disability or other specified condition? Program design can assign the government agency that will be responsible for implementing the program. The choice of agency is a very, very political decision. Does the agency have staff with the skills to carry out the program? Does the agency have too many programs already to take on one more? Does the agency want or need the funding that accompanies the program? Does the agency have a record of successful implementation of other programs? Does this program fit within the agency's mission? Does this program bring jobs to a state that the Member who championed the bill represents, which could be seen as pork-barreling or unduly influencing funding decisions? Members are elected to represent the US not just their own constituencies. However, since House members are elected for two-year terms, they always are mindful of the folks back home and try to convince constituents that they are working in the constituents' behalf, which often involves bringing programs and money to their districts.

Influencing Policies and Legislation through Informatics

Politics is the process of persuading a person to accept your perspective and take action on bills, policies, and programs that you support. We all practice politics at some time. Did you ever try to convince your parents to buy you something or allow you to go somewhere that you thought they might not approve? You used political means to make your point. Politics is using communications techniques that come naturally to some and must be learned by others.

Lobbyists are experts at encouraging others to act in a predetermined way. Lobbyists use well-honed communications methods such as active listening, clarification ("Did I hear you say . . . "), reframing ("Let's look at it from another perspective"), and even silence. Nurses, physicians, pharmacists, dentists, and psychologists use these methods in their daily practice. Using these skills with legislators and their staff is exactly what lobbying is about. Individuals also can lobby, and healthcare professionals are convincing when they use data from the Member's own district to personalize a story.

Registered lobbyists are employed by organizations to win favor for a particular bill or political position. Federal lobbyists register with the Clerk of the US House of Representatives and the Secretary of the US Senate and must file reports quarterly that list all gifts, travel, and contributions (Registration with the Clerk, 2016). Lobbyists rely on data from many electronic sources to underpin their work. Informatics specialists can help lobbyists find sources and translate statistical data into relevant meaning for members and their staff.

Policy and program evaluation vary depending on how the law or rule is written and the inclination and expertise of the agency head and staff. Often, evaluation either does not take place or reflects a cursory attempt to justify cost. Data obtained from program outcomes are essential for evaluation. Even a cursory examination of data may establish whether or not a program is judged successful.

Example: US National Health Information Technology Policy

The National Health Information Technology Policy (NHITP) is an example of how public and private-sector policies work together. Through the American Recovery and Reinvestment Act of 2009, HIPAA created the Office of the National Coordinator for Health Information Technology (ONCHIT) under the aegis of the Department of Health and Human Services (DHHS). As a result, two federal advisory committees focused on IT were established: the Health Information Technology Policy Committee (HITPC) to develop a framework for a nationwide infrastructure and the Health Information Technology Standards Committee (HITSC) to develop standards, certification, and implementation strategies. These committees gathered together public and private stakeholders who serve as advisors on how to develop and implement a national HIT system. The National Coordinator presented a report to the Congress in 2016 that highlighted the barriers and challenges facing such an undertaking.

The policy process is visible in this example: the idea was put before the Administration but was not high on the agenda. Legislation was passed but as an unfunded mandate. Implementation so far has been sluggish—due to lack of funding? Other DHHS priorities? Lack of a policy entrepreneur? Problems with the Affordable Care Act (ACA)? For the future, will a crisis move the need for a national infrastructure back on the agenda? Will the Congress appropriate funding so that an integrated infrastructure will be developed? Will the advisory committees reach agreement on criteria for standards and certification?

Public policy is incremental. Time is needed to define a problem in a way that policy makers can accept and can begin to visualize possible solutions. Legislation may take several sessions, and drafting regulations for a single program may be very complex, especially when it involves other departments. Implementation often takes years, as bureaucrats refine programs so that the outcomes meet the objectives. Evaluation, unless it is built into the program at the beginning, often is either lost or weak. Persistence is the major requirement for working in the policy arena. So stay tuned as ONCHIT evolves.

Legislation and HIT/Informatics

Healthcare informatics and the associated technologies influence and are impacted by national legislation. Changes in reimbursement for healthcare services can support the use of new informatics strategies, such as electronic data interchange (EDI), support for new healthcare delivery models, validate clinical trials and the use of alternative therapies, improve monitoring of prescriptive practices, and facilitate provision of burden-of-proof evidence. Accurate and complete generation and transmission of diagnostic and billing codes results from the work of informaticists and HIT.

Reimbursement

One of the significant outcomes of legislation involves the issue of reimbursement for services performed. Two major philosophies guide how organizations and physicians are paid: volume-based and value-based.

VOLUME VERSUS VALUE REIMBURSEMENT For many years, US federal policies set payment to hospitals for certain procedures based on how many procedures were completed in a specified time frame. This is known as volume-based compensation. Some diagnostic tests and types of surgeries were reimbursed at higher rates than others, which led to those being used more often.

Proponents of healthcare reform developed a schema known as value-based reimbursement in which diagnostic tests and treatment options were based on the value of those tests and treatments to patient and organizational outcomes. The hope of reformers is to reduce the number of unnecessary or limited-valued tests and treatments. Accountable Care Organizations (ACOs) are examples of entities developed across the public-private sectors in which physicians are reimbursed for coordinated care, and hospitals are paid through fee schedules for physicians (as employees) and per diems or diagnostic-related groups (DRGs) (Berenson, Upadhyay, Delbanco, & Murray, 2016a). The goal is to decrease enterprise costs and improve performance targets that measure quality (Berenson, Upadhyay, Delbanco, & Murray, 2016b).

ELECTRONIC DATA INTERCHANGE Data tracking and retrieval are essential in providing healthcare providers (physicians and healthcare organizations) with useful information. The old system of merely entering paper-based documentation into computers was widespread in the 1970s and 1980s; this highlighted a flaw in both policy and infrastructure when users realized they could not retrieve information that had meaningful use. This term took on major implications in the healthcare industry. For example, a physician may have an e chart for each patient but is unable to access a list of patients with the same diagnoses such as diabetes or congestive heart failure. Many years and much money have produced better systems, but many providers still do not have adequate data exchanges.

The Center for Medicare and Medicaid Services (CMS) has mandated that all providers and insurers submit all claims for reimbursement—for any service or for verification or certification of services—in a consistent format (Department of Health and Human Services, 2014). This order compelled all providers to buy or contract with electronic data interchanges (EDIs) so billing is complete and uniform. When a government agency, such as CMS, prods a lagging healthcare system, this indicates a commitment to reform that has implications for electronic data storage and retrieval and for improved patient care.

HEALTHCARE DELIVERY MODELS The need for accurate and comprehensive data and the principles of healthcare reform have stimulated new models of delivering healthcare. A patient-centered medical home (PCMH) is a model or philosophy that is patient-centered, team-based, coordinated, accessible, and focused on quality and safety (Berenson, et al. 2016b). A team approach and a focus on population health differentiate this model from primary care and specialist care. PCMH practices are being evaluated for efficiency and positive health outcomes; data are imperative in this process.

ALTERNATIVE AND EXPERIMENTAL TREATMENTS AND CLINICAL TRIALS Alternative treatments are those not considered mainstream medical actions and often are not reimbursed by insurance companies. Data may be cited to support a particular treatment; data sources and conclusions must be scrutinized before and during treatment. Developing new treatment approaches and medications takes many years. Clinical trials, a critical element of development, often are supported by research funding, not reimbursement. Accurate and accessible data are absolutely critical during clinical trials. Information systems must capture not only anticipated positive outcomes but also must record trends that may indicate negative patient outcomes. Clinical trials rely on blind, randomized studies and often involve giving patients either a newly developed drug or a placebo. Interpretation of trial results requires astute attention to not only statistical data but to anecdotal data. The latter are qualitative responses from patients, caregivers and family, researchers, and physicians who may note symptoms, reactions, or behavioral responses to the drugs being administered. The informatics specialist should be involved very early in the development of the tools to measure and evaluate statistical and anecdotal data. A knowledgeable, experienced informatics specialist can direct clinical teams on which data to collect, how to collect it, and how and when to interpret it. A robust information system can detect outliers and other data points that may guide researchers to slow, halt, or discontinue a clinical trial. Incomplete data or absent veto points may lead to disastrous effects.

PRESCRIPTIVE PRACTICES The federal Prescriptive Drug Monitoring Program (2016) provides tools for states to collect data about prescription practices. Nearly all state agencies (usually the Boards of Pharmacy) have developed tracking systems. For example, Ohio politicians have been working with pharmacists, physicians, and advanced-practice nurses to strengthen the Ohio Automated Prescription Reporting System (OARRS), due to widespread drug abuse throughout the state. Tracking drug use and prescriptive practices within a state is not enough when drug trafficking crosses many state borders. Informatics specialists must be part of the team that creates tools to reduce and eliminate this social problem by providing expertise in what data to collect, how to collect, how to archive, how to retrieve, and how to interpret the data. Healthcare professionals know the medical and social effects of drug use and abuse but often do not have the skills to develop information systems that can offer data in ways that provide meaningful use.

BURDEN OF PROOF The need to protect patient confidentiality is always juxtaposed with a need to know certain patient information. Is sharing information about a patient among a team of healthcare professionals (and insurers) in direct opposition to privacy? The provider of services shoulders the burden of proof that all criteria required for reimbursement have been met, even those services that were or should have been provided prior to the current practice. For example, in order to obtain reimbursement for treatment in an acute-care hospital, a physician holds responsibility for assuring that a patient has been hospitalized in a freestanding, separate facility before being admitted to a skilled nursing facility. EDI allows patient records to be tracked so the burden of proof can be established. Sharing data in a secure manner will assure better coordination among providers with fewer duplicated services.

Implications of Diagnostic and Billing Codes for HIT and Informatics Practice

Healthcare diagnostic and billing codes can be overwhelming and confusing but are essential to ensuring the success of HIT such as electronic health record systems (EHRSs). Reimbursement for healthcare services is composed of a diagnosis and all of the corresponding treatments used to cure, improve, or monitor that disorder. The International Classification of Diseases (ICD) codes are evolving rapidly to adjust to the growing complexity in medical science, technology, society, and healthcare policy (Moriyama, Loy, & Robb-Smith, 2011). An ICD code consists of a combination of numbers and letters (three-to-seven characters) that designate specific diagnoses, and as the number of digits increases, so does the specificity of the diagnosis. In relation to billing and informatics, the ICD-10 codes, the latest upgrade as ruled by the ACA, categorize an injury or illness and describe in detail the cause, anatomical location, and severity. For example, an ICD-10 code for any injury to a shoulder begins with M75; to denote a right-shoulder injury, the code becomes M75.10; and to further classify the injury as nontraumatic, the code becomes M75.101 (Centers for Medicare and Medicaid Services, 2011). The informatics nurse specialist would be an important asset in analyzing data for healthcare systems.

ACCURACY AND SPECIFICITY The accuracy and specificity of coding directly affects a healthcare organization's billing and reimbursement. Reimbursement for services is essential for the survival of individual healthcare organizations. Accuracy and specificity of coding ultimately relies on the data entered into an EHRS. If a nurse simply documents that the patient has pain in an arm and does not specify duration, intensity, exact location, mechanism of injury, and so on, it becomes increasingly difficult to properly code for a procedure or service, which may lose revenue for the organization. Each piece of data entered into an EHRS should be specific, measurable, and accurate, so it can be compared, audited, and used to show meaningful use. At this point, the informatics nurse would be a valuable asset in training and mentoring personnel on the importance of accurate data entry. This nurse also should be utilized to coach the billers and coders on the nuances of data collection. For example, a misplaced decimal point for a given medical code could have a negative impact on reimbursement. Data collected through EHRSs also assist organizations in increasing quality, safety, and efficiency, which also has an end result of helping healthcare organizations remain open for providing continued care to their communities.

DO-NOT-PAY LIST The Deficit Reduction Act (DRA) of 2006 required that the Centers for Medicare and Medicaid Services (CMS) oversee the Hospital Acquired Conditions-Present on Admission (HAC-POA) Program. The HAC-POA evaluates payment, based on whether there is documented clinical evidence that a condition was present during the hospitalization and if it was noted to be present on admission to the healthcare facility (Snow et al., 2012). If conditions are not properly documented within the EHRS as being present on admission, the condition is assumed to be hospital acquired and, therefore, will most likely fall into the do-not-pay category of CMS reimbursement. Examples of the HAC-POA conditions that CMS has placed on a do-not-pay list include: stage III-and-IV pressure ulcers, falls and trauma, catheter-associated urinary tract infection, vascular-catheter associated infection, surgical-site infection, and deep-vein thrombosis (Centers for Medicare and Medicaid Services, 2015a).

Impact of HIT System Usability

Usability is a term that refers to the quality of a user's experience when interacting with a product, system, software, or other applications. Usability is about effectiveness, efficiency, and overall user satisfaction (Department of Health and Human Services, 2016a). HIT has offered some benefits for healthcare providers, payers, and businesses but still has usability faults that may have negative consequences. Currently, no federal regulation mandates that usability guidelines must be followed when developing new software (Reider, 2014). EHRS-related errors, such as data being lost, incorrectly entered, displayed or transmitted, leads to a loss of integrity and potential errors, harm, or even death (Bowman, 2013). In cases where HIT usability is inadequate, informatics nurse specialists could offer expert knowledge for redesigning software to obtain more meaningful use from the data.

Regulation (Rule-Making) and Implications for Informatics

Introduction: The Federal Regulatory Process

The legislative and regulatory processes are parallel and powerful methods of establishing laws and implementing them through rules (Loversidge, 2016). Federal agencies write rules in an orderly manner. First, a notice of proposed rulemaking (NPR) is published in the **Federal Register (FR)**. The FR is published daily, except for federal holidays. The NPR includes the name of the agency, the language (i.e., a narrative of the intended rule), contacts, and deadline dates for receiving comments.

Comments from the public are invited in the form of phone calls, face-to-face meetings with staff, letters, faxes, and emails. The agency must review all comments, respond to each inquiry, and consider seriously each suggestion. Changes to the proposed rule are noted in the FR as a notice of final rule (NFR). There still are opportunities to amend rules, even after the final rule is published. New data, re-interpretation of data, a change in philosophy about a program, or a change in administration can prompt changes in programs. All changes must go through the original process. The openings for inserting comments are numerous; there are hundreds of agencies and many proposals, so it is imperative to review the FR frequently.

Impact of Specific Rules

HIT use has grown exponentially over the past decade in response to new policies, laws, and regulations for healthcare reform. It is important to understand that each entity listed below has been instrumental in changing how healthcare organizations utilize patient data. While the overall goal of each rule is to improve quality, safety, and efficiency, each rule addresses a different facet of HIT reform.

THE MEDICARE ACCESS AND CHIP REAUTHORIZATION ACT OF 2015 The Medicare Access and CHIP Reauthorization Act of 2015 (MACRA) changed the way providers are reimbursed for services rendered to Medicare beneficiaries. Prior to this reform, healthcare providers were paid according to the sustainable growth rate (SGR) provision, which was estimated by four factors including: percentage change in physician-service fees, percentage change in the average number of Medicare beneficiaries served, an estimated 10-year average-percentage change in real gross domestic product, and percentage of change in expenditures due to changes in healthcare policy. MACRA ended the SGR, created a new framework to reward healthcare providers for providing quality care, and combined existing quality-reporting programs into one system. The goal of MACRA is to drive healthcare reform toward providing improved reimbursement for care, based on value and quality rather than quantity.

The MACRA quality payment program consists of the merit-based incentive payment system (MIPS) and alternative payment models (APMs). MIPS is a new program that combines other incentive programs, such as the physician quality reporting system (PQRS) and the Medicare EHRS, that will be measured based on quality, resource use, clinical-practice improvement, and meaningful use of EHRS technology. APMs offer new ways in which providers will be paid for the services they provide to Medicare beneficiaries. Two payment methods include lump-sum incentives that will begin in 2019 and increased annual payment rates for providers utilizing APMs, beginning in 2026. Currently, provider enrollment is completely voluntary, but the implications of MACRA are vast. Providers who practice under the MACRA and show quality improvement through meaningful use of their electronic health-information technologies will be compensated accordingly, which will elevate the individual success of these providers and the healthcare systems for which they work (Centers for Medicare and Medicaid Services, 2016a).

MACRA regulations were published in the *Federal Register* in May 2016. (Don't let the 900 pages of the NPR put you off—it is organized into sections that address EHRSs, reimbursement, etc.) All comments were accepted and the final rule was released in November 2017. This was an example of a real-life opportunity for informatics nurses to comment on and possibly improve a rule.

THE HEALTH INSURANCE PORTABILITY AND ACCOUNTABILITY ACT The Health Insurance Portability and Accountability Act (HIPAA) of 1996 required the Department of Health and Human Services (DHHS) to develop regulations protecting the privacy and security of designated health information. HIPAA includes a privacy rule and a security rule. The privacy rule established national standards for protecting health information, and the security rule established national security standards for protecting health information being held or transferred in electronic form (Department of Health and Human Services, 2016b). A major goal of the security rule is to protect individuals' health information while ensuring that the healthcare workforce has secure access to that same information through portable devices, such as cell phones, tablets, and/or computers. A key tenet is that protected health information (PHI) must not be disclosed to unauthorized persons. HIPAA violations within healthcare organizations can result in disciplinary action, fines, civil and criminal action, and even termination.

ESIGNATURE As HIT becomes a larger part of healthcare, questions arise regarding the acceptability of electronic signatures (esignature). What is an esignature? Are there federal regulations regarding esignatures? What public policies are there in place to guide healthcare organizations in implementing esignatures? Is the process of electronic signatures valid or acceptable? Electronic signatures are becoming standard in healthcare documentation as the use of EHRSs continues to grow. Healthcare staff are required to log in to their computers with specific user names and passwords that are reset multiple times throughout a year. This log-in can also be used to verify orders entered into a patient's health record, sign a note made by a provider, or authenticate prescriptive entries. Another form of esignatures includes the use of biometrics. Many EHRSs utilize biometric fingerprinting to place orders, administer medications, or verify complete documentation to a record. It is important that healthcare workers keep their log-in information private, completely log out of their computers when not in use, and periodically change their passwords in order to increase the validity and acceptability of the EHRS, including their esignatures (Downing, 2013). Although the Food and Drug Administration (FDA) accepts signatures that are written, scanned, or digitalized, the informatics nurse should be familiar with the FDA regulations for updates regarding electronic signatures.

MEDICARE IMPROVEMENTS FOR PATIENTS AND PROVIDERS ACT In 2008, Congress enacted the Medicare Improvements for Patients and Providers Act (MIPPA), which contained several provisions that changed the Medicare program and allocated federal funding for state-based assistance programs directed at providing outreach to low-income Medicare beneficiaries (Community Living Administration, 2015). Low-income Medicare beneficiaries tend to be sicker than those on the higher end of the Medicare spectrum and often require more services for their treatment. Informatics played a role in MIPPA as it changed the way federal and state agencies shared data. Prior to MIPPA, there was limited coordination between the federal Social Security Administration (SSA), which determines low-income eligibility, and state Medicaid agencies. There are still many hurdles to conquer to streamline the data sharing between the federal and state entities, but since the enactment of MIPPA, millions of individuals have been enrolled into the low-income-subsidy group. The data collected has enabled low-income beneficiaries to gain access to local support agencies, utilize statewide assistance programs, and have greater access to healthcare.

THE AMERICAN RECOVERY AND REINVESTMENT ACT The American Recovery and Reinvestment Act (ARRA) was enacted in 2009 as an attempt to revive the nation's economy, create jobs, and address widely neglected challenges that impact the future. Many of the provisions to the ARRA were directed toward improving healthcare such as reduced COBRA health-insurance premiums, a tax credit for health coverage to encourage greater compliance, and federal funding or incentives for healthcare organizations to upgrade HIT systems. In 2011, healthcare systems began the transition from paper documentation to electronic documentation with the intent to show meaningful use and receive incentives for successful EHRS adoption. Organizations that adopted EHRSs were given funding for the system itself, for staff education, and for evaluation tools to ensure successful implementation. EHRSs have enabled providers to connect, share information, evaluate patient data, and work as a team to obtain higher quality health outcomes for each patient (Adler-Milstein, Everson, & Lee, 2015; Centers for Medicare and Medicaid Services, 2009; Cresswell, Bates, & Sheikh, 2016; Tharmalingam, Hagens, & Zelmer, 2016; Yanamadala, Morrison, Curtin, McDonald, & Hernandez-Boussard, 2016).

The Health Information Technology for Economic and Clinical Health (HITECH) Act is a provision of the ARRA that aimed to ensure that healthcare organizations were not only adopting EHRSs but also validating their implementation by showing meaningful use. HITECH included approximately two billion dollars in funding for loans, grants, EHRS adoption, technical assistance in process implementation, workforce training, and new technology research and development (Centers for Disease Control and Prevention, 2016). Healthcare systems were faced with a momentous job of planning for new technologies, establishing training programs, ensuring competency of basic computer skills, implementing a go-live date once training was complete, and transferring healthcare information from paper documentation into the EHRS. HIT has changed every aspect of healthcare. No longer will a patient room be without some type of electronic device, or staff be without mobile devices equipped with HIT applications, or patients be without immediate access to their healthcare charts through the use of electronic health websites. As new information technologies are implemented within healthcare systems, the specifics of the HITECH Act may change in order to evolve with the technology.

AFFORDABLE CARE ACT In 2010, the Affordable Care Act (ACA) became one of the most significant healthcare-reform acts in the US (Rak & Coffin, 2013). One of the many goals of the ACA was to improve healthcare quality through the use of information technology. The ACA also aimed to ensure affordable healthcare by reducing the cost and increasing the number of individuals insured. The ACA was instrumental in ensuring that healthcare organizations implemented EHRSs and that these records could provide meaningful use to improve upon quality, safety, and efficiency. As the ACA implements new types of healthcare reform, clinical informatics will be needed to measure quality and compliance. Clinical informatics works to assess specific treatment options by providing visibility into how each patient responds to different approaches. The visible data, stored within electronic devices, then can be used to uncover areas for improvement. Clinical informatics provides the power to evaluate data and make necessary improvements to comply with the quality and safety standards set forth by the ACA.

MEDICAID Medicaid is administered by states, according to federal requirements. Medicaid provides health coverage to millions of Americans including low-income adults, children, pregnant women, the elderly, and those living with a disability (Centers for Medicare and Medicaid Services, 2016b). Each state manages the Medicaid provider payment that is usually based on fee-for-service rates or managed care arrangements. Approximately 70% of individuals receiving Medicaid are served through managed care, which means that providers are paid monthly based on specific trending factors and rates. Where informatics is concerned, healthcare providers must be aware of the continually changing supply costs, trending costs for services, advanced technology fees, and coding upgrades in order to produce both higher quality outcomes and increase revenue for the organization.

Accreditation

Legislation and regulation are government (i.e., public) responses to problems. Accreditation agencies, most of which are from the private-sector, also have impact on healthcare. These agencies develop national standards through which reimbursement and quality of care are determined. Documentation is so extensive that robust electronic information systems are required to capture data and issue prompts when standards are not met. Making sure that healthcare agencies and providers document correctly and in a timely manner mandates that a team of billers, coders, programmers, data analysts, and nursing and fiscal officers are competent in their skills and knowledge.

Standards address privacy and confidentiality, uniform definitions, training of users, integration of clinical systems, direct patient information, and comparative data. There are many accreditation agencies but all are intended to help the healthcare agencies keep track of the quality of care provided, patients' and care providers' satisfaction, and safety of care. Public reports are made and the reputation of healthcare organizations is measured against the reports. Organizations with highly rated scores tend to attract qualified professionals who are eager to practice in such organizations.

Seeking accreditation is lengthy and time-consuming. Much effort is expended in compiling data and evaluating internal processes. Most organizations provide a mock accreditation visit prior to an actual visit. This allows all employees to be knowledgeable about what is in the application. Every employee is expected to be able to speak with an accreditation visitor and answer inquiries about the services. Although this expectation puts pressure on individuals, the organization can be assured that it is prepared for the visit. Decisions from the accreditation agency are sent in writing, and the organization has a time frame in which to respond. Accreditation is issued for a specified time and can be re-issued if requirements are met.

Nongovernmental Agencies

THE JOINT COMMISSION The Joint Commission (TJC) is an independent, not-for-profit organization that accredits and certifies approximately 21,000 hospitals and other healthcare organizations nationwide (TJC, 2016). TJC accreditation and certification is recognized as a symbol of quality and reflects an organization's commitment to meeting or exceeding identified performance standards. TJC aims to accredit those facilities working to continuously provide and value safe, effective, high-quality care.

Informatics plays an important role during the accreditation process. TJC members often conduct interviews with frontline staff; complete an on-site visit; and review safety data, incident reports, and adherence to quality standards set by the institution along with many other data sets. This data is only as accurate as the information input into the system. For example, if a safety measure is to perform safety time-outs prior to every surgical procedure and the time-outs are not documented or are documented incorrectly, even one time, the surgical department falls out on that metric and may not pass accreditation.

HEALTHCARE FACILITIES ACCREDITATION PROGRAM The Healthcare Facilities Accreditation Program (HFAP) is authorized by CMS to survey all hospitals for compliance with Medicare Conditions of Participation and Coverage (Centers for Medicare and Medicaid Services, 2015b). The goal of HFAP is to meet or exceed the expectations set forth for CMS compliance. The accreditation process consists of an application, survey, deficiency report, plan of corrective action, and accreditation action. As with TJC, HFAP also conducts an onsite survey that consists of inspecting the facilities, interviewing employees, and reviewing medical records. Inconsistencies or lack of documentation can impede an organizations ability to become accredited which could lead CMS to withdraw reimbursement.

THE ACCREDITATION COMMISSION FOR HEALTHCARE The Accreditation Commission for Healthcare (ACHC) is a nongovernmental, proprietary corporation established to ensure high-level, clearly written standards for in-home aide services (Tavenner, 2015). ACHC is responsible for accrediting healthcare specialties such as home health, hospice, pharmacies, and behavioral-health facilities. ACHC is also a deeming authority for CMS that means that CMS has granted ACHC the power to determine the accreditation guidelines and status for those organizations noted. ACHC must ensure that specific conditions are met, standards are being set and achieved, and that high quality care is being provided. Complete, real-time documentation, whether it is paper or electronic, is essential for providing evidence of adherence to the standards set by the ACHC and CMS. The informatics nurse specialist is expertly prepared to document and oversee documentation of others.

AMERICAN NURSES CREDENTIALING CENTER MAGNET PROGRAM The American Nurses Credentialing Center (ANCC) is a member of ANA Enterprise, which is the overarching organization for the American Nurses Association, American Nurses Foundation, and the American Nurses Credentialing Center (ANA Enterprise, 2016). The ANCC's mission is to promote excellence in nursing and healthcare globally through credentialing programs (American Nurses Credentialing Center, 2016). ANCC programs certify and recognize healthcare organizations for promoting safe, positive work environments, along with several other areas of recognition. The ANCC is of particular interest because the ANCC Magnet Recognition Program recognizes healthcare organizations for quality patient care, nursing excellence, and innovation in nursing practice. Magnet hospitals are famous for meeting and exceeding high standards for safety, quality, and efficiency. Magnet recognition empowers staff to take ownership of their work and to go beyond simply doing a job.

An organization must meet several requirements to be considered for Magnet recognition; these include: nurse education, with a focus on all nursing staff possessing or obtaining a bachelor's degree in nursing; utilizing a shared governance model to promote nurse autonomy; and incorporating evidence-based research into nursing practice to improve outcomes.

Relationships among Entities

The relationship among accreditation decisions, reimbursement, quality of care, and informatics is evident. Accreditation cannot be earned without documentation of relevant data. Reimbursement (the very reason for an organization in a capitalist system) will be in jeopardy if support data are inaccurate, incomplete, or absent. Quality of care depends on healthcare providers making decisions based on evidence, which is often found in integrated data exchanges. Data sharing among providers, organizations, and other relevant and secure entities can contribute to quality care. Informatics specialists must be at the table as decisions are made about computer- and electronic-related systems. These specialists can offer insight, expertise, and wisdom so that information systems are developed, implemented, and evaluated in a useful manner.

Policy Making, Interprofessional Teams, and Informatics

The most recent occurrence in policy making is the philosophy of interprofessional teams. Historically, nurse-related policies were made by nurses; medical policies were made by physicians; pharmacy-related policies were made by pharmacists, and so on. While policies might have been cogent and focused, they did not reflect the cooperation and coordination that occurred in real life between and among professionals or, more than likely, the lack of cooperation and coordination. Education, practice, and research were separate entities among the professions. As healthcare became more complex, and roles became blurred, blended, or shared, the need for joint efforts became more evident and more acceptable.

The Institute of Medicine (IOM) report, *Crossing the Quality Chasm: A New Health System for the 21st Century* (Institute of Medicine, 2001), urged educators to work collaboratively. A later report, *The Future of Nursing: Leading Change Advancing Health* (Institute of Medicine, 2010), predicted financial incentives for care coordination. The Patient Protection and Affordable Care Act (PPACA) required teamwork among healthcare providers by 2014 (Kuramoto, 2014).

Educators tried to share courses among students from related disciplines. Several barriers became obvious. Since nurses are educated in associate and baccalaureate degree programs, and medical students are educated in graduate programs, there was a gap in the level of instruction. When nurses in graduate programs shared classes (e.g., pharmacology) with medical students, the nurses were found to have a much stronger foundation because the nurses brought with them knowledge from practice experience. Finding the level and content needed by all students was a challenge.

Clinicians found collaboration a bit more feasible. Nurses and physicians (especially residents) discovered that hospital rounds focused on patient care and treatment were opportunities to share perspectives. Rounds enhanced respect among participants as each came to understand the other's viewpoint. Research funding that traditionally expected single or single-discipline investigators slowly began to accept and encourage interdisciplinary proposals.

INTERPROFESSIONAL EDUCATION COLLABORATIVE The Interprofessional Education Collaborative (IPEC) was initiated in 2011 by leaders from the American Association of Colleges of Nursing, Association of American Medical Colleges, American Association of Colleges of Osteopathic Medicine, American Dental Association, American Association of Colleges of Pharmacy, and Association of Schools of Public Health. Through a series of conferences and workshops, IPEC developed competencies needed for all healthcare professionals (Interprofessional Education Collaborative, 2018).

Challenges stem from several areas:

- The population is much more diverse than even ten years ago and there is a need for culture-sensitive caregivers.
- The elderly are a fast-growing group, especially those older than 75 years of age. Providers must be knowledgeable about age-sensitive care.
- Workers who are nearing retirement are a huge population expected to have many healthcare problems and will demand services.
- Fragmented care will become more expensive as people experience more complex problems and may need to see a number of providers.
- Predictions indicate there will be a shortage of caregivers such as nurses, physicians, and dentists. Education programs may not want to invest in the complexity of coordinating learning experiences.

Benefits of interprofessional education include:

- Building an environment in which all providers demonstrate respect for each others' education and experience.
- Forming a strong clinical team whose members use tested competencies.
- Attracting providers to healthcare organizations that adopt national standards.
- Improving patient care through collaborative practice that attends to the whole patient, family, and community.
- Increasing public recognition of a caring provider community.

Providing Evidence for Best Practices

One issue absent from some presentations on IP issues is the need to include discussion about informatics. Healthcare teams need data in order to form opinions, diagnoses, and treatment plans. All members of the team should know where to locate data and how to retrieve it. Smart phones with a variety of applications are the most-often used information technology today. Computers are being replaced by phones (even watches) that can access data quickly and securely. Organizations must have policies in place that direct or restrict how current information technology is used. Security and privacy continue to be central to any discussion.

Big data is a term gaining popularity and relevance over the last few years as electronic technologies increase and evolve. In relationship to healthcare, big data refers to the rapidly increasing quantity of clinical data being collected and stored within EHRSs. It is important that healthcare systems be able to analyze the data in order to gain insight into what is currently working for an organization, what is not working, where improvements need to be made. Big data analytics could significantly reduce the cost of healthcare in several areas such as hospital readmissions, adverse events, and treatment optimization for patients with disease processes affecting multiple organ systems. For example, adverse events are those undesirable events that occur without causal effects secondary to medication administration or utilization of implanted medical devices. Adverse events can cause permanent health problems, and in some cases, death. Information technologists have the capability to modify EHRSs to enhance performance, based on big-data analytics for the purpose of quality improvement, that is decreasing the incidence of adverse events. EHRSs can be programmed to alert healthcare professionals of potential drug interactions that may cause an adverse event. Big data has ongoing implications within healthcare that will continue to drive organizations to provide higher quality care, based on the value of services provided.

Ethical Considerations

Ethics means doing the right thing. Robust health-information systems present huge amounts of data that are interpreted by many individuals and organizations. There is always a temptation to skew data to support one's perspective but doing so is an example of unethical use of data. Users who enter, archive, retrieve, interpret, and share data have an obligation to treat the data with utmost security (that is, do not discuss or share with those who do not have legitimate access) and respect. Casual handling of any aspect of healthcare information is unacceptable. Intentional misuse of data is unethical and could lead to civil action. The informatics specialist should instruct all users about the implications of unethical behavior and should be a role model in the proper attention to and use of HIT.

Future Directions

It may seem hard, with all of the changes to healthcare and HIT presently occurring, but try to imagine what the future of healthcare will look like in upcoming decades. Already, there are advancements in HIT policy aimed to address technology advancements in healthcare such as EHRSs, mobile health applications, and software that allow patients to access their records from any electronic device. Digital trackers that record an individual's level of activity, vital signs, and sleep patterns are becoming popular. This technology could eventually be used to improve patient outcomes, with software development that would allow digital trackers to communicate data directly to an individual's healthcare record. Family practices or emergency medicine may move away from traditional office visits and, instead schedule online patient visits with the use of webcams, secure websites, email, and telephone conference. Artificial-intelligence software is emerging as an alternative means of diagnostic imaging to detect when an individual is having a stroke. This type of information technology significantly reduces the time that a patient will go without treatment and potentially increases the patient's outcome. Healthcare is continuously evolving, and HIT is growing exponentially, which means that healthcare legislation, policy, and regulation must progress in order to address all facets of information technology within healthcare.

Case Study

Developing an Information System

A hospital in a small town in middle America has been struggling with an information system intended to store patient records. Problems include: complicated data entry, confusing data organization, and inability to retrieve data that relate to common populations served by the hospital. So far, healthcare providers who have been trained in accessing data include physicians, nurses, and pharmacists. The proprietary system's technicians have been called in as consultants to help to figure out how to work with the system. Identify four priorities for the consultants and propose at least one possible solution for each. Who should have been included in the team that assessed systems before one was chosen? Why?

Case Study

Rules for Hospital Reimbursement

CMS proposed a change in a rule that affects reimbursement to hospitals. Where can you find the Notice of Proposed Rule? What, beside the change, is included in the notice? How can you or your organization provide data to support or oppose the change? How will you go about gathering people inside your organization who have a stake in the change? If you go outside your organization, what other individuals or groups would you talk with? In what ways can you provide input and to whom? If you miss the proposal and read about a final rule, what can you do if you have a difference of opinion or additional data to support your opinion? At what points in the federal process of policy-making could you have intervened? That is, whom would you contact and what data would you provide?

About the Authors

Sunny Biddle MSN, RN has diverse experience in medical-surgical, renal, rehabilitation, oncology, cardiac, and intensive care nursing over the past 10 years at a general hospital in southeastern Ohio. She has worked as emergency department clinical coordinator, circulating nurse in an outpatient surgery center, and Magnet liaison for the outpatient surgery department. She is currently a full-time nursing instructor with the Central Ohio Technical College in Newark, Ohio. She earned a BSN from the University of Toledo (Ohio) and an MSN from Walden University where she is a member of Sigma Theta Tau International.

Jeri A. Milstead, PhD, RN, NEA-BC, FAAN, is an internationally known expert in public policy and the politics of healthcare. Dr. Milstead is the senior author editor with Dr. Nancy Short of *Health Policy and Politics A Nurse's Guide*, 6th ed., and *Handbook of Nursing Leadership: Creative Skills for a Culture of Safety*. She earned a PhD in Political Science from the University of Georgia, an MS and BS, cum laude, in Nursing from The Ohio State University, and a diploma from Mt. Carmel Hospital School of Nursing. She is an active Fellow of the American Academy of Nursing, board-certified as a Nurse Executive-Advanced by ANCC, and a member of Sigma Theta Tau International. She is Professor and Dean Emerita at the University of Toledo College of Nursing. where she was named a "Pioneer" in distance education. She has conducted research and consultation in China, The Netherlands, Jordan, Nicaragua, and Cuba.

References

Adler-Milstein, J., Everson, J., & Lee, S. D. (2015). EHR adoption and hospital performance: Time-related effects. *Health Services Research, 50*(6), 1751–1771. doi:10.1111/1475-6773.12406

American Nurses Credentialing Center. (2016). Accreditation. Retrieved from www.nursecredentialing.org/

ANA Enterprise. (2016). The American Nurses Association unveils the ANA Enterprise. Retrieved from http://nursingworld.org/ANAEnterprise-PressRelease

Bardach, E. (1977). *The implementation game: What happens after a bill becomes a law.* Cambridge, MA: MIT Press.

Berenson, R., Upadhyay, D., Delbanco, S., & Murray, R. (2016a). Accountable care organizations—Integrated delivery systems. Retrieved from www.urban.org

Berenson, R., Upadhyay, D., Delbanco, S., & Murray, R. (2016b). Payment methods and benefit design: How they work and how they work together. Retrieved from www.pcpcc.org

Bowman, S. E. (2013). Impact of electronic health record systems on information integrity: Quality and safety implications. *Perspectives in Health Information Management, 10*, 1–19.

Centers for Disease Control and Prevention. (2016). Meaningful use. Retrieved from www.CDC.gov

Centers for Medicare and Medicaid Services. (2009). Medicare and Medicaid health information technology: Title IV of the American recovery and reinvestment act. Retrieved from www.cms.gov/Newsroom/MediaReleaseDatabase

Centers for Medicare and Medicaid Services. (2011). State Medicaid ICD-10 implementation assistance handbook. Retrieved from www.Medicaid.gov

Centers for Medicare and Medicaid Services. (2015a). Hospital-acquired conditions. Retrieved from www.cms.gov/medicare/medicare-fee-for-service-payment/hospitalacqcond/hospital-acquired_conditions.html

Centers for Medicare and Medicaid Services. (2015b). CMS-approved accrediting organizations contacts for prospective clients. Retrieved from www.cms.gov

Centers for Medicare and Medicaid Services. (2016a). Quality payment program: Delivery system reform, Medicare payment reform, & MACRA. Retrieved from www.cms.gov/Medicare/Quality-Initiatives-Patient-Assessment-Instruments/Value-Based-Programs/MACRA-MIPS-and-APMs/MACRA-MIPS-and-APMs.html

Centers for Medicare and Medicaid Services. (2016b). Overview. Retrieved from www.medicaid.gov/medicaid-chip-program-information/medicaid-and-chip-program-information.html

Cohen, M. D., March, J. G., & Olsen, J. P. (1972). A garbage can model of organizational choice. *Administrative Science Quarterly, 17*(1), 1–25.

Community Living Administration. (2015). Availability of program instruction for MIPPA funds program. Retrieved from www.federalregister.gov/documents/2015/07/07/2015-16509/availability-of-program-instructions-for-mippa-funds-program-title-medicare-improvements-for

Cresswell, K., Bates, D. W., & Sheikh, A. (2016). Six ways for governments to get value from health IT. *Lancet, 387*(10033), 2074–2075. doi:10.1016/S0140-6736(16)30519-0

Department of Health and Human Services. (2014). Medicare Billing: 837P and Form CMS-1500). Retrieved from www.cms.gov/Outreach-and-Education

Department of Health and Human Services. (2016a). Usability evaluation basics. Retrieved from www.Usability.gov/what-and-why/usability-evaluation.html

Department of Health and Human Services. (2016b). The HIPPA privacy rule. Retrieved From www.hhs.gov/hippa

Downing, K. (2013). Electronic signature, attestation, and authorship (2013). *AHIMA Practice Brief*, October 2013. Retrieved from http://library.ahima.org/doc?oid= 107151#.V5ZGBY-cFYc

Institute of Medicine. (2001). *Crossing the quality chasm: A new health system for the 21st century*. Washington, DC: The National Academies Press.

Institute of Medicine (IOM). (2010). *The future of nursing: Leading change, advancing health*. Washington, DC: The National Academies Press.

The Interprofessional Education Collaborative (IPEC). (2018). About IPEC. Retrieved from www.Ipecollaborative.org/About_IPEC.html

Joint Commission (TJC). (2016). About the Joint Commission. Retrieved from www .jointcommission.org/about_us/about_the_joint_commission_main.aspx

Kingdon, J. W. (1995). *Agendas, alternatives, and public policies*. New York: Harper Collins College Publishers.

Kingdon, J. W. (2001). A model of agenda-setting with applications. *Law Review*, M., S. G-D, C., L., 331.

Kuramoto, F. (2014). The Affordable Care Act and integrated care. *Journal of Social Work in Disability and Rehabilitation*, *13*(1-2). doi: 10.1080/1536710X.2013.870515

Loversidge, J. M. (2016). *Government regulation: Parallel and powerful*. In J. A. Milstead, Health policy and politics: A nurse's guide (5th ed.). Burlington, MA: JBLearning, 99–150.

Moriyama, I., Loy, R., & Robb-Smith, A. (2011). History of the statistical classification of diseases and causes of death. Retrieved from www.cdc.gov/nchs/data/misc/ classification_diseases2011.pdf

Prescriptive Drug Monitoring Program. (2016). About the training and technical assistance center. Retrieved from www.pdmpassist.org

Rak, S., & Coffin, J. (2013). The Affordable Care Act. *The Journal of Medical Practice Management*, *28*(5), 317–319.

Registration with the Clerk of the US House of Representatives and Secretary of the Senate. (2016). *LDA guidance revision*. Retrieved from http://lobbyingdisclosures.house.gov

Reider, J. (2014). Usability of EHRs remains a priority for ONC. Retrieved from www .healthit.gov

Snow, C., Holtzman, L., Waters, H., McCall, N., Howpern, M., & Newman, L. (2012). Accuracy of coding in the hospital-acquired conditions present on admission program. Retrieved from www.CMS.gov/Medicare/Medicare-fee-for-service-payment

Tavenner, M. (2015). Notices. *Federal Register*, *80*(12). Retrieved from www.GPO.gov

Tharmalingam, S., Hagens, S., & Zelmer, J. (2016). The value of connected health information: Perceptions of electronic health record users in Canada. *BMC Medical Informatics & Decision Making*, *16*, 1–9. doi:10.1186/s12911-016-0330-3

Yanamadala, S., Morrison, D., Curtin, C., McDonald, K., & Hernandez-Boussard, T. (2016). Electronic health records and quality of care: An observational study modeling impact on mortality, readmissions, and complications. *Medicine*, *95*(18), e3332–e3332.

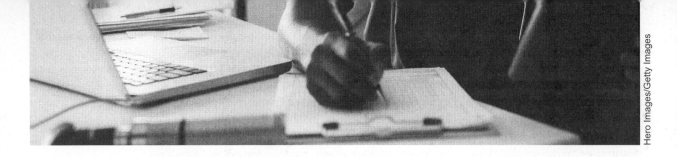

Hero Images/Getty Images

Chapter 7
Electronic Health Record Systems

Rayne Soriano, PhD, RN
Kathleen Hunter, PhD, RN-BC, CNE

 ## Learning Objectives

After completing this chapter, you should be able to:

- Differentiate between electronic health record (EHR), electronic medical record (EMR), and personal health record (PHR).

- Explain the relationship between an EHR and an electronic health record system (EHRS).

- Describe the relationship between *meaningful use* and the adoption and use of the EHR in hospitals, practitioner offices, and other settings.

- Discuss benefits associated with an EHRS.

- Review the current status of EHRSs.

- Discuss future directions for EHRSs.

To improve the quality of care through Health Information Technology (HIT), **electronic health record system (EHRS)** implementation has become a top priority in US hospitals and healthcare organizations, underpinned by national initiatives such as the Health Information Technology for Economic and Clinical Health (HITECH) Act and EHR incentive programs such as Meaningful Use (MU) (Centers for Medicare and Medicaid Services, 2013). Beyond the goal of stimulating the implementation of EHR systems, the MU initiative was developed as an incentive program to assure that EHRSs are used according to standards that achieve quality, safety, and efficiency measures (Centers for Medicare and Medicaid Services, 2013).

Numerous terms have been used over the years to describe the concept of an EHR, leading to confusion about the definitions. EHR has been used as a generic term for all electronic healthcare records and the related systems and recently became the favored term for an individual's lifetime computerized record. In most usage, the term EHR is used to mean both the displayed or printed record and the supporting software system (EHRS). In this chapter,

EHR refers to the patient record, and EHRS is the supporting system. Some other frequently used terms include electronic medical record (EMR), and electronic patient record (EPR), and shared electronic health record (SEHR). In addition to numerous terms, each term has been defined differently by different authors and organizations.

A basic definition of an EHR is a database of an individual's healthcare data during healthcare encounters. An EHRS is the database management software enabling the many functions needed to create and maintain an EHR. Another simple definition is that an EHR is comprised of any patient data stored in electronic form. Other, lengthier definitions build from this premise. Updates to the electronic record are restricted to authorized clinicians and staff. Patients may be shown data in an EHR but do not have control. The EHRS usually includes software to manage: a data repository (the EHR database), practitioner order entry (POE)—also known as computerized practitioner order entry (CPOE)—clinical decision support (CDS), and practitioner documentation.

Kohli and Tan, in 2016, described an **electronic medical record (EMR)** as an early form of the EHR, in which the focus was on bringing together the diagnostic and treatment information for an individual patient within a specific healthcare setting, such as a hospital or an office practice. EMR is still used to refer to a patient's record in a practitioner's office. These EMRs are isolated from other practices and facilities. Data are collected during each patient encounter, and data from prior encounters can be reviewed on demand.

One of the major potential benefits of electronic health information is the ability to engage patients in their care and provide venues to access caregivers virtually, using email and web platforms, providing ease and convenience to the patient. One approach to increasing patient engagement is the **personal health record (PHR)**, which is a collection of patient data controlled by the patient and accessible by patient and providers (Roehrs, deCosta, Righi, & Oleveira, 2017). A **shared electronic health record (SEHR)** is an electronic record system that allows clinicians to access a patient's data and information from the patient's EHRs at different facilities (Rinner, Grossmann, Sauter, Wolzt, & Gall, 2015). The SEHR enables a clinician at the point of care to access a patient's records without the delays of submitting requests and waiting for transmissions.

EHRSs provide users with enhanced versions of the functionality found in traditional paper-based health records. The addition of computer technology and digital data improves and expands on the basic set of functions. Current functionality includes:

- Point of care (POC) access by practitioners.
- Support for multiple users to view data on same patient at the same time.
- Results review (laboratory, pathology, imaging, notes, etc.).
- Quality metrics.
- Dashboards.
- Documentation.
- Electronic communication.
- Order management.
- Patient monitoring in real time.
- Patient summary displays.
- Patient support.
- Medication administration record.

- Population health.
- Bar code medication administration.
- External reference resources.
- Billing (Payne, 2016; Hydari, Telang, & Marella, 2015).

Another concept associated with electronic health record systems is the **continuity of care record (CCR)**. The CCR is a formal technical standard developed by the American Society for Testing and Materials (ASTM) and several other groups (Chen & Liou, 2014). This record is intended to improve continuity and quality of care, including reduction of errors, when clients move between various points of care. The CCR provides a snapshot of a person's current health and healthcare to a provider who does not have direct access to that person's electronic health record. The CCR has been named in the meaningful-use regulations for the exchange of clinical information (Medicare and Medicaid Programs; Electronic Health Record Incentive Program—Stage 2, Final Rule, 2012).

Meaningful Use

The American Recovery and Reinvestment Act (ARRA) of 2009 included the Health Information Technology for Economic and Clinical Health Act (HITECH), which authorized incentive payments to specific types of hospitals and healthcare professionals for adopting and using interoperable health information technology and EHRS. To implement these incentive payments, the Medicare and Medicaid EHR Incentive Programs, in 2011, developed sets of MU criteria (Centers for Medicare and Medicaid Services, 2017).

Meaningful use requires that use of an EHRS results in improved quality, safety and efficiency while reducing inconsistencies in healthcare; increases patients' and families' active involvement in their care; increases the coordination of healthcare; advances the health of the public; and safeguards the privacy and security of personal health data and information (Stimson & Botruff, 2017).

The Centers for Medicare and Medicaid Services (CMS) developed core criteria that defined basic functions EHRSs must demonstrate, including: basic entry of clinical information such as demographic data, vital signs, medications, and allergies; use of several software applications that begin to realize the true potential of EHRSs to improve the safety, quality, and efficiency of care through clinical decision support; and entry of clinical orders with safety measures within the software. In addition to these core requirements, MU included a menu of 10 other EHR tasks from which providers could choose to implement 5 in 2011 to 2012. These tasks included abilities to perform drug formulary checks, incorporate clinical laboratory results into EHRSs, provide reminders to patients for needed care, identify and provide patient-specific health education resources, and employ EHRSs to support the patients' transitions between care settings or personnel (Centers for Medicare and Medicaid Services, 2017).

The Medicare and Medicaid EHR Incentive Programs include three stages with increasing requirements for participation. All providers begin participating by meeting the Stage 1 requirements for a 90-day period in their first year of meaningful use and a full year in their second year of meaningful use. After meeting the Stage 1 requirements, providers have to meet Stage 2 requirements for two full years. In October 2015, CMS published a final rule for Stage 3 of meaningful use, which focuses on the advanced use of EHRS to promote health-information exchange and improved outcomes for patients.

Box 7-1 lists the 14 core requirements for hospitals. In the beginning, the MU requirement was being implemented in stages; however, by 2018, all providers are required to participate in MU (Waldren & Solis, 2016). Stage 1 measures focused on patient movement through the emergency department, stroke care, and treatment of blood clots. CMS has identified the degree of expected compliance to meet each measure. Additionally hospitals must meet 5 of the 10 requirements that are depicted in Box 7-2, although they have the latitude to choose the measures they will adopt from this second list. Stage 1 emphasizes the electronic capture and sharing of health information in coded format, and the use of that information to track conditions and coordinate care.

MU is divided into three stages, each intended to prepare a provider to successfully achieve meaningful use of their EHR system. Stage 1 established the foundation for the program by instituting requirements for the electronic capture of clinical data and by providing patients with electronic access to their health information. Providers who began participating in the program in 2011 or 2012 were eligible to achieve incentive payments totaling up to $44,000 over five years. Providers who started reporting in 2013 or 2014 could achieve up to $39,000 over four years, or $24,000 over three years, respectively. No new incentive payments were provided after 2014 (Resnick, Meara, Peltzman & Gilley, 2016).

Box 7-1   Stage I—Meaningful Use Core Requirements for Hospitals

1. Record demographic information (preferred language, gender, race, cultural background, date of birth, date/cause of death (inpatient setting only)).
2. Computerized provider order entry.
3. Clinical decision support and the ability to track compliance with rule(s).
4. Automatic, real-time drug-drug and drug-allergy interaction checks based on the medication list and allergy list.
5. Maintain an active medication list.
6. Maintain an active medication allergy list.
7. Record and retrieve vital signs (height, weight, blood pressure, BMI, growth charts for ages 2–20 years).
8. Record smoking status for patients 13 years old and older.
9. Mechanisms to protect information created or maintained by the certified EHR technology that include access control.
10. Electronically exchange key clinical information among providers and patient-authorized entities.
11. Supply patients with an electronic copy of their health information upon request.
12. Supply patients with an electronic copy of their discharge instructions upon request.
13. Report required clinical quality measures to CMS.
14. Maintain up-to-date problem lists of current and active patient diagnoses.

SOURCE: Medicare and Medicaid; Electronic Health Record Incentive Program Final Rule. 75. Fed. Reg. 443313. (July, 38, 2010). Retrieved from http://edocket.access.gpo.gov/2010/pdf/2010-17207.pdf

> ## Box 7-2 Menu Set of 10 Optional Stage I Meaningful Use Core Measures
>
> 1. Incorporate clinical lab test results as structured data.
> 2. Generate patient lists by specific conditions to use for quality improvement, reduction of disparities, research or outreach.
> 3. Submit electronic data to immunization registries.
> 4. Submit syndromic public health surveillance data electronically in accordance with applicable law.
> 5. Identify and provide patient-specific education resources.
> 6. Conduct drug-formulary checks.
> 7. Support medication reconciliation.
> 8. Generate summary care records for transition of care/referral.
> 9. Enable electronic submission of reportable lab results.
> 10. Create advance-directive forms for patients 65 years old and older.
>
> **SOURCE:** Medicare and Medicaid; Electronic Health Record Incentive Program Final Rule. 75. *Fed. Reg*. 443313. (July, 38, 2010). Retrieved from http://edocket.access.gpo.gov/2010/pdf/2010-17207.pdf

The State of Meaningful Use

As the environment of implementation and adoption of EHRSs evolved, so has the MU program. On October 6, 2015, the CMS and the ONC updated and released a final rule governing MU through 2018. The new rule eases the requirements in Stage 2 and changes the reporting period for all eligible professionals (EPs) to any consecutive 90 days in 2015. More important, the new rule initiated a fundamental change in MU that will roll the program into a single set of requirements, beginning in 2015 and ending in 2018 (Waldren & Solis, 2016). In order to eliminate the complexity from the original rules, the following standards and objectives were implemented in modified Stage 2 of MU:

- The patient electronic access measure requires patients to view, download, or transmit their health information online. This measure previously required at least 5% of an EP's unique patients to access their records this way during the attesting period but now requires just one unique patient to do so. The objective still requires that at least 50% of unique patients have access to their records, such as through a patient portal.

- The measure requiring EPs to receive secure electronic messaging from patients has undergone a similar change, with the requirement shrinking from at least 5% of patients to at least one patient.

- With the public health reporting requirement, providers are now expected to report two of the three public health reporting measures (the others include syndromic surveillance reporting and specialized registry reporting).

- MU no longer distinguishes between "core" and "menu" objectives. All measures are now required.

- A number of measures have been eliminated from attestation because CMS either determined them redundant or found that EPs are already tracking them at high levels, including:

  - Record patient demographics.
  - Record and chart changes in vital signs.
  - Record smoking status.
  - Provide clinical summaries for patients for each office visit.
  - Incorporate clinical laboratory results as structured data.
  - Generate lists of patients by conditions.
  - Identify patients needing preventive/follow-up care and send reminders.
  - Provide summary of care records for more than 50% of patient referrals or transitions of care and perform at least one successful exchange electronically with another provider (note: EPs must still provide 10% of care summaries through an electronic health record or health information exchange).
  - Record electronic notes in patient records.
  - Provide imaging results consisting of the image itself and any explanations or other accompanying information in the electronic health record.
  - Record patient family history as structured data (Waldren & Solis, 2016).

The third and final stage of MU is planned for implementation in 2018. Stage 3 will contain a single set of criteria focused on the advanced use of EHR systems. CMS recently decided to move away from the staged approach and will require all providers (including first-time participants) to satisfy the objectives and measures of Stage 3 by 2018. Beginning in 2019, the MU program will transition into a new merit-based incentive payment system (MIPS) program established by the Medicare Access and CHIP (Children's Health Insurance Program) Reauthorization Act. The Stage 3 requirements and objectives will be maintained (Resnick et al., 2016).

Another important factor in achieving MU is the level of investment and resources that eligible hospitals (EH) commit to the journey. In a study assessing resources needed to achieve MU Stage 1 in the ambulatory care setting, Shea, Reiter, Weaver, and Albritton (2016) found that having quality improvement teams involved in leading the MU initiative was significantly associated with achieving MU. In a study evaluating the effects of the type of hospitals, Wolf, Harvell, and Jha (2012) used nationally available hospital data to provide a baseline of EHRS adoption rates for hospitals that are ineligible for federal incentives. It compared the use of EHRSs at ineligible hospitals with that at short-term acutcare hospitals. Survey results revealed a wide range in the rates of EHR system adoption by hospital type, including adoption of specific EHR system functions. Researchers highlighted one consistent pattern: compared to short-term acute-care hospitals, ineligible hospitals had lower rates of adoption for each of the 24 individual functions that make up a comprehensive or basic EHRS. In evaluating the state of MU in children's hospitals, Nakamura, Harper, and Jha (2013) found that, out of 126 participating children's hospitals, major teaching hospitals were significantly more likely to have an EHRS. The proportion of children's hospitals with an EHRS increased from 21% (in 2008) to 59% (in 2011). In 2011, 29% of children's hospitals met the 12 core criteria in the researchers' meaningful-use proxy measure. EHRS adoption rates and meaningful use were significantly higher for children's hospitals than for adult hospitals as a whole but similar for children's and adult's major teaching hospitals. Literature has revealed that US hospitals are continuing to invest in the adoption of EHRSs to achieve meaningful use; however, disparities exist with rural and critical-access hospitals. These findings raise questions as to how organizations use EHRSs to assure quality, safety, and efficiency as hospitals face the challenges of EHRS adoption.

In reviewing outcomes associated with achieving MU, studies have been done to review MU's effects on quality, utilization, and management of patient populations. Appari, Johnson, and Anthony (2013) set out to estimate the incremental effects of transitions in EHRS capabilities on hospital process quality in heart attack, heart failure, pneumonia, and surgical-care infection prevention. They found that hospitals transitioning to EHR systems capable of meeting 2011 MU objectives improved in quality, and lower-quality hospitals experienced even higher gains; however, hospitals that transitioned to more advanced systems saw quality declines. In comparing the quality of care between hospitals that achieved MU Stage 1 to those that used EHRSs but did not achieve MU Stage 1, Kern, Edwards, Kaushal, and Investigators (2015) conducted a longitudinal study of primary care physicians and found that no difference in quality was found between those who achieved Stage 1 MU and those who were using EHRSs but had not achieved MU. Overall, more than half of eligible patients received recommended care for 7 of the 9 measures. In evaluating individual measures, there were significant, unadjusted differences within each year between the MU group and the control group, with the MU group providing higher quality of care for five measures including: hemoglobin A1c testing, low-density lipoprotein testing, nephropathy screening, chlamydia screening, and appropriate care for children with pharyngitis. Stimson and Botruff (2017) described how EHRS reports met MU standards but also allowed remote monitoring and improved the quality of care for trauma patients in the emergency department setting.

In evaluating the effects of achieving MU on utilization, Kern, Edwards, Kaushal, and Investigators (2016) performed a cohort study of primary care physicians to determine the effects on healthcare utilization of MU of electronic health record systems compared to typical use of EHRSs without MU. They found that those primary care providers who both used EHRSs and achieved Stage 1 MU provided more efficient care, with 6% fewer primary care visits and 4% fewer laboratory tests. In another study on utilization, Lammers and McLaughlin (2016) evaluated the effects of meeting MU Stage 1 criteria to the expenditures for elderly Medicare beneficiaries. They specifically looked at Medicare expenditures for elderly beneficiaries with four common chronic conditions—chronic obstructive pulmonary disease (COPD), congestive heart failure (CHF), diabetes, and ischemic heart disease (IHD)—since these patients have high healthcare utilization and receive care across multiple providers. They found that an increase in the hospital EHRS penetration rate was associated with a small but statistically significant decrease in total Medicare and Medicare Part A acute care expenditures per beneficiary. An increase in physician EHRS penetration was also associated with a significant decrease in total Medicare and Medicare Part A acute care expenditures per beneficiary as well as a decrease in Medicare Part B expenditures per beneficiary. Another area of MU outcomes explored by DesRoches, Worzala, and Bates (2013) was the association between EHRS adoption and ease of use and physicians' ability to use EHRSs for patient panel management. Out of 1820 primary care physicians surveyed, 43.5% reported having a basic EHRS, while 9.8% met MU criteria. Physicians with EHRS functionalities for panel management reported that these systems varied in ease of use. Approximately one half of physicians with the respective computerized systems reported that they could not or that it was very or somewhat difficult to generate lists of patients by laboratory result, lists of patients who were overdue for care, and reports on quality of care and track referrals. Physicians with an EHRS that met MU criteria were significantly more likely than those not meeting the standard to rate panel management tasks as easy.

While studies evaluating the outcomes of achieving MU on quality, efficiency, and affordability are still emerging, bright spots have revealed that having EHR systems that meet MU criteria can be leveraged to improve the quality of care in patient populations; improve efficiency by eliminating redundancies and automating tasks; and decrease spending in areas where information can easily be accessed versus having to repeat diagnostic tests and procedures. As EHRSs evolve, the goals of using these systems in the most meaningful and optimized way is also shifting from merely utilizing features towards how to best leverage the data and information from EHR systems in order to transform healthcare.

Benefits of EHRSs

The main goal of implementing technologies such as EHRSs is to improve the quality and safety of patient care through benefits such as: improving the accuracy and completeness of patient health information; increasing the speed at which care is provided; enhancing the coordination of care; and increasing transparency of health information for patients and their families. In addition to these benefits, EHRSs can add decision support and flag potentially dangerous drug interactions, verify medications, and reduce the needs for risky tests and procedures. Benefits can be categorized according to general areas, those affecting caregivers, the healthcare system, and consumers of healthcare.

General Benefits

- *Improved data integrity.* Information is more readable, better organized, and more accurate and complete.
- *Increased productivity.* Caregivers are able to access client information whenever it is needed and at multiple convenient locations. This can result in improved client care due to their ability to make timely decisions based on appropriate data.
- *Improved quality of care.* The EHRS supports clinical decision-making processes for physicians and nurses. For example, the clinician can tailor a view of patient information that shows the most recent labs, vital signs, and current medications on one screen or select another view that graphs lab values and vital signs over time. This capability could be used to show renal response to ordered medications or for any number of other scenarios.
- *Increased satisfaction for caregivers.* Caregivers are able to take advantage of easy access to client data as well as other services, including drug information sources, rules-based decision support, and literature searches.

Nursing Benefits

- Facilitates comparisons of current data and data from previous events.
- Supports an ongoing record of the client's education and learning response across encounters or visits.
- Eliminates the need to repeat collection of baseline demographic data with each encounter, saving nursing time.
- Provides universal data access to all who have access to the EHR.
- Improves data access and quality for research (Davis & Haines, 2015).
- Provides prompts to ensure administration and documentation of medications and treatments.
- Improves documentation and quality of care (Hickey, Katapodi, Coleman, Reuter-Rice, & Starkweather, 2017.).

- Facilitates automation of critical and clinical pathways (Campbell, 2016).
- Supports the development of a database that facilitates research, provides information useful to administrators and clinicians, and allows recognition of nursing work in measurable units when used with a common unified structure for nursing language.

Benefits for Healthcare Providers

- Improved eligibility for reimbursement.
- Simultaneous record access by multiple users and promotion of interdisciplinary care (Hansen, Martin, Jones, & Pomeroy, 2015).
- Previous encounters may be accessed easily (King, Patel, Jamoom, & Furukawa, 2014).
- Faster chart access, eliminating waiting for old paper records to be located and delivered from the medical records department.
- More comprehensive information is available (Davis & Haines, 2015).
- Fewer lost records than with paper systems.
- Improved efficiency of billing inclusive of automated charge capture.
- Better reporting tools. Trends and clinical graphics are available on demand.
- Reduced liability through better decision-making and documentation (King at al., 2014).
- Improved reimbursement rates.
- Enhanced decision support through system-generated prompts with preventive care protocols (Hicks, Dunnenberger, Gumpper, Haidar, Hoffman, 2016).
- Enhanced ability to meet regulatory requirements such as the physician quality reporting initiative (Bell & Thornton, 2011).
- Supports pay-for-performance bonuses.
- Early warnings of changes in patient status (King at al., 2014).
- Improved population health.
- Increased efficiencies in workflow.

Healthcare Enterprise Benefits

- Improved client record security.
- Instant notice of authorization for procedures with integration with payer-based health records.
- Strengthened communications.
- Fewer lost records.
- Decreased need for record storage.
- Reduced medical record department costs because pulling, filing, and copying of charts are decreased.
- Improved verification of client eligibility for healthcare coverage.
- Faster turnaround for outstanding accounts with electronic coding and claim submission.
- Decreased need for x-ray film and physical filing, storage, and transport of films.
- Improved cost evaluation based on clinical outcomes and resource utilization data.

- Fewer emergency department visits (Kern et al., 2016).
- Enhanced compliance with regulatory requirements.

Consumer Benefits

- Decreased wait time for treatment.
- Improved access and control over health information.
- Increased use of best practices with incorporation of decision support.
- Improved ability to ask informed questions.
- Greater responsibility for one's own care.
- Increased medication safety (Seibert, Maddox, Flynn, & Williams, 2014).
- Quicker turnaround time for ordered treatments.
- Alerts and reminders for upcoming appointments and scheduled tests.
- Increased use of preventive care.
- Increased satisfaction.
- Greater clarity to discharge instructions.
- Elimination of healthcare disparities (Douglas et al., 2015).

Payer Benefits

- Supports pay for performance as quality measures are gathered (Bardach et al., 2013).
- Supports disease management, lowering costs for expensive diagnoses.

Although benefits of EHR systems affect healthcare systems, providers, and consumers of healthcare, it is important to study the current state of EHR systems in various healthcare settings in order to account for the challenges, barriers, and methods of overcoming them.

Current Status of EHRSs

There are numerous sources reporting rates of EHRS adoption. Not surprisingly, the reported results can vary. EHRS adoption rates in physician office practices are higher in rural areas than in urban areas according to a 2017 study by Whitacre. Analyzing data from a 2012 data set, the author found that urban practices reported an adoption rate of 45% and most rural areas reported adoption rates of 60%. Milstein et al. (2015) analyzed data from a 2014 American Hospital Association survey. These researchers determined that 75% of 3,277 responding hospitals have adopted some form of EHRS. This percentage is an increase of 16% from 2013.

Challenges with Using EHRs

Despite the growing financial incentives, and federal and organizational resources dedicated to achieving hospital environments where EHRSs are used meaningfully, there are still many challenges in using EHRSs. Cifuentes et al. (2015) presented challenges experienced in utilizing EHRSs to integrate behavioral health and primary care workflows including those related to: (1) documenting and tracking relevant behavioral health and physical health information;

(2) supporting communication and coordination of care among integrated teams; and (3) exchanging information with tablet devices and other EHRSs.

Limitations in resources, especially in small, non teaching, rural hospitals also led to variability in using an EHRS (DesRoches et al., 2012). The availability of usable functionality in the system was also associated with variable EHRS use (Rogers et al., 2013).

These variations have led to the continued reliance on paper including work-arounds from the intended use of EHRSs (Cifuentes et al., 2015; Flanagan et al., 2013; Friedman et al., 2013), and hospitals falling behind in adoption and in achieving meaningful use (Wolf et al., 2012; DesRoches et al., 2013).

In studying challenges with EHRS use, Agno and Guo (2013) found challenges with technical features and a lack of technical support for clinicians. While robust in volume, clinical documentation often is highly fragmented, which makes it difficult to learn a complete story about a patient (Effk & Weaver, 2016). Zahabi, Kaber, and Swangnetr (2015) conducted a systematic review and analysis of electronic health record system research since 2000. They focused on usability and safety studies and identified 14 categories of usability issues in EHRSs: failure to follow natural work flows naturalness, lack of consistency, prevention of errors, failure to minimize cognitive load, inefficient interactions, lack of useful feedback, ineffective language use, ineffective presentation of information, and inability to customize a system. Nurses and pre-licensure nursing students also expressed challenges in using EHRSs (Whitt, Eden, Merrill, & Hughes, 2017).

Work-arounds in Accessing Information from the EHRS

Despite the automated features that EHRSs provide, caregivers have used process work-arounds as a means to document and access information to care for patients amidst the complexity and limitations of structural features and applications (Flanagan et al., 2013; Friedman et al., 2013; Rogers et al., 2013). As a result of structural and functional challenges in accessing information, an emerging area of study focuses on these process work-arounds by system users. Work-arounds are variations in procedures and processes created to accomplish work when systems or workflows are deficient or inefficient (Stutzer & Hylton Rushton, 2015). Studies have revealed that common reasons prompting the implementation of work-arounds include: insufficient and inconveniently located data (Friedman et al., 2013); mismatches between the electronic system and real-world workflows (Rogers et al., 2013); resource limitations (DesRoches, Worzala, & Bates, 2013); and disruptions to user workflows (DesRoches et al., 2012; Flanagan et al., 2013). These challenges heightened the need for actual or perceived increases in efficiency, increased awareness of new and important information, better memory queues for old and existing information (Flanagan et al., 2013), and the need to integrate data from paper into the EHRS (Friedman et al., 2013). As a result of these structural barriers, common process work-arounds included double documentation, scanning, limiting EHRS use in certain care areas, manual verification of electronic data, ignoring or disabling EHRS functions, staggering EHRS access (Friedman et al., 2013); use of paper (Friedman et al., 2013); and reliance on using free-text areas in the EHRS (Rogers et al., 2013).

Aside from the structural and system limitations as mentioned above, some work-arounds were found to be related to individual-level barriers to using EHRSs including perceptions of the lack of user control, freedom, flexibility, and ease of use, as found in nurses' use of electronic systems to document care (Rogers et al., 2013).

Considerations When Implementing the EHRS

Information system vendors as well as healthcare providers are aware of the pressing need to develop and deploy EHRS. Compliance with regulatory and reimbursement issues, particularly MU, is a major driver. This requires the use of certified EHRSs or strategies to update existing EHR systems. Development of an electronic infrastructure and the associated cost have been two of the biggest impediments to the creation of a fully functioning EHRS. The principal requirement is that the major participants in the healthcare arena, including healthcare facilities, payers, and physicians, must be linked electronically. This is a costly undertaking. Other issues have included practice issues such as workflow adoption, physician engagement, training and staffing, as well as vendor issues such as lack of vendor support, upgrade challenges, technical challenges, and lack of training support (Heisey-Grove et al., 2014).

ONC-Authorized Testing and Certification

The ONC established a temporary certification program for HIT as a means to facilitate the adoption of interoperable EHRSs capable of meeting MU core requirements. The purpose of the testing and certification program is to provide a way for organizations to become authorized by the National Coordinator to test and certify EHRS technology. Certification, in turn, provides the assurance that adopted EHRS technology is capable of helping organizations meet meaningful use criteria.

Initially only two entities were authorized as ONC-authorized testing and certification bodies (ONC-ATCBs). The list of ONC-ATCBs has since been expanded and is available on the ONC website. ONC issued the final rule to establish the permanent HIT certification program in January 2011. Box 7-3 lists functionality required for EHRS certification; additional functions may be added at future dates.

Electronic Infrastructure

Healthcare facilities, payers, physicians, and nurses all need the ability to access and update the client's longitudinal record. This ability requires linkage of the various information systems that support these stakeholders via a network infrastructure. Agreement must be reached regarding the nature and format of client data to be stored, as well as the mechanisms for data exchange, storage, and retrieval. This means that all participants use common data communication standards. The lack of standards has been a key barrier to establishing this type of electronic connectivity. First and most important is the decision regarding the recognition of a universal client identifier or MPI (master patient index) number, so that all client data can be associated with the correct client. The Social Security number has been widely used for this purpose, but it is unreliable because it may be stolen or inaccurately provided; in addition, some individuals have used more than one number, while others do not have one. Improvements in connectivity alone are not enough to support the EHR. It is also important to include components such as interoperability, comparability, decision support, and POC data capture to achieve a longitudinal electronic record.

Cost

Another impediment to an EHRS is cost. Financial considerations include vendor fees, capital availability, lack of or limited incentive eligibility (Heisey-Grove et al., 2014). Initial and ongoing costs for deploying and maintaining IT systems were cited as the greatest barrier to IT.

Box 7-3 Functionality Required for Certified EHRSs

Function	Inpatient Settings/ Hospitals	Outpatient Settings/ Physician Offices
Record demographic information	X	X
• Preferred language		
• Gender		
• Race		
• Cultural background		
• Date of birth		
Date/cause of death (inpatient setting only)		
Computerized provider order entry	X	X
Clinical decision support and the ability to track compliance with rule(s)	X	X
Automatic, real-time drug-drug and drug-allergy interaction checks based on the medication list and allergy list	X	X
Maintain an active medication list	X	X
Maintain an active medication allergy list	X	X
Record and retrieve vital signs	X	X
• Height		
• Weight		
• Blood pressure		
• BMI		
• Growth charts and BMI ages 2–20 years		
Record smoking status for patients 13 years old and older	X	X
Mechanisms to protect information created or maintained by the certified EHR technology that include access control	X	X
Electronically exchange key clinical information among providers and patient-authorized entities	X	X
Supply patients with an electronic copy of their health information upon request	X	X
Supply patients with an electronic copy of their discharge instructions upon request	X	N/A
Report required clinical quality measures to CMS	X	X
Maintain up-to-date problem lists of current and active patient diagnoses	X	X
Incorporate clinical lab-test results as structured data	X	X
Generate patient lists by specific conditions to use for quality improvement, reduction of disparities, research or outreach	X	X

Function	Inpatient Settings/ Hospitals	Outpatient Settings/ Physician Offices
Submit electronic data to immunization registries	X	X
Submit syndromic public health surveillance data electronically in accordance with applicable law	X	X
Identify and provide patient-specific education resources		
Drug-formulary checks	X	X
Support medication reconciliation	X	X
Generate summary care records for transition of care/referral	X	X
Electronic submission of reportable lab results	X	N/A
Advance directives	X	
Patient reminders for preventive and/ or follow-up care	N/A	X
Provide patients with timely electronic access to their information	N/A	X
Check insurance eligibility electronically	X	X
Submit claims electronically	X	X
Support electronic prescriptions	N/A	X

SOURCE: Medicare and Medicaid; Electronic Health Record Incentive Program Final Rule. 75. *Fed. Reg.* 443313. (July, 38, 2010). Retrieved from http://edocket.access.gpo.gov/2010/pdf/2010-17207.pdf

According to recent CMS estimates, which have not been updated, eligible providers will spend an average of $54,000 to purchase and implement a certified EHRS for their offices and eligible hospitals will spend an average of $5,000,000 for purchase and installation; those figures do not include annual maintenance costs (Harris, 2010). Furthermore, the development of the electronic links forming the infrastructure is costly, and the allocation of fiscal responsibilities is difficult. Until the introduction of MU incentives, most of the expense for EHRS development has been underwritten by each individual provider, hospital, or healthcare enterprise. Links to other facilities and agencies are rare and for the most part limited to provider–payer arrangements.

Vocabulary Standardization

Standardization of clinical terms used in patient records facilitates interoperability as it ensures a common understanding of terms. Standardized languages make it possible to generalize research findings across settings, countries, and cultures; compare patient outcomes; facilitate communication with other disciplines and delivery systems; and showcase nursing's contributions to healthcare. Despite these clear advantages, adoption of standard nomenclature has been slow. The increased acceleration of EHRS adoption can be used as an opportunity to realize the benefits associated with standardized nomenclature for the entire healthcare sector as well as for nurses who could use the power of standardized nursing nomenclatures to demonstrate contributions made by nurses. In-depth discussion of standardized nomenclature takes place in Chapter 15.

Security, Privacy, and Confidentiality

Security and confidentiality concerns are critical considerations in EHRS development and use. Even as EHRS adoption increases, security and privacy concerns remain (Furukawa et al., 2014). The EHR system must be configured to allow access only to those who have been identified as authorized users. The system must authenticate the user's identity with user IDs and passwords and possibly biometrics. HIPAA considerations include the need to be able to provide the client, upon request, with a log of caregivers who have accessed his or her chart. In addition, client information should not be available to anyone without the client's approval. Data that are communicated via the Internet must be encrypted. Firewalls must be in place when data are sent and received via the Internet to safeguard data integrity. Meaningful use requirements also include measures to protect patient information that strengthen HIPAA requirements. Preservation of the client's privacy is one of the most basic and important duties of the healthcare provider. Because one of the key attributes of an EHRS is the ease of data sharing, the client's privacy rights must be guarded by all who have access to the record.

Data Integrity

Data integrity can be compromised in three ways: incorrect entry, data tampering, and system failure. In general, data integrity can be improved by implementing security measures, including the use of audit trails, as well as the development of detailed procedures and policies.

INCORRECT DATA ENTRY The client data found in an EHRS are only as accurate as the person who enters them and the systems that transfer them. Therefore, critical information, such as allergies and code status, should be verified for accuracy at each encounter. This will allow the correction of data entry errors and screen for changes that have occurred in client status. This is especially crucial because data may be entered or modified from many different encounters in the healthcare arena, such as hospitals, clinics, and home care visits. Data integrity is also compromised if an interface is not receiving or sending data correctly. When corrections to the data in the electronic record must be made, data must be corrected in multiple areas. The data in the initial system must be corrected, as well as any receiving systems. For example, if information is incorrect in the hospital information system, it must be corrected there. Any other systems that derive information from this, such as physician office systems and ancillary systems, must also be updated. This may involve correction using interface transactions or manual intervention. Some systems may not allow automated correction, which means that a person must make changes.

DATA CORRECTION An effective audit trail procedure permits the tracking of who entered or modified each data element, allowing appropriate follow-up measures. Policies need to be in place for the correction and updating of data, particularly when erroneous data is discovered.

Master File Maintenance

The development and maintenance of master files and data dictionaries is critical to preserving data integrity. Careful attention to initial development of the files, including documentation, will ensure that data are accurate and communicate valid information. Periodic review and validation of master files, at least annually, is necessary to maintain current and accurate data.

SYSTEM UPDATES AND MAINTENANCE The robust nature of today's technology requires frequent system updates and maintenance in order to comply with new regulations and/or organizational needs. In the clinical setting, this can be disruptive and lead to issues with data integrity. Scheduled system maintenance is a common occurrence with most EHRSs and may require the clinician to revert to paper forms and alternate communication methods if the downtime is lengthy. Major system updates can change the database structure and cause loss of important information unless version control is carefully monitored. Downtime policies and procedures need to be developed and communicated to ensure appropriate steps are taken to enter lost data due to system updates or maintenance.

SYSTEM FAILURE Hardware and software malfunctions, such as a system crash, may result in incomplete or lost data. Once the problem has been resolved, it may be necessary to verify the client data that could have been affected. It may then be necessary to append paper records or manually enter data once the system is restored. Downtime procedures and disaster recovery plans should be developed during the initial EHRS implementation process and updated on an ongoing basis in preparation for potential system failure. These documents should outline the roles, responsibilities, policies, and procedures necessary to continue business as usual while recovering a failed system.

Ownership of the Patient Record

Currently, paper medical records are the property of the institution at which they are created. This institution is responsible for ensuring the accuracy and completeness of the record. With the development of EHRSs, however, ownership issues become more complex. Because many providers use the same data, it is unclear who actually owns them and is responsible for maintaining their accuracy. Because the data are shared and updated from many sites, decisions must be made regarding who can access the data and how the data will be used. In addition, it must be determined where the data will actually be stored. With meaningful use requirements, mechanisms must be in place to allow patients timely access to their data as well as provide electronic copies of their records, which helps to ensure that patients "own" information and can take steps to correct errors or omissions. As EHRSs become more prevalent, a movement towards granting patients access to view their providers' electronic documentation called *Open Notes* has emerged, and initial studies have shown improved patient engagement, improved relationships with providers, and fewer concerns expressed (Bell et al., 2016; Esch et al., 2016).

Legal Aspects Related to Online Documentation

The move toward EHRSs brings forth new legal issues and highlights old ones. Maynard (2010)noted that the rules of discovery for lawsuits are rapidly changing as healthcare moves to the EHRS. Federal law has been amended to address the discovery of electronically stored information. Many states have also updated their laws in this area. In a study conducted by Saleem et al. (2009)—one that is still relevant—in a Veterans Affairs Medical Center with a fully implemented EHRS, persistent use of paper work-arounds was found; these were categorized into 11 different types. Saleem et al., concluded that that there were occasions when paper was an important tool that assisted healthcare personnel to perform their work, but in other cases, paper work-arounds circumvented the intended use of the EHRS resulting in potential gaps in documentation as well as possible errors. Another documentation issue with EHRSs comes into play when there are multiple data entry sites—such as hospitals, clinics, physician offices—and the question of who is ultimately responsible for updating key information as it becomes known. For example, if a patient exhibits or reports an allergic reaction when visiting a physician, who should enter that change into the EHRS? Also, how will the mix of unstructured data from physician offices that do not have EHRSs be integrated into an EHRS? And what might be the implications of important unstructured data present in an era of increased automation? Many of the issues related to discoverable information have not been fully addressed as yet and will require new areas of expertise.

Future Directions

Since its inception, the benefits associated with EHRSs are being realized from various aspects of the healthcare system. With the updates to meaningful use, providers and healthcare organizations will hopefully benefit from clearer guidance and the elimination of complexity from the initial standards. The increased emphasis upon patient engagement and empowerment will change the way healthcare consumers and practitioners interact along with the prevalence of mobile device use paving the way for virtual means of interaction with the healthcare team. Individual consumers will have greater responsibility for managing their own health with tracking and benchmarking information at their fingertips.

Payne et al. (2015) provided a comprehensive summary describing five key areas with recommendations in each in order to take EHRSs to a higher level by 2020:

- Simplification and Increased Speed of Documentation
  - Decrease the data entry burden on the clinician.
  - Separate data entry from data reporting.
  - Enable systematic learning and research at the point of care during routine practice, including a better understanding of the costs (in time) and benefits (to care delivery, research, and billing) of different approaches to capturing and reporting clinical data.

- Refocus Regulation
  - Focus on (1) clarifying and simplifying certification procedures and MU regulations, (2) improving data exchange and interoperability, (3) reducing the need for re-entering data, and (4) prioritizing patient outcomes over new functional measures.
  - Support novel changes to and innovation in EHR systems through changes in reimbursement regulations.

- Increase Transparency and Streamline Certification
  - In order to improve the usability of EHRSs and patient safety, to foster innovation, and to empower providers and EHRS purchasers, how an EHRS vendor satisfies certification criteria should be flexible and transparent.
  - In order to improve usability and safety and to foster innovation, healthcare organizations, providers, and vendors should be fully transparent about unintended consequences and new safety risks introduced by health IT systems, including EHRSs, as well as best practices for mitigating these risks.

- Foster Innovation
  - EHRS vendors should use public, standards-based APIs and data standards that enable EHRSs to become more open to innovators, researchers, and patients. These standards should support extensions and innovations from both the academic informatics community as well as from innovators inside and outside traditional health IT communities.

- In 2020, EHRSs must support effective person-centered care delivery
  - Promote the integration of EHRSs into the full social context of care, moving beyond acute care and clinic settings to include home health, specialist care, laboratory, pharmacy, population health, long-term care, and physical and behavioral therapies.

As electronic health record systems become hardwired in hospitals and healthcare organizations, there is a growing need to try and leverage the big data generated from clinical documentation across many organizations. The challenge in moving from electronic documentation to the next level goes beyond what was once moving from paper to electronic systems. In developing new models of care to support the Triple Aim goals, electronic systems must also evolve to not only work across the continuum of care but to also capture more than just vital signs, assessments, and clinical values but also social determinants of health. In doing so, the number of variables increases in creating predictive algorithms to not only include clinical data but social and contextual data about patients' lives. With the emergence of precision medicine and the use of genetic information in care delivery and healthcare analytics, there are growing opportunities to reach higher levels of information gathering as well as synthesizing information for individual and population health needs.

Summary

- The electronic health record (EHR) houses individual healthcare encounter data under the control of the provider.
- An electronic health record system (EHRS) refers to the database management software enabling the functions needed to create and maintain an EHR.
- The electronic medical record (EMR) preceded the EHR bringing together information within a specific setting initially for a single encounter or visit.
- The personal health record (PHR) is a collection of patient data controlled by the patient that may be accessible to providers.
- The EHRS offers additional functionality to enhance safety and patient management.
- The continuity of care record (CCR) provides a snapshot of a person's current health and care for a provider who does not have access to their EHR as a tool to improve continuity and quality of care.
- The American Recovery and Reinvestment Act (ARRA) of 2009 included the Health Information Technology for Economic and Clinical Health Act (HITECH) and financial incentives to encourage adoption of EHRSs, digitalize and collect patient health information for the purpose of improved outcomes through associated learning. The Medicare and Medicaid EHR Incentive Programs operationalized this initiative.
- The Medicare and Medicaid EHR Incentive Programs implemented meaningful use requirements in three stages with increasing requirements for each.
  - Stage 1 required electronic capture of clinical data.
  - Stage 2 called for patients to view, download, or transmit their health information online, and for the capability for secure messaging between providers and patients, and reporting public health measures. Requirements for percentages of participation were later modified.
  - Stage 3, slated for implementation in 2018, focused on the advanced use of EHRS to promote health-information exchange and improved outcomes for patients.
- Research evaluating EHR systems that meet MU criteria suggest improvements in outcomes and decreased expenditures.

- Benefits associated with EHRSs include improved data access and integrity, productivity, quality of care, greater satisfaction, improved eligibility for reimbursement, decision support and alerts, improved workflow, enhanced compliance, safety, and improved tracking and benchmarking for individual and population health.
- The majority of facilities and physician offices now have some form of EHRS.
- Remaining challenges to using EHRS include:
  - Integration of behavioral health and primary care workflows.
  - Information exchange.
  - Limited resources.
  - Work-arounds.
- Work-arounds are variations in procedures and processes created to accomplish work when systems or workflows are deficient or inefficient which can, and frequently do, defeat positive features such as safety.
- EHRS implementation considerations include:
  - Compliance with requirements including ONC Certification for MU, as well as other regulatory and accreditation demands.
  - The creation of the electronic infrastructure, necessary policies and procedures to provide access to patient information.
  - Funds for purchase costs, improvements, ongoing maintenance and support.
  - Standardization of terms.
  - Security, privacy, and confidentiality.
  - Measures to ensure data integrity including creating and maintaining master files and data dictionaries.
  - Backup options.
  - Ownership of patient information.
- Future use of EHRSs will continue to evolve to better support and engage consumers in their care and provide big data to support a learning healthcare system (LHS).

Case Study

Your community hospital is exploring the purchase of an EHRS. The chief nursing officer wants you, the informatics nurse, to educate the nurse leaders about potential benefits and detriments of an EHRS as well as implementation issues. Where would you begin and what key concepts would you share?

About the Authors

Rayne Soriano earned his PhD in Nursing Science and Healthcare Leadership from the University of California at Davis. He has helped with 20 EHR implementations, served as Manager of Clinical Informatics, Kaiser Permanente National IT and Patient Care Services, and works with Medicare Operations leaders to transform healthcare using data, technology, and performance improvement methods. Dr. Soriano chaired the Exemplar Workgroup for TIGER (Technology and Informatics Guiding Educational Reform) and is adjunct faculty at Chamberlain College of Nursing MSN program.

Kathleen Hunter graduated from Church Home & Hospital and served with the Army Nurse Corps. She earned her BSN, MS in nursing, and PhD at the University of Maryland. Nursing informatics is her area of practice. Dr. Hunter has taught online for several years. Her contributions to nursing informatics include starting the MSN informatics track at

Chamberlain College, leadership roles, and research on nursing informatics competencies. Dr. Hunter is a Professor with the Chamberlain MSN Program and has been recognized as an American Academy of Nursing Fellow.

References

Agno, C. F., & Guo, K. L. (2013). Electronic health systems: Challenges faced by hospital-based providers. *Health Care Management, 32*(3), 246–252. doi:10.1097/HCM.0b013e31829d76a4

Appari, A., Eric Johnson, M., & Anthony, D. L. (2013). Meaningful use of electronic health record systems and process quality of care: Evidence from a panel data analysis of US acute-care hospitals. *Health Services Research, 48*(2 Pt 1), 354–375. doi:10.1111/j.1475-6773.2012.01448.x

Bardach, N. S., Wang, J. J., De Leon, S. F., Shih, S. C., Boscardin, W. J., Goldman, L. E., & Dudley, R. A. (2013). Effect of pay-for-performance incentives on quality of care in small practices with electronic health records: A randomized trial. *Journal of the American Medical Association, 310*(10), 1051–1059.

Bell, B., & Thornton, K. (2011). From promise to reality achieving the value of an EHR. *Healthcare Financial Management, 65*(2), 50–56.

Bell, S. K., Mejilla, R., Anselmo, M., Darer, J. D., Elmore, J. G., Leveille, S., . . . Walker, J. (2016). When doctors share visit notes with patients: A study of patient and doctor perceptions of documentation errors, safety opportunities and the patient-doctor relationship. *BMJ Quality & Safety,* 26(4), 262–270. doi:10.1136/bmjqs-2015-004697

Campbell, N. (2016). Electronic SSKIN pathway: Reducing device-related pressure ulcers. *British Journal of Nursing, 25*(15 Suppl), S14–26. doi:10.12968/bjon.2016.25.15.S14

Centers for Medicare and Medicaid Services. (2013). Meaningful use. Baltimore, MD: Centers for Medicare and Medicaid Services. Retrieved from www.cms.gov/Regulations-and-Guidance/Legislation/EHRIncentivePrograms/Meaningful_Use.html.

Centers for Medicare and Medicaid Services (2017). Electronic health records (EHR) incentive programs. Retrieved from www.cms.gov/Regulations-and-Guidance/Legislation/EHRIncentivePrograms/

Chen, H., & Liou, Y. (2014). Performance evaluation of continuity of care records (CCRs): Parsing models in a mobile health management system. *Journal of Medical Systems, 38*(10), 117. doi:10.1007/s10916-014-0117-y

Cifuentes, M., Davis, M., Fernald, D., Gunn, R., Dickinson, P., & Cohen, D. J. (2015). Electronic health record challenges, work-arounds, and solutions observed in practices integrating behavioral health and primary care. *Journal of the American Board of Family Medicine, 28 Suppl 1,* S63–72. doi:10.3122/jabfm.2015.S1.150133

Davis, M. F., & Haines, J. L. (2015). The intelligent use and clinical benefits of electronic medical records in multiple sclerosis. *Expert Review of Clinical Immunology, 11*(2), 205–211. doi:10.1586/1744666X.2015.991314

DesRoches, C. M., Audet, A. M., Painter, M., & Donelan, K. (2013). Meeting meaningful use criteria and managing patient populations: a national survey of practicing physicians. *Annals of Internal Medicine, 158*(11), 791–799. doi:10.7326/0003-4819-158-11-201306040-00003

DesRoches, C. M., Worzala, C., & Bates, S. (2013). Some hospitals are falling behind in meeting 'meaningful use' criteria and could be vulnerable to penalties in 2015. *Health Affairs, 32*(8), 1355–1360. doi:10.1377/hlthaff.2013.0469

DesRoches, C. M., Worzala, C., Joshi, M. S., Kralovec, P. D., & Jha, A. K. (2012). Small, nonteaching, and rural hospitals continue to be slow in adopting electronic health record systems. *Health Affairs, 31*(5), 1092–1099. doi:10.1377/hlthaff.2012.0153

Douglas, M. D., Dawes, D. E., Holden, K. B., & Mack, D. (2015). Missed policy opportunities to advance health equity by recording demographic data in electronic health records. *American Journal of Public Health, 105 Suppl 3,* S380–388. doi:10.2105/AJPH.2014.302384

Effk, J. A., & Weaver, C. A. (2016). Spring cleaning—The informatics version. *Online Journal of Nursing Informatics, 20*(2), 7.

Esch, T., Mejilla, R., Anselmo, M., Podtschaske, B., Delbanco, T., & Walker, J. (2016). Engaging patients through open notes: an evaluation using mixed methods. *BMJ Open, 6*(1), e010034. doi:10.1136/bmjopen-2015-010034

Flanagan, M. E., Saleem, J. J., Millitello, L. G., Russ, A. L., & Doebbeling, B. N. (2013). Paper- and computer-based work-arounds to electronic health record use at three benchmark institutions. *Journal of the American Medical Informatics Association, 20*(e1), e59–66. doi:10.1136/amiajnl-2012-000982

Friedman, A., Crosson, J. C., Howard, J., Clark, E. C., Pellerano, M., Karsh, B. T., . . . Cohen, D. J. (2013). A typology of electronic health record work-arounds in small-to-medium size primary care practices. *Journal of the American Medical Informatics Association, 21*(E1). doi:10.1136/amiajnl-2013-001686

Furukawa, M. F., King, J., Patel, V., Hsiao, C. J., Adler-Milstein, J., & Jha, A. K. (2014). Despite substantial progress In EHR adoption, health information exchange and patient engagement remain low in office settings. *Health Affairs, 33*(9), 1672–1679. doi:10.1377/hlthaff.2014.0445

Hansen, A. G., Martin, E., Jones, B. L., & Pomeroy, E. C. (2015). Social work assessment notes: A comprehensive outcomes-based hospice documentation system. *Health & Social Work, 40*(3), 191–200.

Harris, C. M. (2010). *An overview of the meaningful use final rule.* Retrieved from www.himss.org/content/files/MU_Final_Rule_Overview_PPT.pdf

Heisey-Grove, D., Danehy, L. N., Consolazio, M., Lynch, K., & Mostashari, F. (2014). A national study of challenges to electronic health record adoption and meaningful use. *Medical Care, 52*(2), 144–148. doi:10.1097/MLR.0000000000000038

Hicks, J. K., Dunnenberger, H. M., Gumpper, K. F., Haidar, C. E., & Hoffman, J. M. (2016). Integrating pharmacogenomics into electronic health records with clinical decision support. *American Journal of Health-System Pharmacy, 73*(23), 1967–1976. doi:10.2146/ajhp160030

Hickey, K. T., Katapodi, M. C., Coleman, B., Reuter-Rice, K., & Starkweather, A. R. (2017). Improving utilization of the family hstory in the electronic health record. *Journal of Nursing Scholarship, 49*(1), 80–86. doi:10.1111/jnu.12259

Hydari, M. Z., Telang, R., & Marella, W. M. (2015). Electronic health records and patient safety. Communications of the *ACM, 58*(11), 30–32.

Kern, L. M., Edwards, A., Kaushal, R., & Investigators, H. (2015). The meaningful use of electronic health records and health care quality. *American Journal of Medical Quality, 30*(6), 512–519. doi:10.1177/1062860614546547

Kern, L. M., Edwards, A., Kaushal, R., & Investigators, H. (2016). The meaningful use of electronic health records and health care utilization. *American Journal of Medical Quality, 31*(4), 301–307. doi:10.1177/1062860615572439

King, J., Patel, V., Jamoom, E. W., & Furukawa, M. F. (2014). Clinical benefits of electronic health record use: national findings. *Health Services Research, 49*(1 Pt 2), 392–404. doi:10.1111/1475-6773.12135

Kohli, R., & Tan, S. S. (2016). Electronic health records: How can IS researchers contribute to transforming healthcare?. *MIS Quarterly, 40*(3), 553–574.

Lammers, E. J., & McLaughlin, C. G. (2016). Meaningful use of electronic health records and Medicare expenditures: Evidence from a panel data analysis of US health care markets, 2010-2013. *Health Services Research.* doi:10.1111/1475-6773.12550

Maynard, K. G. (2010, Jan–Feb). Trends and issues with electronic discovery of medical information. *Physician Executive.* Retrieved from http://findarticles.com/p/articles/mi_m0843/is_1_36/ai_n48840395/

Medicare and Medicaid Programs; Electronic Health Record Incentive Program—Stage 2 Final Rule. *Federal Register.* 53968. (September 4, 2012). Retrieved from: www.gpo.gov/fdsys/pkg/FR-2012-09-04/pdf/2012-21050.pdf

Milstein, J. A., DesRoches, C. M., Kralovec, P., Foster, G., Worzala, C., Searcy, T., Jha, A. K. (2015). Electronic health record adoption in us hospitals: Progress continues, but challenges persist. *Health Affairs, 34* (12), 2174–21801

Nakamura, M. M., Harper, M. B., & Jha, A. K. (2013). Change in adoption of electronic health records by US children's hospitals. *Pediatrics, 131*(5), e1563–1575. doi:10.1542/peds.2012-2904

Office of the National Coordinator for Health Information Technology (ONCHIT). (2011). Certification programs. Retrieved from http://healthit.hhs.gov/portal/server.pt/community/healthit_hhs_gov__certification_program/2884

Payne, T. H. (2016). The electronic health record as a catalyst for quality improvement in patient care. *Heart, 102*(22), 1782. doi:http://dx.doi.org.proxy.chamberlain.edu:8080/10.1136/heartjnl-2015-308724

Payne, T. H., Corley, S., Cullen, T. A., Gandhi, T. K., Harrington, L., Kuperman, G. J., . . . Zaroukian, M. H. (2015). Report of the AMIA EHR-2020 task force on the status and future direction of EHRs. *Journal of the American Medical Informatics Associaton, 22*(5), 1102–1110. doi:10.1093/jamia/ocv066

Resnick, C. M., Meara, J. G., Peltzman, M., & Gilley, M. (2016). Meaningful use: A program in transition. *Bulletin of the American College of Surgeons, 101*(3), 10–16.

Rinner, C., Grossmann, W., Sauter, S. K., Wolzt, M., & Gall, W. (2015). Effects of shared electronic health record systems on drug-drug interaction and duplication warning detection. *Biomed Research International, 2015.* doi:10.1155/2015/380497

Roehrs, A., da Costa, C. A., Righi, R. R., & de Oliveira, K. F. (2017). Personal health records: A systematic literature review. *Journal of Medical Internet Research, 19*(1), e13. doi:10.2196/jmir.5876

Rogers, M. L., Sockolow, P. S., Bowles, K. H., Hand, K. E., & George, J. (2013). Use of a human factors approach to uncover informatics needs of nurses in documentation of care. *International Journal of Medical Informatics, 82*(11), 1068–1074. doi:10.1016/j.ijmedinf.2013.08.007

Saleem, J. J., Russ, A. L., Justice, C. F., Hagg, H., Ebright, P. R., Woodbridge, P. A., & Doebbeling, B. N. (2009). Exploring the persistence of paper with the electronic health record. *International Journal of Medical Informatics, 78*(9), 618–628

Seibert, H. H., Maddox, R. R., Flynn, E. A., & Williams, C. K. (2014). Effect of barcode technology with electronic medication administration record on medication accuracy rates. *American Journal of Health-System Pharmacy, 71*(3), 209–218. doi:10.2146/ajhp130332

Shea, C. M., Reiter, K. L., Weaver, M. A., & Albritton, J. (2016). Quality improvement teams, super users, and nurse champions: a recipe for meaningful use? *Journal of the American Medical Informatics Association, 23*(6), 1195–1198. doi:10.1093/jamia/ocw029

Stimson, C. E., & Botruff, A. L. (2017). Daily electronic health record reports meet meaningful use requirements, improve care efficiency, and provide a layer of safety for trauma patients. *Journal of Trauma Nursing*, 24(1), 53–56. doi:10.1097/JTN.0000000000000262

Stutzer, K., & Hylton Rushton, C. (2015). Ethics in critical care. Ethical implications of workarounds in critical care. *AACN Advanced Critical Care*, 26(4), 372–375. doi:10.1097/NCI.0000000000000107

Waldren, S. E., & Solis, E. (2016). The evolution of meaningful use: Today, stage 3, and beyond. *Family Practice Management*, 23(1), 17–22.

Whitt, K. J., Eden, L., Merrill, K., & Hughes, M. (2017). Nursing student experiences regarding safe use of electronic health records: A pilot study of the safety and assurance factors for EHR resilience guides. *CIN: Computers, Informatics, Nursing*, 35(1), 45–53. doi: 10.1097/CIN.0000000000000291

Wolf, L., Harvell, J., & Jha, A. K. (2012). Hospitals ineligible for federal meaningful-use incentives have dismally low rates of adoption of electronic health records. *Health Affairs*, 31(3), 505–513. doi:10.1377/hlthaff.2011.0351

Zahabi, M., Kaber, D. B., & Swangnetr, M. (2015). Usability and safety in electronic medical records interface design: A review of recent literature and guideline formulation. *Human Factors*, 57(5), 805–834. doi:10.1177/0018720815576827

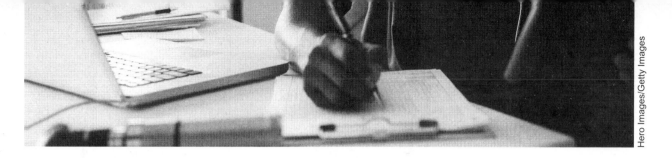

Hero Images/Getty Images

Chapter 8
Healthcare Information Systems

Carolyn Sipes, PhD, CNS, APN, PMP, RN-BC

and Jane Brokel, PhD, RN, FNI

Administrative information systems (AIS)

After completing this chapter, you should be able to:

- Differentiate between clinical information systems (CIS) and administrative information systems (AIS).

- Describe two or more applications for each type of system: CIS and AIS.

- State one format for representing healthcare knowledge.

- Discuss the definition and potential benefits for practitioners or patients of smart technology.

An **information system**, at its simplest, is a combination of computer hardware and software that can process data into information to solve a problem. The terms **healthcare information system** and **hospital information system (HIS)** both refer to an information system used in a healthcare enterprise. The healthcare enterprise is most usually an acute-care hospital but can be a group of related hospitals and healthcare settings. A HIS typically comprises two major types of information systems: clinical information systems and administrative information systems. **Clinical information systems (CISs)** are large, computerized database management systems that support several types of healthcare activities, including provider/practitioner order entry, results retrieval, documentation, and decision support, across locations (a.k.a., a distributed system). **Administrative information systems (AIS)** support client care by managing financial and demographic information and providing reporting capabilities. This category includes client management, financial, coding, payroll, human resources, and quality assurance applications. Figure 8-1 shows the relationships between various components of a hospital information system.

Clinical and administrative information systems may have applications designed to meet the needs of a specific department(s) or organizational function(s), or the systems may have applications intended to support all organizational departments and functions. Either clinical or administrative systems can be implemented as standalone systems, or they may work with other systems to provide information sharing and seamless functionality for the users.

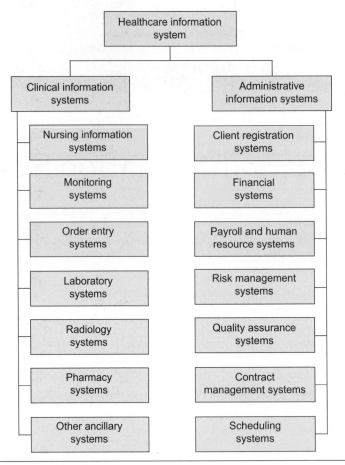

Figure 8-1 • Relationship of the healthcare information system components.

Any one healthcare enterprise may use one or several of the CIS and AIS applications but may not use all of them.

While expensive to purchase, implement, and maintain, the potential benefits of healthcare information systems are expected to offset these costs. These potential benefits include improving healthcare quality, efficiency, and use of guidelines; and reducing both the incidence and associated costs of medication errors and adverse drug events (ADE) (Campanella et al., 2015).

Clinical Information Systems

Clinical information systems (CISs) focus on management of clinical (patient) data and information as compared to administrative information systems. They enable practitioners and patients to be involved in acquiring, reviewing, and using data at various points of care. Clinical information systems include many applications that integrate and use the information obtained from other applications and healthcare devices. The clinical information systems provide the infrastructure to bring these applications together so healthcare professionals may have functional use of the data, information, and knowledge that is stored and/or collected for an electronic health record. Some applications that integrate within clinical information systems are described in the following paragraphs. Many of these functional applications collect and share data useful in clinical decision support applications.

Computerized provider (or practitioner) order entry (CPOE) facilitates the process of selecting scripted orders that include precise start-and-stop times, timing of orders, and much more detail. Prior to electronic ordering, patient care orders were often missing details on route, dosing, timing, and indication; fixing these gaps required significant investigation in order to execute the requested orders. The CPOE applications support the prescribers' decisions to enter orders and immediately share the orders with appropriate health professionals who execute the orders and the departments that need to dispense, schedule, or immediately deliver services to patients. Ideally, this application allows integration of nursing orders with physician orders; if so, all orders can be viewed together. The application may include team-designed evidence-based order sets or care sets and may connect orders to links that provide descriptions, context, and current evidence to support decisions for ordering a test, medicine, or intervention.

Results-reporting applications facilitate the sharing of laboratory values and results from other diagnostic tests within the electronic health records for clinicians to view. The values can be displayed in different formats along with associated reference ranges to help in the interpretation of values.

Electronic documentation is provided through electronic health record systems (EHRSs) and other applications reported here. Electronic documentation enhances the traditional paper-based documentation through the EHRSs' capabilities of rapid movement of data, data-and-information sharing simultaneously from multiple locations, presenting data in multiple formats (often customized to particular groups or individuals), and removing the challenge of interpreting handwriting. Structured templates, free text, dictation, and video formats may be used for data entry. Electronic documentation also supports the use of controlled terminologies.

Laboratory-information systems (LISs) provide functionality to receive requests, schedule the tests, and track specimen collection and trajectory through the appropriate laboratory. The transmission of test results is accompanied by referenced knowledge for accurate interpretation of the findings. Current LISs permit the display of values over time to show trends and ranges. When the values are critical, processes are in place to ensure the relevant practitioners are notified, and documentation of the notification is timed and captured.

Radiology-information systems (RISs) have functionality to receive requests; schedule imaging, including people, rooms, and equipment; provide patient-focused information that helps patients prepare for scheduled diagnostic imaging, manage image storage, and store and report the radiologists' interpretations. **Picture archiving and communication system (PACS)** applications support the wide-spread use of digitized medical imaging for x-rays, magnetic resonance imaging (MRI), computerized tomography, and ultrasound. A PACS is designed specifically for storage, retrieval, presentation, and sharing of digital images. These images may be viewed simultaneously by multiple healthcare team members and electronically transmitted to remote locations.

Pharmacy information systems (PISs) combine administrative and patient-care functions. On the administrative side, functions may include inventory control, billing, and preparation of documentation such as patient profiles, medication labels, and fill lists. Clinical functions address order entry (or receipt of orders from a CIS), tracking of drug dispensing, alerting practitioners and pharmacists of prescription errors and potential interactions, patient education, and providing access to clinical information (El.Mahalli, El-Khafif, & Yamani, 2016).

Physiological monitoring systems are applications that obtain and store real-time data about various physiological (versus anatomical) aspects of a patient. Karunanithi's article in 2010 on physiological monitoring is an informative and still relevant discussion of this topic.

Monitoring is done to track changes in the monitored parameter from a baseline. Aspects that can be monitored today include basic vital signs, arterial blood pressure, intracranial pressures, cardiac rhythm and waveform trends, fetal heart rate, pulse oximetry, continuous video EEG monitoring, electromyography, phonocardiograph, and many more (Karunanithi, 2010). Because these applications usually are integrated with a CIS, the data are collected automatically and stored for review and decision-making by healthcare professionals. Devices not directly integrated usually have mechanisms for uploading data into a CIS.

Operating room information systems (ORISs) a.k.a., **surgical-information systems (SISs)** or **perioperative information systems** provide managerial functions to manage the OR case times and assignment of rooms (a.k.a., surgical scheduling), which helps to minimize the costs of unused OR time and the performance of elective cases outside of normal allocated OR time. Patient tracking, perioperative nursing and anaesthesia documentation, tissue tracking, integration of medical devices, and revenue and materials management, and real-time displays of ongoing OR activity are additional functions found in ORISs (A report card on OR info systems, 2011). Current ORISs integrate preadmission testing and scheduling and align nursing and anaesthesia documentation with all stages of the perioperative experience.

Anaesthesia information management systems are separate, specialized applications for the surgical setting. These systems are connected to physiological monitors, anaesthesia machines, other devices, and—ideally—to the facility's clinical information system. Anaesthesia personnel can enter other data into the online anaesthesia record, such as intubation status, induction time, and extubation (Deng & Hickey, 2015).

Critical care information systems (CCISs) incorporate or integrate most of the prior applications as well as interfacing with multiple bedside devices to automatically capture physiological dataand fluid intake and output; facilitating calculation of clinical indices; and helping to organize and manage the large volume of data assessments to reduce diagnosis and treatment time (Ehteshami, Sadoughi, Ahmadi, & Kashefi, 2013). Remote support for critical care practitioners can be found in many facilities. This support is provided by a team of expert nurses and physicians, working at a distance, who have access to the CCIS and to cameras, speakers, and microphones placed in each patient room. If a nurse or doctor has a question, or the remote staff identify an emergent problem, two-way communications and problem-solving are engaged.

Clinical decision support systems (CDSSs) (a.k.a., computerized decision support systems) are applications that support healthcare practitioners in making patient-care decisions. A CDSS combines one patient's specific data, available because of integration with the facility CIS, with up-to-date clinical knowledge to generate recommendations or guidelines for that particular patient (Moja, L., Friz, H. P., Capobussi, M., Kwag, K., Banzi, R., Ruggiero, F., et al., 2016). The clinical knowledge is applied through using modeling, data-processing techniques specific to medical data, and methods of artificial intelligence. Results of CDSS action include clinical guidelines and reminders; drug-dosing support; and alerts for drug allergy, drug-drug interaction, and drug-laboratory interaction (Castaneda et al., 2015). A critical element in decision support systems is making sure the knowledge base being used can grow in order to provide up-to-date reasoning (Gurupur & Gutierrez, 2016).

Knowledge Representation

In a still-relevant article, Davis, Shrobe, and Szolovits (1993) explained that, as a concept, knowledge representation refers to methods for presenting something from the real world; a specific knowledge representation is a substitute or surrogate for a real thing. Formalized, systematic methods for representing knowledge facilitate communication, reasoning, and decision-making. Standardized nomenclatures, such as the Systematized Nomenclature of Medicine (SNOMED), Current Procedural Terminologies (CPT), and Nursing Interventions Classification (NIC) are examples of textual knowledge representations for concepts in medicine and nursing. Bowen and Evans (2014) noted that visual symbols and metaphors are knowledge representations that support visual thinking (e.g., the double helix of DNA). The development of health-related knowledge representations is a formal process that includes clinical experts representing specialties and healthcare professionals who understand the science, research evidence, and presenting of information for interpretation and comprehension.

Administrative Information Systems

Administrative information systems support client care by managing administrative, financial, and demographic data and information and providing reporting capabilities that support the overall functions of an organization. In contrast to clinical systems, the administrative systems include client-management services such as registration and scheduling, coding for billing, financial, payroll, human-resources, and quality-assurance and risk-management systems.

Registration and Scheduling Systems

The client **registration and scheduling system** is critical to the effective operation of many other systems within the healthcare setting. The system applies predetermined rules for determining how resources and client information should be used to schedule a particular type of appointment.

This system collects and stores all client identification and demographic data, which is verified and updated at the time of each visit. Today, with mobile devices and patient kiosks, patient scheduling offers many opportunities for patients to self-schedule and cancel appointments, receive text reminders of appointments, and complete registration-intake forms online before arriving for the scheduled appointments. After the appointments, patients can access test results and other communication through a patient portal. With integrated, cross-department EHRSs, if patients do not have mobile devices or other access to a portal, healthcare staff can effectively and quickly obtain the information once the patient has arrived for the appointment. Increased use of information technology increases productivity and the potential ability to see more patients. The data for the management of patients crosses to the CIS, where patient information combines to include client care and billing. The benefits associated with using a registration-and-scheduling system include increased staff productivity, increased client satisfaction, and cost savings to the organization.

An **admission/discharge/transfer (ADT) system** is used in healthcare organizations to support the process of providing client care. This system is integrated with other administrative and clinical systems and tracks a patient's activities and location from hospital or clinic admission through any and all transfers within the facility and, finally, through discharge.

Patient Acuity/Staff Scheduling

In the past, patient-acuity levels and complexity-of-care information was labor intensive to collect and evaluate and not timely when staffing schedules needed to be done quickly. Today, there are a number of information systems that can instantly provide data to be analysed, trended, and accessed to create staffing models that address evolving acuity levels. These systems have the capability to calculate acuity levels and complexity by scanning clinical documentation; for example, scanning the minutes of care provided and resources required to complete care.

Financial Systems

Financial systems, the first information systems implemented in healthcare-delivery organizations, are integrated with registration systems and ensure that patients' demographic data and insurance information could be accessed to charge for services provided and receive reimbursement. As the sophistication of information technology increased, it became possible to charge patients automatically once a clinical service was completed. For this reason, all other information systems were typically built around financial systems.

Risk-Management Systems

A **risk-management system** enhances an organization's ability to identify potential risks and develop strategies to deal with them. In addition to vendor systems that include risk-assessment software packages, professional organizations, such as the Healthcare Information and Management Systems Society (HIMSS), as well as the Department of Health and Human Services (2014) provide tools to conduct reviews as well as training on how to conduct a risk assessment and mitigate threats.

One of the first risk assessments needed is a review of the organization's security, which is required by the HIPAA Security Rule and the Center for Medicare and Medicaid Services (CMS) Meaningful Use Incentive Program. Due to the need to understand an organization's security, Wright et al. (2015) developed and piloted a self-assessment instrument, using clinical decision support (CDS) functionality, for assessing a healthcare organization's ability to mitigate malpractice risk. Seven organizations conducted the self-assessment based on malpractice data and found they could mitigate risk and prevent loss using CDS assessments. If loss does occur and a risk-management system is in place, the loss can be tracked back to the point of origin to pinpoint and address specific issues and liabilities. Both small and large organizations benefit from risk-management systems. Increasingly, features in these systems include dashboard views; regular emailing of reports; and the ability to manage policies, claims, litigation, and other insurable risk information.

Payroll and Human-Resources Systems

Human-resources information systems come with a variety of software, including processes for tracking, depending on the organizational needs. The systems can provide tracking mechanisms from attendance—including vacation, time sheets—tracking for payroll purposes; health benefits, including insurance information; and career development. The goal of such a system is to connect, track, and provide data within one system.

Quality Assurance Systems

Employing the use of a **quality-assurance (QA)** or continuous-quality-improvement (CQI) system is a way of checking that the organization is continuously improving what it does and how it does it. This is done through continuous monitoring and evaluation of performance and through the collection and processing of data and other evidence. The capability to track quality defects and documents, control user access, track software versions and revisions, and provide training depends on organizational needs, and the availability and functionality of a QA or CQI system. The systems can also manage audits; track compliance with permits, licensing, and legal requirements; monitor and control identified issues as a risk-management function, and track emergency responses.

Contract-Management Systems

Contract-management (CM) software provides invaluable assistance to organizations to better manage their resources and improve efficiency. Healthcare institutions typically have multiple contracts with third-party payers as well as with vendors and various suppliers. CM software provides greater efficiencies and effective time savings, thereby, reducing costs as well as reducing risks because documents can be better tracked and audited. Basic functions include tracking, storage, and retrieval of key documents with the ability to quickly access needed information. CM software supports contract creation, report capability, eprocurement, alerts, and notifications on key business events, and can even support automation of the entire contract process.

Summary of Administrative Systems

Various administrative systems may be used in healthcare. Box 8-1 provides a brief review of many of these systems; some of these were described here.

Smart Technology

The advent of EHRs has made it easier to access data and to enter data one time and see it flow across systems from the first patient engagement until the patient is seen by a provider at the point of care. From this point, patient information is gathered; orders are written and entered into the electronic system; and then moved seamlessly to areas such as scheduling, laboratory, or pharmacy, eliminating steps for both the patient and provider. These features when used with other technology that can support, patient care, are often referred to as smart technology.

Box 8-1   Administrative Information Systems Used in the Healthcare Setting

- Financial systems provide the facility with accounting functions. Accurate tracking of financial data is critical for enabling the organization to receive reimbursement for services.
- Payroll and human resource systems track employee time and attendance, credentials, performance evaluations, and payroll-compensation information.
- Contract-management systems manage contracts with third-party payers.
- Risk-management systems track and plan prevention of unusual occurrences or incidents.
- Quality-assurance systems monitor outcomes and produce reports that are used to guide quality improvement initiatives.
- Physician-management systems support patient registration, scheduling, coding, and billing in the physician's office and may support results retrieval. These systems also provide better protection of patient privacy than paper records.
- Executive-information systems provide administrators with easy access to summarized information related to the financial and clinical operations of the organization.
- Materials-management systems facilitate inventory control and charging of supplies.

What Is Smart Technology?

Smart technology is the functionality behind the scenes that provides the capability of the electronic system to send real-time messages to all of the various areas required during a patient visit, where providers document the visit, order the medications while also checking alerts for errors, schedule appointments, and generate bills, to name just a few of the functions of an EHRS. All of this is done because the different systems are tied or interfaced together so the electronic messages can cross systems. For example, if a particular system is not interfaced, messages such as an order for x-ray will not flow or follow the workflow from where the order was placed by the provider in the patient record to the radiology system.

Benefits for Clinicians

Smart technology can benefit clinicians. An advantage of sending real-time messages from the patient point of care increases efficiencies for clinician and patients alike. It can increase communication between care providers as information is more quickly transmitted. For example, clinicians can receive an alert that a specific medication is due or late, eliminating errors of omission. Alerts also send messages that a particular task, such as a dressing change, may be due. When completed, the tasks are quickly documented in the mobile computer system in the patient's room. A provider can receive an alert if the medication has already been ordered, thus eliminating duplicate medication orders. An alert can inform the provider of the potential for a drug-drug interaction with an order. Further, smart technology includes **bar code-scanning** capability where the patient's armband is scanned as well as the medication pulled from the medication cart. If there is no match of patient-to-medication, the medication cannot be given.

With any EHRS, the organization's leadership selects the functionality required and can choose to eliminate some functionality such as medication alerts. For example, medication-alerts functionality would not be beneficial if providers would routinely override the alerts, due to **alert fatigue**, too many alerts, or other factors. There are many capabilities within a system's design that can be very beneficial for all clinicians and that will potentially decrease workload and increase efficiencies, if they are used properly.

Benefits for Patients and Families

Smart technology can benefit patients through improved efficiencies such as dramatically decreasing wait-times for patients to be seen. Today, a patient may arrive to an appointment and be greeted in the lobby by someone from registration/scheduling who is carrying a tablet device. This registrar/scheduler collects the patient's name, date of birth, and a few other demographics; confirms the appointment and department; and sends the patient on in less than three to four minutes. With the increased use of information technology, there is increased productivity and potential for providers to see more patients and benefits to patients by not having to wait in long lines to check-in and register before being seen.

In the hospital, patients access tablet computers in their rooms to order meals as they wish, as well as other items, such as extra blankets, water, or other needs. Patients can also send and receive messages to and from family members. They can select educational materials to explain a new diet, explain a procedure and follow-up requirements, as well as post their own questions. A plan of care may be posted, with information regarding expectations of scheduled tests. Patients can be monitored electronically for vital signs without the interruptions necessitated by a clinician coming into the room to use a manual device to take a reading.

Current Topics in Healthcare Information Systems

This section brings information on the concept of big data, obstacles and risks to keeping information systems current, and costs of maintaining functional HISs,

Big Data

Currently, a main concern with the increasing numbers of organizations implementing EHRSs, is the huge amounts of data—known as **big data**—being collected without the knowledge or processes in place to properly analyze and utilize it. This includes patient data, such as x-rays, pharmacy, and therapy data, as well as other research information. Currently, this data resides in unstructured databases with much of it inaccessible because it is not categorized in ways understood by current systems; therefore, it cannot be retrieved. The need is great for better understanding of methods to retrieve data, and implementation of structured data management systems is now a priority for many organizations.

Obstacles and Risks

A consideration with maintaining current information technology is the age of many computer systems. For example, when an older, slower system cannot handle large volumes of information and data movement during peak work periods nor additional users on the system at the same time, it may cause the system to become inaccessible, which is also known as **downtime**. When this happens, procedures are implemented that all must use, which often includes reverting back to documenting on paper until the system can be fixed and brought back up. This disruption causes major obstacles since data is not readily accessible, orders cannot quickly flow to appropriate departments, and there may be duplicate orders and documentation when the system does come back up because there are both paper and electronic versions of the same items.

Costs

Implementing and maintaining computer systems is very expensive, as they must be upgraded every two to three years with new software and hardware to keep them functioning properly and accurately and with increased speed. Systems also need to be optimized, meaning if a particular function was put aside during the original implementation to wait until the next phase, it is now time to add that functionality. Adding this delayed functionality can cause problems because the added functionality must be correctly interfaced with the current system, which is now two to three years older. The best approach is to optimize quickly, within a few months after the original system has been implemented.

The areas discussed above—current state of health IT, obstacles, risks, and expenses—are only a few examples of the many topics that apply to information systems and information technology in health care. Today's healthcare world is rapidly changing to meet increased and evolving demands. In the future, these topics may not be applicable as described, as they may totally change the way we consume healthcare.

Future Directions

The health IT research agenda of the Agency for Healthcare Research and Quality (AHRQ) (Dimitropoulos, 2014) identifies advances in healthcare information technology expected to emerge in the near future. These include advanced decision support tools, analysis of big data, display and communication of health data, use of health IT to support distributed care models and improve efficiency, and health IT safety monitoring and testing. The AHRQ will prioritize funding for research and demonstration projects in these areas.

An innovation under development for CDS is a process of translating guidelines from a narrative form to semi formal forms that are machine-interpretable. The result is an ability to use a CDS across multiple EHRS and in diverse care settings (Mardon et al., 2014).

A few of the administrative information system applications and functionality used today were discussed above. The overall goal of these applications is to increase usability and efficiencies and decrease workload for clinicians. The future holds even more promise. A few examples of recent and unfolding developments are discussed in the following paragraphs.

Advancement of smart technology includes smart wearable devices, which range from wristbands, bras, contact lenses, braces, and clothes with smart buttons. The wearable devices have the potential to increase patient mobility and provide telehealth home-health monitoring systems where clinicians can closely monitor chronic conditions such as diabetes, and congestive heart failure. Khan et al. (2016) discussed how advances in wireless technology—when composed of silicon-based, low-powered electronics—have the potential to interface with skin to monitor vital signs such as temperature, heart rate, blood pressure, pulse oxygenation, and blood glucose.

Other wearable devices can be in the form of T-shirts that have sensors embedded in the fabric capable of capturing cardiac and respiratory signs, which can transmit data to snap-fastener terminals that connect to an external device such as a Holter monitor (Trindade et al., 2016).

With closer monitoring, detrimental changes in patients' conditions can be quickly managed before they get out of hand. The data from wearable devices can be sent back for analysis using the Internet, which is transformational for healthcare and has analysis capabilities based on the technology of **cloud computing**. Alerts from the wearable devices regarding a patient's condition can quickly be sent to cloud computing, collected, then sent on to an external system. With real-time tracking and alerts that support quick interventions to a patient's condition, improved outcomes can be realized for both treatments and disease management. Rapid sharing of data and information will increase patient satisfaction, as well as decrease healthcare costs through decreased hospital admissions and shorter stays.

According to Meyyappan (2016), researchers in biomedical engineering have been working on a system for early diagnosis and prevention to mitigate and prevent debilitating illness, which will help reduce healthcare spending overall. The system, known as a **lab-on-a-chip** has "point of care diagnostics for the routine monitoring of health-related vital information and status of chronic diseases as well as the detection of contagious diseases in settings outside of the hospital or clinic" (Meyyappan, 2016, p. 4).

Liao, Leeson, and Higgins (2016) discussed needs of the aging population and presented a **wireless body area network (WBAN)**, which is a specialized communication network that integrates miniature sensors/devices in the human body to enable the remote monitoring of the vital signs of patients, that can transmit information to care providers using the Internet. Other sensors implanted in the in the body can also measure pacemaker function and other data. On-body sensors, usually put on clothes or portable devices, can gather and transmit heartbeat frequency, electrocardiograph (EKG) data, and other information.

Ahanathapillai et al. (2015) discussed the development of a **wrist wearable unit (WWU)**, also known as an android smart-watch, to monitor the physical activity of people older than 60-years old. The device would continuously measure activity levels, such as step counts, and recognize a change in health status. The data is sent over the Internet to a system where data is collected, stored, and processed. Their research indicates this type of a system is more reliable than self-reported measurements.

Vettoretti et al. (2016) presented research related to how continuous glucose monitoring (CGM) sensors used today remain inaccurate. From their research, they found a way to greatly improve the accuracy of CGM by evaluating signals from sensors that used a new calibration method. The improved performance of CGM impacts diabetes technology research including improving the accuracy of the artificial pancreas.

According to Li and Diamandis (2016) recent advances in medical diagnostics can transform medicine as we know it today. Consumers wishing instant health information can test themselves where or whenever they chose by using smartphones integrated with microfluidics and microelectronics. The authors caution this functionality is in development stages. Evidence that these advances are successful in preventing or detecting diseases is currently lacking.

Ma et al. (2016) studied possible uses of a self-powered biomedical monitor that does not use an external power source. The monitor is a flexible, implantable triboelectric active sensor (iTEAS) that can provide real-time continuous monitoring of multiple clinical signs, including cardiac arrhythmias such as atrial fibrillation and ventricular premature contraction. It can also monitor respiratory rates by analyzing variations of the output peaks of the iTEAS, and blood pressure can also be estimated by calculating the velocity of blood flow with the aid of a separate arterial pressure catheter.

In summary, the examples above provide a small glimpse into the future of what we can expect using smart technology. The advances in medicine, healthcare, and technology are limitless.

Summary

- A healthcare information system is actually comprised of multiple, interfaced computer systems that are used to support clinical care and administrative functions.
- While clinical or administrative systems can stand alone, the ability to share information with other information systems provide greater benefits for clinicians and patients.
- Clinical information systems (CISs) focus upon the acquisition, review, and use of patient data. Functions may include order entry, results-reporting, scheduling, and documentation.
- Clinical information systems may be specific to certain areas such as the laboratory, radiology, or pharmacy, or to particular patient populations such as perioperative or critical care settings.
- The Picture Archiving and Communication System (PACS) facilitates storage, transmission, and sharing of medical images. including x-rays, magnetic resonance imaging (MRI), computerized tomography, and ultrasound.
- Clinical decision support systems use patient-specific data and up-to-date clinical knowledge to provide guidelines and alerts to aid clinicians.
- Administrative systems can include registration and scheduling; tracking through admission, transfer and discharge; patient acuity and staff scheduling; financial or accounting systems; risk management; payroll and human resources; quality assurance; and contract management functions.
- Smart technology provides behind the scenes functionality with cumulative benefits for patient safety and improved efficiencies.
- Current areas of interest in healthcare information systems include big data, aging technology, and controlling the high costs associated with the implementation and maintenance of HIT.

- Emerging areas in HIT include advanced decision support tools, greater use of big data, display and communication of health data, HIT to support new care models, and closer examination of HIT safety.
- Increased numbers and types of wearable devices for consumers are becoming available, changing the way patients are monitored, and supporting the delivery of more services in the community.

Case Study

Take an inventory of the information systems in your organization, through your own observations and conversations with staff and leaders. Compare your list with the systems described in this chapter. How would you rate the information-technology status of your organization?

About the Authors

Dr. Sipes teaches nursing informatics at Chamberlain College of Nursing. She has more than 30 years of experience in management, consulting, and teaching that includes national and international implementation of electronic health records (EHRs). She holds project management professional (PMP) certification through the Project Management Institute (PMI), holds eight Epic clinical systems certifications, is board certified by the American Nurses Credentialing Center in Nursing Informatics (RN-BC), and is an ANCC Nursing Informatics Content expert.

After completing her doctorate, she worked as a research scientist for a major pharmaceutical company where she designed the first Tolerability of Medication Assessment tool (TOMA) and presented the research at the international World AIDS Research conference. Dr. Sipes has published and presented extensively and authored the book, *Project Management for the Advanced Practice Nurse.*

Dr. Brokel served on the executive committee and advisory council from 2009–2016 to guide the development, implementation and operations for the Iowa Health Information Network. She teaches family nurse practitioner students online for Simmons College and is adjunct faculty for the University of Iowa College of Nursing. Dr. Brokel is an active practicing nurse clinician and advocate for identifying future information solutions to coordinate better care for pediatric clients at home and in schools.

References

A report card on OR info systems. (2011). *OR Manager*, 27(7), 17–19.

Ahanathapillai, V., Amor, J., Goodwin, Z., & James, C. (2015). Preliminary study on activity monitoring using an android smart-watch. *Healthcare Technology Letters*, 2(1), 34–39. doi: 10.1049/htl.2014.0091

Bowen, T., & Evans, M. M. (2014). What does knowledge look like? Drawing as a means of knowledge representation and knowledge construction. *Education for Information*, 31(1/2), 53–72. doi:10.3233/EFI-150947

Campanella, P., Lovato, E., Marone, C., Fallacara, L., Mancuso, A., Ricciardi, W., & Specchia, M. L. (2016). The impact of electronic health records on healthcare quality:

A systematic review and meta-analysis. *European Journal of Public Health, 26*(1), 60–64. doi:10.1093/eurpub/ckv122

Castaneda, C., Nalley, K., Mannion, C., Bhattacharyya, P., Blake, P., Pecora, A., & Goy, S. A. (2015). Clinical decision support systems for improving diagnostic accuracy and achieving precision medicine. *Journal of Clinical Bioinformatics, 5*(4). doi: 10.1186/s13336-015-0019-3

Davis, R., Shrobe, H., & Szolovits, P. (1993). What is a knowledge representation? *AI Magazine, 14*(1), 17–33.

Department of Health and Human Services. (2014). Security risk assessment tool (SRA tool). Retrieved from www.healthit.gov/providers-professionals/security-risk-assessment-tool

Deng, F., & Hickey, J. V. (2015). Anesthesia information management systems: An underutilized tool for outcomes research. *AANA Journal, 83*(3), 189–195.

Dimitropoulos, L. (2014). *Health IT research priorities to support the health care delivery system of the future.* (AHRQ Publication No. 14-0072-EF). Rockville, MD: Agency for Healthcare Research and Quality.

Ehteshami, A., Sadoughi, F., Ahmadi, M., & Kashefi, P. (2013). Intensive care information system impacts. *ACTA Informatics Mdicine, 21*(3), 185–191.

El. Mahalli, A., El-Khafif, S. H., & Yamani, W. (2016). Assessment of pharmacy information system performance in three hospitals in eastern province, Saudi Arabia. *Perspectives in Health Information Management, 13*(Winter), 1–25.

Gurupur, V. P., & Gutierrez, R. (2016). Designing the right framework for healthcare decision support. *Journal of Integrated Design & Process Science, 20*(1), 7–32. doi:10.3233/jid-2016-0001

Karunanithi, M. K. (2010). Physiological monitoring. *Studies in Health Technology and Informatics,* 151, 207–218.

Khan, Y., Ostfeld, A. E., Lochner, C. M., Pierre, A., & Arias, A. C. (2016). Monitoring of vital signs with flexible and wearable medical devices. *Advanced Materials, 28*(22), 4373–4395. doi: 10.1002/adma.201504366

Li, M., & Diamandis, E. P. (2016). Technology-driven diagnostics: From smart doctor to smartphone. *Journal of Critical Reviews in Clinical Laboratory Sciences.* 53(4), 268–276. doi: 10.3109/10408363. 1149689. 2016.1149689

Liao, Y., Leeson, M., & Higgins, M. (2016). Flexible quality of service model for wireless body area sensor networks. *Healthcare Technology Letters, 3*(1), 12–15. doi: 10.1049/htl.2015.0049

Ma, Y., Zheng, Q., Liu, Y., Shi, B., Xue, X., Ji, W., et al. (2016). Self-powered, one-stop, and multifunctional implantable triboelectric active sensor for real-time biomedical monitoring. *Nano Letters* Article ASAP *16* (10), 6042–6051. doi: 10.1021/acs. nanolett.6b01968

Mardon, R., Mercincavage, L., & Johnson, M., et al. (2014). *Findings and lessons from AHRQ's clinical decision support demonstration projects.* (AHRQ Publication No. 14-0047-EF). Rockville, MD: Agency for Healthcare Research and Quality.

Meyyappan, M. (2016). Nanotechnology in biosensing. *IEEE Nanotechnology Magazine, 10*(3), 4. © 2016. doi: 10.1109/MNANO.2016.2572241

Moja, L., Friz, H.,P. Capobussi, M., Kwag, K., Banzi, R., Ruggiero, F., & Bonovas, S (2016). Implementing an evidence-based computerized decision support system to improve patient care in a general hospital: The CODES study protocol for a randomized controlled trial. *Implementation Science, 11*(1), 1–10. doi:10.1186/s13012-016-0455-x

Trindade, I. G., Machado da Silva, J., Miguel, R., Pereira, M., Lucas, J., Oliveira, L., et al. (2016). Design and evaluation of novel textile wearable systems for the surveillance of vital signals. *Sensors (Basel)*, *16*(10), 1573. doi: 10.3390/s16101573

Vettoretti, M., Facchinetti, A., Del Favero, S., Sparacino, G., & Cobelli, G. (2016). Online calibration of glucose sensors from the measured current by a time-varying calibration function and Bayesian priors. *IEEE Transactions on Biomedical Engineering*, *63*(8), 1631–1641. doi: 10.1109/TBME.2015.2426217

Wright, A., Maloney, F. L., Wien, M., Samal, L., Emani, S., & Zuccotti, G. (2015). Assessing information system readiness for mitigating malpractice risk through simulation: Results of a multi-site study. *Journal of the American Medical Informatics Association*, *22*(5), 1020–1028. doi: 10.1093/jamia/ocv041

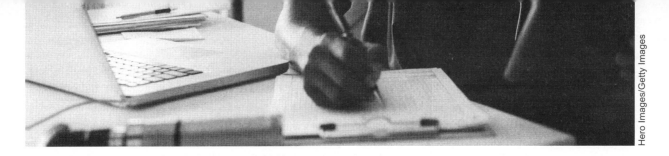
Hero Images/Getty Images

Chapter 9

Strategic Planning, Project Management, and Health Information Technology Selection

Carolyn Sipes, PhD, CNS, APN, PMP, RN-BC

 ## Learning Objectives

After completing this chapter, you should be able to:

- Define strategic planning. Discuss the value of strategic planning in health information technology (HIT), and explain why is it important.

- Describe how strategic planning is related to an organization's mission, scope, vision, goals, and objectives.

- Understand the relationship between strategic planning for information systems and planning for the overall organization.

- Explain the importance of assessing the internal and external environments during the planning process.

- Understand the importance of developing a timeline during the planning phase of strategic planning.

- List tools or processes that may be used to evaluate the outcome of and provide feedback about the planning process.

- Describe two functions in the project management process that must be considered during the HIT selection activity.

- List two skills a nurse informaticist must possess in order to apply best practices in HIT selection.

- List two methods used to manage change—using change theory—when planning a new project.

- Discuss one consideration for the future of project management.

In 2009, the $787 billion American Recovery and Reinvestment Act (ARRA) included $19.2 billion to increase the use of the electronic health record systems (EHRS) by providers and hospitals through the Health Information Technology for Economic and Clinical Health Act (HITECH) through Medicare and Medicaid incentives. This has spurred tremendous energy toward the implementation of these information systems, requiring extensive planning and reworking of many healthcare organizations and their strategic plans. The big initiative to implement electronic health (EHRSs), and then assess how they were being used in a meaningful way has changed significantly since it was introduced. The Centers for Medicare and Medicaid Services (CMS) announced in January 2016 that it will be ending the meaningful use EHR Incentive Program in 2016 (Slavitt, 2016).

However, health information continues to be captured and used, and a key consideration now is to determine what to do with the old data. Some say we have entered the era of big data and with this era comes a need to understand the best way to maintain the integrity and quality of health information as new systems are planned and approved.

Overview of Strategic Planning

This chapter defines and discusses the value of strategic planning when a health information technology (HIT) system is being considered. It defines the different components needed for a successfully functioning information management process, as well as the phases of a **systems development life cycle (SDLC)** and **project management life cycle (PMLC)**, which are concepts used in managing projects. This chapter explains how nurse informaticists (NIs) can provide valuable information regarding how a system should be designed to meet their needs, and addresses the necessity for understanding and managing a project and the changes that occur with the implementation of a new system. Examples of nursing informatics roles are provided, as well as suggestions for future directions in HIT.

Project and Strategic Planning

Project planning and **strategic planning** for the management of information is a critical first step in any planning process to determine what an organization wants in the future, in order to plan how and where to collect and utilize health data; when the guidelines and framework are followed, it increases potential for the project to succeed (Nickols, 2016). The **Project Management Institute (PMI)** is the organizing and certifying organization that defines the standards and methodologies for organizing work into structured processes and formats. According to the PMI, the methodologies for project management are scientifically proven, providing a systematic and disciplined approach to project design, execution completion, and evaluation (Project Management Institute, 2014). Regardless of an organization's size, the processes remain the same and must be deployed consistently. Omitting even one step can lead to overall project failure.

The planning process starts after leadership and stakeholders make a decision that the current system must be upgraded or built new, fully replacing the legacy or old system. **Stakeholders** are those who have a vested interest in the new project; because it will impact them in some way, they are involved at some level in the decision-making process. Once a decision has been made to upgrade or replace the current system, a plan is initiated after a review and analysis of the current status, objectives, and strategies of the business, or review of future state—what might be. Using a process known as **SWOT analysis** (strengths, weaknesses, opportunities, and threats) will help identify gaps in the current system, as well as potential opportunities if a new or updated system is implemented (PlanWare, 2016).

The plan must be detailed as it will help lay the groundwork and guidelines for the project, using a step-by-step process documented in various documents such as the scope and charter for the project. The project may directly impact daily practice or have a financial impact for the whole organization; whatever the reason, each stakeholder will want to be included in the decision-making process.

Strategic planning is an outcome of strategic thinking. To think strategically requires continual assessment and application of new business acumens. The goal is to use these insights to reinforce a company's place in the industry. Thinking strategically must come before the team can move on to strategic planning (Perkins, 2012). Strategic thinking includes spending much needed time assessing the costs of what a new or upgraded system will entail, which may be a substantial cost. In the past, when cost was not well considered, organizations had to cut resources and or even merge with a more profitable, larger organization in order to survive. Strategic planning provides the focus for how a vision will be achieved. Successful strategic plans require the identification of a single vision, and a single mission that fits within that vision, with all activities designed to meet the identified mission.

Components of a strategic plan include developing the project plan, which includes a scope and charter document, goals, objectives, project timeline, team selections with roles and responsibilities, and a work-breakdown structure. It also includes risk management, communication plans, change-management processes, implementation, monitoring and control strategies, a list of final deliverables, final close processes with evaluations, and finally, knowledge transfers. Many of these same terms are also congruent with the SDLC terminology (to be explained later in this chapter).

In today's digital world, use of information systems and technology has become even more critical for organizations as it helps to more efficiently and effectively run the daily business at higher levels, and, in addition, is used to collect data needed in decision making at all levels of the business (Altameem, Abeer, & Nuha, 2014). With that said, the strategic planning process for information management is the most critical issue facing decision making for information systems. The strategic planning process is initiated when the organization realizes and approves needed changes, such as upgrading or even adding a new system. The next step would be to identify the goals—based on the organization's vision and mission—for achieving the planned or needed change. For example, suppose a healthcare enterprise plans to purchase a client-monitoring system to be used throughout its facilities. Other organizational changes—such as plans for construction, unit relocation, and infrastructure upgrades, including computer wiring and cabling, and updating the client care information systems in general—may have initiated the plans for obtaining the monitoring system. Important questions to ask as decisions are made are will the technology solve a serious and urgent problem; is it needed (Hayes, Inc., 2016)? The decisions must be justifiable to leadership. Once administrators realize the need for careful, strategic planning for the monitoring system, they must identify the measureable goals of the plan. These goals should be developed in accordance with the mission and goals of the organization.

As first steps, when the final consensus is made that a new or updated system is required, key leadership will define goals and measureable objectives that the new system will need to meet, and begin to develop a plan outlining specifics. This planning includes categorizing by must- haves needed now versus the nice-to -haves, which can wait until the optimization phase.

Examples of goals and rationales for the system and the functionality they must meet are discussed next. Each goal is followed by a brief explanation of how it applies to an exemplar medical center when selecting a new client monitoring system.

- *To support business and clinical decisions.* Data management supports better decision making by providing timely and accurate information. In the example of planning for a new client monitoring the system, a driving force behind these plans is the need to provide healthcare providers with accurate and complete data regarding a client's condition.

- *To make effective use of emerging technologies.* New technologies can create administrative efficiencies and attract providers and clients. A perfect example of this can be seen with the use of handheld and other wireless devices to collect, view, and transmit patient information from the point of care. The Internet and ehealth represent other developments that have changed access to and delivery of healthcare; because patient results can be made available online from any location, patients can become more connected to their healthcare, patient questions can be addressed, and decision making can be informed. These developments must be included in the strategic planning process as they can change familiar processes from a known system to an unknown workflow, which may cause anxiety and confusion.

- *To enhance the organization's image.* The effective use of information technologies enhances how the organization is perceived by providers, clients, the community, and other external groups. This is especially critical in these times of competitive healthcare. For example, achieving state-of-the-art technology for cardiac monitoring provides efficient and effective client care. Patients are often looking for the latest technology when making healthcare choices.

- *To promote satisfaction of market and regulatory requirements.* Effective information-system strategic planning must include those issues related to meeting market and regulatory requirements, such as ehealth, payer requirements, The Joint Commission guidelines, the National Quality Forum (NQF), client confidentiality, and data security. For example, when selecting a monitoring system, it is also important to determine that the system complies with safety regulations such as protection against damage from defibrillation.

- *To be cost-effective.* Cost-effectiveness is achieved when redundancies are eliminated. In the monitoring system example, this advantage is evident. If all of the critical care and monitored bed areas in the enterprise use the same monitoring system, training is cost-effective, because nurses need be trained on only one system to work in any monitored area of the hospital. Other cost benefits are seen in the need to maintain only one type of backup monitor for replacement of nonoperational equipment, as well as increased efficiency for the biomedical technicians who must maintain the monitoring equipment.

- *To provide a safer environment for patients.* There is a strong initiative for patient safety at this time. A number of organizations, including government agencies, regulatory bodies, consumer groups, and professional organizations, are looking into ways to improve patient safety.

Information Management Components

According to McGonigle and Mastrian (2015), information is data that has been organized and then managed using knowledge. Information management systems are typically computer systems used for managing four primary components, which include software, hardware, health or business data, and the network, as well as project management processes and project teams, including stakeholders. Furthermore, an information system is represented as networked components, which, when coordinated and interfaced, can be used to first process, and then, finally, create information (Neumann Sobernig, & Aram, 2014).

The American Nurses Credentialing Center (ANCC) (American Nurses Credentialing Center, 2014) described important tasks to know when selecting a clinical system. Knowledge of hardware, such as smart devices, tablets, laptops, small-footprint computers, and multi-function devices, is important to understand, especially for anyone wishing to become NI certified. Other essential skills include knowledge of software appropriate to device type as it is used in different clinical scenarios (e.g., mobile computing and barcode medication administration). Finally, NIs need to have skills and knowledge to recommend solutions for both software and hardware enhancements and upgrades that will support nursing workflows. Understanding this information is also important for achieving the ANCC certification as a nurse informaticist. The test content outline (TCO) is available on the ANCC website as a study tool.

Software refers to the applications and programs that are used by hardware to process information and data. Hardware is the computer used for input and output, as well as the peripheral devices, such as the keyboard, monitor, and printer, which are all used to work with and organize data and information. Data is input into databases so that it can be analyzed and organized into functional information, using such applications as Microsoft Access and Excel. Once analyzed and organized, reports and other documents can be created from the output. The network provides a means for connecting all computers into one, which is known as the "system." The four components described previously make up what is known as the "platform," which the IT department uses to manage data and information.

As the strategic planning process continues, much time (as much as three to four months) must be spent on vendor and system selection assessments, because this is an area where substantial funding is required. Often, the costs run into the hundreds of millions of dollars for an enterprise system; system upgrades cost less as they occur in smaller phases. Enterprise systems are large organizations that have different operating systems across a number of facilities that can share the same databases to support multiple functions. Box 9-1 lists a number of key assessments that must be completed during the vendor and system selection process.

The term open source (OOS/FS) is defined as free, publicly available software governed by a license that defines the terms and limitations of use—Open Source Initiative (OSI). Advantages and disadvantages of both open and closed source systems are discussed later.

Open source definition: The distribution terms of open-source software must comply with the following criteria:

- Free redistribution
- Source code
- Derived works
- Integrity of the author's source code
- No discrimination against persons or groups
- No discrimination against fields of endeavor
- Distribution of license
- License must not be specific to a product
- License must not restrict other software
- License must be technology neutral.

Box 9-1 Checklist when Developing the Strategic Plan for Functionality of an IT System

- Does the system use open architecture?
- Is the system based on personal computer, client/server, thin client, or Internet technology?
- Does it support the use of a variety of devices such as PDAs, iPods, iPads, tablets, and other means for entry or retrieval of data?
- Does it follow human–computer-interaction (HCI) design standards?
- Does the software comply with HL7 standards for interfaces?
- Does the database incorporate SNOMED, LOINC, and other terminology standards?
- Does the system sufficiently safeguard individual patient data from unauthorized users?
- Does the system allow the user to query aggregate data and produce online reports?
- Does it support performance measurement?
- Does it support a customized view or the ability to customize functions?
- Can it support expansion of features, increased numbers of users, and/or records?
- Does it allow the use of evolving technologies, such as smart cards, optical disks, interface engines, wireless technology, integrated services digital network (ISDN) communication, ehealth or ecommerce, video conferencing, telemedicine, and fiber-optic networks?
- Does it support a paperless/wireless environment?
- How much will it cost for purchase, installation, training, and ongoing support?
- Have criteria been developed to measure successful implementation?

According to Damico (n.d.), closed source programs refer to proprietary or commercial software, such as Microsoft Outlook, which is owned and sold by an organization where the purchaser pays for the right to use, but does not own, the program. It is distributed through a variety of retail channels including the owner's website. If the program is in the form of shareware, a fully functional version of the program can be installed and run with a time limit, after which it will become disabled.

Disadvantages, including issues of quality, reliability, and security of both open and closed systems, must be a key consideration. Considerations include: how mature is the program, was it built by volunteers where maintenance and technical support might be a problem, was it tested properly, what are the cost and interoperability issues, are licenses free and unlimited, and how secure is the program?

Continuing to finalize the strategic IT plan for a new system and after an initial review and elimination process, an invitation for a request for information (RFI) and request for proposal (RFP) from the vendors are sent out. Questions to ask during the initial elimination process include those that address issues other than product functionality. For each of the following assessment questions, there are additional questions that can be found in EHR-focused documents on the HealthIT.gov website in the section titled How to Implement EHRs. Two helpful documents are (*EHR demonstration scenario evaluation and vendor questions* (National Learning Consortium, 2013), and *Step 3: Select or Upgrade to a Certified EHR* (National Learning Consortium, 2014). The summary of possible vendor assessment questions and examples include:

Questions about the company	How long has your company been in business? How many employees do you have?
Questions about the product	Is your software sold modularly or does it need to be purchased as a complete package?
What functions are available?	Can you add functionality as the need grows?
Pricing questions	How are the licenses issued? Concurrent user versus per practitioner?
Interface questions	Can your software interface with practice management systems and lab systems? Is there an added cost for these interfaces?
Implementation questions	Will your company assume all aspects of implementation (i.e., hardware and software)?
Ongoing support questions	What is the frequency and depth of upgrades?
Technical/maintenance questions	What personnel and qualifications do I need to support and operate this system?

After the number of vendors have been narrowed down, site visits are made before final selection. During the site visit, other assessments include:

How reliable is the system? How much downtime do you experience?

What is the response time?

How is the system backup accomplished? And how frequently is this done?

Are there any problems with information exchange with other information systems?

How do customizations or enhancements get made to the system (in-house or by vendor)?

How much training was required for users to learn the system?

What do you like most about the system?

What things would you like to change about the system?

What features would you like to see added to the system?

How is information access restricted, and how is security maintained?

What have your experiences been with vendor support?

Is it easy to generate reports, and can they be customized easily to meet user needs?

What problems are you trying to solve?

What would you do differently if you could go back in time?

More tools and templates, including contract questions, RFP, and pricing templates needed for vendor selection, can be found on websites, such as HealthIT.gov, including the Vendor Evaluation Matrix Tool, a tool which consists of 58 assessment questions that should provide answers from evaluation by functionality/usability and prioritizing vendors. Each vendor is scored on a scale from 1 (poor) to 5 (excellent) on each of the prioritized items, then ratings are tallied at the end for a total score.

One Vendor versus Best of Breeds

Further concepts to consider are defined as one vendor versus best of breed, which refers to using only one specific vendor for all desired functionality or selecting the best technology from a number of vendors. The advantages of one vendor limits issues of interoperability across the system and it provides a standardized, performance.

The disadvantages include lack of competition, so it may not be the best of all systems, the organization may be locked in to a certain system due to contracts, and there may be no access to the latest and greatest technology because the vendor cannot keep up. Best of breed provides the advantage of access to the latest and greatest technology. The disadvantages require expertise of the IT team to understand all of the different vendors' technology in order to maintain the system. Interoperability is a huge issue as there are few consistent standards between vendors that meet different organizations' criteria.

Configurability

What does configurability mean? When referring to software, it means the way it can be adapted or changed to meet a user's needs, within limits. For example, Epic systems provide a basic package, or standard software package, that is easily configurable to meet some of the customer's needs. Issues arise when the customer might want to go beyond the standard package and add to or customize the system, which typically is not flexible or configurable in the future. A lesson learned with a new vendor early in the vendor's growth was the error of customizing many of their applications for individual customers only to find later the customized software could not be upgraded but had to be completely redone or replaced.

Interoperability

Interoperability is the ability to exchange information across systems. For example, an old legacy system interacting/interfacing with a new system so that data and information flow from one to the other. Considerations include questions such as, what would need to be done to create an application that would support moving data and information across systems, or interacting across systems? To support interoperability, any newly designed system would need to be able to connect with both old and new systems, different systems, and software applications in order to exchange data and information across all systems.

Ease of Use/Usefulness of Systems

Ease of use refers to how easy the system is to use when inputting information into an electronic health record or other electronic documents. How many clicks does it take to get to the area where information is entered, and how easy are the directions to follow? Other considerations with usability include user satisfaction, user experience, and skill levels.

With reference to usability of information systems, ease of use is a key consideration when building an application for an EHRS—how easy is it for the end users to use, enter and retrieve information and other functions needed to accomplish their work tasks? How long does it take to learn the functionality? Anytime a new system is implemented or upgraded, there needs to be consideration for the learning curve, or the time it will take end users to adapt to and efficiently, effectively, and competently use the system. This process can be enhanced with training, super users support, and even providing a playground environment where users can use the new system without making mistakes in the live system.

Usefulness, on the other hand, is how well the system meets the needs of the user. Would it make the job easier in terms of accessing the data needed in a job? Do the end users find it useful in making their jobs more effective and efficient? When these criteria are perceived by the end users, there will be a greater chance of user acceptance.

Planning at the Project Level—The Project Management Process

Once the strategic plan described previously, has been approved and in place, and the vendor selection process is complete and agreed on by the organization, the actual project management process begins. The next step is to start developing documents for the first of the five phases of the PMLC: design/plan, implementation, monitoring and control, evaluation, and lessons learned with knowledge transfer. Phase one of the project management cycle—design/plan—includes the creation and development of the tools needed to manage the project: scope and charter documents, which guide how the system will be implemented and what officially can and cannot be done, then evaluated including adding metrics to monitor measures of success progress.

According to Sipes (2016), the scope document is an official document that details how the project will be managed and what the project requirements are. It further defines what can and cannot be done officially. The scope document will address an opportunity or problem the organization is trying to address or solve (see Box 9-2). Whether the project is large or small, the same process and documents will need to be used as a guideline. Included in the scope document are the goals and objectives for the project as they are developed to meet the mission and vision of the organization. Both scope and charter documents are required by leadership, because they fall under different members' responsibilities, so there will be some duplicate information. The documents define who is involved at this level, such as the stakeholders—many times, these are the same people who were involved in strategic planning (previously discussed)—or others including practitioners and other end users. In the charter, project participants' roles, responsibilities, and time requirements are defined, as well as the estimated hours, members, and expected deliverables.

Box 9-2   Example of Project Scope Content

Organization name

Title of project

Scope document name/number/priority level

Project manager

Sponsor

Mission statement

Vision

Measureable project objectives

Justification of project

Implementation strategy

Project resources

Completion date

Measures of success

Assumptions

Constraints

Approvals: sponsor, project manager, and owner

Final document approved and signed off by executives

These official documents include the organization's mission and vision statements; the project plan must be congruent with these statements as well as include the overall strategy. As the plan is developed, the guideline of the five Ws (who, what, when, where, why) and H (how), described by Sipes (2016) for developing measurable objectives, is useful. It includes high-level strategic plans, as well as other areas of planning in the organization. When using this guideline, the who, what, when, why, and how of the plan should incorporate longer-term goals of the project.

The mission is the purpose or reason for the organization's existence, and represents the fundamental and unique aspirations of the organization that differentiates it from others. The mission is often conveyed in the form of a mission statement that broadly declares what a business aspires to be by telling the organization's personnel and customers who they are and what they do. The mission statement should incorporate meaningful and measurable criteria. The mission statement is an important tool when used to guide the planning process and should resonate with those involved with the organization, including key stakeholders. The mission statement should be one of the first things considered when evaluating a strategic decision. The vision statement is a future-oriented, high-level view of what an organization would like to become. The vision statement is often the first consideration in strategic planning. An example of a vision statement may include statements such as:

ABC Medical Center will strive to:
- Be the hospital of choice for patients, physicians, and employees in our area because of our preeminent patient care and teaching programs.
- Be recognized as a technology leader in our region.
- Be the academic center of choice for residents and healthcare professionals.
- Be a prominent community member known for meeting the healthcare needs of the entire community through incomparable patient care and wellness programs.

Sponsors and stakeholders are identified in the scope and charter, as well as in the strategic plan discussed earlier. Regardless of the level—from end users to senior management—there must be agreement and collaboration in all project decision-making, as stakeholders can make or break a project. Furthermore, decisions should be made based on the business needs of the organization, which are the first components to be identified. Finally, the key to strategic planning is not only creating the plan, but also executing, maintaining, and evaluating the project once it is implemented.

The goals and objectives in all formal documents must be specific and include detailed metrics with projected due dates for implementation, as well as owners for specific tasks and closure of the project. The final approved scope document provides the guidelines for the project. If items and tasks fall outside of what has been documented and officially approved, it is referred to as scope creep—unapproved change, which can cause serious delays or even project failure. Box 9-2 depicts an example of content found in a scope document. Box 9-3 shows content commonly found in a project charter.

The SDLC previously mentioned is a conceptual model in project management using terminology and descriptions of tasks that need to be completed in each phase of a project. In the literature, descriptions of the both SDLC and PMLC processes include anywhere from four to six phases; steps in the process, depending on the work breakdown, is defined by the organization. However, the main phases that need to be accomplished when implementing a project include design, initiation/planning, implementation, closeout, and evaluation. Within these phases, the 16 components of a strategic plan identified previously must be included for whichever term the organization is using—SDLC or PMLC—for the project to be successful. Overall, the life cycle concepts provide the timelines and framework for managing a

---

Box 9-3 **Example of Project Charter Content**

Title of project

Objective of project

Population to be served

Services to be provided

Justification of project

Scope statement summary

Project participants

Executive Steering Team:

Names	Titles	Department

(List each team, steering, work group, team governance)

Project Teams:

Names	Titles	Department

Roles, responsibilities

Time requirements; estimated hours/member

Define expected deliverables

Final approval and sign off by executives

---

project. The process is initiated following a gap analysis of an existing IT, or legacy, system, and completion of workflow.

As the scope and charter are developed, a gap analysis of the existing information management methods (including current information systems—also known as, legacy systems) should be conducted, which helps to define and support the rationales for the project. Workflows are analyzed, looking at the current state—what is occurring now and might not be working. This is compared with—the future state—what is desired and planned for in the project.

During phase one, the timeline for the project start and its projected finish is developed. This document is designed to provide a quick overview of due dates, week-by-week and month-by-month, with tasks to be completed and major milestones outlined. This is also a great way to communicate projected deadlines to the team.

Phase one is the time for team selection. As teams are formed, applications are reviewed for the level of expertise and skills needed, which is based on an assessment of the new system requirements and functionality. Team resources include the end users, physicians, nurses, pharmacists, and others, such as IT, who have knowledge and expertise of system functionality and what the new workflows should look like. Many times, consultants with years of experience and expertise are brought in to work with the organization's employees, who are not as skilled, to help support and educate team members as they learn how to work with and develop the system. Consultants will also build functionality and specific applications for the system as well. This process can get a project moving more quickly rather than waiting for employees to be trained and develop the needed skills.

Other key considerations include evaluation of resource availability. If teams are shared across several projects, which is seen in organizations that use project management offices (PMOs) instead of dedicated project managers, it may lead to one project being delayed over another, depending upon the project priority. At first, it may look like a great way to monitor expenses, but 99% of the time projects are not on time due to unforeseen issues or tasks inadvertently overlooked. When resources have been assigned to a delayed project that is overdue for completion, there is a domino effect for all other projects aligned and ready to start utilizing the same resources. The best approach is to get a commitment for a budget to cover all resources for the one project until it is complete.

Phase two of project management requires the creation of a document known as the work breakdown structure (WBS). Here, the tasks defined in the scope, as well as all duties, are broken down into specific work packages, and are then assigned to each team's members who will be responsible for completion of that task. From the WBS, the Gantt chart is developed with an owner for each specific task, subtask, and due date with start and end dates. During this phase, defining the level of detail is more important than meeting a time constraint to complete documents, because any omission can lead to costly project delays or even failure. With the necessary detail, the Gantt chart will also function as the resource—human and technology—management plan and schedule. The communication plan is developed in this phase. It must include information on how each upper-leadership shareholder, including the chief executive officer (CEO), chief information officer (CIO), chief nursing officer (CNO), and chief nursing informatics officer CNIO (also known as the C suite), as well as other team members, will receive communication and updates on the project status and issues, and what form it will take. The risk assessment and management plan is critical to the project and is developed during this phase. In this plan, risks are documented and tracked; assessment of the risks are marked as high, medium or low; determinations are made on how each risk will be managed and the priority of each risk. For example, if the risk is labelled as high, it will need to be monitored more frequently until the risk is lowered or completely resolved. Finally, all risks, after review and prioritization, are assigned an owner who will be responsible for tracking decisions to make sure they reach a resolution.

As part of the phase two development process for the project plan, an understanding and plan for change and change management must be included. As progress and final decisions are made for a new or upgraded system, a key strategy to consider is how current staff will accept the future changes. With change, many different behaviors can be observed, including resignations, resistance, and feelings of loss similar to Kubler-Ross stages of grief or the Grief Model (Cleverism, 2015). Two other frequently used models are Lewin's change model from 1950, and Kotter's change management theory (2016). Organizations that do well managing change by beginning to educate staff early about needed requirements and modifications, will find little resistance and chaos because these changes were anticipated. A key first step to managing change well is to bring staff together and explain the new workflows and how these workflows will impact and improve their day-to-day practice. For example, one of Kotter's eight stages is to "create a sense of urgency," which begins to motivate people so that they understand the need for a new or upgraded system. It is important to assure staff that jobs will not be lost (if this is truly the case), and that the new workflows will enhance and make their jobs more efficient and effective.

To manage change at the staff level, it is important to put a framework and guidelines in place that will add structure and consistency to the change process and, thereby, reduce anxiety. Sipes (2016) refers to the Katzenbach Center studies, which identified ten principles to use as a framework when implementing change. Two of the key principles include to first "lead with culture, determining where the resistance is," and then, engage all levels of employees (as cited in Aguirre & Alpern, 2014).

Additional Katzenbach Center survey findings are noted here:

- 84% said that the organization's culture was critical to the success of change management.

- 64% saw it as more critical than strategy or operating models. However, change leaders failed to address culture, including overcoming cultural resistance.

- Additionally, 76% reported that executives failed to take account of or ignored existing culture when designing the transformation, leading to the company's inability to sustain change over time (as cited in Aguirre & Alpern, 2014).

The change management process at the organizational project management level includes setting up a **change control board (CCB)**. While the project plan may be viewed as a "living" document with the need to be updated continually, it must be monitored to prevent scope creep. Any requests for changes or issues are brought before the board at least monthly and more frequently within 30 to 60 days of go-live for the new system. The CCB is responsible for monitoring, assigning owners, notifying all stakeholders, and resolving of all issues, including such items as requested changes in the scope and charter, the project plan, or other official documents. The process includes completion of formal, documented change request forms with dates, actions taken with rationale and resolution of changes or issues, and then formal approval by all members of the CCB.

A final process in phase two that must be accomplished, but is often cut too short due to time constraints, is a **functional test** to make sure all databases are working as designed. Other testing methodologies and rationales, such as user acceptance, integration, and unit testing, are discussed in other chapters of this text.

The Informatics Nurse's Role as Project Manager

As noted in Sipes (2016), a report by the Health Resources and Services Administration (HRSA) stated that management and implementation of an EHRS requires skills in leadership and direction of the project team that few possess. Furthermore, many nurses view the concept of project management as foreign and not applicable to anything they might do. In fact, the **NI** in the role of project manager (PM) follows a process that is very similar to the nursing process. The concepts are similar; for example, the five steps of the nursing process and the five phases of project management both include the first step of assessment, in which analysis of what is and what is needed occurs. Step two/phase two, developing the care plan and the project plan, are completed similarly as well. The final three steps/phases for both the nursing process and project management include implementing the plan, monitoring outcomes, and the final evaluation and lessons learned with knowledge transfer.

Phases one and two of project management, design/initiation and developing the project plan, were reviewed previously. The next phase of project management, phase three, is to implement the plan that has been developed and approved by an official sign-off by leadership. For an EHRS implementation, as the system goes live, it is time to apply all of the tools previously developed in phases one and two. Phase three implementation can take several weeks or even months to go live if the organization is very large, such as at a regional medical center with many outlying clinics and other facilities. During the implementation phase, the system go live occurs when all of the new applications and functionality are accessible to the end users who will begin to enter patient data into the system. During phase three, the system will be monitored and controlled closely using the tools developed in phase two to make sure all functions are accurate and functioning well, such as the ability to access and record medications or treatments, as well as create records/reports and track all patient tasks. According to the Project Management Institute (2013), regardless of the organization's size, the processes for project implementation remain the same and must be deployed consistently for each phase. If one step is omitted, it can lead to overall project failure. Additionally, the tools developed in phase one and two must be utilized as the process moves forward as both detailed tracking tools, and as a means of officially documenting what is and is not working within sub-phases of implementation.

As the NI assumes the PM role, providing oversight for the five phases of an EHRS implementation, other attributes become obvious, such as developing the ability to facilitate communication between IT and nurses and other healthcare providers. For example, when the first EHRSs were developed, they were created solely by IT without input from nurses regarding needed workflows. This led to many project failures when nurses and physicians realized that the workflows and functionally did not meet their practice workflows, and subsequently refused to use the systems. Currently, NIs work well in the PM role. They provide much needed facilitation between IT, nursing staff, and other departments. Through this process, they are also advocates for improving patient safety and satisfaction.

Essential Skills in Other Advanced Nurse Practice Roles

Today, differing levels of informatics skills and project management are common in most new job descriptions at an advanced level of practice for nurses and other healthcare providers. A partial list of specific advanced practice roles and skills are discussed next.

The American Nurses Credentialing Center (ANCC) outlined core abilities necessary for a nurse administrator, including the ability and experience to use management skills, to manage change, and to communicate effectively. The Association for Perioperative Registered Nurses (AORN) lists needed skills, such as an ability to assess, plan, implement, evaluate, and document care (PM skills) in addition to critical thinking skills. These same attributes and required skills are also listed in job descriptions for clinical nurse specialists (CNS) and nurse practitioners (NP), along with many other requirements. These skills are important to doctoral students and doctorate of nursing practice (DNP) graduates as they not only provide patient care but are also required to apply practice management skills.

The role of the chief nursing informatics officer (CNIO) has been mentioned as a key decision maker in the strategic planning process, and aligned information technology strategic planning activity. One of the newest and fastest-growing roles to emerge in recent years is that of the CNIO and it may be modeled on the chief medical informatics office role. The CNIO is the most senior nursing informatics executive and functions as a bridge between nursing and the IT department through critical relationships with the CEO, chief informatics officer (CIO), and chief nursing officer (CNO). Depending on the needs and structure of an organization, the CNIO position may be one that has a horizontal or dotted line linkage to the CNO and the CIO.

The key responsibility of CNIOs is to capitalize on their nursing informatics knowledge and project management skills. The role encompasses an understanding and integration of multiple computer, information, analytical, and nursing science skills in order to manage, as well as strategically and operationally lead, stakeholders of the interprofessional healthcare team in decision-making to achieve organizational outcomes. The CNIO uses these skills when focused on the design, planning, and implementation of health information systems, and when managing the adoption of other supporting clinical initiatives.

To summarize, a partial list of skills needed by all roles defined here (as well as others not listed) include:

- Organizational and management skills
- Clinical re-engineering
- Change management
- Work processes support
- Information management
- Time management
- Resource management
- Leadership
- Communication skills
- Strategic planning
- Decision making and decision support
- Problem solving
- Budget development and cost monitoring (Sipes, 2016, p. 29).

All of the skills listed previously, as well as others, are required of a PM and are listed in the American Nurses Association (ANA, 2015) *Nursing Informatics: Scope and Standards of Practice* functional areas for the informatics nurse specialist (INS) and for NIs as well.

Future Directions

The process for developing strategic plans was described earlier, including the tools and stakeholders required in the decision-making process. Federal agencies use much of the same standard format to develop their strategic plans, which are required by government. With the Affordable Care Act (Patient Protection and Affordable Care Act, 2010) as a driving force, the Department of Health and Human Services (DHHS) developed a strategic plan for fiscal year 2014 to 2018, based on various initiatives defined in the ACA. The strategic plan defines how it will address many evolving health and human services issues. As discussed previously, a strategic plan defines its mission, goals, and metrics as outlined in the management documents—the scope and charter. As a web document, it is a "living" document, and is frequently updated to reflect changes in strategies, actions, and goals. The DHHS strategic plan provides priorities and targets for accomplishment, and next steps that are tracked as part of the project management process.

In addition to the DHHS plan, there is also a Federal Health IT Strategic Plan for fiscal years 2015 to 2020 (Office of the National Coordinator for Health Information Technology, 2015). This strategic plan includes the following listed goals, which can be found on the HealthIT.gov website for strategic plans:

- Strategic goal 1: strengthen healthcare
- Strategic goal 2: advance scientific knowledge and innovation

- Strategic goal 3: advance the health, safety, and well-being of the American people
- Strategic goal 4: ensure efficiency, transparency, accountability, and effectiveness of DHHS programs

Within each of the goals are more specific sub-goals, which outline how the goal should be accomplished, including emphasis on project management and informatics skills. The rationale for the HealthIT.gov goals goals listed previously is explained next:

> (the) federal government intends to apply the effective use of information and technology to help the nation achieve high-quality care, lower costs, a healthy population, and engaged individuals. This Plan focuses on advancing health IT innovation . . . to modernize the US health IT infrastructure
>
> (Office of the National Coordinator for Health Information Technology, 2015, p. 5)

The goals defined in the Federal Health IT Strategic Plan for 2015 through 2020 have many detailed subcategories and serve as driving forces to move health IT forward through 2020 as described in the following:

> the infrastructure will support dynamic uses of electronic information that facilitate and expedite the transformation of data to information, information to knowledge, and knowledge to informed action . . . infrastructure implementation will fortify cultural shifts necessary to strengthen collaborative relationships for improving health/ health care, research, and innovation.
>
> (Office of the National Coordinator for Health Information Technology, 2015, p. 5)

While the overall goal is to improve the infrastructure of HIT, it also speaks to the need for developing project management and informatics skills described previously.

Summary

- Strategic planning is the development of a comprehensive long-range plan for guiding the activities and operations of an organization. Strategic planning is an ongoing process.
- As a "living" document, the strategic plan is one of the most important factors in the selection and design, and more specifically, implementation of information systems, because the plan can save valuable resources over time and ensure that the needs of the enterprise are met, even as changes occur.
- The strategic plan supports the mission, scope, vision, goals, and objectives of the organization.
- The mission is the purpose for the organization's existence and represents its unique aspects.
- Strategic planning is guided by upper-level administrators and stakeholders including the CEO, CIO, CNO, and CNIO.
- Strategic planning involves the following steps: identification of the need for change, definition of goals and scope, scanning of external and internal environments, data analysis, identification of potential solutions, selection of a course of action, implementation, and evaluation and feedback.
- The selection and implementation of an information system occurs through a well-defined process called the life cycle of an information system. Descriptions of both SDLC and PMLC processes include anywhere from four to six phases, depending on the organization structure.
- The needs assessment and gap analysis process is often initiated when a deficit in the current method of manual or automated information handling is recognized.

- The system selection steering committee is an essential component of the assessment and selection process; leadership and other stakeholders may impact the success or failure of the project.
- The project management process provides a framework that can improve the likelihood of project success.
- Passage of the ACA is a driving force for the development of HIT innovations and infrastructure.

Case Study

Consider ways in which what you have learned about project management might be applied to an experience in your life such as planning a wedding, buying a house, or selecting a college. Can you identify advantages over processes that you have used previously? If so, what might those be? What, if anything might you do differently if you were to apply project management to the process, and why? How will knowledge of project management change how you handle future projects?

About the Author

Carolyn Sipes, PhD, CNS, APN, PMP, RN-BC, teaches nursing informatics at Chamberlain College of Nursing. She has more than 30-years experience in management, consulting, and teaching, which includes national and international implementation of electronic health records (EHRs). She holds project management professional (PMP) certification through the Project Management Institute (PMI), holds eight Epic clinical systems certifications, is board certified by the American Nurses Credentialing Center in Nursing Informatics (RN-BC), and is an ANCC Nursing Informatics Content expert.

After completing her doctorate, she worked as a research scientist for a major pharmaceutical company, where she designed the first Tolerability of Medication Assessment tool (TOMA) and presented the research at the international World AIDS Research conference. Dr. Sipes has published and presented extensively and authored the book, *Project Management for the Advanced Practice Nurse.*

References

Aguirre, D., & Alpern, M. (2014). *10 Principles of leading change management; time-honored tools and techniques.* Retrieved from www.strategy-business.com

Altameem, A. A., Abeer, I. A., & Nuha, A. A. (2014). *Strategic information systems planning (SISP). Proceedings of the World Congress on Engineering and Computer Science* 2014 Vol I. Retrieved from www.iaeng.org/publication/WCECS2014/WCECS2014_pp168-170.pdf

American Nurses Credentialing Center. (2014). Test content outline. Retrieved from www.nursecredentialing.org/Documents/InformaticsCertification/TestContentOutlines-TCO2014

American Nurses Association. (2015). *Nursing informatics: Scope and standards of practice* (2nd ed.). Silver Spring, MD: Nursebooks.org.

Cleverism. (2015). Major approaches & models of change management. Retrieved from www.cleverism.com/major-approaches-models-of-change-management/

Damico. (n.d.). Open vs. closed source. Retrieved from www.damicon.com/resources/openvsclosed.html

Hayes, Inc. (2016). Making healthcare technology decisions with limited evidence: 10 questions to ask. Retrieved from http://evidence.hayesinc.com/making-healthcare-technology-decisions-with-limited-evidence

McGonigle, D., & Mastrian, K. (2015). *Nursing informatics: The foundation of knowledge* (3rd ed.). Burlington, MA: Jones Bartlett, Inc.

National Learning Consortium. (2013). EHR demonstration scenario, evaluation, and vendor questions. Retrieved from www.healthit.gov/providers-professionals/ehr-demonstration-scenario-evaluation-and-vendor-questions

National Learning Consortium. (2014). Step 3: Select or upgrade to a certified EHR. Retrieved from www.healthit.gov/providers-professionals/ehr-implementation-steps/step-3-select-or-upgrade-certified-ehr

Neumann, G., Sobernig, S., & Aram, M. (2014). Evolutionary business information systems. *Business and Information Systems Engineering,* 6(1), 33–36. doi:10.1007/s12599-013-0305-1

Nickols, F. (2016). Strategy, strategic management, strategic information, and strategic thinking. Retrieved from www.nickols.us/strategy_etc.pdf

Office of the National Coordinator for Health Information Technology. (2015). Federal health IT strategic plan for FY 2015-2020. Published by U.S. Department of Health & Human Services. Retrieved from www.healthit.gov/sites/.../9-5-federalhealthitstratplanfinal_0.pdf

Patient Protection and Affordable Care Act, 42 U.S.C. § 18001. (2010).

Perkins, L. (2012). 3 essential steps to thinking strategically. Retrieved from www.inc.com/lauren-perkins/three-essential-steps-to-thinking-strategically.html

PlanWare. (2016). Business planning papers: Developing a strategic plan. Retrieved from www.planware.org/strateagicplan

Project Management Institute. (2013). *A guide to the project management body of knowledge (PMBOK guide), foundational standards.* (5th ed.). Newtown Square, PA: Project Management Institute

Sipes, C. (2016). *Project management for the advanced practice nurse.* New York: Springer.

Slavitt, A. (2016). CMS to end meaningful use in 2016. Journal of American Health Information Management Association. Retrieved from http://journal.ahima.org/2016/01/13/cms-to-end-meaningful-use-in-2016

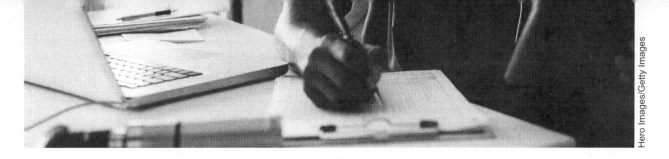

Chapter 10

Improving the Usability of Health Informatics Applications

Nancy Staggers, PhD, RN, FAAN

 ## Learning Objectives

After completing this chapter, you should be able to:

- Distinguish among the terms user experience, human factors, ergonomics, human–computer interaction, and usability.

- Describe the goals of usability and its three axioms.

- Analyze the impacts of poor usability on clinicians' work.

- Identify the major components of human–computer interaction models.

- Compare and contrast methods employed in usability studies.

- Construct basic usability tests for health informatics applications.

"The dumbest mistake is viewing design as something you do at the end of the process to 'tidy up' the mess, as opposed to understanding it's a 'day one' issue and part of everything."

TOM PETERS

Good usability is critical for the adoption and safe use of health-informatics products. All informaticists need a suite of skills to conduct usability tests, whether the focus of their work is health information technology (HIT) design, development, implementation, use, or evaluation. Concepts about usability guide informaticists in creating and purchasing technologies that users find effective, efficient, and satisfying to use. This chapter presents definitions of major terms—user experience, human factors, ergonomics, human-computer interaction (HCI) and usability—along with usability goals and principles. Examples of current usability issues are given and benefits of incorporating usability into HIT are described. HCI frameworks are offered for guidance on conducting usability tests. Usability-test design and methods are explained using examples of actual usability studies performed in health settings. After reading this chapter, health informaticists will be able to design and conduct usability tests to determine the effectiveness, efficiency, and/or satisfaction with HIT.

Introduction to Usability

Usability problems are a global issue for contemporary HIT. Classic and recent HIT evaluations showed unintended consequences and new errors with HIT due to usability issues (Ash, Sittig, Dykstra, Campbell, & Guappone, 2009; Hardmeier, Tsourounis, Moore, Abbott, & Guglielmo, 2014; Koppel et al., 2005; Slight et al., 2016). In 2015, The Joint Commission (TJC) issued an alert about HIT-related sentinel events. After evaluating 3,375 previous adverse event reports, TJC found 120 were HIT-related (The Joint Commission, 2015) for user interface, workflow, and communication issues. Members of the Health Information and Management Systems Society (HIMSS) User Experience (UX) committee completed a national project in 2016 to understand nurses' HIT pain points (HIT User Experience Committee, 2016; Staggers, Elias, Makar, Hunt, & Alexander, 2016), finding that extensive documentation requirements, care transitions, and lack of HIT integration were significant issues for nurses in all sites and across all vendors. Other examples of usability issues include the difficulty nurses and physicians have finding critical information and developing the big picture of the patient (HIT User Experience Committee; Staggers, et al. 2016; Stead & Lin, 2009). Lastly, electronic medication-administration records (eMARs) created potential patient safety issues because nurses were not able to efficiently organize medications for their groups of patients or easily see missed medications (Guo, Iribarren, Kapsandoy, Perri, & Staggers, 2011; Staggers, Iribarren, Guo, & Weir, 2015). Clearly, usability is linked to patient safety as well as practitioner efficiencies.

The costs of poor usability are substantial even without catastrophic errors. Usability issues can result in:

- Decreases in productivity.
- Errors.
- Treatment and decision delays.
- Extreme user frustration.
- Underutilization of systems.
- Deinstallations.
- The need for extra support personnel to install and maintain systems.
- Covert and overt resistance to applications and.
- The need for substantial funding to redesign and remedy problems (Healthcare Information and Management Systems Society, 2011).

Fortunately, these kinds of issues can be ameliorated by employing usability principles and practices (Carayon, Xie, & Kianfar, 2014). The uptake of these principles has been slow in healthcare, but vendors and healthcare organizations are beginning to understand the value of usability as a strategic asset, and design HIT products to better fit the way clinicians think and work.

Potential Benefits of Incorporating Usability Techniques into HIT Applications

Well-designed systems can improve individuals' performance to increase patient safety, reduce errors, increase productivity, and improve cognitive support. Readers are referred to a publically available HIMSS user experience white paper outlining usability maturity and return on investment for organizations when usability is incorporated into organizations (HIMSS Usability Task Force, 2011). Besides individual benefits, the paper outlines organizational efficiencies due to decreased maintenance, training, and development costs.

UX and usability techniques allow informaticists to identify and solve issues with information technology. More importantly, usability methods address *why* users are having those problems. Issues can then be addressed before the technology is released or with redesign after release. Two examples illustrate the potential of these techniques. Researchers employed usability techniques to create novel designs for integrating physiologic data in a graphic object (Drews & Westenskow, 2006; Wachter et al., 2006). The new design provided integrated, at-a-glance pictorial data to show clinicians the changes in patients' physiologic parameters. These graphics are now incorporated into vendors' products as an adjunct to numeric data displays. Another example is the design and testing of new displays for ICU nurses after researchers performed a comprehensive study of nurses' tasks and cognitive requirements (Koch et al., 2012).

Every health informaticist should be educated in usability techniques to promote more usable HIT. The remainder of this chapter provides background material as well as the knowledge and skills to conduct usability tests.

Definitions of Terms and Interrelationships of Concepts

User Experience

When we use the term **user experience**, or UX, we use a classic definition to mean all aspects of a user's interaction with a service, system, or HIT product (Kuniavsky, 2003). Formally, the term was defined as perceptions and responses resulting from the use (or anticipated use) of a product, system, or service by the International Organization for Standardization (ISO), 9241-11 (Human Factors and Ergonomics Society, 2012; International Organization for Standardization, 1998). UX can be a range of experiences from walking into a bank to creating HIT designs that fit into complex ecosystems with many interacting users, such as enterprise electronic health record systems or EHRSs (Schaffer, 2010). A high-quality user experience in any venue requires collaborative work from multiple disciplines, such as engineering, graphic and industrial design, interface design, psychology, and domain experts in the discipline at hand (HIMSS Usability Task Force, 2011.).

Human factors, ergonomics, HCI, and usability are all embedded within the broader concept of UX. Usability overlaps both ergonomics and HCI, and usability, ergonomics, and HCI all edge into UX.

Human Factors

The term **human factors** describes the interactions between humans and tools of all kinds. Human factors is a broad term that can include topics, such as the design of motorcycle controls to fit human hands and feet, or an evaluation of how work is performed within the layout of a hospital room in an intensive care unit (ICU). A most readable and classic text about the need for human factors in the design of common objects was written by Donald Norman (Norman, 1988).

Ergonomics

Ergonomics is concerned with human performance as it relates to the physical characteristics of tools, systems, and machines as is indicated in a classic HCI textbook (Dix, Finlay, Abowd, & Beale, 2004), where the focus is on designs for safety, comfort, and convenience. The term ergonomics is often used interchangeably with human factors in Europe, but less so in the United States. Ergonomics can address the design of a cooking utensil to fit a human hand, the design of computer chairs to promote comfort and safety, and/or the intuitive operation of drinking fountains. A healthcare example is purchasing an electronic device that is not too bulky or heavy for nurses to use in patient care.

Human–Computer Interaction

Human–computer interaction (**HCI**) is the study of how people design, implement, and evaluate interactive computer systems in the context of users' tasks and work (Dix et al., 2004). HCI blends psychology and/or cognitive science, applied work in computer science, sociology, and information science into the design, development, purchase, implementation, and evaluation of applications. Sample HCI topics include:

- The design of menus in a patient-controlled analgesia device.
- User satisfaction with a patient portal.
- Users' perceptions about the effectiveness of the design of clinical documentation.
- The meaning of icons.
- The design and evaluation of applications or systems to support groups of people.
- Principles of effective web design.
- Social issues in computing, such as dropping an individual from your virtual group.
- Functional allocation of work between humans and computers.
- User modeling, such as cognitive analyses of users.

Usability

Usability is a subset of HCI and one of its major components. The term usability is often used interchangeably with HCI. More formally, the classic definition is given by the international technical standard titled ISO 9241-11. Usability focuses on specific users and their goals for a specific context. It is the extent that a product can be used by users in their particular context to achieve their goals with effectiveness, efficiency, and satisfaction (International Organization for Standardization, 1998). That is, a usable product is one that allows users to achieve specific goals with a product in a specific context. Usability is multidimensional, including topics such as:

- Using a mHealth application safely, efficiently, and effectively.
- How well HIT supports the way users think and work.
- The effort needed to learn a system.
- How easy it is to remember how to use technology after time has elapsed.
- User satisfaction with any product.
- How long it takes to enter clinical notes after a patient visit or how to arrange simultaneous documentation during a visit.
- How to design error-free/error-forgiving interactions.
- Seamless fit of an information system to the task(s) at hand.

Ease of use is a rather vague notion that can imply many factors, from having a suitable screen layout and easy navigation in a system to understanding what the system is doing during interactions and having appropriate language for users within a particular context.

A health informaticist can assist in determining which aspects contribute to a usable product in given settings.

The Goals of Usability

The broad goals of usability are promoting acceptance and use of systems through improved effectiveness (including safety), efficiency, and satisfaction. These goals are achieved by optimizing the use of interactive systems and software, developing new kinds of applications to support specific work, and promoting job optimization with the use of HIT. A user interface can effectively disappear if a system is designed well. This allows users to focus only on the task at hand rather than tending to the technology itself.

Usability experts cite three main goals of HCI and usability: effectiveness; efficiency; and user satisfaction. Effectiveness is related to the usefulness of a technology in completing desired goals. It includes completeness, accuracy, and flow of information; that is, how well the function matches a user's cognitive flow of information, the flow of information among a group of users, and/or the optimal allocation of functions between human and computer.

Of course, in life-critical systems, such as a fetal-uterine monitor or medication orders, the safety of the application is paramount. For example, the accurate transfer of physiological monitoring data to an information system in labor and delivery, or the accurate display of patient medications in eMARs, is imperative.

The efficiency of systems deals with the expenditures of resources, where resources are time, productivity, error rates of users, or the costs of the system, to the organization in terms of value of the product compared to the purchase price, little-used options, or redesign of applications. Learnability is related to productivity, because better-designed systems can take less time to learn and remember.

A classic way user satisfaction can be assessed is by measuring user perceptions about the efficiency or effectiveness of interactions with the system. Users' perceptions about usability and the perceived benefits of using systems are components of satisfaction and can enhance application acceptance and use.

The Axioms of Usability

HCI authors agree on three classic axioms of usability, often called user-centered design processes, or UCD (Dix et al., 2004; Rubin & Chisnell, 2008):

- An early and central focus on users in the design and development of systems.
- Iterative design of applications.
- Systematic usability measures or observations of users interacting with information systems.

Researchers published these principles in the 1980s (Gould & Lewis, 1985). They remain pertinent and widely quoted today. An early and central focus on users means understanding users in-depth. Informaticists will want direct contact with users early and often throughout a design or redesign process. Iterative design means having rounds of design and allowing users to evaluate prototypes to determine their effectiveness and efficiency. One design is never sufficient (Nielsen, 1993). Typically, at least three rounds (or more) are necessary. Users are central to determining requirements. Once a design is available, informaticists work with users to determine issues with effectiveness and efficiency. Major usability problems can then be corrected by developers. Design and evaluation occurs in a recurring cycle. Authors stress the need for structured and systematic observations, even empirical assessments, of users as they interact with technology.

Usability and the System Life Cycle

Most authors focus usability discussions nearly exclusively on application development. However, usability axioms and user-centered design methods apply to all phases of the system's life cycle: the selection, purchase, customization, and fielding of contemporary systems. Moreover, these principles can be applied to the purchase of all products, not just electronic health records or traditional HIT applications. Thus, assessing the usability of products during purchase is paramount. Informaticists can construct time-efficient usability assessments to compare and rate products, as will be discussed later. Informaticists can perform usability tests by understanding local users, tasks, and environments. This can be critical to selecting a product and being able to customize it to its intended environment.

Human–Computer Interaction Frameworks

Human–computer interaction frameworks provide broad guidance for health informaticists to understand major elements of usability projects and usability testing. These frameworks guide health informaticists in completing user-centered design processes, usability tests, IT-adoption evaluations, and usability research. The frameworks can guide advanced usability tests from a theoretical level. In this section, we will provide an overview of existing frameworks and describe an example of one framework—the Staggers Health Human–Technology Interaction Framework.

Examples of Human–Computer Interaction Frameworks

A number of frameworks and models are available to describe the relationships between users and computer or technology interactions (Ammenwerth, Iller, & Mahler, 2006; Johnson, Johnson, & Zhang, 2005; Staggers, 2001; Yusof, Kuljis, Papazafeiropoulou, & Stergioulas, 2008; Zhang & Butler, 2007). Three well-known frameworks are explained briefly: TURF or uFURT, CoCom or Joint Cognitive Systems, and SEIPS (now in version 2.0).

TURF TURF was originally called UFuRT for user, function, representation, and task analyses. The model asserts that system knowledge is distributed across multiple users who have differences in expertise and cognitive characteristics. TURF includes a task-analysis portion to describe steps in tasks and interactions (Zhang & Butler, 2007; Zhang & Walji, 2011). However, how interactions mature is not considered a part of this framework.

JOINT COGNITIVE SYSTEMS Since the early 1980s, Woods and Hullnagel (2006) promoted a concept called cognitive systems engineering. This notion grew from the realization that sociotechnical systems—that is, complex technologies embedded within social systems—were increasingly complex, system failures were rampant, and simple HCI models did not account for interacting issues. Instead of more traditional HCI models, these authors propose a cyclical model for joint cognitive systems, called a contextual control model, or CoCom. The model is based upon users' planning and action with feedback and feedforward loops. Users are part of the whole model, and the influence of a context is direct. The distinctions of the CoCom model compared to others include that humans anticipate actions, and human behavior is seen as a plan versus single actions. Joint cognitive systems and the CoCom model imply that information is shared or distributed among humans and technology.

SEIPS 2.0 SEIPS 2.0, or systems engineering initiative for patient safety, incorporates human factors using three higher-level concepts: configuration, engagement, and adaptation (Holden et al., 2013). This model is useful for thinking about work systems and the performance of work in a sociotechnical environment. It is constructed at a much higher level of abstraction than typical HCI frameworks.

Existing frameworks are helpful but may be inadequate because they are incomplete. Frequently missing elements include (1) interactions among disparate users, (2) listing the setting or context, and (3) a developmental time for interactions. Context is critical because designs for one unit, say a rehab unit, will not fit the work of an ICU. Authors need to consider the context of the interaction within a particular unit, profession, organization, and/or social setting (Despont-Gros, Mueller, & Lovis, 2005) as well as broader concepts, such as the design of the work (Zhang & Butler, 2007). The developmental-time element allows informaticists to consider designs for both inexperienced and expert users of a particular application (Despont-Gros et al., 2005; Staggers, 2001). Critical elements for health informaticists to consider are a user's or group's characteristics, interactions, tasks (work), information, selected technology and its characteristics, the context, and development over time. The following section organizes these elements into a framework for health informatics.

The Staggers Health Human–Computer Interaction Framework

The Staggers health human–computer interaction framework builds upon initial work (Staggers & Parks, 1992, 1993) outlining a dyad of a nurse interacting with a computer. An expanded HCI framework (Staggers, 2001) extended the framework to groups of providers, patients, and other health consumers, and provider/patient interactions. Readers should note that the framework can be applied to any information technology interactions so the term computer can be interpreted broadly (Staggers, 2014).

In this framework, interactions are centered on information exchange among elements. All components act in a system of mutual influences of humans and computers (or information technology) as impacted by context and time. Provider, patient, and computer actions are a result of respective characteristics. Interactions occur within a context(s), and the interactions mature and change over time.

Humans or information technologies can initiate interactions. The initiator sends information to the user interface for viewing; for example, sending an alert to a provider's mobile device about an abnormal laboratory result for a patient in a surgical unit. From the interface, the information is processed through either the technology according to its characteristics (software and hardware) or humans according to their characteristics (expertise, age, and cognitive characteristics). The recipient then reacts to the information; for example, a provider would acknowledge the alert on the user interface and then access other functions and information to act on the alert. Technologies or humans receive the new information and process it according to their characteristics. As these iterative cycles continue, humans and computers act according to defined characteristics. Goals and outcomes are implicit in interactions.

Patient, Provider, and Computer Behaviors

Behaviors are observable and measurable actions. Examples include navigating in an EHR or, from the technology perspective, displaying requested information on a user interface. Behaviors are influenced by characteristics and by other framework elements, such as context, defining a repertoire of available behaviors.

USER INTERFACE ACTIONS A user interface (UI) allows humans and computers to cooperatively perform tasks with specific goals. User interface actions are often displayed as data or information, sound, or other observable or detectable elements. Technology-user interface actions are related to specific characteristics of embedded software and respective hardware. For instance, a provider requests data about a patient's previous encounter. The result, an interface action, is intimately related to the application software and hardware characteristics such as the elegance of the program, the complexity of the system, and speed of system and network.

CHARACTERISTICS OF PATIENTS, PROVIDERS, AND COMPUTERS Characteristics, such as human memory or attention, are attributes that are measurable but not always immediately observable. Other human characteristics could include a patient's knowledge about using his or her personal health record, age, profession, education, or frustration level. Human characteristics are a particular focus of human factors and usability. Computer (or information technology) characteristics are attributes programmed into software and related existing hardware such as accessible random-access memory, storage space, and processor power. Computer characteristics are distinct from user interface actions. Characteristics include programming attributes that determine information to be directed to the user interface while the user interface actually displays the information according to the user interface and technology characteristics.

THE TASK AND INFORMATION EXCHANGE PROCESS Either humans or computers begin the process by entering and retrieving information to complete a specific task. For example, providers may access the latest evidence about diabetes care from a highly rated app. A nurse, pharmacist, and physician cooperate in completing a medication-reconciliation process for a patient across inpatient and ambulatory records. Each task includes an explicit or implicit goal; even if the actions are to explore the system, a goal is still embedded in the process. Some behaviors and characteristics are outside any one particular task because each task accesses only a subset of all available behaviors and characteristics for elements in the framework.

HEALTH CONTEXT Interactions are contained with a context. This environment may be an actual or virtual setting; for example, a conference room for change-of-shift report on an inpatient unit or virtual work space for a team of researchers in disparate locations. The context can include more abstract elements such as cultural or political contexts, norms or mores, and associated ergonomics features such as noise. Human–technology interactions are influenced by the characteristics of these contexts. Thus, a handoff between two providers using an EHR on a quiet night shift clearly is different than a handoff on a busy unit with call bells, cell phones, and patient alarms interrupting the activity.

DEVELOPMENTAL TRAJECTORY The interactions of humans and computers (or other information technology) move along a developmental trajectory over time. Progressing in this way allows the interactions and information exchange to change over time. New human and computer technology characteristics can influence the interaction because new information is displayed and exchanged as the process matures (or degrades), according the mutual influence of elements, characteristics, and behaviors. This component of the framework is critical for the health informaticist because it acknowledges the influence of human experience and practice with technology. The informaticist will assure that naïve users—those using a selected technology for the first time—require distinct designs compared to users practiced with the application. Likewise, novices and experts need different features such as prompts and menus versus hot keys, respectively. Informaticists will know that users' initial responses to a particular design will be distinct from those practiced with it. Therefore, both perspectives are important to usability testing and design creation.

The important point for this section is that using a theoretical structure can assist informaticists in thinking about HIT adoption, usability, and the conduct of usability studies. A theoretical structure also provides an organized way of thinking about how users interact with information technology. This understanding can be applied to systems selection, design, implementation, and evaluation.

Usability Methods

UX researchers have a unique set of methods for assessing usability, and they use research techniques such as typical qualitative and quantitative designs and methods. Readers may wish to view explanations of usability-research methods available at www.usability.gov. A sample of common usability methods is discussed here. Classic references are used to provide an accurate portrayal of these foundational usability methods.

Heuristic Evaluation

Nielsen recommended a divergence away from large-scale usability studies to those with reduced numbers of users, early prototypes (even paper), and an evaluation-inspection method done by experts. He titled these "discount usability methods" (Nielsen, 1993, 1994); these are a staple in UX research. They can be completed by any health informaticist and offer economies of time, effort, and cost. Also, they can be completed at any time during the system life cycle even well after the information technology is installed.

A heuristic is a rule of thumb. **Heuristic evaluations** compare applications against accepted guidelines or published usability principles. Heuristic evaluations can reveal both major and minor usability problems that concentrate on two of the three usability goals: efficiency and effectiveness. Heuristic evaluations are typically completed by usability experts, although any informaticist can complete a heuristic evaluation after modest training. Nielsen recommends three to five experts. Each completes an independent assessment by interacting with the application and assigning usability problems to heuristic categories. The lists are consolidated, and severity scores (see Table 10-1) are assigned. The resulting lists gives designers clear problems to fix.

Several lists of usability heuristics are available (Nielsen, 1994; Shneiderman & Plaisant, 2010; Zhang, Johnson, Patel, Paige, & Kubose, 2003). Zhang et al., (2003) combined two previous guidelines into 14 heuristics, called the Nielsen-Shneiderman heuristics, and used them to evaluate infusion pumps. They found a large number of heuristic violations, some of which could contribute to medical errors. Their 14 adapted heuristics and their definitions are in Table 10-1. Once health informaticists understand the gist of each heuristic, they may evaluate any health-information technology for conformance to the heuristic categories in any phase of the system life cycle.

In addition to discount techniques, UX researchers use other methods to understand users, their tasks/goals, and usability issues with HIT.

Table 10-1   Nielsen-Shneiderman Heuristics and Severity Rating Scheme

Heuristic Category	Definition
Consistency and standards	Consistency across all aspects of the information technology such as methods of navigation, messages and actions, meaning of buttons, terms, and icons. Congruence with known screen-design principles for color, screen layout. Consistency with International Organization for Standardization (ISO) usability guidelines.
Visibility of system state	Users understand what the system is doing and what they can do with the information technology through messages, information, and displays.
Match between system and world	The information technology matches the way users think, using appropriate information flow, typical options users need, and expected actions by the system.
Minimalist	No superfluous information is presented. System-and-screen design are targeted to the primary information users need. Progressive disclosure is used to display details of a category of information only when needed. The exception can be designs for expert users, where screen density is preferred (Staggers, 1993).
Minimize memory load	The amount of information and tasks users have to memorize to adequately use the information technology is minimized. Sample formats for data input are used.
Informative feedback	The information technology provides prompt and useful feedback about users' interactions and actions.
Flexibility and efficiency	Individuals' needs can be addressed through tailoring and customizing. This includes novice and expert capabilities; for example, type-ahead and hot-links.
Good error messages	Users are told what error occurred and how to recover from the error. Messages are not abstract or general (e.g., Action not allowed). Error messages are precise and polite and do not blame the user.
Prevent errors	Catastrophic errors must be prevented; for example, medication orders with doses well above the usual range, or inadvertently deleting an order set.
Clear closure	Users should know when a task is completed, and all information is accepted.
Reversible actions	Whenever possible, actions and interactions should be able to be undone (within legal limits in electronic health records).
Use the users' language	The information technology uses language and terms the targeted users can comprehend and expect. Health terms are used appropriately.
Users in control	Users initiate actions versus having the perception that the information technology is in control. Surprising actions are avoided such as the user ending up in unexpected places, or loud sounds with errors.
Help and documentation	Help for users is provided within the context where actions occur (context-sensitive). Help functions are embedded throughout the application.
Severity Scale Rating Element	**Definition**
0—No usability problem	No need to correct the issue.
1—Cosmetic problem	Correct the issue only if extra time and fiscal resources allow, lowest priority.
2—Minor problem	Annoying issue with minor impact. Low priority to fix.
3—Major usability problem	Issue with major impact to use or training or both. Important to fix. Considerations are the numbers and kinds of users impacted by a persistent problem. Example: Orders on a patient summary are truncated when printed.
4—Usability catastrophe	Severe issue that must be corrected before product release. Example: An IV-pump button turns off the whole pump versus just one intended channel.

SOURCE: Based on Zhang, J., Johnson, T. R., Patel, V. L., Paige, D. L., & Kubose, T. (2003, February-April). Using usability heuristics to evaluate patient safety of medical devices. *Journal of Biomedical Informatics*, *36*(1–2), 23–30.

Task Analysis

This method is one of the most well-known collections of techniques in HCI and usability. The generic term, task analysis, can mean a focus on cognitive processes, observable user actions, or the interaction of a user(s) with a system. Task analysis is a systematic method to understand what users are doing or required to do with information technology. It focuses on tasks and behavioral actions between users and information technologies (Sweeney, Maguire, & Shackel, 1993). Conceptually, task analysis is the process of learning about and documenting how ordinary users complete actions in a specific context. It often involves interviewing and observing users in usability laboratories or, ideally, at their actual work sites. Task analysis is particularly useful for determining users' goals when they interact with HIT.

After observations and interviews, informaticists may record user actions in flowcharts that include task descriptions. Detailed references are available for performing task analyses (Hackos & Redish, 1998). Sample outputs from task analyses might include: a narrative of user characteristics; workflow diagrams to depict tasks and flow; descriptions of use cases; grouping information that can be used to fuel design ideas; and videotapes of users as they interact with a system using Morae software, asking users to perform specific tasks.

Task analyses are helpful in identifying task completeness, the correct or existing incorrect sequencing of tasks, accuracy of actions, error recovery, and task allocation between humans and information technologies. Task analysis can be used throughout the system life cycle to determine user requirements for design or redesign, or to identify usability issues for complex events, such as determining who in an ambulatory clinic is responsible for attending to alerts that go to various practitioners, for assessing the match of a prototype to users' methods of work, or for determining the impact of a system on workflow.

Often, task analysis is used to identify problems, whether this is early in the system life cycle or after installation. For example, researchers videotaped nurses as they interacted with an installed eMAR in an inpatient clinical-information system. Then they observed nurses perform medication tasks in several acute-care units (Staggers, Kobus, & Brown, 2007). The researchers created a task-flow diagram of medication tasks and also delineated deficiencies with the current application. A novel prototype eMAR was created after the task analysis and evaluated.

COGNITIVE WALKTHROUGH This method is a type of task analysis. Cognitive walkthrough consists of a detailed review of a sequence of real or proposed actions to complete a task in a system (Dix et al., 2004). It compares a developed user interface design (which is actually the designer's model of the tasks) to the users' understanding or model of the work to be done (Cockton, Woolrych, & Lavery, 2008). The method uses think-aloud techniques to elicit users' thought processes while using an actual product. Users, experts, or even designers step through the actions in an application and check for potential usability problems, such as the ease to learn the system through exploration versus formal training. Four questions are asked (Dix et al., 2004):

- Will the users try to achieve the correct action? If the user is to view a patient's recorded vital signs in a EHRS, will the user know what to do first (e.g., access a list of patients)?

- Will users be able to notice that the correct action is available? If the user is to pick an item off of a menu, the user probably will figure out this action easily. If an icon or image of a person is shown, will the user know this is to be selected?

- Once users find the correct action on the UI, will they know it is the right action for the effect they want? If there is a menu item labeled "patient list," the user should know to select that item. A menu item labeled "PL" may not lead the user to the correct action.

- After the action is taken, will users understand the feedback they get? After selecting the patient list, the user will know the action was correct if a dialogue box states "patient list elected," followed by a list of patients. No feedback and a delay in presenting the patient list will be less useful.

A cognitive walk-through can include audio or video taping, allowing a structured evaluation for informaticists to record findings and track problems. Categorizing problems can help designers determine priorities for application changes, especially before product release. Informaticists can also better understand users' tasks by identifying specific goals and actions for the particular task. Cognitive walkthroughs are often used early in the system life cycle to identify issues with prototypes and initial designs. They can also be used as an evaluation technique for established systems to identify usability problems and elements critical for information-technology redesign. For example, researchers in a classic study (Kushniruk, Patel, Cimino, & Barrows, 1996) used cognitive walkthroughs and think-aloud protocols to describe physicians' cognitive-information processing as they used information systems. They analyzed video recordings that included details about the physical settings and social context coupled with physicians' thought processes, and searched for key words to determine frequencies of behaviors, problems in interpreting a UI, and/or describing tasks.

Think-Aloud Protocols

Another common method in usability and HCI is a **think-aloud protocol**. In this technique, users talk aloud as they interact with an application. First, an informaticist determines a specific set of tasks for users to complete. An evaluator observes and records actions using one of the following: videotaping, audiotaping, paper notes, automatic capture of keystrokes, and/or user and evaluator paper and pencil diaries or logs (Dix et al., 2004). The result is a record of actions or a protocol which is then analyzed.

This method is commonly used in the design, redesign, development, or evaluation of applications at any time in the system life cycle. It allows a detailed examination of the specified tasks, in particular to uncover major effectiveness issues. Analyzing the products from this method can be time-consuming. Think-aloud methods may be used, and are often used, in conjunction with other usability methods. An example is a study of patients' interactions with a mHealth application for managing diabetes (Georgsson & Staggers, 2016a). Researchers asked patients to talk aloud during interactions and videotaped them. This method was compared to others in its ability to generate usability problems; think-aloud and observations generated more usability data than interviews or questionnaires.

Contextual Inquiry or Focused Ethnographies

Ethnography is a method from anthropology and sociology that includes fieldwork and analysis of people in cultural and social settings. Researchers describe the person of interest's point of view, focusing on experience and interactions in social settings rather than the actions themselves (Dourish & Button, 1998). **Contextual inquiry** is a generic term that means the informaticist interacts with users in their actual sites or field settings. Researchers concentrate on individuals' points of view—their experiences and interactions in social settings—rather than on just the actions of those individuals (Hammersley & Atkinson, 2007; Viitanen, 2011). In these techniques, the informatics researcher is an observer and not a participant in the setting. Detailed descriptions are generated with an emphasis on tools (artifacts), work-arounds, and other usability issues. In UX and elsewhere, contextual inquiry is a focused description of users' experiences, from their point of view, in their own settings.

Contextual inquiry and ethnographies are important to understand how HIT impacts workers and work. In a set of classic studies, Ash and colleagues used this method extensively to understand the impacts of computerized provider order entry (CPOE) in acute-care facilities (Ash, Sittig, Dykstra, Campbell, & Guappone, 2007; Ash et al., 2009; Ash, Sittig, Poon, et al., 2007). Their observations were complemented by interviews and focus groups. They found numerous unintended consequences of CPOE to include new work and more work, workflow issues, system demands, communication, emotions, and dependence on the technology. While not always feasible, informaticists are wise to observe users in their actual settings whenever possible. This provides depth of understanding of HIT use and usability issues.

Usability Questionnaires

Informaticists can assess users' perceptions of usability with short questionnaires. At least two examples of this type of questionnaire are available: the QUIS or Questionnaire for User Interaction Satisfaction (Norman, Shneiderman, Harper, & Slaughter, 1998) and the SUS or System Usability Scale (Bangor, Kortum, & Miller, 2008). The QUIS addresses users' perceptions of an information system for areas such as overall reaction, terminology, screen layout, learning, system capabilities, and other subscales such as multimedia applications. The instrument demonstrates adequate psychometric evaluations for internal consistency reliability and construct validity. QUIS subscales can be mixed and matched to fit the application at hand. For example, nurses completed the QUIS in five to ten minutes and indicated the new design had good usability (Staggers et al., 2007).

The SUS is commonly used outside healthcare but is being employed more often in usability studies for HIT. In fact, UX professionals consider the SUS an industry standard; it has been used widely on a variety of products outside of and internal to healthcare (Bangor et al., 2008; Sauro, 2011). The SUS is a publicly available, ten-item scale developed in 1986 by John Brooke at Digital Equipment Corporation (Bangor et al., 2008).

Usability Tests

How do you conduct a usability test? When do you perform one? Do you have to be an expert or a researcher to conduct a usability testing? This section answers these questions. Generally, usability tests are systematic and structured examinations of the effectiveness, efficiency, or satisfaction of any component in a HCI framework(s). For instance, a usability study could be done to describe the satisfaction and usability issues with a new CPOE application targeted to emergency-room providers (Zafar, Gibson, Chiang, & Staggers, 2010), or a usability test might evaluate the time on task and errors patients make when they use a mHealth application to manage their Type-2 diabetes (Georgsson & Staggers, 2016b).

Usability tests can be informal or formal, simple or complex, and use a few individuals or a large number and variety of users. The exciting part of usability is that informaticists can derive rich details about application usability using only a few participants. Likewise, usability researchers can design sophisticated studies combining usability precepts with traditional experimental, or mixed-methods, research designs. The type of usability study an informaticist conducts is dependent upon a number of factors, including where the assessment is targeted within the systems life cycle, desired outcome of the study, and available resources including time, people, and money.

Usability tests can be done at any point in the system life cycle, from clarifying users' requirements; to initial design or redesign using paper prototypes or simple computerized applications; to iterative prototype development, system selection, product customization; to evaluating the impact of a system during and after installation. *Usability experts recommend usability tests early and often.* Studies are divided in this section into formative and summative tests; that is, early in development and when development is nearly complete. Informaticists can match these types of studies to the constraints of available resources, the position in the system life cycle, and outcomes needed.

Formative Usability Tests

Formative usability tests can help determine or clarify determination of users' requirements, and assess the adequacy of a design or redesign earlier in the systems' life cycle. Formative usability tests are completed as ideas are beginning to be coded or when redesign of a fielded product is needed.

SIMPLIFIED USABILITY TESTS USING EARLY PROTOTYPES Nielsen's (1993) discount usability techniques include the use of small numbers of users; typically, an early prototype (even paper) and the think-aloud protocol described earlier. Nielsen advocates the use of qualitative methods early and often during any design or redesign process. He recommends having five users talk aloud or think aloud as an observer watches and records any issues. The process can detect as much as 60–80% of design errors (Nielsen, 1994). Later research confirmed that as few as five-to-eight users are sufficient for most early usability tests (Dumas & Fox, 2008).

DETERMINING USER NEEDS AND REQUIREMENTS This type of usability is typically conducted at the beginning of the system life cycle or redesign cycle to elicit users' characteristics, task activities, work design, interactions among users and tasks in specific environments, and particular needs related to the context of interactions. Usability tests can be conducted with fairly limited resources but, depending upon the scope of the project and complexity of the elements, may consume a more substantial amount of time and effort. Assessments and exploratory work answer these kinds of questions (Rubin & Chisnell, 2008):

- What are basic activities in this context?
- How do users cognitively process information, and what information processing can be supported by information technology?
- What special considerations should be made for users in this environment?
- What attributes need to be in place for an initial design?

An example is determining requirements for an application to support nurses during change-of-shift report. This cognitively intense time period includes determining information about the users (novice, expert; oncoming nurse or nurse giving report; whether nurses had the patient before), the interactions (what information is typically exchanged), the technology (paper, mobile, or stationary device), the context (the type of patients usually seen on this unit; the mandates from the organization such as the use of CPOE), and the developmental component (novice or expert clinical-documentation user).

A health informaticist could observe nurses giving report, taking notes about the computer functions they access, if any; audiotape the report and analyze information typically conveyed; and listen to nurses' responses to questions about whether shift report should be computerized. From this analysis, preliminary requirements can be developed. Such a study is available that analyzed the content and context of shift report for medical and surgical units (Staggers, Clark, Blaz, & Kapsandoy, 2011, 2012).

EXPLORATORY TEST This type of usability study is conducted early during development or redesign after very basic or preliminary designs are created. These can be paper-based. Because exploratory tests occur early in the development process, few programming resources are committed to the project and changes are easier to effect. The objective of an exploratory test is to evaluate the effectiveness of the emerging design concepts being assessed (Rubin & Chisnell, 2008) and a small number of participants can be used. Typical questions are:

- Is the basic functionality of value to users?
- Is basic navigation and information flow intuitive?
- How much computer experience does a user need to use this module?

Exploratory tests can be informal and require extensive interaction between informaticists and users. The major usability goal of interest is *effectiveness*. Informaticists have users perform common tasks with the prototype or step through paper mockups of the application. They may use think-aloud, observation, and audio-video-recordings. Informaticists strive to understand *why* users are behaving as they do with the application rather than how quickly the prototype completes a task. The informaticist is interested in finding cognitive disconnects with basic functions, finding missing information or steps, and assessing how easily users understand the task at hand once it is represented by designers.

ASSESSMENT TEST Another type of usability test is conducted early or midway into the development of an application, after the organization and general design are already determined (Rubin & Chisnell, 2008). This kind of test can be economical in terms of time and resources, depending upon the complexity of design and targeted users. An assessment test appraises lower-level operations of the application, stressing the efficiency goals of the product (versus effectiveness), and how well the task is presented to a small number of users. Questions during this test might include:

- How well can users perform selected tasks?
- Are the terms in the system consistent across modules?
- Are operations displayed in a manner that allows quick detection of critical information?

During an assessment test, users perform common tasks on a system with a coded prototype. Some quantitative measures of the interaction, such as error rates, are captured and analyzed. Think-aloud methods can also be used to elicit issues. Information-technology designers use iterative processes—typically three rounds of design—to eliminate major usability issues.

Summative Usability Tests

Usability testing can be as advanced as an informaticist or researcher wants, depending upon the desired results, resources, and the location of the design in the system life cycle. Typical usability testing includes validation and comparison tests but can be combined with any suitable research design. Summative testing is often completed against benchmarks and objective measures. For summative tests, at least 15 users are recommended (Virzi, 1992). Table 10-2 outlines sample measurements for summative usability tests.

VALIDATION TEST Late in the system design cycle, a validation test can be conducted. Using a more mature product, a validation test assesses how this particular product compares to a predetermined standard, benchmark, or performance measure (Rubin & Chisnell, 2008). A second purpose can be to assess how all the modules in an information-technology application work as an integrated whole. Questions for a validation test might be:

Table 10-2 Taxonomy of Usability Measures

Usability Focus	Usability Measures
User behaviors (performance)	Task times (speed, reaction times)
	Percentage of tasks completed
	Number and kinds of errors
	Percentage of tasks completed accurately
	Time and frequency spent in any one option
	Number of hits and amount of time spent on a website
	Training time
	Eye tracking
	Facial expressions
	Breadth and depth of application usage in actual settings
	Quality of completed tasks (e.g., quality of decisions)
	Users' comments (think-aloud) as they interact with technology
	System setup or installation time, complexity of setup
	Model of tasks and user behaviors
	Description of problems when interacting with an application
User behaviors (cognitive)	Description of or system fit with cognitive information processing
	Retention of application knowledge over time
	Comprehension of system
	Fit with workflow
User behaviors (perceptions)	Usability ratings of products
	Perceptions about any aspect of technology—speed, effectiveness
	Comments during interviews
	Questionnaires and rating responses—workload, satisfaction
User behaviors (physiologic)	Heart rate
	EEG
	Galvanic skin response
	Brain-evoked potentials
User behaviors (perceptions about physiologic reactions)	Perceptions about anxiety, stress
User behavior (motivation)	Willingness to use system
	Enthusiasm
Expert evaluations (performance)	Model predictions for task performance times, learning, ease of understanding
	Observations of users as they use applications in a setting to determine fit with work
Expert evaluations (conformance to guidelines)	Level of adherence to guidelines, design criteria, usability principles (heuristic evaluation)
Expert evaluation (perception)	Ratings of technology, informal or formal comments
Context (organization)	Economic costs (increased full-time equivalent positions for the helpdesk for a new application)
	Support staff, training staff for application or technology
	Observations about the fit with work design, workflow in departments, organizations, networks of institutions
Combined	Video-and audio-taping users as they interact with an application and capturing key-strokes. Can capture any combination of the above.

SOURCE: From Taxonomy of Usability Measures by Staggers, N. in Health Care Informatics: An Interdisciplinary Approach by Sheila P. Englebardt and Ramona Nelson. Copyright © 2001 by Elsevier.

- Can 80% of the users retrieve the correct radiology test within 15 seconds of interacting with the system?

- Does the product adhere to the usability principles defined by Nielsen (1994) or Dix et al. (2004)?

- Are there major or catastrophic usability issues with an electronic medication administration record?

Validation tests are typically more structured and preclude extensive interactions with informaticists or developers. An informaticist determines the specific benchmarks or standards before the test begins. Methods for a validation test can be similar in rigor to those in an experimental study, or they might be an assessment against criteria made before the testing begins (a hospitalist should be able to access a patient's full medication list in less than two seconds, for example). A validation test could also be useful in a system-selection process as decision makers could use it to decide how a new vendor fares against pre-set benchmarks and supports critical tasks such as medication barcoding or decision support within CPOE.

COMPARISON TEST Informaticists can conduct comparison studies anywhere in the system life cycle. Comparison tests can be used to assess different information technologies or compare the elegance of designs from two vendors for chemotherapy protocols. Comparison tests can consume time and other resources. The major objective of this usability test is to determine which application or information technology is more efficient or effective (Rubin & Chisnell, 2008). The design can be informal exploratory or assessment tests or a formal design with objective outcome measures such as time-on-task and errors. Designs are more easily compared if the designs are substantially different from one another.

Steps in Conducting Usability Tests

Readers of this text are likely to be expected to conduct usability tests. Excellent, step-by-step guides are available (Healthcare Information and Management Systems Society, 2009; National Institute of Standards and Technology, 2011; Rubin & Chisnell, 2008). When conducting a usability test, informaticists should consider these five steps:

- *Define a clear purpose.* The specific purpose will guide readers in determining the type of study, the details, and methods required. Is the purpose to define user requirements for clinical documentation for team members in a busy rehabilitation hospital? Select a vendor's system to support practitioner activities in an orthopedic center? Evaluate the effectiveness of a newly designed telehealth system? Each of these purposes is distinct and will point to selecting differing designs and methods for completion. For example, if the purpose relates to an assessment of a redesign of a CPOE module for the emergency-department practitioners or a mHealth application, an exploratory test may be indicated.

- *Assess constraints.* Informaticists are always faced with study constraints—time; resources; availability of the software to be evaluated; availability of other equipment such as video cameras, testing labs, or users themselves, especially if the users are physicians or other specialists. These kinds of constraints may drive a section of or even the whole usability test. For example, if the goal is to evaluate an application to support transplant surgeons, these busy surgeons may not be willing to spend time in a usability test lasting more than 30 minutes.

- *Use an HCI framework to refine each component.* Assess each component of the framework and match to the purpose of the study. Which users are most appropriate? What are representative, common tasks? What element of the tasks is of interest? What information needs to be exchanged; for example, between physicians and nurses during a phone call about a patient issue? What information-technology characteristics are needed and which actions? What setting or context? Will a naturalistic setting help determine exactly how an application will be used, or will a laboratory be used to control typical interruptions? What is a representative time in the developmental trajectory, or is there more than one? If the informaticists are doing a comparison study using a new and old version, how will equivalent practice be assured? The latter is a typical mistake for new usability testers. Be sure to examine this component carefully to ensure a valid comparison. The most important point is to remember that multiple tests are needed for each product being designed or redesigned.

- *Emphasize components of interest.* Informaticists will want to control some framework components and emphasize others for testing. With experimental or other more-rigorous tests, readers will want to ensure that they are measuring only what they want to know in a particular test. For example, if the purpose is to compare the efficiency (speed) of a user interface for robotic-assisted surgeries, informaticists will want to control for equivalency in computer processors, type of users, and context. In other usability studies, informaticists may wish to test a whole team of users in the complexity of their real environments; for instance, to determine the time constraints for clinical documentation during and after a code in an acute-care unit.

- *Match methods to the purpose, constraints, and framework assessment.* Selecting methods occurs after the previous steps. Early in the system life cycle, or for example, when little is understood about why users declined to use a module designed for perioperative care, a method that produces rich results would be selected—a think-aloud protocol, a contextual-inquiry observation with clarifying questions, or a cognitive walkthrough. If the purpose of the usability study is to validate a near-final design for a patient portal, completing a validation test using interaction-task times and errors with patients may be more appropriate. Once the method is selected, the informaticist puts all these pieces into action and conduct the study. The following examples show usability studies for a heuristic evaluation, requirements determination, and a comparison usability test.

Example of a Heuristic Evaluation

The purpose of this discount usability test was to determine whether an eMAR used by Veterans' Administration nurses conformed to heuristic evaluation (HE) categories (Staggers et al., 2015). The constraints for this study were time and lack of robust funding for observations. The team chose the HE method because of the constraints and because this descriptive study would add to knowledge about eMARs, an understudied and critical topic. Three nurse informaticists were trained in HE techniques, completed training on this eMAR, and defined typical tasks for medication planning and administration. These experts followed typical HE methods by completing their assessments separately and meeting to resolve any differences. A consolidated list of heuristic violations was created and given severity ratings. A lengthy list of usability issues was created to guide future redesign.

Example of a Requirements Determination Usability Study

Researchers completed a study to begin requirements determination to support nurses' thinking and activity planning during change-of-shift report: a highly complex and cognitively intensive period. Nurses going off-shift synthesize information about patients and communicate it to nurses coming on shift (Staggers et al., 2012). Constraints included having research funding to observe and interview about 25 participants. The authors chose the type of study (requirements determination) and methods (qualitative) to obtain rich details about the complex process. The HCI framework guided the authors to think about requirements for different nurses—experts and novices, types of units, and types of nurse such as per diem. The task component guided thoughts about different methods of giving report such as face-to-face and bedside reports. The authors sampled widely across medical-surgical units to assure various nurses and reports were included in the test. The researchers used contextual-inquiry observations, audio recording and taking field notes on five medical-surgical units, 93 handoffs, and 26 nurses. They found few nurses used an electronic handoff form, preferring paper; nurses need at-a-glance information; and nurses modified paper tools for individual needs. These findings resulted in requirements for future electronic handoff forms (Staggers et al., 2011).

Example of a Comparison Study

The purpose of this study was to determine whether nurses performed more efficiently and effectively and had improved user satisfaction with a new user interface for orders' management compared to an older interface. Performance measures were task time, errors, and user satisfaction (Staggers & Kobus, 2000). The major constraint in this study was the availability of busy nurses at the tertiary-care center. The tasks and interactions were planned to minimize the amount of time to 45 minutes to minimize time away from patient care. The HCI framework guided the test. Identical computers were used to test both interfaces. These were disconnected from the local-area network to assure that system network loads did not affect processing times. Tasks were real-world nursing orders that any nurse could understand, and the tasks were the same across designs. Only clinical nurses were included in the study. The environment was a quiet room away from patient-care units and distractions. The developmental trajectory was considered in this study to assure that results were not impacted by practice time. Based on pilot work, 40 tasks for each interface allowed nurses to become practiced with each user interface. Tasks, keystrokes, and errors were captured by computer. The QUIS was administered after each interface. Each nurse interacted with both interfaces, but the order of interface presentation was randomized. The results showed a significant difference for all three variables—performance speed, errors, and user satisfaction for the new design.

Future Directions

Clearly, current interest will continue to create solutions to HIT usability problems. Several major EHRS vendors now employ UX researchers, so user-centered design techniques are becoming more common. With the wide-spread EHRS installations and the increase in mHealth applications, usability is critical enough that accelerated expansion in the future is imperative.

Informaticists will face even more complexity in system design and concomitant usability issues. New users, such as increasing numbers of health consumers, patients, and interacting groups of users, will need to be accommodated. New types of information—in particular genetic and nanomaterials—will create layers of complexity beyond current sociotechnical-system issues.

As information technology disappears into everyday action and objects, ubiquitous computing may become a reality. Informaticists focused on usability will likely have challenges and novel solutions for ubiquitous computing in the future.

Computer-supported cooperative work for empowered patients deserves more attention in the future. This area focuses on people as they act in their normal lives, including work lives. Support of tasks becomes intertwined with patterns of group behaviors as reflected by social or situational contexts. Examples here include the growth of groups of people as they act in virtual worlds, create health blogs, and work in virtual teams. Designing for usability is just beginning; its future is assured.

Case Study Exercise

Your facility has a history of adopting HIT that is not well received or used by the staff. Leaders recently determined that mHealth applications for patients with chronic conditions such as diabetes and heart disease will be developed in the near future. In your role as an informatics nurse, what actions would you take to ensure usability is incorporated into the development process to assure better adoption and use?

SUMMARY

- Current usability issues in health information technology (HIT) applications include unintended consequences and new errors, high costs associated with unusable systems, increased maintenance issues, and reduced practitioner productivity.
- The term *usability* is often used interchangeably with *human–computer interaction (HCI)*. More formally, usability is the extent to which a product can be used by specific users in a specific context to achieve predefined goals with effectiveness, efficiency, and satisfaction.
- Usability goals include creating HIT for improved user efficiency, effectiveness, and satisfaction. HIT outcomes include improved patient safety and decision making.
- Three axioms of usability or user-centered design principles are an early and central focus on users in the design and development of systems, iterative design of applications, and systematic usability measures.
- HCI frameworks include the major elements of patients, practitioners, technology, context, tasks, information, interactions, and a developmental trajectory.
- Usability tests are systematic and structured examinations of the effectiveness, efficiency, or satisfaction of any component or interactions in the HCI framework(s).
- Usability tests can be done at any point in the system life cycle, although experts recommend they be done early and often. Informaticists need to match the type of study to the constraints of available resources.
- Any informaticist can learn and conduct discount usability tests, using usability inspection techniques, small-scale prototypes, and reduced numbers of users.
- Usability tests vary from scaled-down studies and methods that offer economies of time and effort such as heuristic evaluations to more detailed tests comparing applications against benchmarks.
- Common usability methods include heuristic evaluations, think-aloud protocols, task analysis, cognitive walkthroughs, contextual inquiries, focused ethnographies, and usability questionnaires.
- Five steps for planning and conducting usability tests include:
  - Definition of purpose
  - Assessment of constraints
  - Use of an HCI framework to refine each component
  - Emphasis on components of interest
  - Matching methods to the purpose, constraints, and framework assessment.
- Expanding interest in usability, increased complexity of systems, ubiquitous computing, and computer-supported cooperative work ensure a role for informaticists in assessing usability in the future.

About the Author

Nancy Staggers, PhD, RN, FAAN is an international expert in clinical informatics. Her background includes leading enterprise EHR projects in Department of Defense and elsewhere, writing on foundational NI topics and having a research program on improving HIT usability. She received the designation as a NI pioneer in 2006 and received the Virginia K. Saba award from AMIA for her NI career in 2013.

References

Ammenwerth, E., Iller, C., & Mahler, C. (2006). IT-adoption and the interaction of task, technology and individuals: A FIT framework and a case study. *BioMed Central, 6*(3), 1–13.

Ash, J. S., Sittig, D. F., Dykstra, R., Campbell, E., & Guappone, K. (2007). Exploring the unintended consequences of computerized physician order entry. *Studies in Health Technology and Informatics, 129*(Pt 1), 198–202.

Ash, J. S., Sittig, D. F., Dykstra, R., Campbell, E., & Guappone, K. (2009). The unintended consequences of computerized provider order entry: Findings from a mixed methods exploration. *International Jounal of Medical Informatics, 78 Suppl 1*, S69–76. doi:S1386-5056(08)00133-0 [pii]. 7y10.1016/j.ijmedinf.2008.07.015

Ash, J. S., Sittig, D. F., Poon, E. G., Guappone, K., Campbell, E., & Dykstra, R. H. (2007). The extent and importance of unintended consequences related to computerized provider order entry. *Journal of the American Medical Informatics Association, 14*(4), 415–423. doi:M2373 [pii]. 10.1197/jamia.M2373

Bangor, A., Kortum, P., & Miller, J. T. (2008). An empirical evaluation of the system usability scale. *International Journal of Human-Computer Interaction, 24*(6), 574–594.

Carayon, P., Xie, A., & Kianfar, S. (2014). Human factors and ergonomics as a patient safety practice. *British Journal of Quality & Safety, 23*(3), 196–205. doi:10.1136/bmjqs-2013-001812

Cockton, G., Woolrych, A., & Lavery, D. (2008). Inspection-based evaluations. In A. Sears & J. Jacko (Eds.), *The Human-Computer Interaction Handbook: Fundamentals, Evolving Technologies and Emerging Applications*, (2nd ed., pp. 1172–1188). New York: Lawrence Erlbaum.

Despont-Gros, C., Mueller, H., & Lovis, C. (2005). Evaluating user interactions with clinical information systems: A model based on human-computer interaction models. *Journal of Biomedical Informatics, 38*(3), 244–255. doi:S1532-0464(04)00171-6 [pii] 10.1016/j.jbi.2004.12.004

Dix, A., Finlay, J. E., Abowd, G. D., & Beale, R. (2004). *Human-computer interaction* (3rd ed.). Essex, England: Prentice Hall, © 2004.

Dourish, P., & Button, G. (1998). On "technomethodology": Foundational relationships between ethnomethodology and system design. *Human-Computer Interaction, 13*, 395–432.

Drews, F. A., & Westenskow, D. R. (2006). The right picture is worth a thousand numbers: Data displays in anesthesia. *Human Factors, 48*(1), 59–71.

Dumas, J. S., & Fox, J. E. (2008). Usability testing: Current practice and future directions. In A. Sears & J. Jacko (Eds.), *The Human-Computer Interaction Handbook: Fundamentals, Evolving Technologies and Emerging Applications* (2nd ed., pp. 1129–1149). New York: Lawrence Erlbaum.

Georgsson, M., & Staggers, N. (2016a). An evaluation of patients' experienced usability of a diabetes mHealth system using a multi-method approach. *Journal of Biomedical Informatics, 59*, 115–129. doi:10.1016/j.jbi.2015.11.008

Georgsson, M., & Staggers, N. (2016b). Quantifying usability: An evaluation of a diabetes mHealth system on effectiveness, efficiency, and satisfaction metrics with associated user characteristics. *Journal of the American Medical Informatics Association, 23*(1), 5–11. doi:10.1093/jamia/ocv099

Gould, J., & Lewis, C. (1985). Designing for usability: Key principles and what designers think. *Communications of the ACM, 28*(3), 300–311.

Guo, J., Iribarren, S., Kapsandoy, S., Perri, S., & Staggers, N. (2011). Usability evaluation of an electronic medication administration record (eMAR) application. *Applied Clinical Informatics, 2*(2), 202–224. doi:10.4338/ACI-2011-01-RA-0004

Hackos, J. T., & Redish, J. C. (1998). *User and task analysis for interface design.* New York: John Wiley & Sons.

Hammersley, M., & Atkinson, P. (2007). *Ethnography: Principles in practice* (Vol. 3rd ed.). London: Routledge.

Hardmeier, A., Tsourounis, C., Moore, M., Abbott, W. E., & Guglielmo, B. J. (2014). Pediatric medication administration errors and workflow following implementation of a bar code medication administration system. *Journal of Healthcare Quality, 36*(4), 54–61; quiz 61–53. doi:10.1111/jhq.12071

Healthcare Information and Management Systems Society (HIMSS). (2009). *Defining and testing EMR usability: Prinicples and proposed methods of EMR usability evaluation and rating.* Retrieved from www.himss.org/ResourceLibrary/GenResourceDetail. aspx?ItemNumber=39192

HIMSS Usability Task Force. (2011). *Promoting usability in health organizations: Initial steps and progress toward a healthcare usability maturity model.* Healthcare Information and Management Systems Society. Retrieved http://s3.amazonaws.com/rdcms-himss/files/production/public/HIMSSorg/Content/files/HIMSS_Promoting_Usability_in_Health_Org.pdf

HIT User Experience Committee. (2016). *Contemporary nursing UX issues & proposed solutions. A view from the experts.* Healthcare Information & Management Systems Society. Retrieved from www.himss.org/contemporary-nursing-ux-issues-proposed-solutions

Holden, R. J., Carayon, P., Gurses, A. P., Hoonakker, P., Hundt, A. S., Ozok, A. A., & Rivera-Rodriguez, A. J. (2013). SEIPS 2.0: A human factors framework for studying and improving the work of healthcare professionals and patients. *Ergonomics, 56*(11), 1669–1686. doi:10.1080/00140139.2013.838643

Human Factors and Ergonomics Society (HFES). (2012). Definitions of human factors and ergonomics. Retrieved from www.hfes.org/Web/EducationalResources/HFEdefinitionsmain.html#govagencies

International Organization for Standardization (ISO). (1998). ISO 9241–11. Retrieved from www.usabilitynet.org/tools/r_international.htm#9241–11

Johnson, C. M., Johnson, T. R., & Zhang, J. (2005). A user-centered framework for redesigning health care interfaces. *Journal of Biomedical Informatics, 38*(1), 75–87. doi:S1532-0464(04)00153-4 [pii]10.1016/j.jbi.2004.11.005

Koch, S. H., Weir, C., Haar, M., Staggers, N., Agutter, J., Gorges, M., & Westenskow, D. (2012). Intensive care unit nurses' information needs and recommendations for integrated displays to improve nurses' situation awareness. *Journal of the American Medical Informatics Association, 19(4),* 583–590. doi:amiajnl-2011-000678 [pii]. 10.1136/amiajnl-2011-000678

Koppel, R., Metlay, J. P., Cohen, A., Abaluck, B., Localio, A. R., Kimmel, S. E., & Strom, B. L. (2005). Role of computerized physician order entry systems in facilitating medication errors. *Journal of the American Medical Association, 293*(10), 1197–1203. doi:293/10/1197 [pii]. 10.1001/jama.293.10.1197

Kuniavsky, M. (2003). *Observing the user experience: A practitioner's guide to user research*. San Francisco: Morgan Kaufmann Publishers (Elsevier).

Kushniruk, A., Patel, V., Cimino, J. J., & Barrows, R. A. (1996). Cognitive evaluation of the user interface and vocabulary of an outpatient information system. *Proceedings of the AMIA Annual Fall Symposium*, pp. 22–26.

National Institute of Standards and Technology. (2011). Technical evaluation, testing and validation of electronic health records (NISTIR 7804). Retrieved from www.nist.gov/healthcare/usability/

Nielsen, J. (1993). *Usability engineering*. Cambridge, MA: AP Professional.

Nielsen, J. (1994). Heuristic evaluation. In J. Nielsen & R. L. Mack (Eds.), *Usability inspection methods* (pp. 25–62). New York: John Wiley & Sons, Inc.

Norman, D. (1988). *The psychology of everyday things*. New York: Basic Books.

Norman, K., Shneiderman, B., Harper, B., & Slaughter, L. (1998). Questionnaire for user interaction satisfaction, version 7.0. Retrieved from http://lap.umd.edu/quis/

Rubin, J., & Chisnell, D. (2008). *Handbook of usability testing: How to plan, design and conduct effective tests*. New York: John Wiley & Sons, Inc, 2008.

Sauro, J. (2011). Measuring usability with the system usability scale (SUS). Retrieved from www.measuringusability.com/sus.php

Schaffer, E. (2010). Is usability different than the user experience? *HFI Connect: User Experience for a Better World*. Retrieved from http://connect.humanfactors.com/profiles/blogs/is-user-experience-different

Shneiderman, B., & Plaisant, C. (2010). *Designing the user interace: Strategies for effective human-computer interaction* (5th ed., pp. 74–76.). Boston: Addison-Wesley.

Slight, S. P., Eguale, T., Amato, M. G., Seger, A. C., Whitney, D. L., Bates, D. W., & Schiff, G. D. (2016). The vulnerabilities of computerized physician order entry systems: A qualitative study. *Journal of the American Medical Informatics Association*, 23(2), 311–316. doi:10.1093/jamia/ocv135

Staggers, N. (2001). Human-computer interaction. In S. Englebardt & R. Nelson (Eds.), *Information technology in health care: An interdisciplinary approach* (pp. 321–345). Harcourt Health Science Company.

Staggers, N. (2014). Improving the user experience for health information technology. In R. Nelson & N. Staggers (Eds.). *Health informatics. An interdisciplinary approach*, 2nd. ed. Chicago: Mosby(pp, 352-269).

Staggers, N., Clark, L., Blaz, J. W., & Kapsandoy, S. (2011). Why patient summaries in electronic health records do not provide the cognitive support necessary for nurses' handoffs on medical and surgical units: Insights from interviews and observations. *Health Informatics Journal, 17*(3), 209–223. doi:17/3/209 [pii] 10.1177/1460458211405809

Staggers, N., Clark, L., Blaz, J. W., & Kapsandoy, S. (2012). Nurses' information management and use of electronic tools during acute care handoffs. *Western Journal of Nursing Research, 34*(2), 153–173. doi:0193945911407089 [pii]. 10.1177/019394591 1407089

Staggers, N., Elias, B., Makar, E., Hunt, J., & Alexander, G. (2016). Identifying nurses' health IT pain points and solutions: Preliminary findings. *Lecture Notes in Computer Science*, (9737 2016)7, 203–214. Springer.

Staggers, N., Iribarren, S., Guo, J. W., & Weir, C. (2015). Evaluation of a BCMA's electronic medication administration record. *Western Journal of Nursing Research*, 37(7), 899–921. DOI: 10.1177/0193945914566641

Staggers, N., & Kobus, D. (2000). Comparing response time, errors, and satisfaction between text-based and graphical user interfaces during nursing order tasks. *Journal of the American Medical Informatics Association, 7*(2), 164–176.

Staggers, N., Kobus, D., & Brown, C. (2007). Nurses' evaluations of a novel design for an electronic medication administration record. *CIN: Computers, Informatics, Nursing, 25*(2), 67–75.

Staggers, N., & Parks, P. L. (1992). Collaboration between unlikely disciplines in the creation of a conceptual framework for nurse-computer interactions. *Proceedings of the Annual Symposium on Computer Applications in Medical Care*, 661–665.

Staggers, N., & Parks, P. L. (1993). Description and initial applications of the Staggers & Parks Nurse-Computer Interaction Framework. *CIN: Computers, Informatics, Nursing, 11*(6), 282–290.

Stead, W., & Lin, H. (2009). *Computational technology for effective healthcare: Immediate steps and strategic directions.* Washington, DC: National Academies Press.

Sweeney, M., Maguire, M., & Shackel, B. (1993). Evaluating user-computer interaction: A framework. *International Journal of Man-Machine Studies, 38*, 689–711.

The Joint Commission (TJC). (March 31, 2015). Safe use of health information technology. Retrieved from www.jointcommission.org

Viitanen, J. (2011). Contextual inquiry method for user-centred clinical IT system design. *Studies in Health Technology and Informatics, 169*, 965–969.

Virzi, R. A. (1992). Refining the test phase of usaiblity evaluation: How many subjects is enough? *Human Factors, 34*, 457–468.

Wachter, S. B., Johnson, K., Albert, R., Syroid, N., Drews, F., & Westenskow, D. (2006). The evaluation of a pulmonary display to detect adverse respiratory events using high resolution human simulator. *Journal of the American Medical Informatics Association, 13*(6), 635–642. doi:M2123 [pii] 10.1197/jamia.M2123

Woods, D. & Hollnagel, E. (2006). Joint cognitive systems: Patterns in cognitive systems engineering. Boca Raton, FL.: CRC Press.

Yusof, M. M., Kuljis, J., Papazafeiropoulou, A., & Stergioulas, L. K. (2008). An evaluation framework for health information systems: Human, organization and technology-fit factors (HOT-fit). *International Journal of Medical Informatics, 77*(6), 386–398. doi:S1386-5056(07)00160-8 [pii] 10.1016/j.ijmedinf.2007.08.011

Zafar, N., Gibson, B., Chiang, Y., & Staggers, N. (2010). *A usability evaluation of Cerner FirstNet at the University of Utah Hospital.* Paper session presented at NLM Informatics Training Conference 2010, University of Colorado Anschutz Medical Campus, Boulder, CO.

Zhang, J., & Butler, K. A. (July 22–27, 2007). *UFuRT: A work-centered framework and process for design and evaluation of information systems.* Paper session presented at HCI International 2007, Beijing, China.

Zhang, J., Johnson, T. R., Patel, V. L., Paige, D. L., & Kubose, T. (2003). Using usability heuristics to evaluate patient safety of medical devices. *Journal of Biomedical Informatics, 36*(1-2), 23–30. doi:S1532046403000601 [pii]

Zhang, J., & Walji, M. F. (2011). TURF: Toward a unified framework of EHR usability. *Journal of Biomedical Informatics, 44*(6), 1056–1067. doi:10.1016/j.jbi.2011.08.005

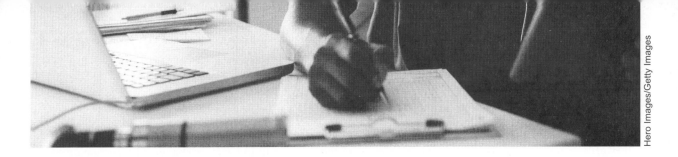

Chapter 11
System Implementation, Maintenance, and Evaluation

Sue Evans MSN RN-BC

 ## Learning Objectives

After completing this chapter, you should be able to:

- Discuss the significance of change in a culture.

- Describe the barriers to implementation.

- Illustrate ways that implementation-committee members are selected.

- Review the importance of establishing a project timeline or schedule.

- List the decisions that must be addressed when performing an analysis of hardware requirements.

- Discuss the "go-live" process and identify the components involved in planning for it.

- Identify variables that must be considered in the testing process.

- Summarize several common implementation pitfalls.

- Explain the significance of providing ongoing system and technical maintenance.

- Provide examples that show the cyclical nature of the information system life cycle.

- Explain the role of the nurse informaticist in the implementation and evaluation processes.

Chapter 9 discussed the first two phases of the life cycle of an information system. This chapter explores system implementation and maintenance, which make up the third and fourth phases. It also touches upon the evaluation process.

System Implementation

System implementation requires change. In fact, introducing an innovation is similar to tossing a pebble in a quiet pond. Inevitably, that single stone generates ripples across the pond. The ripples impact other aspects of the pond, resulting in more change. This section presents changes required for a system implementation.

Changing a Culture

Once people in an organization no longer feel comfortable with the current state of the organization's service culture and begin to believe that fundamental change in how the organization designs and delivers care is crucial to raising the level of quality, they start to feel activated and begin to move toward change (Coplan & Masuda, 2011). Having said that, the only thing we can be certain of is that change is constant. In a classic work that remains relevant today, Kotter (1996) described the journey of change in his model, as one that includes defined steps to achieve a change in culture at the organizational level. People resist change for many reasons, and understanding these reasons and accepting their existence is paramount to the success of the implementation process. There are other theories, models, and sciences that contribute to a successful organizational shift that the informatics nurse should also be familiar with. These include, but are not limited to, Rogers' diffusion of innovation theory, and implementation science (Leeman, Birken, Powell, Rohweder, & Shea, 2017; Nilsson, Borg, & Eriksen, 2014; Rogers, 1983). Boxes 11-1 and 11-2 provide some basic information on each.

Implementation of health information technology (HIT) is one-third technology and two-thirds organizational culture and work process. Successful electronic health record system (EHRS) implementations devote significant time and resources to planning efforts that examine and redesign clinical workflow. Analysis of current workflow helps an organization more easily integrate technology into care delivery processes (Detwiller & Petillion, 2014). Process redesign does not require expensive consultants or software, but it does require significant

---

Box 11-1 **Rogers' Diffusion of Innovation Theory**

This widely used theory clarifies the necessary steps for acceptance of innovation. Diffusion refers to the process by which an innovation is communicated within a social environment over time. Diffusion is a five-step process consisting of the following phases:

- Knowledge
- Persuasion
- Decision
- Implementation
- Confirmation.

Movement from phase to phase may vacillate, and different levels of an organization may exhibit different phases at any one time. It is useful to classify individuals or groups by their rate of acceptance of innovation as:

- Innovators
- Early adopters
- Early majority
- Late majority
- Laggards.

SOURCE: Herbert, V., & Connors, H. (2016). Integrating an academic electronic health record: Challenges and success strategies. *CIN: Computers, Informatics, Nursing. 34*(8), 345–354; Kaminski, J. (Spring 2011).Diffusion of Innovation Theory Canadian Journal of Nursing Informatics, 6(2). Retrieved from http://cjni.net/journal/?p=1444

> **Box 11-2 Implementation Science**
>
> Study of methods, interventions, and variables to integrate research findings and evidence into practice
>
> Fairly new field
>
> Definition may vary by type of research and setting
>
> Underlying intent is to identify barriers and facilitators to successful implementation
>
> Examines individuals and organizations
>
> Has its own dedicated journal, *Implementation Science*, devoted to research relevant to healthcare
>
> **SOURCE:** Implementation Science. (n.d.) About. Retrieved from https://implementationscience.biomedcentral.com/about

staff time and effort. Investing in process redesign on the front end of EHRS projects will significantly pay off in the end.

Form an Implementation Committee

Ideally, the implementation phase is planned prior to the purchase of the system. Once the organization has purchased the information system, the implementation phase continues. A project leader is identified, and a team of hospital staff is selected to support the project, forming a working committee. This leader is one who will not only be instrumental in all planning phases of the project but will also play a key role in the gap analysis, which is key to implementation. One important consideration in choosing the project manager is to ensure that this role is filled by a nurse leader. A nurse overseeing the implementation project will ensure aspects relevant to all disciplines are addressed. Often, it is the nurse leader who has the clear vision necessary to make changes relevant to patient care, provide insight into the nursing process and nursing workflow, and coordinate the implementation plan into a feasible process. This leader must have the ability to maintain a strong relationship with all members of the implementation team. If it is not possible to have a nurse in this position, the chief information officer, strategy officer, a non-nurse informatics specialist, project manager, or a consultant experienced in this area may serve in this capacity. It is important, however, that the project leader be involved in the entire selection and implementation process and possess strong leadership and communication skills. This ensures that the project leader has a firm understanding of the vision, goals, and expectations for the information system. The leader should be one who is supportive of change and can keep the implementation process moving forward. One of the keys to ensuring the product meets the needs of the end users is to utilize not only nurse leaders, but also to include end users, not only for initial input, but for validating workflows. Only after reviewing and addressing end user needs should an information system be fully implemented. Recruiting efforts should focus on people who display the characteristics that support effective group dynamics and represent all key stakeholders. According to Kaminski (2011) using Kurt Lewin's principles for guiding change is an important step to gaining early adopters who will ultimately make the change a success. In addition, the project leader should facilitate the development of effective group dynamics. This is the stage where a working knowledge of conflict management is beneficial to the success of not only the group, but the overall success of the project as well.

Any effort that involves the implementation of an information system for nurses (or that will be used by nurses) should include an informatics nurse specialist or informatics nurse. These individuals are uniquely qualified to communicate the needs of clinical staff

---

Box 11-3 Characteristics of a Successful Implementation Committee

Individual Members

- Buy into the need for a new system and processes
- Communicate openly
- Demonstrate patience with other members
- Are players
- Are task and goal-oriented
- Acknowledge individual and group accomplishments
- Nurture fellow team members
- Provide suggestions and feedback from peers on current process
- Possess a high degree of critical thinking skills and ability to "think outside the box"

Group Characteristics

- Work toward a common goal
- Work to establish regular, effective meetings
- Encourage members to teach and learn from one another
- Develop its members' skills
- Build morale internally
- Resolve conflicts effectively
- Show pride in its accomplishments
- Represent all disciplines in the decision-making process

---

to information-services personnel and have a working knowledge of regulatory and system requirements, strategic plans, and budgetary constraints. Informatics nurse specialists and informatics nurses are qualified to identify current problems or issues, and help to choose or develop a solution. This nurse becomes the important link between clinical personnel and the analysts tasked to build the system. The committee members and organizational issues are every bit as important as the technology itself when implementing a new information system. Box 11-3 lists some characteristics of a successful implementation committee:

An effective project leader lays the groundwork for the implementation committee by helping the committee identify the goals for the implementation. At the primary level, the groundwork includes the mission, objectives, and outcomes. At the secondary level, it includes the benefits and outcomes. The project leader also helps to prioritize what is emergent, urgent, important, and supportive. The project leader plays a vital role with identifying assignments and responsible parties, training decisions, metrics for monitoring system operation, maintenance, reliability, and usability.

Plan the Installation

The initial work of the implementation committee is to develop a comprehensive project plan or timeline, scheduling all of the critical elements for implementation. This plan should address what tasks are necessary, the scope of each task, who is responsible for accomplishing each element, start and completion dates, necessary resources, and constraints. At this point in the project, it is necessary for the project leader to set goals and realistic expectations for both individuals and the group. An excellent way to keep everyone up to date on the current state of the project is to utilize a large wall to put up a "paper timeline." If you intend to use charts to communicate progress to the team, one that is particularly helpful is the Gantt chart. A visual plan helps keep everyone on track and understanding where others are in the project. This also allows the project leader accessibility to the overall progress at a quick glance. Table 11-1 shows a sample template for a system implementation.

Questions asked at this stage focus on the background of the project, its goals, sponsor, key stakeholders, benefits, and budget. Clear definition of this phase of the project requires time, energy, and lots of good communication. Failure to adequately address this phase jeopardizes successful implementation. Project-planning software may be helpful in developing the project timeline (or schedule) and a hierarchical arrangement of all specific tasks. This type of plan is referred to as a work breakdown structure (WBS). The idea behind this process is to subdivide a complicated task into smaller tasks until a level is reached that cannot be further subdivided. At that point, it is usually easier to estimate how long the small task will take, and how much it will cost to perform, than it would have been to estimate these factors for the higher levels (Heagney, 2016). After the project is defined, it is imperative to work on team building and planning for control and execution, review, and exit. Inadequate attention to these phases can also jeopardize implementation success.

The committee members should first become familiar with the information system they will be implementing, which can be accomplished in several ways. The vendor can provide on-site training, hospital staff can receive training at the vendor's corporate centers, or third-party consultants may be hired. Vendor training should provide the opportunity to continue to update the skills of the committee members—who may ultimately be the employees—and to subsequently use them as a resource throughout the implementation process. Once committee members have acquired an understanding of how the system functions, they will have the knowledge needed to analyze the base system as delivered from the vendor. Ideally, the following issues are addressed during system selection, but should be considered by the implementation committee before the system is installed, in the event that clarification or changes are necessary.

- *The technology.* It is important to consider whether the technology that is used is current and can be upgraded easily or is already obsolete. It is also necessary to have a good match between the system and the needs of the area.

- *Vendor standing.* Committee members need to consider vendor history of similar projects, as well as financial solvency of the vendor for long-term service and dialog with other customers to determine their implementation issues and resolution.

Table 11-1 Sample Template for a System Implementation Timeline

Miles tone	Person Responsible	Estimated Start Date	Completion Date
Phase 3: System implementation			
Develop implementation committee			
Analyze hardware/software requirements			
Develop training documents			
Develop training guidelines			
System and integrated testing			
Preload preparedness			
Provide user training			
Go-live event			

- *Vendor compliance with regulatory requirements.* System customization for regulatory compliance can be expensive. It is essential to determine vendor responsibility for federal and state regulatory compliance.

- *Integration with other systems.* It is important to establish how easily the selected information system exchanges information with other major systems, such as medical records and financial systems. One important detail to keep in mind is improved technology and users' increasing knowledge. As each information system is implemented, the skills of the end user become more pronounced, and the users are constantly challenging the system to do more. This increased desire for new and improved functionality makes it paramount to choose a system that can be easily integrated with other systems.

- *Use for different types of patient accounts.* Does the system work equally well for inpatient, outpatient, and emergency-care encounters? An important aspect to consider when planning the implementation is the ease with which a product can be used in various departments throughout the hospital. This is why it is extremely important to include all disciplines in the decision-making process during implementation planning. Often a group focuses on the needs most closely resembling their own care delivery specializations, and frequently forgets that the system must be functional for all patient-care areas, not just inpatient areas. For example, staff in an outpatient setting (e.g., family practice clinics) will focus on their information-management needs, which will have similarities and significant differences from information-management needs in intensive care units.)

- *Electronic health record system support.* Does the organization and its leadership support the electronic health record system? Can the computer system interface with other hospital applications?

- *Remote access.* Does the product permit secure access to patient data from all locations, particularly remote sites?

- *Clinician support.* Does the product support patient care?

The next step is to decide whether this system should be used as-is or be customized to meet the specific needs of the organization. This decision will act as the implementation strategy that will guide the committee through the implementation process. Regardless of which implementation strategy is followed, the committee must next gather information about the data that must be collected and processed. Consideration must be given to the data that is pertinent to each function and available to the user for entry into the system. A function refers to a task that may be either performed manually or automated; some examples include order entry, results reporting, and documentation. The identification of the present processes used throughout all clinical areas is termed workflow, while determining how these processes might be improved is known as workflow optimization. This critical step is often forgotten in the implementation process. If adequate time and resources are not allocated to this phase of the project, critical steps and processes are overlooked. This part of the project is best led by the nurse project manager with input from all disciplines. This workflow-optimization team will utilize the technique of gap analysis to identify changes in workflow from system implementation that will require changes to the present process. It is the responsibility of this part of the committee to validate the future design with a prototype application that will increase user acceptance of or decrease resistance to the new system. The output of the system should also be examined. For example, the format and content of printed requisitions, result reports, worklists, and dashboard displays of data and managerial reports must be evaluated. Once decisions have been made regarding system design and modification related to specific work flows, the appropriate department heads should approve these specifications before the actual changes are made. At this stage of the implementation, it is important to include not only director-level personnel, but staff as well (Cresswell, Bates, & Sheikh, 2013; Shea et al., 2014). Given sufficient time for an in-depth review of the prototype, the staff will develop a clear vision as to what will work. The staff can then challenge the proposed conversions if they do not see them as positive changes or see changes that will result in major workflow interruptions. If groups meet to review new system requirements and adjustments made prior to implementation, delays can be avoided. Numerous changes delay implementation of the system and drive up costs.

At this point, the identified changes should be made to the system in the test environment. The test environment is one copy of the software where programming changes are initially made. After any changes are made, the software must be tested to ensure that the changed elements display and process data accurately and do not disrupt system functioning. Before this can be accomplished, the implementation team and all responsible managers must agree on a test plan. This includes determining long-term goals and what must be tested. Testing is best accomplished by following a transaction through the system for all associated functions. In some cases, vendors provide a significant cost reduction in product purchases if the buyer is willing to beta test the product. Beta testing occurs on-site under everyday working conditions. This crucial testing phase is needed to allow the end users to see the project in an environment close to the live environment, in order to determine its feasibility and usability. Software problems are identified, corrected, and retested. This follows alpha testing, which is an intensive examination of new software features. An example of this testing procedure might be to enter a practitioner's order for an x-ray into the system for a particular client. The correct creation of the requisition is verified. Transmission of the request to the radiology department is verified. Next, the system is examined to verify that the results of the x-ray are entered for this client with a correct time stamp. Both the retrieval of the online results and the printed-report content should be verified. Finally, the system should be checked to make certain that the appropriate charges have been generated and passed on to the financial system.

It is important to realize that the test environment is not exactly the same as the live environment, because the live environment is much larger and more complex. As a result, the findings of the system test may not always indicate how well the system will perform in the live environment. To help ensure that testing is valid, it is essential to involve more than a handful of persons from the IT staff, the implementation committee, or a quality-assurance group. It is strongly recommended that staff-level personnel be involved in script testing. Script testing is the crucial milestone in implementing a new health IT system, such as an EHR. Script testing determines if the system build supports your workflows and staff members have appropriate system access to perform their tasks. If your comprehensive script testing is a success, then your system implementation will be successful. Script testing is conducted in four phases: Unit testing is performed within an application to confirm the application workflows are supported by the new information system. Integrated testing is a complex workflow encompassing multiple applications. System testing tests the entire system as one entity to ensure the entire system is working properly. User acceptance testing is an independent test performed by end users prior to accepting the product (Schwable, 2016). These individuals are able to question the reality of a situation and determine the validity of the proposed test. They can often recognize issues during the testing that may not be evident to IT staff. Box 11-4 summarizes some tips to ensure successful testing.

Analyze Hardware Requirements

A separate group of tasks related to the analysis of hardware requirements must also be addressed during the implementation phase. These tasks should be initiated early in the

---

Box 11-4 Tips to Ensure Successful Testing

Plan ahead. Thorough testing requires sufficient time, human input, and, sometimes, dedicated space and equipment.

Determine functions/features that will be tested. This will help to identify necessary human resources, levels of testing, and expected deliverables.

Establish expected end products or deliverables. These will be included in test scripts and serve to measure success. Incorporate testing at the function/feature (unit), integration, system, and user acceptable levels.

Identify how testing will be managed. Some organizations contract for consultant expertise, especially if there is a lack of experience with any part of the testing process.

Construct detailed test scripts. With healthcare scenario-based, step-by-step test scripts, ensure that the system is used as designed and provide precise documentation in the event that issues occur.

Elicit buy in from administrators to free staff for participation. Successful testing requires input from end users to create test scripts and conduct testing, but cannot take place unless staff and administrators are committed to the process.

---

implementation phase and continue simultaneously while system design and modifications are being completed. Some of these items include the following.

- *Network infrastructure.* The determination of network requirements, cable installation, wiring and access points, and technical standards should be initiated early in the implementation phase. The processing power, memory capacity of network components, and anticipated future needs must be addressed by the technical members of the implementation committee or other information-services staff. Extensive changes to network configuration are expensive and should be avoided whenever possible; although developments in technology and algorithms promise greater flexibility to handle functions, such as digital imaging and archiving, and telemedicine, they place high demands on the network even when using wireless technology (Misra, Ghosh, & Obaidat, 2014; Reddy & Venkata Krishna, 2015).

- *Type of workstation or mobile device.* The system may be accessed via a number of different devices. These may include a networked personal computer (PC), thin client, or a wireless or handheld device, such as a smartphone or laptop. The committee must investigate the advantages of each option and make recommendations regarding the types of hardware for purchase and installation. Once a decision has been made regarding the type of workstation, the appropriate number of devices per area or department must be determined. An essential step in this process of device investigation is to conduct a device fair where staff can actually work with several devices that are being considered. They can evaluate the ease of use of the device and its functionality, and provide significant feedback to the committee regarding recommendations for use. These events not only yield important information, but also promote staff engagement and buy in.

- *Workstation-location strategy.* A related workstation decision is the strategy for locating and using the hardware. Several options are available. Point of care devices are located at the site of client care, which is often at the bedside, especially in the emergency department, delivery room, operating room, and radiology. Another strategy involves a centralized approach, where workstations are located at the unit station. A third option is to use handheld or mobile devices that may be accessed wherever the staff finds it most convenient.

- *Hardware-location requirements.* The areas where the equipment is to be placed or used must be evaluated as to the adequacy of electrical receptacles, cabling constraints, and/ or reception-and-transmission capabilities. In addition, work areas may require modifications to accommodate the selected hardware. Another major consideration is the need to protect health information from casual viewing, while facilitating caregiver-patient communication.

- *Printer decisions.* Printer options should be examined, although print needs have decreased. The de facto standard is laser-printer technology, although dot-matrix technology is still used, and ink-jet printers may suffice in low-traffic locations. Other decisions focus on features such as the number of paper trays and fonts. Printed output requires the same considerations for protecting privacy and confidentiality of information.

Develop Procedures and Documentation

Comprehensive procedures for how the system will be used to support client care and associated administrative activities should be developed before the training process is begun. In this way, training may include procedures as well as hands-on use of the system. One approach is to examine the current nursing policy-and-procedure documents, and to incorporate new policies and procedures related to automation. Policies that are controlled by regulatory bodies must be rewritten to reflect new technology and care-delivery systems. There must be a clear understanding of who will take on the enormous task of categorizing the policies and making the necessary changes prior to go live. Changes to policies and standards must be approved by designated authorities. During training, information should be included on procedures used in the event that the system is not running (downtime), either for reasons of scheduled maintenance or unforeseen circumstances. Scheduled downtime allows for the implementation of changes in the system. Unscheduled downtime may occur with server, application, network, or electrical problems. It may be beneficial to develop separate documentation that includes the downtime procedures and manual requisition forms, and to place these in an easily identifiable and accessible location. It is crucial that support staff maintain these downtime forms, because system upgrades may necessitate the use of new forms to coincide with electronic versions of documentation. A process must be in place to ensure these are up-to-date at all times. The analysis of a system's downtime process and guidelines for documentation is critical prior to a go live. Failure to address these steps can lead to user frustration and failure of the implementation.

System user guides should also be developed at this point, including downtime processes. These documents explain how to use the system and the printouts that the system produces (Saba & McCormick, 2015). It is important that the educational team develop an end user resource that can be used as a quick-reference guide. Job aids should also be developed to help the end user determine his or her new role in the electronic world. Another good reference to develop is frequently asked question (FAQ) lists that can be utilized by all staff. These tools reassure the end user, and can also alleviate some calls to the help desk during the initial stages. One important aspect of documentation is the development of a dictionary of terms and mapping terms from one system to another. This ensures that everyone has a clear definition of terms and uses them in the same way. Data dictionaries do not contain actual data, but rather list and define all terms used and provide bookkeeping information for managing data. Data dictionaries help to ensure that data are of high quality.

Testing

The process of testing includes the development of a test plan, the creation of test scripts, system testing, and integrated testing. An effective test plan cannot be created until screens and pathways are finalized, and policies and procedures are determined. Otherwise, the plan must be revised one or more times. You can never start the testing process too early. The identification of an analyst whose sole job is to create the test scripts is key to the success of this part of the project. The test plan prescribes what will be examined within the new system, as well as all systems with which it shares data. Successful testing requires the involvement of staff who perform day-to-day work, because they are aware of the current process and expected outcomes. The test plan should include patient types and functions seen in the facility. A review of test results is done to identify whether functions are completed without error. Problem areas should be tested again before the person responsible for that area indicates approval and signoff. After system testing, integrated testing can start. Integrated testing looks at the exchange of data between the test system and other systems to ensure its accuracy and completeness. While testing is critical to success, it never identifies every defect. The ultimate test begins during the cutover to the production environment, where defects never before identified can be uncovered.

Provide Training

Once all modifications have been completed in the test environment, a training environment should be established. A training environment is a separate copy of the software that mimics the actual system that will be used. Many organizations populate the training database with fictitious clients and make this database available for formal training classes during the implementation process and for ongoing education.

A key aspect of this part of the project is the designation of a training-management specialist or educational champion. This person has the sole responsibility for the planning, executing, controlling, and closing of project tasks for educating users to take advantage of workflow and system benefits (Coplan & Masuda, 2011; Paramkusham & Gordon, 2013). Once identified, this key individual conducts a training-needs assessment to determine exactly what is needed in terms of resources and time necessary for the training. A training need is a description of the specific instructions each user requires to improve skills to use the new system and perform new workflows.

In preparation for designing the training plan, the following is a guide for doing the assessment:

- Observe user behavior to monitor current workflow patterns.
- Meet with all managers to gather feedback on their specific training needs and concerns.
- Conduct a strengths, weaknesses, opportunity, and threats (SWOT) analysis to gain insight into the specific needs of the end users.
- Administer a survey to ascertain end users' level of computer usage.
- Analyze the survey results and other data collected during this process.
- Formulate the training plan.

The training plan includes a description of the target audience, the audience's level of computer literacy, the curriculum, schedule of training dates and times, resource allocations, and training deadline.

An assessment of the target audience's computer knowledge is crucial to the overall success of training. It is vital to provide basic entry-level education on computer skills and realize the various levels of expertise to expect during training.

Classroom instruction requires dedicated instructors, as well as sufficient proctors to assist with technical difficulties encountered to avoid interfering with the flow of the class. Training is most effective if the training session is scheduled at a time independent from the learners' other work responsibilities and at a site separate from the work environment. This allows the learner to concentrate on comprehending the system without interruptions. Although this is the best scenario for learning, it presents a logistical challenge for managers, related to scheduling. With very careful planning, however, the obstacles can be overcome to allow training to take place for all personnel in a timely manner.

An essential part of the training plan is the designation of an educational champion. The selection of this individual should occur early in the design phase to allow time to develop the educational plan for the project. This champion should work closely with all unit and department leaders, as well as maintain contact with the implementation team; this will ensure that the timeline is maintained. Any difficulties in the training plan need to be communicated to the implementation team to allow adjustments to be made to avoid a delay in the go live. It is extremely important to insist that training be mandatory for all staff. The emphasis on training is essential if training is to be effective and, ultimately, the implementation successful. Planning for the training must include the following resources:

- Classrooms.
- Instructors.
- Computers.
- Training scripts to teach the classes.
- Time.

When planning the class schedule, it is imperative to remember that training needs to occur 24/7. An aspect that often gets overlooked is that nurses and other hospital personnel do not all work during the day; therefore, not all classes should be Monday through Friday during daylight hours. The allocation of computers in the training room is vital, as it is essential that students learn hands-on, thus requiring the availability of a computer for every student.

Another important aspect of training is the timing of the classes. It is important to allow training time for not only end users, but super users as well. Super users are very important to the implementation process in the departments and must be relied upon heavily for their expertise. Because of this increased responsibility, super users need to have additional training to become proficient in this new system.

In addition, learners should have a place to practice after the formal classroom instruction. If at all possible, a training domain should be made available in all departments to allow staff to play in a safe environment. Learning is enhanced when students have the opportunity to utilize the new skills they have learned, and the training domain provides this opportunity. The use of a training domain has implications that impact training. IT personnel need to maintain this site and plan for possible errors arising from student errors. Even though such errors impact training and increase the demands on the implementation team, this is an extremely important part of training.

One of the most important aspects of training is to be able to provide feedback to the students on concerns or questions raised during the classroom training. It is important to allow students to feel they are in a safe environment and understand that their input and opinions about this new system are valued. Students lose trust in the instructor if they feel threatened or not valued.

During the training phase of implementation, it is vital to stress to the end user the importance of confidentiality, security, and patient privacy. An EHR provides easy access to patient data, and can create unsafe and unethical situations. The student must understand the implications of accessing data that should not be accessed. They need to understand that if they have a need to access a patient chart to provide care, this is acceptable; however, it is also imperative they understand how their access can be tracked and time stamped. This understanding is extremely important to emphasize at the beginning of training.

Go-Live Planning

The committee determines the go-live date, which is when the system will be operational and used to collect and process actual client data. It is important to choose this date very early in the project, as this is the date that will guide development of the system. A more successful training plan will be developed by starting at the end point (go live) and working backwards. At go live, the production environment is in effect. The **production environment** is a term that refers to the time when the new system is in operation. Some of the necessary planning surrounding this event includes the following.

IMPLEMENTATION STRATEGY An overall implementation strategy should include:

- Transfer of data from the old system to the new system
- Establishment of user- and system-support procedures
- Development of short- and long-term evaluation procedures to monitor impact and effectiveness of the new system
- Creation of a change-control procedure to assure that all changes to the new system are documented and carried out properly.

The committee determines whether implementation will be staggered, or occur all at once. An example of a staggered-implementation strategy may be to go live in a limited number of client units; the remaining units are scheduled to go live in groups staggered over a specified time frame. The term **rollout** is sometimes used to refer to a staggered, or rolling, implementation. Another option for implementation is a big-bang implementation, also known as an all-at-once implementation. This occurs when a complete system goes live across an entire organization on a specific date and time.

The decision on timing of an implementation is made at the beginning of the planning process. This decision drives the plan and enables the organization to begin promoting its decision. A factor to keep in mind when making this decision is to ensure the organization has a fully committed senior-management staff as well as a strong physician champion. The implementation process will be received in a more positive light if the drive comes from the top down, as well as from the bottom up. All parties need to be clear on the vision and promote the positive aspects of the project, as well as maintain a grasp on reality and understand the push back that is going to happen because of the change in process. Additional considerations for the committee follow:

- *Conversion to the new system.* Decisions must be made regarding what information will be back loaded, or preloaded, into the system before the go-live date. This decision includes identification of who will perform this task and the methodology used to accomplish it. Plans for how orders will be back loaded must be developed. For example, a "daily × 4 days" order for a complete-blood-cell count should be analyzed to determine how many days will be remaining on the go-live date. This number should be entered when the backload is performed. Back loading may be needed to create accurate worklists, charges, or medication-administration sheets. Plans for verification of the accuracy of preloaded data should be considered.

- *Developing the support schedule.* It is often necessary to provide on-site support around the clock during the initial go-live or conversion phase. Support personnel may include vendor representatives, information-system staff, and other members of the implementation committee. Staff must be involved in this support aspect and, therefore, staffing allowances are very important at this implementation stage. This, again, is where senior managers need to show their presence, especially at the physician level. A clear understanding of exactly what is expected of the staff during the go live needs to be communicated effectively and consistently to avoid major conflicts, which could interrupt patient care.

- *Developing evaluation procedures.* Satisfaction questionnaires and a method for communicating and answering questions during the go-live conversion should be provided. These questionnaires must provide the implementation team with truthful feedback on how the end user is accepting the change. In the surveys, it is important to ask open-ended questions as well as pointed answer questions to allow staff to vocalize some of their barriers to using the new system

- *Developing a procedure to request post go-live changes.* Priority must be given to required changes for making the system work as it should. Additional changes should go before the implementation committee or hospital steering committee to determine necessity. This process helps to keep costs manageable.

System Installation

Once the production system is turned on, users are expected to switch from manual procedures or their prior information system. Generally, it takes users longer to perform tasks during this transition period until they become acclimatized to changes in workflow and the new system. This can cause stress, frustration, and treatment delays. Adequate support staff must be available 24/7 at the point of care to help users through this process for the first few weeks until they become adept at its use. Typically, this is a time that unforeseen problems will surface; these might include users who did not receive training, access issues, system errors, and failure of the system to perform as designed in all cases.

Part of the planning includes what type of on-the-job training will be available once the system is turned on. The expectation should be clear that if training has not occurred, staff should not work. This expectation needs to be supported so others will not have their work impacted simply because their peers did not receive proper training. Support staff at the point of care can quickly resolve issues on-site or refer them to appropriate information-services staff for follow-up.

Common Implementation Pitfalls

There are several common pitfalls with system implementation. Perhaps the most common is an inadequate understanding of how much work is required to implement the system, resulting in underestimation of necessary time and resources. If the initial timeline is not based on a realistic estimate of the required activities and their scope, the implementation process may fall behind schedule. Therefore, it is necessary to fully investigate the impact of the system and control the scope of the project in the early stages of planning.

A major consideration when planning the implementation is the number of hours needed to devote to the development of the project. Team members must be relieved of current jobs and duties to be able to fully commit to the venture.

Another serious problem that may occur during implementation is that of numerous revisions during design activities, creating a constantly moving target. This is known as scope creep or feature creep. Scope creep is the unexpected and uncontrolled growth of user expectations as the project progresses. Feature creep is the uncontrolled addition of features or functions without regard to timelines or budget. As needed, customizations and modifications are identified, it is imperative that the appropriate department heads approve and sign off on them before programming changes are made. Frequent changes can become very frustrating for the technical staff and result in missed deadlines. Ultimately, this can be very expensive and emotionally draining for the implementation team.

The amount and type of customization that is done to the information system can also result in problems. To guide the implementation team, the implementation strategy must address the degree of customization that will be done. One strategy is using the system as delivered by the vendor, with minimal changes. The advantage of this strategy, which is often called the vanilla system, is an easier and quicker implementation. In addition, future software upgrades may be implemented with greater ease and speed. The disadvantage of using this system is that user workflow may not match the system design.

The opposite implementation strategy is to fully customize the information system so that it reflects the current workflow. Full customization of the information system features and functions is more extensive than cosmetic changes to the look of screens or user views, which do not change how the underlying system works. Full customization may seem appealing but its disadvantages include a complicated, lengthy, and expensive implementation process, and complications when system-software upgrades are needed. Customization may require extensive programming effort before upgrades can be installed. As a result, the present trend in the hospital information systems industry is to recommend use of the vanilla systems as delivered by the vendors.

Other common pitfalls include failure to consider annual maintenance contracts and related costs, providing insufficient dedicated resources to the implementation committee, and a hostile culture. The vendor's purchase price for a system is only a portion of overall costs. Vendors charge additional fees for annual technical support, customization, and license fees. These charges are levied on the size of the institution or the number of users, which may or may not be concurrent. Additional costs may include hardware; operating or report software needed to support the system; site preparation; uninterrupted power systems; installation; and ongoing operating costs such as maintenance, supplies, personnel, and upgrades. Project success is impeded by a hostile culture, resistance to change, and refusal to see the benefits of the technology being implemented.

There may also be problems with testing. These problems can include poorly developed test scripts, inadequate time to retest problem areas, and the inability to get other systems to exchange data with the test system. Inadequate testing can lead to unpleasant surprises at the time of rollout or go live. The development of the test scripts needs to be a work in progress. Although the basic learning concepts must be consistent, it is important to be able to adapt the material to varied class makeups. Not all students in the class will grasp the material quickly, making adjustments to the class necessary. It is also vital to make changes when concepts may not be clear to the students and suggestions are made as to how to improve the content.

All too often, training suffers from inadequate allocation of time and resources. The training environment should mirror the testing environment, as well as the later production environment. Design may not be completed when training starts, which creates a negative impression of the system as well as confusion among end users.

Finally, it is important to continually reinforce the concept that the implementation and the information systems are owned by the users. If the users feel no ownership of the system, they may not accept the system or use it appropriately, nor will they provide feedback regarding potential system improvements. Factors that can result in a lack of buy in include a lack of communication, insufficient support, and inadequate training for users and IT staff. All stakeholders should receive frequent communication via newsletters, posters, banners, buttons, and informational meetings. Staffs seem to become more engaged in the process if they are part of the process from the beginning. They will view this new change with much anticipation and often fear, but given the opportunity, they will embrace the challenge. Input from all stakeholders must be solicited and evaluated. It is important to work with the vendor to resolve issues rather than assign blame. Consider whether the scope of the project was clearly defined, with responsibilities assigned and parties empowered to perform their jobs; and whether project milestones were defined and tracked.

User Feedback and Support

One important aspect of maintenance is communication. Soon after the go-live event, feedback from the implementation evaluation should be acted on in a timely manner. This is usually the first aspect of system maintenance to be addressed. The results should be compiled, analyzed, and communicated to the users and information-services staff. Any suggested changes that are appropriate may then be implemented. An important avenue for staff to convey concerns or question processes is through suggestion boxes that are reviewed daily to ascertain user adoption and competency at this stage of implementation.

Continued communication is imperative for sharing information and informing users of changes. Communication can be accomplished in a variety of ways. For example, an electronic newsletter or printed announcement can be sent to the users, on either a regular or an as-needed basis. System messages can be displayed on the screen or printed at the user location. Focus groups or in-house user groups can be formed for discussion and problem solving.

Another form of user support is the help desk. The **help desk** provides round-the-clock support that is usually available by telephone as well as email. Most organizations designate one telephone number as the access point for all users who need help or support related to information systems. The help desk is usually staffed by personnel from the information-systems area who have had special training and are familiar with all of the systems in use. Often, they are able to help the user during the initial telephone call. If this is not possible, the help desk may refer more complex problems or questions to other staff who have specialized knowledge. The help desk should follow up with the user and provide information as soon as it is available. It is expected that end users will become very frustrated if they feel no one is there to support them during a time of crisis. Often, users just want the reassurance that someone will be able to walk them through a problem. The biggest problems during go live occur with sign-on and passwords, as well as with users who missed training or may not remember how to sign on to the system.

Visibility of the support staff in the user areas is another important form of support. By making regular visits to all areas, the support staff is able to gather information related to how the system is performing and impacting the work of the users. In addition, users have the opportunity to ask questions and describe problems without having to call the help desk.

System Maintenance

Maintenance is the term used to describe the period of time during which new behaviors (i.e., work flows and processes) are solidified. Engaging end users in the process of making change—in this case, in implementing an EHRS—is critical. The result is often that users in the maintenance phase are not attended to, and easily slip back into old ways while no one is noticing. To successfully maintain the change to an EHR system, regular monitoring, continued celebration of positive results, and immediate course correction, where necessary, is critical to avoid workarounds or a return to old ways.

Ongoing system maintenance must be provided in all three environments: test, training, and production. This enables programming and development to continue in the test region without adverse effect on the training or production systems. Therefore, training can continue without interruption, and the training environment can be upgraded to reflect programming changes at the appropriate time. Actual client data and workflow will not be affected in the production system until the scheduled upgrade has been thoroughly tested in the test environment.

Requests submitted by users can provide input for upgrading or making necessary changes to the system. For example, a user might request changes to standard physician orders, such as a request to delete some lab tests to contain costs, or nursing documentation related to regulatory issues or The Joint Commission recommendations, such as adding advanced-directives documentation. The requesters must provide a thorough explanation of the desired changes, as well as the reason for the request. One method of facilitating this communication is to develop a request form, to be completed by the requesting users and submitted to the information-services department. On receiving this form, the information-services staff should determine if the change is feasible and should consider whether any alternative solutions exist.

Technical Maintenance

A large portion of ongoing maintenance is related to technical and equipment issues. This maintenance is the responsibility of the information-services department. Some examples of technical maintenance include:

- Performing problem solving and debugging.
- Maintaining a backup supply of hardware, such as monitors, printers, cables, trackballs, and mice, for replacement of faulty equipment in user areas.
- Performing file-backup procedures.
- Monitoring the system for adequate file space.
- Building and maintaining interfaces with other systems.
- Configuring, testing, and installing system upgrades.
- Maintaining and updating the disaster-recovery plan.
- Update security protections.
- Secure off-site storage usage, services, and availability.
- Review software and hardware warranties.

System Evaluation

The conclusion of the systems development life cycle (SDLC) includes evaluation. Aspects of evaluation have been presented throughout this chapter. Along with the evaluations done throughout the system life cycle, formal evaluations are needed when the implementation phase is completed. The following is a summary of the usually performed evaluations. Types of evaluation are operational, technical, financial, social, and cultural. Box 11-5 includes some key points to consider for each type of evaluation. Findings may lead to the start of a new cycle.

The Role of Informatics Nurse and Informatics Nurse Specialist

Nurses have historically gathered and interpreted data. All nurses use data and information to generate useful knowledge to care for their patients. This increased knowledge base in today's nursing workforce is the catalyst for moving nursing and information technology into the future.

Nurse informaticists provide credibility for IT projects. The ability to fulfill these responsibilities is largely dependent upon a supportive environment created at the executive level. Implementation of information technology is a very political process, particularly in the cost-controlled, healthcare-delivery systems of today. The success of an electronic health record system also relies on how usable the software is for clinicians, and a thorough usability evaluation is needed before implementing a system within an organization. Not all nurses have the knowledge and skills to perform extensive usability testing; therefore, the informatics nurse specialist plays a critical role in the process. As technology and software become more sophisticated, usability principles must be used under the guidance of the informatics nurse specialist to provide a relevant, robust, and well-designed electronic health record to address the needs of the busy clinician (Rojas & Seckman, 2014).

Case Study

You are the informatics nurse specialist (INS) at a local hospital, which is a 300-bed community hospital. You have been a nurse at this facility for 10 years and in the role of an informatics nurse specialist for three years. The hospital is implementing an EHRS, and you have been asked to assume responsibility for the development and management of a training plan to prepare end users for go live. Although the hospital is implementing the EHRS for all disciplines, you will only be responsible for developing a training plan for nurses. This responsibility/role will require you to perform a gap analysis to determine nurses' educational needs in order to transition them from the current state of paper documentation to the future state of documentation using an EHRS. As the INS, you will need to identify the resources you will need, such as rooms, equipment, and so on, as you begin to develop your training plan. The hospital has 400 full-time nurses and 300 part-time and casual nurses. There are 2 training rooms that have 15 computers in each room. Your informatics team consists of two other informatics nurses and one IS specialist. An estimation of eight to ten training hours will be needed for each nurse to prepare them in using the newly developed EHR. The entire hospital is currently using paper to document all levels of care. The estimated date for going live with the new system is one year from now. Discuss your analysis of the training needs and determine the best plan for your facility. Explain your rationale for the chosen plan and outline pitfalls to successful implementation.

Summary

- Change is the only constant. It is important to consider the impact of change on the organization.
- One important aspect of information-system implementation is the development of an effective implementation committee comprising the informatics specialists and clinical and technical representatives.
- The first task for the committee is the development of a timeline for system-implementation activities; the second task is staying with it.
- The implementation strategy must be determined by the committee. This strategy may call for using the information system as it is delivered by the vendor, or significantly customizing the system to match the current work needs.
- Identified modifications are made to the software in the test environment, so that actual client data and workflow are not affected.
- The following hardware considerations must be addressed during the implementation phase: servers, types of workstation devices, hardware locations, printer options, and network requirements.
- User procedures and documentation are developed during the implementation phase and provide support to personnel during training and actual use of the information system.

- Training is a key element for a successful information-system implementation.
- Careful consideration must be given to planning the go-live conversion activities to minimize disruptions to client care.
- The implementation committee must be aware of the common pitfalls and problems that may negatively affect the implementation process.
- Maintenance—an ongoing part of the implementation process—includes user support and system maintenance.

Box 11-5 Types of Evaluations

Aspects of evaluation have been presented throughout this chapter. Along with the evaluations done throughout the system life cycle, formal evaluations are needed when the implementation phase is completed. The following is a summary of the usually performed evaluations.

Types of Evaluations	Key Points
Operational	Determining if the planned objectives were met. Questions to ask include: • Does production system meet planned requirements? • Is there potential for growth and improvements? • What lessons were learned from project? • Have business processes improved? • Which potential benefits were achieved?

Technical	Determining if the system operates correctly:
	• Utilization
	  • Use of a particular resource over time.
	  • The times that a particular resource is used.
	  • Impact of the resource's use on the system.
	• Problem analysis
	  • In-depth, systematic analysis and assessment of reported or observed problems or issues.
	  • Proposal of possible solutions.
	• Current-state analysis
	  • Proactive testing of combinations of system functions (such as how well clinical documentation works; how much it is being used).
	  • Determining if users are using functions correctly and according to published standards of performance.

Financial	Determining of the economic impact of the system: • Cost-benefit analysis—weighing the total expected costs versus the total expected benefits of one or more actions in order to choose the most profitable option. • Emphasis on choosing from some set of alternatives makes this analysis more appropriate for the planning stage. • Be cautious when evaluating a decision already made and acted on. • Consider productivity, quality of care, and task performance. Most of these are amenable to quantitative measurement. • Return on investment (ROI)— how effectively a business uses its capital to generate profit; the higher the ROI, the better. • Calculating ROI involves two parts: knowing what to measure and understanding how to quantify the value of those measurements into actual dollars. • For the SDLC, examine the cost of the system; the costs of selection, planning, and implementation; and the cost reductions (tangible and intangible) after implementing the system.
Social and Cultural	Determining if the system is actually beneficial to end users: • Focus—Decide what you are going to evaluate. Are you going to examine the process you used, the solution you chose, or both? The methods and questions might vary. • Include all levels of users. • Clarify what you want to measure and how to measure. • Look beyond immediate problem feedback and consider impacts of changes. • Careful framing of inquiry items, be as specific as possible, and include open-ended inquiries. • Timing depends upon what you are going to measure, and how well you think the implementation has gone.

- The information-system's life cycle is a continuous cyclical process.
- The INS plays a critical role in the evaluation of new technology.

About the Authors

Sue Evans MSN RN-BC is an Informatics Nurse II at the University of Pittsburgh Medical Center East and adjunct faculty for Thomas Edison State University and Chatham University. She retired at the rank of Major from the United States Army Reserve having served as a nurse. During her 40 year nursing career she has also been an active participant in informatics groups sharing her expertise with others.

References

Coplan, S., & Masuda, D. (2011). *Project management for healthcare information technology*. New York: McGraw Hill.

Cresswell, K. M., Bates, D. W., & Sheikh, A. (2013). Ten key considerations for the successful implementation and adoption of large-scale health information technology. *Journal of the American Medical Informatics Association*, 20(E1), E9–E13.

Detwiller, M., & Petillion, W. (2014). Change management and clinical engagement. *CIN: Computers, Informatics, Nursing*, 32(6), 267–273.

Heagney, S. (2016). *Fundamentals of project management* (5th ed.). New York: Work Smart.

Kaminski, J. (Winter, 2011). Theory applied to informatics—Lewin's change theory. *CJNI: Canadian Journal of Nursing Informatics*, 6(1). Retrieved from http://cjni.net/journal/?p=1210

Kotter, J. P. (1996). *Leading change*. Boston: Harvard Business School Press.

Leeman, J., Birken, S. A., Powell, B. J., Rohweder, C., & Shea, C. M. (2017). Beyond "implementation strategies": classifying the full range of strategies used in implementation science and practice. Implementation Science, 121-9. doi:10.1186/s13012-017-0657-x

Misra, S., Ghosh, T. I., & Obaidat, M. S. (2014). Routing bandwidth guaranteed paths for traffic engineering in WiMAX mesh networks. *International Journal of Communication Systems*, 27(11), 2964. doi:10.1002/dac.2518

Nilsson, L., Borg, C., & Eriksen, S. (2014). Social challenges when implementing information systems in everyday work in a nursing context. *CIN: Computers Informatics Nursing*, 32(9), 442-450.

Paramkusham, R. B., & Gordon, J. (2013). Inhibiting factors for knowledge transfer in information technology projects. *Journal of Global Business & Technology*, 9(2), 26–36.

Reddy, C. P., & Venkata Krishna, P. (2015). Ant-inspired level-based congestion control for wireless mesh networks. *International Journal of Communication Systems*, 28(8), 1493. doi:10.1002/dac.2729

Rogers, E. M. (1983). Diffusion of Innovations (3rd ed.). New York: The Free Press.

Rojas, C., & Seckman, C. (2014). The informatics nurse specialist role in electronic health record usability evaluation. *CIN: Computers, Infomatics, Nursing*, 32(5), 214–220.

Saba, V. K., & McCormick, K. A. (2015). *Essentials of nursing informatics*, (6th ed.). New York: McGraw-Hill.

Schwable, K. (2016). Project human resources management. In *Information Technology Project Management*, (8th ed., pp. 344–383), Boston: Cengage Learning.

Shea, C. M., Reiter, K. L., Mose, J., Weiner, B. J., Weaver, M. A., McIntyre, M., & ... Malone, R (2014). Stage 1 of the meaningful use incentive program for electronic health records: A study of readiness for change in ambulatory practice settings in one integrated delivery system. *BMC Medical Informatics & Decision Making*, 14(1), 1–14. doi:10.1186/s12911-014-0119-1

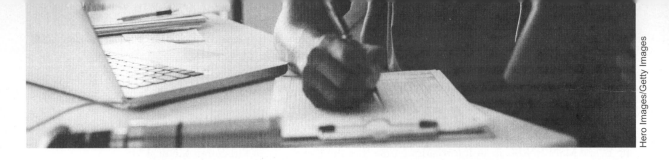

Chapter 12
Workforce Development

Diane Humbrecht, DNP, RN

Brenda Kulhanek, PhD, MSN, MS, RN-BC

 ## Learning Objectives

After completing this chapter, you should be able to:

- Discuss privacy and confidentiality issues related to health information technology training.

- Provide the rationale for introducing information policies during training.

- Recognize the factors that would lead to selection of a specific training-delivery method.

- Examine resources for health information technology training.

- Weigh models used to evaluate training.

- Describe the rationale for training on backup procedures.

Workforce Population

Proficient use of health information technology (HIT) is essential to efficient and quality patient care. Developing a healthcare workforce to effectively utilize HIT requires computer literacy and skills, effective training of system use, and solid understanding and integration of policies and procedures into the training and end user practice. Strong computer literacy is positively correlated with increased satisfaction with computer systems in healthcare (Alasmary, Metwally, & Househ, 2014).

By 2030, the baby-boomer generation will officially be over the age of 65, thereby increasing the demand to increase the healthcare workforce (Auerbach, Staiger, Muench, & Buerhaus, 2012). The United States will need an additional 35% more healthcare workers to support the ratio of healthcare providers to total population (Institute of Medicine, 2008). The National Council of State Boards of Nursing (NCSBN) and The National Forum of State Nursing Workforce Centers (The National Forum) released results of the 2015 National Nursing Workforce Survey (Budden et al., 2016; National Council of State Boards of Nursing, 2016). This study provided a comprehensive picture of the registered nurse

(RN) and licensed practical nurse (LPN) 2015 workforce. Approximately 79,000 nurses participated in the study between June 2015 and July 2015. Researchers were able to trend data based on their last survey, completed in 2013. Two trends identified were a growing number of male RNs and an emergence of a more diverse workforce. Interestingly, the study results showed the work setting has evolved beyond the bricks and mortar of acute-care hospitals due to the increasing use of information technology. Almost half of the participants in the study reported providing some type of nursing care using telehealth technologies.

Nursing informatics has evolved into an important part of the healthcare system and plays a critical role in the development, implementation, evaluation, and enhancement of HIT systems (Hussey & Kennedy, 2016). The Healthcare Information and Management Systems Society (HIMSS) conducted a nursing-informatics workforce survey in 2014. The survey found the nurse informaticist "continues to play a crucial role in the development, implementation, and optimization of clinical applications" (p. 1). The survey results also suggest nurse informaticists have a solid education background, citing a 24% increase in post graduate degrees. Almost half of the respondents (46%) have at least seven years of informatics experience and over half (57%) are satisfied or highly satisfied with their career choice in informatics.

It is important to recognize that nurse informaticists traditionally support the informatics needs of the healthcare workforce (Table 12-1) in a variety of settings (Table 12-2); therefore, they need to have strong workflow-analysis skills to support leveraging information technology to support the diverse healthcare-workforce team.

Table 12-1 Healthcare Workforce Requiring Informatics Support

Healthcare Workforce	
Physicians	Speech-Language Pathologists
Advanced Practice Registered Nurses	Massage Therapists
Physician Assistants	Dietitians and Nutritionists
Registered Nurses	Medical and Health-Services Managers
Licensed Practical and Licensed Vocational Nurses	Medical Secretaries
Dentists, General	Medical and Clinical Laboratory Technologists
Dental Hygienists	Medical and Clinical Laboratory Technicians
Dental Assistants	Cardiovascular Technologists and Technicians
Pharmacists	Nuclear-Medicine Technologists
Veterinarians	Diagnostic Medical Sonographers
Chiropractors	Radiologic Technologists
Optometrists	Emergency Medical Technicians and Paramedics
Opticians, Dispensing	Dietetic Technicians
Clinical, Counseling, and School Psychologists	Pharmacy Technicians
Mental-Health Counselors	Psychiatric Technicians
Rehabilitation Counselors	Respiratory-Therapy Technicians
Substance Abuse and Behavioral-Disorder Counselors	Surgical Technologists
Healthcare Social Workers	Medical Records and Health-Information Technicians
Mental Health and Substance-Abuse Social Workers	Medical Assistants
Physical Therapists	Pharmacy Aides
Physical Therapist Assistants	Personal-Care Aides
Physical Therapist Aides	Home Health Aides
Occupational Therapists	Nursing Assistants
Respiratory Therapists	Psychiatric Aides

SOURCE: Data from Area Health Resource File, 2015.

Table 12-2 Settings Requiring Informatics Support

Healthcare Settings	
Hospitals	Hospice
Long-Term-Care Facilities	Community Health Centers
Home Health Care	Psychiatric, Rehab, and Children's Hospitals
Health Clinics	Primary Care
Ambulatory Services	Urgent-Care Centers

SOURCE: Based on Area Health Resource File, 2015.

Workforce Population Current Knowledge and Skills

HIT has been deemed essential for improving quality of care, patient safety, and process efficiencies for all health professionals (American Academy of Nursing, 2015). Improving the patient experience and the health of populations while reducing the cost of healthcare is a common theme for informaticists who are leveraging information technologies to support practice. Efforts are being made to improve work environments though initiatives such as the American Academy of Nursing's Technology Drill Down program. However, nurses struggle with the lack of interoperability, which prevents them from becoming proficient in the use of information technologies (Clancy et al., 2014). The American Nurses Association (ANA) incorporated informatics competencies into their 2008 publication on the scope and standards of nursing-informatics practice (2015). A Delphi study, now considered a classic resource, was used to identify informatics competencies for novice and experienced nurses, as well as informatics nurse specialists and nurse informatics innovators (Staggers, Gassert, & Curran, 2001). More recently, Abdrbo (2015) studied nursing informatics and patient-safety competencies in nursing students (third or fourth year) compared to nursing interns (graduate nurses fulfilling an internship for one year). He found both groups had equal proportions of individuals who completed an informatics course, and both groups reported equal competencies. However, the nursing students felt they played a greater role in clinical informatics than the interns. Interns had higher scores for applied informatics. Abdrbo recommended all baccalaureate nursing programs have a core informatics course instead of an elective.

Devising a Workforce Development Preparation Plan

The Health Information Technology for Economic and Clinical Health (HITECH) Act addressed barriers to health information technology and HIT's potential to improve safety and quality in the healthcare setting (Sheikh, Sood, & Bates, 2015). Part of the act addresses the need for a well-trained healthcare workforce to implement the known science and best practices of electronic health-record system adoption. In order to develop a workforce plan, one must understand the needs of the educators who train the workforce. Using the funds granted through the HITECH Act, the Office of the National Coordinator for Health Information Technology (ONCHIT) was able to fund selected curriculum development centers (CDCs) to develop curricula for use in health IT training programs based in community colleges. While the materials were well received, pilot testing illustrated the complexity of developing HIT curricula for a diverse workforce. ONC recommends that HIT initiatives be approached from an implementation-science perspective. One size does not fit all learners; therefore, a mix of models is necessary to complete a workforce-development plan.

Implementation science focuses on understanding how change takes place (Fisher, Shortell, & Savitz, 2016). There are four main groups of variables that act together to influence the adoption of innovations: the external environment, the structure of the organization, the characteristics of the innovation, and the processes used.

The most influential domain is related to the characteristics of the innovation being implemented at an organization. If adoption does not occur, individuals will resist the intervention, potentially leading to failure. In order to drive adoption, health professionals need to be engaged early in the process to help them understand the value of HIT solutions (Zimlichman et al., 2012).

Informatics nurse specialists need to understand how the external environment influences the internal environment when putting a plan together. Electronic medication reconciliation is an example of how information technology can fail or provide a false sense of security as patients cross the continuum of care. Lack of interoperability between information systems forces clinicians to work in a variety of systems that support an EHRS. Changes made to medications in one system are not necessarily shared electronically with other systems, placing patients at risk to have an incorrect current medication list and, potentially, leading to a medication error.

The structure of the organization and the individuals involved with the intervention or implementation process must be evaluated by the informatics nurse specialist. Organizational culture can play a big role in the success or failure of implementing an innovation. When implementing change, sabotage is always a risk, as clinicians do not necessarily want to change from their routines of working in a complex, high-risk environment. Emotions start to take over, and goals and objectives are easily overlooked. Informatics nurse specialists need to take a structured approach to being aware of emotions; modifying emotional reactions is a skill known as emotional intelligence (EI) (Savel & Munro, 2016). Using EI throughout the workforce-development plan and implementation can help clinicians function at their highest potential. The ability model defines a set of four EI skills: (a) identification of emotions in self and in others; (b) the ability to reason using emotions; (c) the ability to comprehend emotions; and (d) the ability to control emotions in self and in emotional conditions (Codier & Odell, 2014). An implementation-science approach helps take a variety of models and blends them together to help gain an understanding how change will successfully take place.

Identification of Educational Needs

An educational-needs assessment is an effective way to determine the educational opportunities for improving patient care and clinician processes, and is a requirement for organizations on the journey to American Nurses Credentialing Center Magnet designation (Winslow, 2016). A needs assessment can easily be obtained via a survey, either to a specific specialty or throughout the organization. The needs assessment should focus specifically on a topic of interest related to organizational goals and objectives. For example, if the organization is implementing an EHRS, the questions may focus on computer usage and comfort, knowledge of specific terms, workflow analysis, environment, and data analytics. Understanding the needs of the end users is an important focus. Education and process changes should be based upon known needs, but also on anticipated predictable new needs.

VOICE OF THE END USER Subject-matter experts (SMEs) are identified at the beginning of a project. They are people who are considered knowledgeable in their specialty, work well with others in the workforce, and embrace change. These experts work closely with the project team to ensure new processes fit into end users' workflow, or make suggestions on changes to increase workflow efficiency and predict impediments to patient care. SMEs become the voice of the end users by acting as the bridge between the end user and members of the project team.

Setting Goals and Objectives

Goal alignment is defined as linking individual goals with organizational goals. Alignment of priorities leads to increased performance. It is imperative to have clear goals and related objectives with any workforce-development plan. Individuals are more likely to be driven to achieve goals if they understand what is expected of them (Wilson, 2016). Goals should be measurable in order to determine success or failure. Objectives are actionable steps defined for each individual goal. In order for a project to be successful, the overall vision and work effort must be fully defined. This is achieved by breaking down the project into small, manageable, and actionable portions based on the project's objectives.

Identifying the Scope of Efforts

With well-defined goals identified, the work on the process change begins. Projects are complicated. They consist of many moving parts and deliverables that need to meet specific time lines. **Project scope** is a defining metric that can help keep the project on a focused path. The scope of the project is defined through clear goals and outcome metrics. The scope provides the roadmap for project planning and execution. The project scope must be clear, with measurable outcomes. Without a clear focus, scope creep can occur, leading teams to feel overburdened with daunting challenges, and potentially ending in disastrous results (University Alliance, 2014). As additional requests are made during the project, project-team members can check those requests against the project scope; if the new idea is outside of the scope, it can be revisited after the completion of the original project.

At times, scope creep happens because of something identified during the project that was overlooked or underestimated, and may now put the project at risk. The team must re-evaluate and prioritize the project scope to ensure success. For example, during implementation of a new EHRS, consideration for **device integration** in the critical-care units was overlooked. A project-team member brought the concern of the critical-care nurses to the team, as the nurses felt this lapse would greatly impact their workflow, especially during a critical event, such as the resuscitation of a patient. The project team now needs to weigh the risk of patient harm versus the risk of adding additional work outside of the original scope of the project. If the risk leans to potential for patient harm, the scope of the project may be broadened or adjusted to ensure a successful implementation.

Safeguards for Privacy and Confidentiality

Adult learners perform best when training is based in the context of real-life application, including realistic names, healthcare settings, and health problems (Furlong, 2015; Hoyt, Adler, Ziesemer, & Palombo, 2013; Rashleigh, Cordon, & Wong, 2011). A **training environment** is a carefully planned replica of the HIT that will be used in actual practice. The training environment ideally should contain realistic patient-and-practice scenarios that mimic the real patient-care setting. Case studies and patient scenarios provide an excellent method for application of concepts. However, privacy and security of protected health information must be considered during training development and delivery, and care must be taken to disassociate any patient scenarios from information that could link the episode back to an actual patient. A well-designed computer-training environment will comply with organizational confidentiality and privacy policies and ensure that no identifiable patient information is included during training (Lee, Moy, Kruck, & Rabang, 2014).

Development of a realistic training database can be labor-intensive. Some organizations are able to copy actual patient records into a training database and remove patient identifiers, producing a very realistic training environment. Care must be taken to ensure that identifying information is removed not only from discrete data fields but from demographic information, such as phone numbers, and from any free-text areas within a chart. Keeping this in mind, the amount of work involved in scrubbing actual patient data for training use versus entering simulated patient data into a training database may be similar.

During instructor-led training, the instructors may be familiar with some of the patients or scenarios used in the training environment. Care must be taken to ensure that no actual patient information is revealed during the training process, and that no actual patient scenarios that can identify a real patient are discussed within the training room; learners should clearly understand that information used to create a training database cannot be linked to an actual patient, and students are able to integrate the privacy and confidentiality safeguards and principles into their own practice following training.

Introducing Information Policies

The number of HIT policies and procedures continues to expand to accommodate the many nuances of its use and abuse. Organizations should have policies and procedures governing secure system access, use of patient-health information, use of personal devices, system downtime, and equipment cleaning. Policies and procedures are best introduced during training so they can be integrated into the context of workflow. In addition, policies can support expected behavioral requirements and provide the basis of disciplinary action for lack of adherence. The training environment should be designed to replicate the live clinical system to support policy references and examples.

Policies addressed during training can include:

- *Patient privacy and security*—Healthcare is dependent on an open relationship and communication between the patient and the healthcare practitioner. The patient must be able to trust that information shared with providers will remain confidential and secure. A lack of trust can result in decreased information sharing, and can result in a less-than-full picture of health status and behaviors of the patient (Bova et al., 2012; Brady, 2011; Murray & McCrone, 2015). In order to support this relationship of trust, organizations are required, by regulation, to protect patient information (Dooling, 2012; Peterson, 2012; Rights, T. O. f. C., n.d.). A chart-access policy addresses the user ability to access a patient's healthcare record on a need-to-know basis, such that only persons directly involved in the care of a patient may access this information. Many health-information systems are able to block a caregiver's access to patient records that have not been assigned to that particular caregiver, without that caregiver documenting the reason for the access. Additionally, a patient-focused, privacy-and-security policy should address proper storage and disposal of paper-and-electronic documents containing protected patient information.

- *Downtime*—This policy addresses the procedures to follow during planned and unplanned information-system downtime, and may include the specific paper forms to be completed during this time or the alternate electronic database that must be used. The policy may also specify timeframes for when certain actions must be completed or when forms should be used or not used. Downtime procedures should be introduced at the time of training and reviewed on a routine basis with end users.

- *Email*—Email is a valuable time-saving tool for communication that can also provide opportunities for breaches of patient privacy and security (McGraw, Belfort, Pfister, & Ingargiola, 2015; Murphy, 2000). Email policies should include indications and encryption requirements for outgoing email containing patient information, or alternate procedures for sharing patient information with approved recipients.

- *Cleaning and care of equipment*—HIT equipment can become a vector for disease if not properly cleaned. In addition, use of the wrong cleaning products can damage the hardware. Cleaning policies will specify when and how equipment should be cleaned.

- *Information downloading and uploading*—Downloading or uploading information into the computer systems of an organization represent a security risk that includes misuse of patient information and violation of patient privacy, as well as the opportunity for malicious applications to infect the organizational system. Although many organizations have configured individual computers so that universal serial bus (USB) devices and disk drives cannot be accessed, a policy provides an additional level of safeguard.

- *Password security*—The lack of password protection can produce unauthorized access into secured health information and the potential for user fraud if one user is able to access a system, patient chart, and functionality of a role through password theft. Password policies not only stipulate protection of personal passwords, but also may define the length and complexity of a password and the frequency of password changes.

- *Pictures and cameras*—Most people carry smartphones with camera functionality. When staff have access to this technology while providing patient care, the potential exists for photos to be taken and shared that violate the patient's right to privacy. Camera policies are designed to eliminate unauthorized photographs, while providing the use requirements for appropriate use of photos for patient activities, such as wound documentation.

- *Removing devices from secured areas*—Many data breaches occur when mobile computing devices are removed from secured areas and are then lost or stolen, resulting in potential access to patient information, which may include names, addresses, social security numbers, and other information. Device policies cover both the portability of organizational devices and data protection, as well as specifications for software that can be used to wipe data from devices that go missing.

- *Screen security*—Computers used for patient care are often located in areas where patients, families, and others can view protected patient information if the screen is not secured from view. Screen security policies address the timing of screen lock, the use of screen guards, and other aspects of security that protect patient information from casual or purposeful snooping.

- *Smartphones*—Smartphones are often used for communication during patient care, and many organizations allow staff to carry personal smartphones on their person during work hours. Smartphone policies provide boundaries and guidelines around the use of personal or company-owned phones, including camera use, texting, and disinfection.

- *Social media*—Several recent cases of improper disclosure of patient information on a social-media site have drawn the attention of the media (Polito, 2012). Social-media policies govern the use or non-use of social media for staff, and often expand to cover patient and family use as well.

- *System-error correction*—Errors can be made during electronic charting, and error mitigation and correction is covered by policy, which may include the proper methods to change erroneous information, the timeframe allowed for correction, and the error-correction escalation process.

- *Use of home equipment*—Because of the risk to patient privacy and security, organizations have implemented policies around the use of home equipment, such as personal laptop computers, personal tablets, and personal phones.

Prior to the end of training, learners will be provided with their personal system identifiers and passwords, which are typically accompanied by confidentiality agreements that require signatures. Integrating policies and procedures into the training process can add context to proper use of HIT and reinforce the consequences of improper use.

Target Technology and Related Competencies

Information technology (IT) is a broad topic. It includes technology involving the development, maintenance, and use of computer systems, software, and networks for the processing and distribution of data. The field of HIT is rapidly growing in areas traditionally not involving clinical informaticists. However, since the information technology is intersecting with clinical teams, nurse informaticists are sought to be part of a variety of teams evaluating and implementing the new technology.

Information Systems beyond Clinical Documentation

Electronic health record systems are much more than the documentation provided by clinicians. The integration of multiple information systems is key to viewing the complete legal healthcare record. Take a planned surgical case as an example of the complexity of the EHRS and the multiple modules used to help ensure the patient travels though the health system safely. The outpatient record documents the patient history and need for the surgical procedure. The patient is registered in the registration module for all downstream systems to identify the patient as pre registered to have surgery on a given day. In order for the patient to move forward in the electronic system, a preapproval for the surgery must be obtained from the insurance company and documented in the financial system. Once this is completed, the patient can be scheduled in the operating-room (OR) scheduling system to synchronize with the registration that was completed earlier. The patient now needs preoperative documentation from nursing staff and anesthesiology. Upon arrival for surgery, the patient is admitted through the registration system. Documentation of the patient's arrival is displayed on a large OR-based tracking board for everyone to view. The patient travels through the perioperative arena as the nurses, physicians, anesthesiologist, and technicians document the journey. In some areas, device integration has been established, which automatically feeds vital information to the EHRS. The patient is recovered and discharged to home, with homecare follow up. The visit is coded and billed. The homecare agency gets insurance approval to visit the patient, documents the visit in the homecare EHRS, bills for the visit, submits the bill, and tracks the agency-nurse's travel and visit time. To follow up on the details of the surgery, the patient can log into a personal health portal from the comfort of home. This is an example of potential touch points and systems that need to be maintained, enhanced, and upgraded. These touch points all involve information technology that needs informatics-nurse input on building, testing, implementation, and support.

Bedside Technologies

- Information technology at the point of care is becoming common.

  - Televisions in patient rooms now act as learning centers for the patients. Disease-specific education is automatically assigned to the patient, based on clinical documentation. The televisions are interactive and have interfaces to document viewing of the lesson and post-test in the patient's EHR.
  - Call-bell systems help communicate what a patient may need. Instead of a light and alarm to summon the nurse to the patient room, the call bells can now send specific text messages to patients' care providers, such as "I am in pain" or "I need something to drink," helping care providers anticipate and prioritize their response to the call bell.
  - Smart beds help reduce patient complications. These beds have the ability to turn patients, provide pulmonary toileting, initiate alarms based on patient movement to help prevent falls, reduce pressure points, and gather clinical data, such as patient weights.
  - Smart pumps aid the nurse in delivering intravenous medications by signaling an alert if a rate is outside of set defined parameters.
  - Audiovisual (AV) monitors are deployed to the rooms of patients at high risk for falls. Instead of having a technician sit with each patient, multiple patients can be remotely monitored via AV monitors at a central location. This device offers bi-directional communication and alarms to alert the nurse if a patient is at imminent risk for falling.
  - An electronic intensive-care unit (EICU) is a trend that initially began to help care for critically-ill patients in rural hospitals that did not have access to intensivists. It was proposed as an alternative solution to allow critical-care nurses and physicians to monitor ICU patients off site (Kowitlawakul, Baghi, & Kopac, 2011). Rooms are equipped with AV and physiological-monitoring equipment that interfaces to a remote location for continual monitoring and analysis by specialty trained nurses and physicians who alert and guide care providers in real time of any critical patient concerns.

Bedside technologies continue to grow; they interface with smart phones and other devices to improve communication and, ultimately, patient care. Nursing informatics plays an important role in developing, evaluating, implementing, and enhancing information technology. Leveraging nursing-informatics skills to bring the latest information technology successfully into the workflow of clinicians has been demonstrated to be best practice.

Wearable Technology

Wearable technologies (wearables) are not new, but are becoming more affordable and readily available. Patients are proactively choosing to wear new technologies or download applications to track their own data, before doctors even think to prescribe wearables as potential preventative measures. Children with geriatric loved ones are seeking new solutions to keep their loved ones healthier and safer. Wearables are part of the solution. Wearables may be the popular Apple Watch, or other innovations, such as socks that sense movement; underwear that detects moisture; radio-frequency devices to track a loved ones' locations because they are confused and wander; or necklaces that have a charm that rests on a person's chest, containing an implanted stethoscope to detect the early sounds of a wheeze before it progresses into a full-fledged asthma attack.

Nurses need to consider how this type of information technology will impact their practice. This type of technology requires data storage and surveillance. An informatics nurse can help to identify areas where data can be stored and accessed so as to develop workflows that support routine surveillance of these wearables, including creating indicators to prioritize some types of patient interaction with a clinician.

Education Methods

Training and education are often used interchangeably; however, the purpose, approach, and outcomes of these two methods of delivering information are quite different. Education is associated with the development of a theoretical and knowledge-based foundation intended to prepare the learner for understanding and applying concepts (Pignataro et al., 2014; Van Melle et al., 2014). An example of this are physicians who attend medical school to gain foundational knowledge, and then participate in residency training to gain skills in the application of knowledge and information (Bray, Kowalchuk, Waters, Laufman, & Shilling, 2012; Crofts et al., 2015). Training provides the skills needed to perform a task (Chen et al., 2015; Guppy-Coles et al., 2015). The ability to utilize HIT in practice requires a training approach to identify, develop, and utilize skills needed in the application of learning (Forsberg, Swartwout, Murphy, Danko, & Delaney, 2015; Schaeffer, 2015). Training can be provided without the concepts found in education, and education can be provided without the skills application found in training.

Due to the applied nature of HIT, provision of skills training plays a critical role in adoption and maximized use of HIT (Dastagir et al., 2012; Peck, 2013; Sorensen, 2013; What training resources are available for electronic health record implementation?, n.d.). Nurses, physicians, allied healthcare professionals, and healthcare support staff must become skilled in both the use of computer technology and the use of health-information systems; effective training is a key piece of this process (IT training, 2009; Kulhanek, 2011; Simon et al., 2013). Although training plays a critical role in the successful use of HIT, it consumes a large portion of a technology-implementation budget. There are numerous training-delivery methods, and costs for training differ for each method. Carefully matching training needs, end user characteristics, organizational resources, and training budgets to the best training-delivery method can help to manage and control training costs.

INSTRUCTOR-LED TRAINING Classroom or instructor-led training (ILT) is delivered by an instructor to an audience of learners who are present in the classroom or connected via AV technology. Development of ILT content requires the least amount of work hours, averaging around 100 hours of development per hour of delivered instructional content (Kapp & Defelice, 2009), but does not include time needed to prepare the information technology for training. Development of instructional content can include resources, such as manuals and handouts, the facilitator guide, sign-in sheets, learner exercises and scenarios, class evaluations, and notes pages.

ILT provides a kinetic learner experience, which requires both computer hardware and a training database that mirrors the actual information-technology environment. ILT provides an opportunity for learners to interact and ask questions during the training process and can be a useful tool for change management (Celia & Rebelo, 2015). ILT is often the most expensive training-delivery method; costs include, not only trainer and material costs, but also end user wages, technology, and facilities. Costs for ILT include:

- *Trainers.* Trainers are responsible for the delivery of ILT, and spend time in learner assessment, preparation for training, and formative and summative training evaluation, and may also be accountable for training development, communication, and scheduling.

- *Support staff.* Support staff may be used for printing, collating, and preparation of training materials for each class session, scheduling and tracking end users, and managing class attendance, room logistics, and any refreshments for the class.

- *End users.* Employees attending ILT may be salaried or hourly. With careful scheduling, salary costs for training may be paid as a regular workday. Scheduled development should be flexible so that overtime is avoided for hourly employees. Training schedules should be published far enough in advance so that managers and supervisors can plan for training needs and replacement staff.

- *Technology.* A training classroom that mimics the real information-technology environment will include computer monitors, keyboards, and other equipment for each end user in the class. In addition, each learner will need access to any peripheral devices such as bar-code scanners. This equipment may need to be purchased or leased for training purposes, and costs will include the time and labor for set up and testing.

- *Replacement staff.* Coverage is needed for patient care or other duties while a regularly scheduled employee is attending training. Salary costs for training will include both the replacement employee performing patient care, and the employee attending training.

- *Facilities.* Organizations may not have the available facilities to host ILT classes that would support a quality learning experience. Space may need to be acquired at off-site locations, such as hotel training rooms or conference centers. Costs for these facilities, which may require daily setup and cleanup, are included in training costs.

- *Materials.* Learners attending ILT may be supported with binders, paper manuals, handouts, assessments, job aids, and evaluation forms. Training-material needs must be identified, stock ordered, and the final product prepared for classroom use.

- *Instructional designers.* The design and development of training may be performed by instructional designers, who are specialists in instructional and learning theory, and training best practices. Instructional designers work with subject-matter experts to develop training content and materials so that trainers deliver the content. Costs for training-materials development by professional instructional designers may be less than the costs associated with paying high-salary healthcare staff to perform this function.

Because ILT is designed to be presented to a live audience, this method of training is best suited for a larger-scale training effort. HIT undergoes frequent updates and changes, making it difficult to repeat ILT training on a regular basis for newly hired employees. Large amounts of effort must be focused on ensuring that materials, and the training environment, continue to reflect the system and processes that are used in the live clinical setting.

The key to the success of ILT is the training schedule. Schedules need to accommodate all staff work shifts and include make-up sessions for those not able to attend the regularly scheduled classes. Training schedules for ILT must be developed and communicated early in the planning process so that leaders can accommodate vacations and staffing levels during training. Class length is dependent on the amount of content to be delivered. Sessions can range from one to eight hours and, if scheduled during patient care shifts, replacement staff will be needed for adequate coverage. Classes scheduled before or after work shifts may contribute to decreased concentration and lack of attention to the training due to fatigue, resulting in decreased learning and retention of content.

Training should be delivered as close to the implementation date as possible; when training is delivered too early, the end users will not retain information. The ideal timeframe for training is to deliver content no more than a month before implementation (Peck, 2013). The most successful training strategies make use of dedicated training days and times, when participants are not scheduled for clinical shifts, and expectations about class attendance are communicated and reinforced at the highest levels of leadership (Simon et al., 2013).

Training in a classroom requires suitable accommodations with enough space for the end users, technology, any included peripheral devices, and a screen and projector for the class to view, as well as space for the instructor to stand and move about. If suitable space is not available within an organization, the training rooms may need to be rented, as noted earlier. If space is rented, additional resources will be needed to deliver, set up, and test the training equipment prior to class. Wireless connections will need to be present and reliable, and facilities will need to include adequate parking, restroom and break facilities, and security—so equipment left overnight is safe.

As noted earlier, information technology used in training should include the same computers, keyboards, monitors, processes, and peripheral equipment that will be used in the clinical environment. The training environment may be created using real patient data copied into the training environment and cleansed of any patient-identifiable information. The process of copying live information into the training environment may need to be completed or refreshed just prior to when training begins to reflect the latest functionality in the software applications. If the clinical system changes, or is updated during training, the training environment should be updated as well to reflect the most accurate processes. The log-in process should be similar to the real log-in process, and end users should receive and test their personal log-in IDs and passwords at the end of the training session, necessitating the need to connect with the live clinical system from the training classroom.

Trainers can be employees of the organization who are either involved in education or function as super users. Trainers may also be contracted from vendors or training organizations, who are either involved only in delivering classroom instruction, or the entire training design-and-development process. Vendor trainers may train internal-organization trainers who will then conduct the end user classes. Just as staff must be scheduled for training, a schedule must be created for trainers, so all shifts and classes are accommodated. Depending on the knowledge level and experience of the end users, classes may require multiple trainers—one to present the materials and one or more to assist end users who might have questions or get lost during the instruction.

Most often, trainers are responsible for developing the training data, consisting of realistic patient-care scenarios, which is loaded into the training environment. The training data must meet the learning needs of all of the disciplines and roles represented by employees attending training. Learning needs or issues may emerge during each class, and trainers must have a plan to address or document issues, and communicate these with other trainers and training designers to improve ongoing classes. It may be helpful to establish a method or location for trainer communication and updates, such as a wiki site, group email, or intranet folder.

Training data must be comprehensive enough to address the needs of all learning scenarios presented during training, and enough examples must be present for multiple classes to use fresh examples each day. Data includes de-identified patient, employee, and physician databases; student log-in IDs and passwords; orders for procedures, communication, and medications; system alerts; and admission documentation, test results, and other care documentation for the training patients. The training database should also include alerts, error messages, and decision-support tools seen in the live clinical environment. Development and maintenance of the training database will require collaboration between the training and information-system teams. Trainers must be included in information-system, project-change communication to ensure that all production, application, and environment changes, such as code and software updates, are reflected accurately within the training environment.

The transfer of learning from the classroom to practice is supported by activities designed to keep staff engaged through hands-on practice and problem solving (Adams, 2000; Brady,

2011; Furlong, 2015; Gardner & Rich, 2014). Realistic patient scenarios are first presented using a step-by-step demonstration, followed by hands-on replication of the activity. Scenario-based training places learning into the context of patient care by presenting an end-to-end process, such as a client admission through discharge, which is broken down into smaller learning segments, each building on the prior segment to support completion of the entire scenario.

Ideally, scenarios should be designed to trigger the alerts, error messages, and decision-support notifications that are seen in the live clinical production environment. The scenario method of training supports the various learning-style preferences of the end users through auditory instructions, visual demonstrations, and kinesthetic replication of the presented process (Anderson, 2007; Chai, 2006; Middleton, 2012). Improved learning retention and validation of skills can be accomplished by including exercises into each segment of training. This allows the end users to work through a scenario independently after proceeding through the guided phase of training and through the presentation of specific problems, requiring the end users to access help resources and other tools to resolve the presented issues.

Classroom training is a high-cost, labor-intensive means of end user training that is best used for large-scale software implementations that require a large amount of knowledge dissemination, as well as interaction with and support of end users during learning. One risk of classroom training is there may be variation in the training delivered by different instructors, which can result in inconsistent training results. Classroom training is also difficult to continue for new employees. However, instructor-led training can allow for the flexibility needed when there are frequent changes to a new software application that cannot be taught using other training methods.

ELEARNING A lower-cost training alternative that can be used alone, or in combination with other training-delivery methods, is provided by eLearning, which is the presentation of learning content through information technology, such as a computer or handheld device (Hainlen, 2015a, 2015b). It is developed using applications that can provide content and interactivity; some applications are able to realistically simulate processes seen in the EHRS and other HIT. It also allows for asynchronous training: end users can access training when they are ready and able to learn. The effectiveness of eLearning as a training delivery method equal to ILT is supported by research (Ahlers-Schmidt, Wetta-Hall, Berg-Copas, Jost, & Jost, 2008; Buckley, 2003; Hall, 2015; McLoughlin & Lubna Alam, 2014). This modality can be used as an adjunct to other learning-delivery methods by providing an opportunity for pre-learning and preparation for validation of knowledge.

Development of eLearning requires an instructional designer with a specialized skill-set. Instructional designers work with SMEs to develop a curriculum, identify key learning outcomes, and validate workflows and processes. Each hour of eLearning that is produced typically takes from 100 to 150 hours to develop (Kapp & Defelice, 2009). Costs for the development of eLearning include the time of the instructional designer, the time of SMEs, the cost of the eLearning application, and any specialized software or hardware needed to produce the finished eLearning product, such as video encoders or professional recording microphones and editing software.

Applications for eLearning can range in price from a few hundred dollars for PowerPoint to several thousand dollars for applications such as Adobe Captivate, Lectora®, or Articulate. For professional eLearning development, a specialized computer with enhanced memory and graphics, along with a large high-definition monitor, may be required. Despite the higher costs of acquiring eLearning-development technology, the learning materials are easily reusable with little to no maintenance, providing an ideal tool for training new employees. In addition, employees are often able to complete eLearning during slower periods in a regularly scheduled shift, eliminating the need for replacement staff during class or for overtime pay. Many learning-management systems can track the time that end users spend in each learning module, their completion rates, and their quiz or test scores. Test questions can be randomized to reduce or eliminate issues of dishonesty, which can occur with unmonitored learning evaluation.

A well-designed eLearning program will contain elements that engage the end user through interactive simulations, activities, questions that check knowledge, sounds, and motion (McLoughlin & Lubna Alam, 2014). It may be tempting to include all of the bells and whistles available in an eLearning application into the training; however, research shows that unnecessary images, motion, colors, and other features can cause cognitive overload and decrease learning (Blayney, Kalyuga, & Sweller, 2015; Fraser et al., 2012). In a seminal work, Clark and Mayer (2008) noted that including both audible voice and written words in eLearning decreases learning and increases cognitive overload. Clark and Mayer noted that information obtained through either the ears or the eyes as spoken words or pictures, are processed in a single area of the memory system, which can attend to only one input at a time.

Applications for eLearning can typically be viewed on any computer with access to the learning-management system (LMS) where the eLearning content is housed, and many applications are scalable for viewing on a mobile device. End users may have difficulty viewing eLearning content on computers in patient-care areas if the computers do not contain sound cards or plug-ins that support the other application. Prior to release, eLearning modules should be tested on a variety of computers to ensure that end users have an optimal training experience.

eLearning is less flexible than classroom training, and frequently updating training modules to reflect system changes is not recommended. For this reason, development of eLearning content requires a broader approach to training than classroom training does. SMEs play an important role in the development of effective content. Rather than providing simulation of every detail for every step in a process, SMEs can identify key steps in a process, eliminating the smaller transition steps that are intuitive to the end user and are subject to frequent changes. eLearning can realistically simulate HIT, allowing the end user to see, hear, and perform actions based on realistic patient scenarios. Using this technology, end users can also repeat sections of training if desired or proceed faster through areas where they are familiar. If eLearning is used as an adjunct to classroom training, modules can familiarize end users with system functionality and basic processes, paving the way for shorter classroom time that is focused on the application of learning.

Developing eLearning content requires instructional designers with specialized skills, and the input of SMEs to design learning that focuses on the most important aspects of HIT processes. Due to the inflexibility of eLearning applications once developed, care should be taken to present key concepts, rather than all parts of a process. Evaluation, which will be discussed later, can be used to ensure that eLearning design is accurate, and that end users are demonstrating the desired learning objectives upon completion of the learning.

SELF-GUIDED LEARNING Although not frequently used, self-guided learning is a training-delivery method that utilizes text-based training manuals or materials that the end user can follow to learn a new system or process. Costs to produce a self-learning guide can range from stapled copies of paper or digital training manuals on the low end of cost, to professionally printed and bound manuals on the high end of cost. Learning guides can be a useful resource as staff are initially learning to use HIT, but are best used for limited changes rather than full-system implementations.

Drawbacks to self-guided training include:

- Little-to-no ability to monitor compliance with training.
- Quickly outdated printed materials unless electronic versions are available.

- Lack of control of printed materials: outdated resources may surface years later to guide incorrect processes.
- No instructional interaction with end users.

Due to the static nature of the content with this training-delivery method, best uses should be limited to short job aids for new functionality or for reminders on how to complete infrequently performed tasks in the HIT system.

JUST-IN-TIME TRAINING Just-in-time training is a method often preferred by physicians and other providers who are reluctant to spend time in a training classroom or viewing eLearning that is perceived as not relevant to their job function, preferring to incorporate their learning into daily practice (Catapano, 2012). Training delivered this way enables the physicians to place the process in the context of their daily patient-care activities, and, with a few repetitions of a process, they often feel comfortable performing it on their own. Just-in-time training results in greater efficiency and less non productive time for busy physicians and other providers, does not require classroom or scheduling resources, and supports greater adoption of information technology through training that is targeted to the immediate needs of the learner.

Just-in-time training involves the use of a trainer or super user who can be physically present with the providers to walk them through the processes they feel they need to understand, at the time they are completing the processes. Just-in-time training, however, may result in excessive downtime for trainers, with short periods of time when many providers need assistance simultaneously. Resources can be maximized by assigning these trainers to tasks that can be performed in patient-care areas, such as monitoring user reports, or auditing charts while waiting to assist providers with questions and training needs. Although the expertise of just-in-time trainers is strongest around physician workflows and processes, these trainers can also assist clinical staff with questions and workflow while in patient-care areas.

Additional drawbacks to this training method include gaps in training: the physician seldom sees the entire flow of a process and all of the steps involved from beginning to end. In addition, this type of training does not allow for problem-solving or addressing system alerts, or providing guidance as seen in a carefully planned class.

Blended Learning

Blended learning combines elements of several different training-delivery methods in order to maximize learning and application, while minimizing expensive time spent in a classroom. The blended-learning training model utilizes independent web- or print-based instruction as preparation for an interactive instructor-led training that focuses on integration of concepts, learned by the end user during the independent study, into the context of practice. The classroom portion of this training model can be used to validate skills, present practice scenarios, provide discussions that stimulate critical thinking, and reinforce knowledge gained during the independent portion of training. Costs for blended learning are typically less than classroom training, due to a decreased or eliminated requirement for replacement staff. Blended learning is more easily replicated for training incoming staff on an ongoing basis, due to the reusable materials that support independent study.

Adjunct Training Materials

Training can be supported by a variety of adjunct resources, including job aids; email reminders; ongoing training tips; easily accessible audio-video clips; and the ongoing presence of trainers and super users in work areas, department meetings, and other locations where caregivers gather. For tasks that are complex, infrequently used, or where accuracy is critical, printed job aids provide an additional level of support (Martin, Silas, Covner, Hendrie, & Stewart, 2015). Care should be taken to keep job aids and reference materials to a minimum, because end users will have difficulty locating and accessing these documents in a newly paperless environment where there may be little space for storing paper documents. Critical job aids can be laminated and affixed to computers so that they are readily available when needed.

Specific types of job aids are correlated with the types of information and task needs. As an example a task that must be completed in a particular sequence should have a job aid that depicts each step. When sequence does not matter a checklist is adequate. Other types of job-aids include decision tables, flow charts, and reference sources. Job aids may also be developed in response to practice gaps that are identified after EHRS training and implementation (Lear & Walters, 2015). Over time, the need for job aids, and the presence of the materials in patient-care areas, will decrease. Care should be taken to keep electronic copies of adjunct training materials easily accessible to staff hired after the initial system implementation, and to periodically review materials to ensure that they accurately reflect current system processes.

Training is most effective when the hardware, software, and training environment closely match what will be used in the clinical setting. Development of training content, the technology, and resource materials used to support training requires close collaboration between educators, informaticists, and those managing and updating the HIT system used in production.

Training staff to use HIT is critical to its successful use. Training can be time-consuming and expensive, necessitating careful consideration of all training-delivery options in order to match training to the situation and need. In addition to matching the training-delivery method with the training need, there is some evidence to suggest that certain groups of learners learn best under certain training conditions. New research suggests that rather than a one-time process, training should be regularly offered, and repeated approximately every three years to address declining perceptions of benefits; this helps to improve quality (Juris Bennett, Walston, & Al-Harbi, 2015).

Training Resources

According to the HIMSS EMR adoption model, 93.6% of US hospitals have adopted an EMRS that includes nursing documentation (HIMSS Analytics, 2016). As the initial rush of system implementation winds down, some training resources are now available that offer the chance to reuse content. The federal government, HIT or EHRS vendors, training-development vendors, and professional organizations all provide some form of educational content. Certain professional organizations such as HIMSS, AMIA, and ANIA promote instructional best practices for maximized learning outcomes.

Professional organizations with a focus on training and development provide a rich variety of resources and support for trainers and instructional designers. These organizations include the Association for Talent Development, the International Society for Performance Improvement, and the Association for Nursing Professional Development, most of which offer memberships at a reasonable cost.

The Association for Talent Development (ATD) (2016) is a professional organization that provides networking, research, and resources for professional training and development practitioners around the world. Just as healthcare has best practices and evidence-based care, training and instruction is based on theories and research that provide training best practices. ATD is focused on research and education that supports trainers, instructional designers, and talent-development practitioners with the latest evidence and resources that guide and support best practices for instructional development and delivery. The organization provides courses and certifications in learning design, eLearning, training, and other topics. It also hosts regular webinars and training events, as well as a yearly conference, eLearning resources, publications, and events held at local ATD chapters.

The International Society for Performance Improvement (ISPI) focuses primarily on human performance improvement by examining the most cost-effective interventions that influence human behavior, including training. Courses offered by ISPI look at all aspects of human performance improvement rather than just the development and delivery of training.

The Association for Nursing Professional Development (ANPD) focuses on the specialty of nursing professional development in order to enhance healthcare outcomes. ANPD provides rich experiential resources, links to additional resources, and the opportunity to communicate and collaborate with other clinical educators.

The federal government and some educational institutions provide open-source training materials focused on HIT and the regulatory environment driving change. These materials are useful for providing background and rationale for specific EHRS and information-technology functions within an organization. The Department of Health and Human Services, in collaboration with the Office of the National Coordinator, has developed a complete set of curricula designed to facilitate growth of the HIT workforce (Department of Health and Human Services, 2016). The current curriculum is undergoing an update, which should be available in late 2016 or early 2017. Additional workforce-training materials, such as the Open Learning Initiative launched by Carnegie Mellon University, can provide publicly available content that can be integrated into specific training programs.

An HIT or EHRS vendor may offer training for a client organization through the train-the-trainer method. Using this training method, the vendor trains select internal trainers, who then provide training for all of the end users. The vendor may provide the instructional curriculum, the organization may customize content provided by the vendor, or the organization may develop all of the content internally. Vendor training typically reflects a generic and standard use of information technology, not the customizations and workflow processes used within a specific organization. Customization of curriculum and workflow is often necessary to align the training with the work processes used in an organization.

Many training-development organizations have emerged since the explosion of EHRS implementations. These organizations specialize in providing instructional design, training, and support services to organizations with training needs. These vendors will work with SMEs within an organization to develop custom training that matches the workflow and functionality of the information technology. Training vendors can produce professional quality eLearning that can meet training needs for several years, while eliminating the need to develop internal expertise in the development of eLearning.

Although there are many resources available to produce HIT training, customized work is necessary in order to accurately capture the workflow and functionality of an organization's EHRS. Professional organizations provide resources that support the development and delivery of training by using evidence and best practices. Publicly available HIT workforce-training materials are available on the Internet, and the detailed and customized training that is needed for learning to use an EHRS is available through vendors and training-development organizations.

Evaluating Success

HIT training should focus on producing end users who are competent in using selected information technology, with the assumption that proficiency will occur over time with use. Successful training programs incorporate formative and summative evaluation to determine the effectiveness of the training program, and students' success at accomplishing learning objectives. A training program without evaluation can result in a large expense with little to no benefit. Evaluation should be planned when training is designed and developed.

Formative Evaluation

Formative evaluation assesses the effectiveness of the selected training-delivery method, the content, and the success of the training design to meet the needs of the learners (Flora & Marquez, 2015; Holden et al., 2015; McGowan, Cusack, & Poon, 2008). Formative evaluation can be conducted by involving SMEs and naïve end users in a systematic review of the training content at certain points in the development process. Tools used for formative evaluation can include focus groups, pre- and post-tests after content review, and evaluation of the ability to use the EHRS after completion of the draft version of the training materials.

Formative evaluation can also be conducted during the training process. Review of post-training evaluations and tests may highlight a pattern of learning that points to a gap in the training curriculum, the training-delivery method, or even the instructor. When conducted early in the training process, formative evaluation of training will allow for rapid, on-the-fly changes that increase the effectiveness of ongoing training.

Summative Evaluation

Summative evaluation assesses the success of the training program in enabling students to meet the learning objectives. Summative evaluation can be used to demonstrate reactions to training, knowledge gained during training, application of training on the job, the value of the training program to stakeholders and the business, and ultimately, to determine the return on investment of the training program.

REACTION EVALUATION Evaluation of response, or reaction to training, is the most commonly used method of summative evaluation. In this evaluation, the learners provide immediate feedback about how they liked the training program, how effective the training program was, and the perceived relevance to the work of the learners. Reaction evaluation can help to identify areas for improvement with instructors, class length, content delivery, and other logistics. However, Phillips and Stawarski, in their classic work, noted there is no evidence that a positive reaction to a learning program will result in successful application of learning on the job (2008). Learners can enjoy a training program and never apply the learning to their daily work. When learners are asked a question in an evaluation, there is the expectation that something may change as a result of the time and effort the learner puts into providing feedback. Be careful to only ask questions around items that you have the power to change. A question about the training room might elicit great feedback; however, the trainer may have little to no ability to change the size or other specifics of the training facilities.

KNOWLEDGE EVALUATION Knowledge evaluation is the assessment of how the learner has gained new information and knowledge during the training session. This type of information is typically collected during and immediately after training, using methods such as quizzes, post-tests, return demonstrations, or completion of presented scenarios. Although the learner will not be successful without the acquisition of knowledge during training, gaining knowledge alone does not correlate to successful application of knowledge (Phillips & Stawarski, 2008). The ultimate goal of any HIT-training program is to produce an effective on-the-job application of learning.

APPLICATION EVALUATION Collection of data used to evaluate the application of learning can occur both during the training session and a period of time after training, when the learner has had the opportunity to apply the knowledge gained in a real-life setting. Application-evaluation data requires more effort and time to collect, and may require chart audits and system reports designed to capture workers' use of key functionality. Very few organizations evaluate the application of learning due to the time and effort needed to collect this information; however, application evaluation and correction measures are the best way to ensure accurate and efficient use of health information technology.

BUSINESS EVALUATION The business evaluation, or value evaluation, examines the impact of training on the business of healthcare. This type of evaluation can be difficult to collect in a healthcare environment because the benefits of HIT training are difficult to separate from the benefits of the implementation of the information technology itself, and the impact on quality, error rates, and other business measures. More information about business evaluation can be found in these two classic models: Phillips training ROI model (Phillips & Phillips, 2008) and the Kirkpatrick four levels of evaluation model (Kirkpatrick & Kirkpatrick, 2006).

RETURN ON INVESTMENT The final level of training evaluation focuses on determining the value, or cost of each dollar spent on training for an EHRS implementation project—the return on investment (ROI). Data collection includes all of the summative evaluation data, all of the costs of training, any financial business impact as the result of training, and any intangible benefits, such as user- or patient-satisfaction scores. For more information on the ROI process, the Phillips training ROI model is presented in detail in the ROI Fundamentals series (Phillips & Phillips, 2008).

Training evaluation can provide information to improve training content and delivery methods through formative evaluation, while summative evaluation is used to evaluate the success of the training program in meeting the learning objectives. Learning objectives should be written prior to training development and used to guide both the development of the training materials and content, as well as the evaluation of the success of the training program.

When Information Technology Fails (Training on Backup Procedures)

Education on downtime procedures is necessary so staff are able to continue providing safe patient care and other clinical operations without access to HIT systems. In addition to providing information on where to locate data, how to communicate, and where to document when a system is unavailable, downtime procedures must also include parameters for when data is to be entered back into the computer system.

The latest generation of healthcare workers includes staff who have never used paper to manage patient care. One of the benefits of HIT is that information is contained in one location that is accessible from diverse remote locations. When a downtime event results in documentation of information on paper, the electronic document becomes an incomplete record, which may be missing information that is key to patient care and safety. Even the most reliable HIT system will occasionally experience both planned and unplanned downtime. Downtime planning should include:

- Forms for alternate documentation.
- Alternate sources of data.
- Communication processes.
- Data to be reentered into the chart after downtime—and, who will do the entry.
- Schedule for routine downtime drills.
- Policies and procedures.

- Schedule for planed downtimes that has the least impact on care.
- Methods for storing and accessing backup data.

Future Directions

Proficient use of HIT is dependent on effective training for all members of the workforce. As HIT progresses, advances in training technology keep pace. Just as healthcare strives to utilize best practices and evidence in the provision of care, best practices and evidence exist for training design and delivery. Sources, such as The Association for Talent Development and the Department of Health and Human Services, contain resources that can be easily accessed and implemented to guide training.

In the future, HIT training may need to be considered as an ongoing process, that includes updates on technology and workflow changes. Training in the future may be less disruptive to patient care when supported by the latest training delivery methods. Sustaining a culture of safety requires competent understanding and use of health information technology.

Summary

- Proficient use of HIT is imperative for the delivery of safe, efficient, quality patient care.
- Nurse informaticists play a major role in the development, implementation, and optimization of clinical applications, which include preparing the workforce to use HIT.
- Development of a workforce development plan requires an understanding of the needs of the educators who will train the workforce, how change takes place, how the external environment impacts the internal environment, and organizational culture.
- A workforce development plan requires identification of learning needs, subject-matter experts, goals and objectives, and the scope of the effort.
- A realistic training environment requires work to create and maintain, and facilitates learning.
- Training is an ideal time to introduce policies relevant to maintaining patient privacy and security of personal health information (PHI), system-downtime procedures, appropriate use of email and computer resources, equipment-cleaning protocols, password management, camera use, removal of devices from secure areas, social-media use, information security, error correction, and use of personal devices.
- Workforce development entails more than educating healthcare workers on how to use EHRs; it entails the entire spectrum of HIT they will use to perform their duties.
- The terms training and education are often used interchangeably, but differ in approach; education relies upon the development of a theoretical and knowledge-based foundation to help the learner understand and apply concepts. Training provides skills needed to perform a task.
- Training is not only critical to the successful use of HIT, but also consumes a large portion of a technology-implementation budget.
- Training approaches vary but may include: instructor-led training, eLearning, self-guided learning, just-in-time training, and blended learning. Costs for each method vary.
- Matching training needs, end user characteristics, organizational resources, and training budgets to the best training-delivery method can help to manage and control training costs.
- Adjunct training resources, such as job aids, email reminders, ongoing training tips, and easily accessible audiovisual clips, as well as the ongoing presence of trainers and super users in work areas, can support training efforts.

- The US government, software and training-development vendors, and professional organizations all provide some form of educational resources that can be tapped to maximize learning outcomes, even though training must be customized to reflect workflow and functionality at individual organizations.
- Formative and summative evaluation to determine the effectiveness of training is important to ensure successful HIT use.
- Evaluation should consider the effectiveness of the selected training method, content, and training design to meet the needs of the learners.
- Formative evaluation can identify gaps in training curriculum, delivery method, or with the instructor to provide corrective measures that ensure overall success.
- Summative evaluation can include user feedback, as well as knowledge, application, and business evaluation.
- User feedback is the most commonly used form of summative evaluation, although positive user feedback does not guarantee successful application.
- Knowledge evaluation is often used during or immediately after training to determine knowledge gained; quizzes, post-tests, return demonstrations, and completion of presented scenarios are frequently used measures.
- Application evaluation may be done both during and after training, but is more labor- and time-intensive to collect even though it may provide the best measure of training success.
- Business evaluation can be difficult to determine due to other variables, such as benefits associated with the new technology itself; return on investment (ROI) looks at all costs associated with training measured against positive business impact and intangible benefits, such as user- or patient-satisfaction scores.
- It is critical to include training on backup procedures so staff are able to continue providing safe patient care and other clinical operations without access to HIT: many current healthcare workers have never used paper to manage patient care, nor have they been without the safeguards provided with HIT.

Case Studies

1. Interprofessional Team

A hospital implemented an interprofessional patient electronic health record. All clinicians now document on the same flowsheet in shared areas. Both respiratory and nursing document lung assessments and interventions in the same place on the patient record. Traditionally, this documentation had been completed independently in a siloed health record. Each discipline had their own section for respiratory assessments and interventions. At 8 pm, the nurse documents that the patient's respiratory assessment is within defined limits (meaning normal). At 8:30 pm, the respiratory therapist documents the patient is mildly short of breath with an intermittent inspiratory wheeze. The respiratory therapist does not verbally communicate this to the nurse, thinking the nurse will see the respiratory therapist's assessment and intervention in the EHR. The next nursing assessment for this patient is not due until midnight.

What may be the end result of relying solely on the EHR for communication within the interprofessional team? Is there a way for an informatics specialist to display critical assessments differently to gain the attention of all clinicians?

2. Decision Support and Adoption

The Center for Medicare Services (CMS) requires all patients over the age of 65 who are admitted to the hospital to be screened to determine if they need the pneumonia vaccine. The assessment could be as simplistic as documenting if the vaccine is indicated—relying on a clinician's memory to evaluate the need for an assessment. However, a more innovative approach would be to provide decision-support to the clinician at the point of care. Pulling the age into the electronic vaccine assessment from patient demographics prompts the assessment. The components of the assessment pull from the electronic health record (EHR), or have dropdowns to select specific criteria-based answers. Once the assessment is complete, the clinician sees if the vaccine is indicated, and an automatic order is placed on the electronic medication-administration record scheduling the vaccine to be administered.

What more could be done to provide decision support for the end user so that the perception of the assessment is easy and intuitive?

3. Medication Reconciliation

A heart-failure patient is readmitted to the hospital 30 days post initial admission for shortness of breath. The hospital system has disparate EHRs. The outpatient, emergency room, and inpatient areas are all on different EHRs, which are not integrated. Upon the initial admission, the home-medication list is documented, but incorrect. The correction was made on the inpatient medication reconciliation page and transferred to the patient's discharge instructions, which was faxed to the primary-care physicians, who then noted and made the change in their EHR. Upon readmission, the emergency-room record lists the home-medication list.

What potential risks can you identify? Is there a way to resolve them?

4. Emotional Intelligence

As a nurse informaticist, you are showing subject-matter experts portions of documentation involving a falls risk-assessment screening. The group is diverse and has many opinions on the tool that should be used to screen patients. Some of the staff are extremely passionate on what tool should be used as it was what has always been used. You feel yourself starting to get emotional as well.

What would you do in this situation to keep it under control?

5. End User Needs

The IT department has completed an assessment on all units regarding placement of computers for the upcoming implementation of the EHR. Staff were not involved. However, the decision was made to place computers in every patient room to support the implementation. When nursing informatics learned of this decision, they decided to complete an end user needs-assessment to ensure this was the right decision. The assessment focused specifically on computer accessibility to support real-time point of care documentation in a variety of settings. The assessment identified that different departments, such as med/surg verses critical care, have different needs.

How would you, as a nurse informaticist, approach a new solution and approach to the IT department?

(Continued)

6. Scope Creep	A project team is in the process of implementing bar scanning for medication administration. Someone on the team suggests that scanning be expanded to include breast milk for newborns in the neonatal intensive-care unit. The original scope was to implement bar code scanning for medications only. By adding this to the project plan, many additional tasks need to be completed to ensure the breast milk has a bar code placed on the bottle (workflow), the scanner can read the bar code (process), new tasks need to be built in the EHR (build), and the nurse is able to document the administration on the electronic medication-administration record (process). Although this may not seem like a lot of additional work, every addition distracts the project team from the original project plan and scope. **How should this be discussed with the project team? List the pros/cons.**
7. Failure due to Lack of Integration	Your patient is preregistered for surgery. The register calls the surgery scheduler to let them know the date and time. This is documented in the surgical system. The patient has to cancel due to a family emergency. They call the registrar to let them know. The registrar does not communicate this with the surgical scheduler, assuming they will see the registration change. Because the two systems are not integrated, there is no communication to the perioperative system that anything has been changed. The patient remains on the OR schedule as a case, but never arrives, costing the hospital significant time and money to correct. **Could this communication breakdown have been avoided? If so, how?**
8. Registration Error	One of the cardinal rules of healthcare is to ensure a patient is registered correctly. An incorrect registration—whether it be a duplicate or on an incorrect patient record—could have extreme effects. Twin boys see the same primary physician. Both have had tests at a local hospital. They have different first names; however, they share the same last name and date of birth. The registrar asks one of the patients for his name and date of birth. The record displays prior information. The registrar choses the other twin accidently. The patient goes on to have abnormal results, which are reported back to the wrong twin. Not only is this a HIPAA breach, but it is also potentially an omission of important information that needs to get to the correct patient, and be removed from the incorrect record. Utilizing present day technology to fix this issue is not an easy task, especially regarding the downstream effect it may have on other electronic systems with automatic feeds. **How can this be more streamlined and error proofed?**

About the Authors

Diane Humbrecht, DNP, RN is the Chief Nursing Informatics Officer at Abington Jefferson Health. She serves on the American Nursing Informatics Association Board to promote the role of Nursing Informatics. She also works as an adjunct professor teaching informatics to DNP candidates.

Brenda Kulhanek, PhD, MSN, MS, RN-BC is the AVP of Clinical Education for HCA in Nashville, TN. She has served on the board of the American Nursing Informatics Association since 2012, and currently fills the role of President Elect. Dr. Kulhanek is an adjunct and visiting professor for graduate and post-graduate nursing informatics programs at Walden University and Chamberlain College of Nursing.

References

Abdrbo, A. A. (2015). Nursing informatics competencies among nursing students and their relationship to patient safety competencies: Knowledge, attitude, and skills. *CIN: Computers, Informatics, Nursing, 33*(11), 509–514.

Adams, S. J. (2000). Improving safety instruction and results: Five principles of sound training. *Professional Safety, 45*(12), 40.

Ahlers-Schmidt, C. R., Wetta-Hall, R., Berg-Copas, G., Jost, J. C., & Jost, G. (2008). Evaluating program effectiveness: Creating a reliable and valid tool. *Journal of Continuing Education in Nursing, 39*(3), 139–144.

Alasmary, M., Metwally, A., & Househ, M. (2014). The association between computer literacy and training on clinical productivity and user satisfaction in using the electronic medical record in Saudi Arabia. *Journal of Medical Systems, 38*(8), 1–13. doi:10.1007/s10916-014-0069-2

American Academy of Nursing. (2015). Putting "health" in the electronic health record: A call for collective action. *Nursing Outlook, 63*(5), 614–616.

American Nurses Association. (2015). *Nursing informatics: Scope and standards of practice (2nd ed.)*. Washington, DC: Nursesbooks.org.

Anderson, J. (2007). *A conceptual framework of a study in preferred learning styles: Pedagogy or andragogy*. Dissertation Abstracts International, (UMI NO. 3258204). Retrieved from http://proquest.umi.com.library.capella.edu/pqdweb?did=1296096131&Fmt=7&clientId=62763&RQT=309&VName=PQD

Association for Talent Development. (2016). Who we are. Retrieved from www.td.org/About

Auerbach, D., Staiger, D., Muench, U., & Buerhaus, P. (2012). The nursing workforce: A comparison of three national surveys. *Nursing Economics, 30*(5), 253–260.

Blayney, P., Kalyuga, S., & Sweller, J. (2015). Using cognitive load theory to tailor instruction to levels of accounting students' expertise. *Journal of Educational Technology & Society, 18*(4), 199–210.

Bova, C., Route, P. S., Fennie, K., Ettinger, W., Manchester, G. W., & Weinstein, B. (2012). Measuring patient-provider trust in a primary care population: Refinement of the health care relationship trust scale. *Research in Nursing & Health, 35*(4), 397–408. doi:10.1002/nur.21484

Brady, D. S. (2011). Using quality and safety education for nurses (QSEN) as a pedagogical structure for course redesign and content. *International Journal of Nursing Education Scholarship, 8*(1), 1–18. doi:10.2202/1548-923X.2147

Bray, J. H., Kowalchuk, A., Waters, V., Laufman, L., & Shilling, E. H. (2012). Baylor SBIRT medical residency training program: Model description and initial evaluation. *Substance Abuse, 33*(3), 231–240. doi:10.1080/08897077.2011.640160

Buckley, K. M. (2003). Evaluation of classroom-based, web-enhanced, and web-based distance learning nutrition courses for undergraduate nursing. *Journal of Nursing Education, 42*(8), 367–370.

Budden, J. S., Moulton, P., Harper, K. J., Brunell, M. L., & Smiley, R. (2016). The 2015 national nursing workforce survey. *Journal of Nursing Regulation*, S2.

Catapano, J. (2012). Tying credentialing to health care technology. *Physician Executive, 38*(6), 42–46.

Celia, A., & Rebelo, D. (2015). Sustaining the human experience in a high tech environment: EMR implementation. *MEDSURG Nursing, 24*(2), 8–9.

Chai, K. T. (2006). *Improving online post licensure registered nursing education: Relating learning style and computer and information literacy to success.* Dissertation Abstracts International. (DAI-B 68/01)

Chen, T. C., Hamlett-Berry, K. W., Watanabe, J. H., Bounthavong, M., Zillich, A. J., Christofferson, D. E., & . . . Hudmon, K. S (2015). Evaluation of multidisciplinary tobacco cessation training program in a large health care system. *American Journal of Health Education, 46*(3), 165–173. doi:10.1080/19325037.2015.1023475

Clancy, T. R., Bowles, K. H., Gelinas, L., Androwich, I., Delaney, C., Matney, S., Sensmeier, J., & Westra, B. (2014). A call to action: Engage in big data science. *Nursing Outlook, 62*(1), 64-65. http://dx.doi.org/10.1016/j.outlook.2013.12.006

Clark, R., & Mayer, R. (2008). *elearning and the science of instruction* (2nd ed.). San Francisco: John Wiley & Sons, Inc.

Codier, E., & Odell, E. (2014). Measured emotional intelligence ability and grade point average in nursing students. *Nurse Education Today, 34*(4), 608–12. Published by Elsevier Inc, © 2014. doi:10.1016/j.nedt.2013.06.007

Crofts, J. F., Mukuli, T., Murove, B. T., Ngwenya, S., Mhlanga, S., Dube, M., & . . . Sibanda, T. (2015). Onsite training of doctors, midwives and nurses in obstetric emergencies, Zimbabwe. *Bulletin of the World Health Organization, 93*(5), 347–351. doi:10.2471/BLT.14.145532

Dastagir, M. T., Chin, H. L., McNamara, M., Poteraj, K., Battaglini, S., & Alstot, L. (2012). Advanced proficiency EHR training: Effect on physicians' EHR efficiency, EHR satisfaction and job satisfaction. In *AMIA Annual Symposium Proceedings*, pp. 136–143.

Department of Health and Human Services. (2016). Curriculum development centers program: Providers and professionals. Retrieved from www.healthit.gov/providers-professionals/health-it-curriculum-resources-educators

Dooling, J. A. (2012). It's about the patient: Engagement through personal health records and patient portals. *Journal of Health Care Compliance, 14*(3), 33–34.

Fisher, E. S., Shortell, S. M., & Savitz, L. A. (2016). Implementation science: A potential catalyst for delivery system reform. *JAMA: Journal of the American Medical Association, 315*(4), 339–340. doi:10.1001/jama.2015.17949

Flora, M. S., & Marquez, S. (2015). Formative evaluation of a master of public health curriculum. *Medical Education, 49*(5), 519–520. doi:10.1111/medu.12702

Forsberg, I., Swartwout, K., Murphy, M., Danko, K., & Delaney, K. R. (2015). Nurse practitioner education: Greater demand, reduced training opportunities. *Journal of the American Association of Nurse Practitioners, 27*(2), 66–71. doi:10.1002/2327-6924.12175

Fraser, K., Ma, I., Teteris, E., Baxter, H., Wright, B., & McLaughlin, K. (2012). Emotion, cognitive load and learning outcomes during simulation training. *Medical Education, 46*(11), 1055–1062. doi:10.1111/j.1365-2923.2012.04355.x

Furlong, K. (2015). Learning to use an EHR: Nurses' stories. *Canadian Nurse, 111*(5), 20–24.

Gardner, A., & Rich, M. (2014). Error management training and simulation education. *Clinical Teacher*, *11*(7), 537–540. doi:10.1111/tct.12217

Guppy-Coles, K. B., Prasad, S. B., Smith, K. C., Hillier, S., Lo, A., & Atherton, J. J. (2015). Evaluation of training nurses to perform semi-automated three-dimensional left ventricular ejection fraction using a customised workstation-based training protocol. *Journal of Clinical Nursing*, *24*(11/12), 1479–1488. doi:10.1111/jocn.12666

Hainlen, L. (2015a). Case in point: Elearning saves money in EHR implementation. Retrieved from www.td.org/Publications/Blogs/Healthcare-Blog/2015/02/Case-in-Point-ELearning-Saves-Money-in-EMR-Implementation

Hainlen, L. (2015b). Does elearning really save money in EHR implementations? Retrieved from www.td.org/Publications/Blogs/Healthcare-Blog/2015/01/Does-ELearning-Really-Save-Money-in-EHR-Implementations

Hall, S. (2015). World Health Organization: eLearning equal to traditional training for healthcare workforce. *FierceHealthIT*. Retrieved from www.fiercehealthit.com/story/world-health-organization-elearning-equal-traditional-training-healthcare-w/2015-01-12

Healthcare Information and Management Systems Society (HIMSS). (2014). HIMSS 2014 nursing informatics workforce survey © 2014. Retrieved from HIMSS.org

HIMSS Analytics. (2016). US EMR Adoption Model. Retrieved from https://app.himssanalytics.org/stagesGraph.asp

Holden, C. A., Collins, V. R., Anderson, C. J., Pomeroy, S., Turner, R., Canny, B. J., & McLachlan, R. I. (2015). "Men's health—a little in the shadow": A formative evaluation of medical curriculum enhancement with men's health teaching and learning. *BMC Medical Education*, *15*, 210–210. doi:10.1186/s12909-015-0489-9

Hoyt, R., Adler, K., Ziesemer, B., & Palombo, G. (2013). Evaluating the usability of a free electronic health record for training. *Perspectives in Health Information Management*, 1–14.

Hussey, P. A., & Kennedy, M. A. (2016). Instantiating informatics in nursing practice for integrated patient centered holistic models of care: A discussion paper. *Journal of Advanced Nursing*, *72*(5), 1030–1041. doi: 10.1111/jan.12927

Institute of Medicine (IOM). (2008). *Retooling for an aging America: Building the health care workforce.* Washington, DC: The National Academies Press.

IT training. (2009). *H&HN: Hospitals & Health Networks.* *83*(4), 40–40.

Juris Bennett, C., Walston, S. L., & Al-Harbi, A. (2015). Understanding the effects of age, tenure, skill, and gender on employee perceptions of healthcare information technology within a middle eastern hospital. *International Journal of Healthcare Management*, *8*(4), 272–280. doi:10.1179/2047971915Y.0000000010

Kapp, K., & Defelice, R. (2009). Time to develop one hour of training. *Learning Circuits*. Retrieved from www.td.org/Publications/Newsletters/Learning-Circuits/Learning-Circuits-Archives/2009/08/Time-to-Develop-One-Hour-of-Training

Kirkpatrick, D., & Kirkpatrick, J. (2006). *Evaluating training programs: The four levels* (3rd ed.). San Francisco: Berrett-Koehler Publishers, Inc.

Kowitlawakul, Y., Baghi, H., & Kopac, C. A. (2011). Psychometric evaluation of the nurses' attitudes toward eICU scale. *Journal of Nursing Measurement*, *19*(1), 17–27. doi:10.1891/1061-3749.19.1.17

Kulhanek, B. (2011). EMR development . . . always be prepared. *Nursing Management*, *42*(12), 24–27. doi:DOI: 10.1097/01.NUMA.0000407575.88737.e8

Lear, C. L., & Walters, C. (2015). Use of electronic nurse reminders to improve documentation: A process improvement for a comprehensive stroke center. *CIN: Computers, Informatics, Nursing*, *33*(12), 523–529. doi:10.1097/CIN.0000000000000199

Lee, A., Moy, L., Kruck, S. E., & Rabang, J. (2014). The doctor is in, but is academia? Re-tooling IT education for a new era in healthcare. *Journal of Information Systems Education, 25*(4), 275–281.

Martin, D. B., Silas, S., Covner, A., Hendrie, P. C., & Stewart, F. M. (2015). Development of a hematology/oncology ICD-10 documentation job aid. *Journal of the National Comprehensive Cancer Network, 13*(4), 435–440.

McGowan, J. J., Cusack, C. M., & Poon, E. G. (2008). Formative evaluation: A critical component in EHR implementation. *Journal of the American Medical Informatics Association, 15*(3), 297–301.

McGraw, D., Belfort, R., Pfister, H., & Ingargiola, S. (2015). Engaging patients while addressing their privacy concerns: The experience of Project HealthDesign. *Personal & Ubiquitous Computing, 19*(1), 85–89. doi:10.1007/s00779-014-0809-9

McLoughlin, C. E., & Lubna Alam, S. (2014). A case study of instructor scaffolding using web 2.0 tools to teach social informatics. *Journal of Information Systems Education, 25*, 125–136.

Middleton, K. G. (2012). Clinical simulation: Designing scenarios and implementing debriefing strategies to maximize team development and student training. *Canadian Journal of Respiratory Therapy, 48*(3), 27–29.

Murphy, G. (2000). Patient-centered email: Developing the right policies. *Journal of AHIMA, 71*(3), 47–54. Retrieved from http://library.ahima.org/doc?oid=106416#.V1XVmhUrIVN

Murray, B., & McCrone, S. (2015). An integrative review of promoting trust in the patient-primary care provider relationship. *Journal of Advanced Nursing, 71*(1), 3–23. doi:10.1111/jan.12502

National Council of State Boards of Nursing (NCSBN). (May 18, 2016). NCSBN and the National Forum publish the 2015 national nursing workforce survey. Retrieved from www.ncsbn.org/9487.htm

Peck, A. (2013). EHR implementation: Training pays dividends. *Medical Economics. 90*(14), 53–56.

Peterson, A. M. (2012). Medical record as a legal document part 1: Setting the standards. *Journal of Legal Nurse Consulting, 23*(2), 9–17.

Phillips, P., & Phillips, J. (2008). *Why and when to measure return on investment* (Vol. 1). San Francisco: John Wiley & Sons, Inc.

Phillips, P. P., & Stawarski, C. (2008). Data collection. In P. P. Phillips & J. J. Phillips (Eds.), *The Measurement and Evaluation Series*. San Francisco: John Wiley & Sons, Inc.

Pignataro, R. M., Gurka, M. J., Jones, D. L., Kershner, R. E., Ohtake, P. J., Stauber, W. T., & Swisher, A. K. (2014). Tobacco cessation counseling training in US entry-level physical therapist education curricula: Prevalence, content, and associated factors. *Physical Therapy, 94*(9), 1294–1305. doi:10.2522/ptj.20130245

Polito, J. M. (2012). Ethical considerations in Internet use of electronic protected health information. *Neurodiagnostic Journal (ASET—The Neurodiagnostic Society), 52*(1), 34–41.

Rashleigh, L., Cordon, C., & Wong, J. (2011). Creating opportunities to support oncology nursing practice: Surviving and thriving. *Canadian Oncology Nursing Journal, 21*(1), 7–10. doi:10.5737/1181912x211710

Rights, T. O. f. C. (n.d.). Summary of the HIPAA privacy rule. *Health Information Privacy.* Retrieved from www.hhs.gov/hipaa/for-professionals/privacy/laws-regulations/index.html

Savel, R. H., & Munro, C. L. (March, 2016). Emotional intelligence: For the leader in us all. *American Journal of Critical Care,* 104. doi:10.4037/ajcc2016969

Schaeffer, J. (2015). An academic approach to EHR training. *For the Record (Great Valley Publishing Company, Inc.), 27*(5), 24–27.

Sheikh, A., Sood, H., & Bates, D. (2015). Leveraging health information technology to achieve the "triple aim" of healthcare reform. *Journal of the American Medical Informatics Association, 22*(4), 849–856.

Simon, S. R., Keohane, C. A., Amato, M., Coffey, M., Cadet, B., Zimlichman, E., & Bates, D. W. (2013). Lessons learned from implementation of computerized provider order entry in 5 community hospitals: A qualitative study. *BMC Medical Informatics & Decision Making, 13*(1), 1–10. doi:10.1186/1472-6947-13-67

Sorensen, D. (2013). Best practices: Training your staff to use your new EHR system. *Medical Economics, 90*(20), 82–82.

Staggers, N., Gassert, C., & Curran, C. (2001). Informatics competencies for nurses at four levels of practice. *Journal of Nursing Education, 4*(7), 303–316.

University Alliance. (2014). Managing scope creep in project management. Retrieved from www.villanovau.com/resources/project-management/project-management-scope-creep/#.WEdIytIrLRZ

Van Melle, E., Lockyer, J., Curran, V., Lieff, S., St. Onge, C., & Goldszmidt, M. (2014). Toward a common understanding: Supporting and promoting education scholarship for medical school faculty. *Medical Education, 48*(12), 1190–1200. doi:10.1111/medu.12543

What training resources are available for electronic health record implementation? (n.d.). *Frequently Asked Questions.* Retrieved from www.healthit.gov/providers-professionals/faqs/what-training-resources-are-available-electronic-health-record-implemen

Wilson, T. (2016). Creating co-accountability for workplace goals. *Leadership Excellence Essentials, 33*(10), 40–41.

Winslow, S. (2016). Multisite assessment of nursing continuing education learning needs using an electronic tool. *Journal of Continuing Education in Nursing, 47*(2), 75–81. doi:10.3928/00220124-20160120-08

Zimlichman, E., Rozenblum, R., Salzberg, C.A., Jang, Y., Tamblyn, M., Tamblyn, R., & Bates, D.W. (2012). Lessons from the Canadian national health information technology plan for the United States: Opinions of key Canadian experts. *Journal of the American Medical Informatics Association, 19* (3), 453–459.

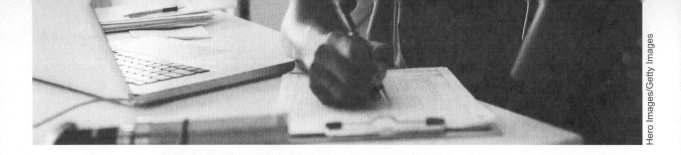

Chapter 13
Information Security and Confidentiality

Ami Bhatt, DNP, MBA, RN, CHPN, CHCI
Patricia Mulberger, MSN, RN-BC

⌄ Learning Objectives

After completing this chapter, you should be able to:

- State the differences between privacy, confidentiality, information privacy, information security, and information consent.

- Describe the processes required to attain security in a computer network.

- Discuss the significance of security for information integrity.

- Recognize potential threats to system security and information.

- Analyze processes to prevent threats to network security, and how to anticipate the threats.

- Discuss the responsibility that nurses have to protect patient information and privacy.

- Review best practices for secure authentication.

- Identify proper disposal techniques for common examples of confidential forms and communication seen in healthcare settings.

- Appraise strategies to ensure that the use of information technology protects the privacy and security of patient information.

- Describe privacy and confidentiality issues with email and social media.

- Identify how the HIPAA security and privacy rules protect personal health information (PHI).

- Examine special considerations related to mobile and wearable technology.

The need for increased levels of security management in organizations continues to grow. With increasing globalization and the increased use of the Internet, information technology

(IT) related risks have multiplied, including identity theft, fraudulent transactions, privacy violations, lack of authentication, redirection, phishing and spoofing, data sniffing and interception, false identities, and fraud attempts. Information system security, integrity, privacy, accessibility, and the confidentiality of personal information are major concerns in today's society as reports of stolen and compromised financial information and healthcare records grow at an increasing rate. The fast-growing and increasingly widespread use of online information technology and electronic business, along with numerous occurrences of information-system penetrations, as well as national and international terrorism, have created a need for better methods of protecting computer systems and the information they store, process, and transmit.

Healthcare information systems are required to provide rapid access to accurate and complete client information for legitimate users, while at the same time safeguarding client privacy and confidentiality. The use of healthcare information systems (HIS) assists us in lowering costs, reducing medication errors, and enhancing productivity, which is needed due to an aging population and a shortage of healthcare professionals (Yang, Kankanhalli, Ng, & Lim, 2013). We must maintain privacy and confidentiality, despite shortages of personnel. As a result, healthcare administrators must implement policies and procedures that protect information, in order to comply with the Health Insurance Portability and Accountability Act (HIPAA) requirements, and to also meet accreditation criteria set forth by the Joint Commission on Accreditation of Healthcare Organizations (1996). These criteria change as technology evolves, and intrusion techniques become more sophisticated. The HIPAA security rule does not specify the utilization of particular technologies (Department of Health and Human Services, 2007); instead, it requires organizations to determine threats and choose appropriate protective measures for information, not only in electronic formats, but in all formats. Protection of client privacy and confidentiality requires an understanding of privacy, confidentiality, information privacy, and system security, as well as potential threats to these issues within an organization. Although there have been numerous improvements in information-technology security capabilities as well as in legal and regulatory standards, breaches of security continue to occur. This fact highlights the need for constant vigilance on the part of an organization's administrators, and all employees, in order to determine threats and implement protective measures for information in all formats. Continuing reports of intrusion and violations of privacy events are clear indications that electronic records are particularly susceptible to compromise on a large scale via loss, theft, or penetration of system safeguards. In the absence of a single, large-scale national authentication infrastructure, information must be protected through a combination of electronic and manual methods. This was corroborated in a systematic review of literature conducted by Rezaeibagha, Susilo, and Win (2015) who analyzed the results of 55 studies using two international standards to identify 13 features essential to safeguard the privacy and security of EHRs. These features represent a combination of technology and policy. But first, a review of key terms and concepts is required, which follows here.

Privacy, Confidentiality, Security, and Consent

While the terms privacy and confidentiality are often used interchangeably, they are not the same. In their discussion of how practitioners need to understand the demands that various forms of technology pose for privacy, Vasalou, Joinson, and Houghton (2015) noted a lack of consensus on the definition of privacy. For the purpose of this chapter the definitions for privacy and confidentiality in the recently revised American Nurses Association (2015a) *Code of Ethics* will be used.

According to the American Nurses Association, "Privacy is the right to control access and disclosure or nondisclosure of information pertaining to oneself and to control the circumstances, timing, and extent to which information may be disclosed" (2015a, p. 9). **Privacy** includes the right to determine what information is collected or shared, how it is used, and the ability to access collected personal information to review its security and accuracy. HIPAA regulations require that healthcare consumers receive clearly written explanations of how facilities and providers may use and disclose their health information.

The American Nurses Association Code of Ethics Provision 3 stresses the nurse's obligation to protect patients from harm. The first interpretive statement for this provision involves the protection of the rights of privacy and confidentiality. Failure to safeguard privacy violates the trust between the nurse and the patient (Winland-Brown, Lachman, & Swanson, 2015). Privacy should be managed in any patient-care setting and every mode.

Personal information identifies a person, or could identify a person. Examples would include name, address, phone number, an email address, and, possibly, photos, videos, and workplace name, as well as opinions and preferences. Such identifying information can potentially allow unauthorized access to healthcare records, financial records, birth records, educational records, credit records, work records, and so on. In an age where identity theft is a real possibility, it is crucial that personal information is managed with caution and security.

Confidentiality refers to a situation in which a relationship has been established, and private information is shared but not disclosed (American Nurses Association, 2015a). In a healthcare environment, confidentiality is an ethical principle and legal obligation that a healthcare professional will not disclose information relating to a patient, unless the patient gives consent permitting the disclosure. Confidentiality is essential for the accurate assessment, diagnosis, and treatment of health-related problems. Once a client discloses confidential information, control over the release of this information lies with the person(s) who access it. Confidentiality is one of the core tenets of healthcare. The ethical duty of confidentiality entails keeping information shared during the course of a professional relationship secure and secret from others. This obligation involves making appropriate security arrangements for the storage and transmission of private information and ensuring that the hardware, software, and networks used for storage and transmission of information are secure, and measures are implemented to prevent the interception of email, instant messages (IMs), faxes, and other types of correspondence that contain private information. Nurses are obligated by the American Nurses Association *Code of Ethics* and state-practice laws to protect patient privacy (Winland-Brown, Lachman, & Swanson, 2015). Inappropriate redisclosure can be extremely damaging, resulting in denial of insurance coverage, harm to reputations and personal relationships, and can even result in job loss.

Most breaches of confidentiality occur as a result of carelessness and can be avoided through rigorous control over client records, and by not discussing clients in public areas or with persons who do not have a need to know. The obligation of confidentiality prohibits healthcare professionals from disclosing information about a patient's case to other interested parties, and encourages them to take precautions with the information to ensure that only authorized access occurs. But the context of healthcare practice makes it difficult to meet the healthcare professional's obligation to protect patient confidentiality. In the course of caring for patients, a healthcare professional will find him- or herself exchanging information about patients with other healthcare professionals. These discussions are often critical for patient care and are an integral part of the learning experience in a teaching hospital. As such, they are justifiable so long as precautions are taken to limit the ability of others to hear or see confidential information. Electronic records are another portal for a breach of confidentiality, and all security measures should be taken.

Information-and- data privacy is the relationship between data collection; information technology; an individual's expectation of privacy; and the legal, ethical, and political issues connected to these relationships. A definition of information-and-data privacy that remains relevant today is the right to choose the conditions and extent to which information and beliefs are shared (Murdock, 1980). Informed consent for the release of specific information illustrates information privacy in practice. Information privacy also includes the right to ensure the accuracy of information collected by an organization (Murdock, 1980). Information-privacy concerns exist wherever personally identifiable information is collected and stored in digital form or any other format. Data-privacy issues can arise with information from a wide range of sources, such as:

- Healthcare records
- Criminal-justice investigations and proceedings
- Financial institutions and transactions
- Genetic traits and material
- Residence and geographic records
- Social networking.

The challenge for information-and-data privacy is to support needed sharing while protecting personally identifiable information. Information-and-data security utilizes software, hardware, and human resources to address this issue.

According to Tajuddin, Olphert, and Doherty (2015), the concept of information security occurs with the realization that information has value and requires protection. This includes the protection of information against threats to its integrity, inadvertent disclosure, or availability. Information systems can improve protection for client information in some ways and endanger it in others. Unlike the paper record that can be read by anyone, the automated record cannot easily be viewed without an access code and privileges. Poorly secured information systems can threaten record confidentiality, because records may be accessed from multiple sites with immediate dissemination of information, making clients vulnerable to the redisclosure of sensitive information. The HIPAA Privacy Rule was created to protect the privacy of people who seek care in the healthcare system. Effective information-security systems incorporate a range of policies, security products, technologies, and procedures. Software applications, which provide firewall protection and virus scanners, are not enough on their own to protect the security of information. A set of policies, procedures, and security systems needs to be applied to effectively deter access to information, and information-system users must make the final determination as to whether they will or will not use the processes and safeguards that have been put into place. Effective information security also requires the realization that information must be secure on information systems as well as the many devices that are used in today's complex healthcare delivery system, including portable devices and smartphones (Chaudhary & Ward, 2014).

Information consent occurs when an individual authorizes healthcare personnel to use and share his or her information based on an informed understanding of how this information will be shared and used for treatment purposes (MITRE Corporation, 2014). Obtaining consent should include making the individual aware of any risks that may exist to privacy, as well as measures implemented to protect privacy. HIPAA has adopted a consent form for the release of health-related information that is intended to protect a patient's privacy. The HIPAA consent form is based on rules and restrictions on who may see or be notified of a patient's personal health information (PHI). These restrictions do not include the normal interchange of information necessary to provide a patient with office services, but attempt to balance these needs with the goal of providing a patient with quality professional service and care (Wulf, 2007). While information consent forms are still largely paper, part of the Office of the National Coordinator for Health Information Technology (ONCHIT) ten-year vision for an interoperable HIT infrastructure calls for electronic management of informed-consent documents.

Information System Security

Information -system security is the continuous protection of both data and information housed on a computer system, and the system itself, from threats or disruption (Park, Chandramohan, Suresh, Giordano, & Kwiat, 2013; Tajuddin, Olphert, & Doherty, 2015). The primary goals of healthcare information-system security are the protection of client confidentiality and information integrity, and the timely availability of information when it is needed. Availability is necessary in today's information-driven world, yet it is constantly challenged as emerging technologies expand traditional security perimeters. Availability is dependent upon survivability.

Park et al. defined survivability as the ability of the information system to "continue its mission even in the presence of damage" (2013, p. 1394). The goals of healthcare-information-system security are best accomplished when security is planned rather than applied to an existing system after problems occur. Planning for security saves time and money, and should be regarded as a form of insurance against downtime, breaches in confidentiality, loss of consumer confidence, cybercrime, liability, and lost productivity. Good security practices are necessary to ensure compliance with HIPAA legislation. Effective security starts with a thorough assessment of assets, risks, and necessary resources; a well-crafted security plan and policy; and a supportive organizational culture and structure. Administrative support is essential to this effort. In addition to being secure, systems must still be easily accessible for legitimate users.

Risks

Risk is a function of the likelihood of a given threat-source exercising a particular potential vulnerability, and the resulting impact of that adverse event on an organization (National Institute of Standards and Technology, 2012). Every component in a network is under attack to some degree at any one time. Potential threats to information and system and device security come from a variety of sources. These can include thieves, hackers, crackers, denial-of-service attacks, terrorists, viruses, snatched websites, flooding sites with fictitious data, power fluctuations that damage systems or data, revenge attacks, fires and natural disasters, human error, and threats barely imagined by most HIT users. The Information Security Forum (ISF), a nonprofit group that studies threats and threat management, issues an annual report on current and evolving threats. Neither the ISF's focus nor its reports are specific to healthcare, but their work is worthy of consideration by information professionals working in healthcare. The ISF's (2016) report, *Threat Horizon 2018*, predicts that threats will worsen, and that organizations risk becoming overwhelmed as they attempt to deal with the rapid proliferation of data, increased regulation, more and more complex technology, and a shortage of prepared HIT workers. The *Threat Horizon 2018* report noted nine key emerging threats grouped by theme; these themes include an increase in threats related to an increased adoption of technology, compromised ability to provide adequate protection, and regulations that fragment security measures or fail to keep abreast of emerging threats. New technologies introduce new threats.

ISF makes specific reference to **Internet of things (IoT)** devices. IoT refers to devices that have embedded microchips, sensors, and actuators that use Internet Protocol (IP) to share data with other machines or software over communications networks. IoT devices are noted as frequently insecure by design, with gaps in current legislation to meet consumer expectations for privacy and security of data (ISF, 2016; Britton, 2016). ISF identified problems with the algorithms used to secure information and increasing numbers of cyberattacks as two other threats related to increased adoption of technology. Identified emerging threats related to compromised ability to provide adequate protection for information and information systems include expansion beyond the capabilities of the organization's security infrastructure, market pressure to retain products with known vulnerabilities, and an exodus by players in the cyber-insurance market as the size and costs related to cyberattacks increase (ISF, 2016). Even as new threats emerge, a report by another IT research and advisory group indicated that the vast majority of vulnerabilities will be those already familiar to IT professionals (Perkins, 2016). Box 13-1 lists some common current threat sources.

Box 13-1   Common Threat Sources to Information and Information System Security.

1. *The insider threat.* Information is stored in files and folders, accessible remotely by large numbers of users. Despite a well-developed security infrastructure, this remains one of the biggest threat sources.
2. *Social networking services.* Sites, such as Facebook, Twitter, and Instagram, provide cybercriminals new opportunities to target unsuspecting users.
3. *Scareware.* Attackers and fraudsters use online pop-ups designed to look like messages from the operating system, warning of a problem or virus infection to coerce users to download a program to correct the problem.
4. *Network and computer operating systems.* Microsoft Windows is widely used worldwide. This massive user base makes it attractive to opportunistic hackers looking to capitalize on vulnerabilities.
5. *Malware attacks.* Cybercriminals are using more creative means to package and deliver malware (viruses, worms, Trojan horses, etc.), especially in emails.
6. *Ransomware.* Perpetrators render a system, or needed information, unavailable until their demands are met.
7. *Smartphones.* The convergence of telecommunications and computing is creating a new target for hackers.
8. *Shadow IT.* This term refers to unofficial practices often devised as workarounds to accomplish the work on hand, but also failing to fall under the official security infrastructure.
9. *Embedded computing.* More devices are connected to and reliant on the Internet. The patchwork of code and protocols that enable this connectivity also support numerous points in vulnerability that include, but are not limited to, the software used. Some common examples in the news include cars that are hacked or stolen through technology loopholes.
10. *Virtualization and cloud computing.* Lower budgets and improvements in distributed computing and high-speed Internet access make cloud computing and virtualization appealing alternatives to costly and complex conventional computing methods, but open alternative paths for intrusion.
11. *Wireless networks (WLANs).* The increase in the use of Wi-Fi networks in healthcare facilities can make patient information and associated information systems vulnerable if not properly secured.

These threats may result in jammed networks, violations to confidentiality, identity theft, information-integrity violations, disruption in the delivery of services, monetary losses, and violation of privacy regulations. Confidential client information may also be exposed through file-sharing applications running on employee workstations, as well as unauthorized access via email, instant messaging, file transfers, and Internet chat sites. For this reason, it is essential to have a real-time threat-management system in place at all times. A threat-management system includes automatic intrusion detection and audit software, as well as security training for all employees. One aspect of security training is the identification of risks and methods to minimize these risks. Professionals can be hired to test a system for vulnerabilities.

Vulnerability is a flaw or weakness in system-security procedures, design, implementation, or internal controls that could be accidentally triggered or intentionally used, resulting in a security breach or a violation of the system's security policy. Vulnerabilities are not merely weaknesses in the technical protections provided by a system; vulnerabilities can be embedded in activities such as the standard operating procedures that system administrators perform, the process that help-desk personnel use to reset passwords, or inadequate log reviews. Vulnerabilities may also occur at the policy level. For example, the lack of a clearly defined risk-management policy may result in a lack of vulnerability scanning.

Viruses, worms, and malicious software are programs that someone writes with the intent to steal information, cause annoyance and mayhem, or conceal other malicious activity he or she is doing. Viruses, worms, Trojan horses, spyware, and rootkits are all forms of malicious software. In general, malicious software may:

- Attempt to reproduce itself automatically and secretly
- Conceal itself from routine forms of detection (e.g., using random file names) and elimination (e.g., turning off your antivirus software)
- Spread itself to other computers via the network, such as by email, unsecured file shares, password guessing, or exploiting security problems on other computers
- Modify the operating system or other legitimate software
- Make copies of itself to writable media (e.g., USB storage devices)
- Send personal information gleaned from the invaded computer back to the maker of the malicious software, or his or her criminal associates, for purposes of identity theft or to collect market data
- Display unwanted advertising banners on websites or in pop-up windows
- Allow malicious individuals to monitor your computer remotely over the network
- Delete, damage, or modify your documents and data files.

Viruses attach themselves to other computer programs. They may, or may not, damage data or disrupt system operations. Some viruses are likened to electronic graffiti in that the writer leaves his or her mark by displaying a message. Infected email and IM attachments are common means to spread malware. Executing, or opening, an attached file spreads the virus to the host computer, which then infects the hard drive. Unfortunately, viruses are frequently widespread by the time of detection. Viruses can also be spread by downloading files from the Internet, visiting certain web pages, and transferring data from infected CDs, DVDs, and flash drives from one computer or network to another. The personal use of the Internet and email when a virus is involved can end up compromising a single computer or the entire network to which it is connected. Viruses may be spread anytime that an infected program is run. Viruses are not the only program types that can damage data or disrupt computing. Other malicious programs include worms, Trojan horses, logic bombs, rootkits, and bacteria.

Viruses, worms, and other malicious viruses are detrimental to the economy because of the loss of productivity and resources required to restore functionality, therefore viral detection and eradication is of the utmost importance. See Table 13-1 for definitions and characteristics associated with each program type.

Although antivirus software can locate and eradicate viruses and other destructive programs, the best defense against malicious programs is knowledge obtained from talking with computer users and experts about problems experienced. Some people are experts in viral detection and eradication. Box 13-2 provides tips for how to avoid malicious programs. If a virus is contained on one machine, it must be isolated and disinfected with antivirus software. Suspect files should be deleted. All backup materials should be considered suspect. It should not be necessary to reformat the hard drive to eliminate the virus(es).

Phishing entails subterfuge in an attempt to steal sensitive information via the Internet, such as credit card or bank account information, online shopping passwords, or personal information such as Social Security numbers or employment details. Phishing can have several phases. In the first phase, the recipient typically receives a phish, or email. The second phase involves the victim following through on what they are asked to do, such as completing a form. Once the recipient completes the information, the hackers now have information that they can use for nefarious purposes. Individuals need to be wary, as phishing sites may look legitimate. A proposed phishing detection approach would be to check hyperlinks in the source code of the email web page, as well as the overall appearance of the website to increase web page security as a simpler alternative to high-cost web security applications (Shekokar, Shah, Mahajan, & Rachh, 2015).

Spam is the use of electronic messaging systems to send unsolicited bulk messages. The most widely recognized form of spam is email, but the term spam can be applied to other media such as IM spam, Usenet-newsgroup spam, web search-engine spam, spam in blogs, wiki spam, online classified ads spam, mobile phone messaging spam, Internet forum spam, junk fax transmissions, social-networking spam, television advertising, and file-sharing

Table 13-1   Characteristics of Malicious Programs

Program Type	Characteristics
Viruses	Require normal computer operations to spread May or may not disrupt operations or damage data
Worms	Named for pattern of damage left behind Often use local-area and wide-area network communication practices as a means to spread and reproduce Usually affect memory and/or hard-disk space
Trojan horses	Appear to do (or actually do) one function while performing another undesired action One common example resembles a regular system log-in but records user names and passwords for another program for illicit use Do not self-replicate Are easily confined once discovered
Logic bombs	Are triggered by a specific piece of data such as a date, user name, account name, or identification, or another event May be part of a regular program or contained in a separate program May not activate on the first run of the program May be included in virus-infected programs and with Trojan horses
Rootkits	Modify the operating system to hide themselves Use worm-like methods to propagate to other computers
Malware	Sends information about the computer, your personal information, or your Internet browsing activities to a third party.
Bacteria	A class of viral programs Do not affix themselves to existing programs

---

Box 13-2   Computer Tips to Avoid Malicious Programs

- Use only licensed software.
- Run the latest version of virus-detection software routinely. Upload updates on a regular basis.
- Use an Internet firewall.
- Never open any file attachment from an unfamiliar source. Malware often comes over in this form.
- Use designated machines to check portable drives, storage media, and software for viruses before use.
- Retain backup copies of original software, work files, and directory structure for each PC. A backup can quickly restore system setup and work.
- Keep a record of all installation information, the operating system, and the make and model of the PC for troubleshooting purposes and to facilitate reinstallation.
- Keep a list of vendors, purchase dates, and serial numbers for all hardware and software items to facilitate virus tracking.
- If a virus is found, send a copy to an expert for tracking purposes.
- Watch for and download software patches that eliminate security problems.
- Ensure that system safeguards have been put into place by IT staff. Safeguards may include programming email servers to reject email containing viruses, policies related to email and IM use, and educating the workforce.
- Stay informed of potential threats.

---

network spam. Because the barriers to entry are low, spammers are numerous, and the volume of unsolicited mail has become extremely high. The costs, such as lost productivity and fraud, are borne by the public and by Internet-service providers, which have been forced to add extra capacity to cope with the volume of spam. Spam threatens security when it serves as a vehicle for the introduction of malware, and when it threatens ready access to information by overloading networks and consuming valuable resources. Email security software can filter out spam. The downside is that this process may result in the loss of a small percentage of legitimate mail. Monitoring email is important to avoid legal liability and maintain network security, employee productivity, and confidentiality of information. Some spam is also dangerous and more complex than just an email.

System Vulnerability

Even the most secure systems can become vulnerable to internal or external threats. This can result from poor or improper system configuration, known and unknown hardware or software flaws, and operational weaknesses in processes or technical countermeasures. The best that can be hoped for is that security strategies will minimize instances of system penetration and minimize damages. One way to reduce attacks is called a penetration test (occasionally called a pentest), which is a method of evaluating the security of a computer system or network by simulating an attack from a malicious source, known as a black hat hacker, or cracker. The process involves an active analysis of the system for any potential vulnerability. According to Nazareth and Choi (2015), information security management should include vulnerability reduction, attack management, and threat deterrence. Barriers to effective security include inadequate resources, money, time, and attention from management;

the complexity of training; and the increasing sophistication of users. Some specific threats to information systems include:

- *Cybercrime.* Cybercrime is now a larger threat than other physical-security problems. Cybercrime commonly refers to the ability to steal personal information, such as Social Security numbers stored on computers. Cyberattackers use widely available hacker tools to find network weaknesses and gain undetected access. Netcrime refers, more precisely, to criminal exploitation of the Internet. Issues surrounding this type of crime have become high profile, particularly those surrounding hacking, copyright infringement, child pornography, and child luring. There are also problems of privacy when confidential information is lost or intercepted, lawfully or otherwise. Inconsistent and inadequate approaches to security risks allow entry. RSA (2014) suggested that cyber-criminals have become more organized and adaptive, and the profitability of the data in question transforms the way they play the game. Combating cyber threats will have to include information sharing to determine the best approach.

- *Opportunists.* Opportunists take advantage of a situation and their access to information for uses not associated with their jobs.

- *Hackers.* Hackers are individuals who have an average, or above-average, knowledge of computer technology, and dislike rules and restrictions. Hackers penetrate systems as a challenge, and many do not regard their acts as criminal. Other hackers, however, break into systems with the intent of obtaining information, creating confusion, destroying files, or gaining a financial benefit. Members of this group are referred to as crackers or black hats.

- *Computer or information specialists.* These individuals are knowledgeable about how networks and computers work and are in an ideal position to commit computer crime and disable systems while avoiding detection.

- *Unauthorized users and over-privileged users.* Although the most common fear is that a system will be penetrated from outside, the greatest threat actually comes from inside sources, namely employees, contractors, consultants, outsourced services, and vendors who view information inappropriately, disrupt information availability, or corrupt data integrity. Such access constitutes unauthorized use and may occur at any level within an organization. Consideration must be given to the access rights accorded to all employees, including system administrators.

Even though healthcare professionals have codes of ethics to maintain client confidentiality, not all professionals act ethically. For this reason, system, safeguards for all users are needed. As healthcare alliances grow and client records become more accessible, the likelihood of unauthorized system access increases. For an individual client, legal protection was limited in the United States until HIPAA compliance became mandatory.

Concern for client confidentiality is not limited to the period in which a client is receiving active treatment. Access to client records may occur after treatment through loopholes that exist in automated systems. These loopholes can be found by curious users and must be corrected as soon as IT staff and administrators become aware of them. One example may be illustrated by the automated system that restricts access to client records during treatment, but allows retrieval of any record or laboratory value after a client is discharged. Healthcare-alliance physicians and office staff often need to see test results after the client's admission, but should only be able to view the results for their clients. This type of problem represents an oversight in the system-design process that must be corrected. Commercial software vendors are now under greater pressure to improve the security of their products as customers use their purchasing power to exert better security demands. The US government has started to stipulate security provisions that vendors must meet to win contracts with the government.

Sabotage

The destruction of computer equipment or data, or the disruption of normal system operation is known as sabotage. IT staff typically have system privileges that would permit this type of destruction, but, in fact, any worker may commit sabotage. Employees who are satisfied, well informed, and feel a vested interest in maintaining information and system security are less likely to perform destructive acts on a system. A positive work environment, a well-defined institutional-ethics policy, and intact security mechanisms help to deter intentional information or system misuse or destruction. As a means to avert this type of threat, consideration should be given to having background checks performed on employees, and all other persons who manage and maintain computer systems or are in a position to misuse information. Insider-threat management is an emerging focus area in information security and operational risk management. The CERT Insider Threat Center at Carnegie Mellon's Software Engineering Institute (SEI) has actively worked to research the issue, as well as solutions to mitigate insider threats (CERT, 2016). The emergence of internal hackers has become more common in organizations. It is important to conduct audit trails and other security measures to prevent any system penetration by an internal intruder.

Errors and Other Disasters

Errors may result from poor design, system changes that permit users more access than they require, failure to follow policies and procedures, poorly trained personnel, the absence of policies and procedures, or poorly written policies and procedures. One example of poor design is when information, restricted during inpatient treatment, is made available to all users after the patient is discharged, whether the users have a need to know or not.

Errors may also arise from incorrect user entries, such as inadvertent selection of the wrong client for data retrieval or documentation. According to Hallman, Stahl, and Ahmadov (2011) data integrity is a major problem that can have horrible effects for an organization. In healthcare, data errors and poor data integrity can make the difference between life and death. An estimated 10% or more of data stored in databases is incorrect. During disasters, manual backup procedures may also compromise information because the primary focus is on maintaining services. One example of this is when paper reports of laboratory findings are not enclosed in envelopes for delivery to client-care units.

Poor Password Management

Additional threats to information and system security come from poor password management, which includes such practices as: sharing passwords, posting log-on IDs and passwords on workstations, leaving logged-on devices unattended, and compromised handheld electronic devices. Poor password management is likely to occur when users have multiple passwords to manage, and it becomes difficult to remember them all. Password-management best practices should be utilized, although more secure methods of authentication are recommended and are increasingly replacing passwords.

Compromised Devices

As more people use personal information devices—such as tablets and smartphones—for job-related tasks and functions, security breaches are moving from the realm of theory to corporate reality. The damages are no longer just personal inconvenience, but can include data theft, private-information broadcasts on the web, significant personal expense, and corporate-network vulnerability. Indeed, as the office is defined less by a physical space and more by the location of its employees at any given time, the security of data held on tablets, and smartphones has become a top concern for chief information officers and IT managers in businesses and organizations of all sizes.

Corporate policies can be written to dictate appropriate use and applications for mobile devices used to access, store, and transmit PHI with the goal of minimizing malware access and transmission to a hospital network, threatening data, PHI, applications, and network security. Recommended practices for the use of mobile devices in these circumstances call for authentication measures, encryption, installation of software that enables remote wiping of data or disabling of devices, no file sharing applications, the installation of a firewall for access to the network, up-to-date security software, physical control of the device, appropriate security when using public Wi-Fi networks, and deletion of all stored information before the device is discarded or reused (HealthIT.gov, 2013).

Security Mechanisms

The security of information and computer systems should receive top priority. Typically, security mechanisms use a combination of logical and physical restrictions to provide a greater level of protection than is possible with either approach alone. This includes measures, such as firewalls and the installation of antivirus and spyware-detection software. These measures should also be reevaluated periodically to determine what modifications need to be made. A simple example of a logical restriction is automatic sign-off after a period of no activity.

Automatic sign-off is a mechanism that logs a user off the system after a specified period of inactivity on his or her computer. This procedure is recommended in all client-care areas, as well as any other area in which sensitive data exist. The level of security provided should reflect the value of the information. Some levels of information may have no particular value and do not need protection from theft, only from unauthorized change. Privacy screens may also be used. They are an economical layer of privacy and protection.

Physical Security

Best practices for physical security are:

1. Lock up the data center and servers.
2. Set up surveillance.
3. Limit access to the data center.
4. Use rack-mount servers.
5. Safeguard workstations.
6. Protect portable devices by limiting access and via encryption.
7. Secure any physical backup media.
8. Disable drives.
9. Protect printers and printouts.

Physical security measures include the placement of computers, file servers, routers, switches, and computers in restricted areas. The server room is the heart of the physical network, and someone with physical access to the servers, switches, routers, cables, and other devices in the server room can do enormous damage. When this is not possible, equipment should be removed or locked.

Physical security is a challenge for remote access. **Remote access** is the ability to use the health enterprise's information system from outside locations, such as a physician's office or home. Secure modems and encryption are particularly useful in conjunction with remote access. As more employees start to work from home, it will be important to ensure security. Employees should sign a confidentiality-and-privacy agreement and complete HIPAA training. As an additional security measure, flash drives or thumb drives should also be encrypted.

Physical security is challenged by the growing use of mobile wireless devices, such as notebooks, tablets, and smartphones, as well as portable storage devices, such as thumb or flash drives. These items may fall into the hands of unauthorized individuals. Security cables, motion detectors, or alarms used with these devices help prevent theft. Secure, lockable briefcases, drawers, or closets should be considered for the storage of devices not in use. In the event that mobile devices are stolen, some measure of protection can be provided by making the boot-up process password protected. The time-out for the screen should also be very short, and ideally less than 60 seconds. Other measures include setting passwords on individual files; storing files in zipped, password-protected folders; and encrypting the hard drive. These actions are not foolproof because hard drives can be removed, decrypted, and copied. Daily backups and portable storage devices, such as an external drive, help to prevent data loss. It is essential to include wireless devices as part of organizational standards, policies, and procedures to ensure that risk management and preventive measures are taken.

Another facet of physical security is introduced when healthcare enterprises provide Internet access within the facility for visitors and patients. Increasingly, this is an expected amenity as it is available in hotels and public places. Individuals who opt to use free wireless connections in public places should employ the following precautions:

- *Look for posted signs that provide the exact name of the hotspot.* This will help to avoid fake networks that are designed to collect passwords, credit card information, and other personal data. Often, connecting to a hospital's free Wi-Fi involves the organization sending a passcode via email or IM to the user requesting connection.
- *Change settings so that permission is required before connecting to a new network.* This measure helps to avoid fake networks.
- *Avoid computer-to-computer networks.* Free wireless networks should be noted as such. Computer-to-computer networks are generally fake networks set up for spurious purposes.
- *Turn off file sharing.* This will keep passersby from accessing stored data.
- *Refrain from online banking or shopping.* These activities should be avoided unless network security can be guaranteed.
- *Do not store passwords on your computer or other mobile devices.* These may be accessed through suspect connections or compromised when the physical device is stolen. Password protection apps can be used to add an extra layer of security.
- *Verify that a PC's software firewall is turned on.*

Public Internet access should not be provided on the same network that is used to transmit secure health data unless extensive measures are used to maintain the security of that data. It is not recommended to conduct online banking with a public Wi-Fi network. The connection is not guaranteed to be 100% confidential.

Authentication

Authentication is the process of determining whether someone is who he or she professes to be. This usually involves a username and a password, but can include other methods of proving identity such as a smart card, retinal scan, voice recognition, or fingerprints. Authentication is equivalent to showing your driver's license or passport at an airport-ticket counter. Several methods of authentication exist, ranging from log-on passwords to digital certificates and public-or-private keys used for encryption and biometric measures. Authentication is one component of identity management (ID management).

ID management is a broad administrative area that deals with identifying individuals in a system and controlling their access to resources within that system by associating user rights and restrictions with an established identity. ID management provides managers with a unique view of the IT environment for each user, which is determined primarily by job function and security concerns. ID management software is available, but it requires more work for what is typically an already overworked IT office. Organizations have to develop a central database to maintain identities, manage the access rights for every user on the network, and enforce a strict policy for how that database will be managed.

Passwords are simply secret alphanumeric sequences, words, or phrases that the user enters into the computer. Password entry may be required after the entry and acceptance of an access code, sometimes referred to as the user name. IT administrators sometimes need this information to problem-solve or reissue passwords. The password does not appear on the screen when it is entered, and it should not be known to anyone but the user and IS administrators. The keys to password strength are length and complexity. An ideal password is long and has letters, punctuation marks, symbols, and numbers. The greater the variety of characters in a password, the greater its strength is. Recommendations for password selection and use are given in Box 13-3. Obvious passwords, such as the user's name, house number, children's or spouse's names, pet names, or dictionary words, are easily compromised.

Box 13-3 Recommendations for Password Selection and Use

- Choose passwords that are at least 12 characters long and include a combination of symbols and numbers. Short passwords are easier to guess.
- Select stronger passwords for higher levels of security.
- Avoid using the same password for more than one application.
- Do not use the browser password-save feature.
- Use combinations of uppercase and lowercase letters, numbers, punctuation marks, and symbols.
- Do not use proper names, initials, words taken from the dictionary, or account names.
- Avoid using family names, street names, or pet names. The hacker may know a lot about you and can guess this information.
- Do not use dates or telephone, license plate, or Social Security numbers.
- Do not store or automate passwords in the computer.
- Change passwords every 60 days or sooner. Set a reminder so this is done.
- Keep passwords private and do not share! It is not realistic to try to remember all of the passwords. Store your passwords in a secure area that only you have access to, and avoid storing the information on your mobile device.
- Use the entire keyboard, not just the letters and characters you use or see most often.

Strong passwords use combinations of letters, numbers, and symbols that are not easily guessed. Software is available to test and eliminate easily compromised passwords before use. Password-management software also provides a better mechanism to store passwords securely, using one master password to access the file, which may be stored encrypted and possibly via the cloud.

Individuals should not share passwords or leave computers logged on and unattended. System administrators must keep files that contain password lists safe from view and copying by unauthorized individuals. One compromised password can jeopardize information and the system that contains it. For this reason, users should not use the same password for access to more than one site or system. Using the same password at various sites reduces security. System administrators need to allow legitimate users the opportunity to access the system, while refusing entry to others. One means to accomplish this is to shut down a workstation after a random number of unsuccessful access attempts and send security personnel to check that area. This information can also be tracked electronically. Although passwords provide considerable system protection, other defenses are still necessary.

Passwords can also be compromised in the following ways:

- Writing them down or sharing them with friends and coworkers.
- Passwords can be guessed, either by a person or by a program designed to try numerous possible combinations in rapid succession. Some systems will request additional information to verify that the user is not a robot.
- Passwords can be transmitted over a network, either in plain text or encoded in a way that can be readily converted back to plain text.
- Passwords can be stored on a workstation, server, or backup media, in plain text or encoded in a way that can be readily converted back to plaintext.

Each of these vulnerabilities makes it easier for someone to acquire the password value and, consequently, pose as the user, whose identity the password protects. Conversely, if passwords are managed securely by users, and if password systems are constructed so as to prevent brute-force attacks and inspection, or decryption of passwords in transit and in storage, passwords can actually be quite secure. These include measures to verify user identity.

Sign-on/log-on access codes and passwords are generally assigned on successful completion of system training. Passwords may be difficult for a user to recall. This leads some people to write passwords down and post them in conspicuous places. This practice should be prohibited. Users who find it necessary to record the dozens of passwords used to access various sites and systems must store them in an area away from the computer and out of casual view. Storing passwords in a file on the computer is a problem, if the device is shared by others, or if the hard drive crashes or is replaced. A file-cleaning utility should be used to permanently erase the drive so that password files cannot be restored. When a file is used to store passwords, it should be encrypted and password protected. Passwords should be regarded as an electronic signature. There is software available to check the strength of a password and it would be useful to test your password with a password checker. A password checker evaluates a password's strength automatically.

Frequent and random password change is recommended as a routine security mechanism. This can be a time-consuming and unpleasant task because it is difficult for users to remember new passwords. There are, however, situations that mandate immediate change or deletion of access codes and passwords, including suspicion of unauthorized access and termination of employees. Codes and passwords should also be deleted with status changes, such as resignations; leaves of absence; and the completion of rotations for students, faculty, and residents. Because information services (IS) staff can view any information in the system, all members of the department should receive new passwords when IS personnel leave. In the event that an IS employee is terminated, department door locks or combinations should be changed as well.

Disadvantages associated with the use of passwords include the following:

- They are typically poorly managed, are frequently forgotten, and often need to be reset by help-desk staff.

- They can be shared or stolen.

- Users often choose very easy passwords.

- Organizations need to force users to change their passwords periodically because users forget to change them.

- The purpose of passwords is defeated when the user sets the browser to remember them on a public computer.

Public key infrastructure (PKI) is a set of procedures that use hardware, software, people, and policies to create, manage, distribute, use, store, and revoke digital certificates (Selvakumaraswamy & Govindaswamy, 2016). PKI is an arrangement that binds public keys with respective user identities by means of a **certificate authority (CA)**. It is a more secure technology than simply using passwords. The term **trusted third party (TTP)** may also be used for certificate authority. PKI uses an encrypted passkey that can be provided to the user in various formats, including a smartcard, token, or wireless transmitter. The passkey provides a secret value that is verified against a registered digital certificate. The user submits the passkey information during the sign-on/log-on process, and the PKI system compares it against the registered digital certificate ID to verify a match. Digital certificates include information about the owner, such as systems that he or she may access, level of access, and biometric measures. Digital certificates provide assurance of the identity, rights, and privileges of the user. Security tokens that resemble key chain fobs are an example of this technology. Tokens strengthen authentication because the user must use both the token and a special personal identification number (PIN) to gain access. PKI can provide a common infrastructure that allows access to multiple delivery systems across an organization or organizations. Despite the value that PKI can provide to enhance the privacy and security of information sent to and from mobile devices it remains little known (Camp, 2015). Some concerns have been expressed that the explosion in digital information use has stressed PKI, highlighting vulnerabilities and the need for greater investment in this area (Grimm, 2016).

BIOMETRICS Scanned employee identification may include a name badge, but generally refers to biometric authentication, which is based on a unique biological trait, such as a fingerprint, voice or iris pattern, retinal scan, hand geometry, face recognition, ear pattern, smell, blood vessels in the palm, gait recognition, or keystroke cadence (Brown, 2012). Biometric technology can be very accurate. Unlike passwords or devices that can be forgotten or stolen, biometric measures are always with the individual, barring major injury, and cannot be lost, stolen, or used without user consent.

Traditionally, the quality of biometric authentication has varied by device and the software used. Fingerprint scanning is a popular biometric employee-identification technique, but may result in a high rate of failure of first-print readings as the number of users increases. This situation may require a second or third reading. Individuals must learn the proper method of placing their fingers into scanners. Skin moisture and temperature also affect the quality of the scan. Very moist or dry skin and cold fingers negatively affect reading. Some readers can be fooled by using tape, gelatin, or other measures. Infection control is a related concern when biometric authentication requires contact. No contact is required to scan the voice or iris pattern, retina, hand geometry, face, ear pattern, smell, blood vessels in the palm, or for gait recognition. Biometric authentication helps organizations to better comply with regulations and reduces the amount of time spent by help staff resetting passwords. The use of biometric measures for authentication is expected to replace password use in the near future.

Other authentication devices include proximity radio systems that detect user badges within a specified distance, picture-authentication packages that use pictures instead of passwords, and digital certificates. Users should have different authentication requirements, depending upon the sensitivity or value of the resources that they access. Authentication can be strengthened by requiring multifactor authentication. Authentication policies should outline acceptable forms of authentication, depending on multiple factors including class of user, type of resources, location, and time of day. The policy must also protect authentication systems from attack and sabotage. Building an authentication policy is one thing, but implementing, managing, and enforcing it is another. Advancements in technology make it possible to use biometric authentication with mobile devices, providing an additional layer of security (Wójtowicz & Joachimiak, 2016).

Firewalls and Other Network Devices

A firewall is a component of a computer system or network designed to block unauthorized access while permitting authorized communications. It is a device or set of devices that are configured to permit or deny network transmissions based upon a set of rules and other criteria. Firewalls can be implemented in either hardware or software, or a combination of both. A typical firewall is a combination of hardware and software that forms a barrier between systems, or different parts of a single system, to protect those systems from unauthorized access. Firewalls screen traffic, allow only approved transactions to pass through them, and restrict access to other systems or sensitive areas such as client information, payroll, or personnel data. There are several types of firewall techniques:

1. *Packet filter.* Packet filtering inspects each packet passing through the network and accepts or rejects it based on user-defined rules. Although difficult to configure, it is fairly effective and mostly transparent to its users. It is susceptible to spoofing, a situation in which IP addresses are forged in order to conceal the identity of the sender.
2. *Application gateway.* Applies security mechanisms to specific applications, such as file transfer protocols (FTP) and Telnet servers. This is very effective but can impose performance degradation.
3. *Circuit-level gateway.* Applies security mechanisms when a transmission-control protocol (TCP) or user-datagram protocol (UDP) connection to the Internet is established. Once the connection has been made, packets can flow between the hosts without further checking.
4. *Proxy server.* Intercepts all messages entering and leaving the network. The proxy server effectively hides the true network addresses.

Multiple firewalls can increase protection. Strong security policies and practices strengthen firewall protection. Once a user has passed through the firewall, controlling access to individual applications takes place elsewhere. Firewalls are not foolproof. Specialists periodically create patches to counter flaws in security software. It is imperative to apply security patches as soon as they become available. Security protocols on network switches and routers also help. Another way to add some additional protection to safeguard information is to segment a network into different levels of security and allow employees access based on their position within the organization. It is also essential to train and remind employees about their role in security. Keeping the system secure is a collaborative effort.

Application Security

Another area of concern is application security, which encompasses measures taken throughout an application program's life cycle to prevent exceptions in the security policy of an application or the underlying system (vulnerabilities) through flaws in the design, development, deployment, upgrade, or maintenance of an application. Application security measures should be used with the client information system and other systems, such as payroll records. Security-testing techniques look for vulnerabilities or security holes in applications. These vulnerabilities leave applications open to exploitation. Ideally, security testing is implemented throughout the entire software development life cycle (SDLC) so that vulnerabilities may be addressed in a timely and thorough manner. Unfortunately, testing is often conducted as an afterthought at the end of the development cycle. Likewise, it is important for employees to sign off when they leave a workstation or computer or are finished using a particular software application, because failure to do so may allow others to use their code to access information. Automatic sign-off has been designed as a security measure when employees fail to properly exit a program or step away from a computer. Some organizations are also using a motion detector. If the computer does not sense that you are in front of it, a screen saver will come up and the user is required to re-enter their password.

Antivirus Software

Antivirus software is a set of computer programs that can locate and eradicate malware, including computer viruses, worms, and Trojan horses. Such programs may also prevent and remove adware, spyware, and other forms of malware from scanned memory sticks, storage devices, individual computers, and networks. The continuous creation of new viruses makes it necessary to update antivirus software frequently. Antivirus software may come preloaded on new computers or be obtained in computer stores or over the Internet. The user must then frequently download updated virus definitions from the vendor's website. Some vendors automatically notify users as new virus definitions become available. Users can set up antivirus software to automatically run a virus check on the PC or server on a scheduled basis in addition to performing random checks. This is recommended for best performance and increased safety. Networked computers are generally set by the administrator to include a virus scan at routine start-up, automatically scan new files, and update antivirus files. Network administrators can also set privileges to prohibit unauthorized file downloads.

Spyware and Ransomware

Spyware is a data-collection mechanism that installs itself without the user's permission. This often happens when a user is browsing the web or downloading software. Spyware can include cookies that track web use, as well as applications that capture credit card, bank, and PIN numbers or other PHI stored on that computer for illicit purposes by an unauthorized person. This is a concern for all healthcare providers because it threatens PHI. No computer that is attached to the Internet is immune.

Clues that spyware has infected a computer include the presence of pop-up ads, keys that do not work, random error messages, and poor system performance. Because of the security threat that this represents, spyware detection software should be utilized.

Ransomware is a type of malware that is being used more frequently. Ransomware hijacks user files, encrypts them, and then demands a ransom or payment for the decryption key. Additionally, the criminals hold the information until they are paid with currency that cannot be traced, such as eGold, bitcoins, or web money. The criminals contact the victims to let them know what payment is expected for release of the decryption key. In 2016, hackers disabled the information system of a hospital in Southern California demanding money. The hospital paid the hackers $17K in ransom in order to restore normal operations (Conn, 2016). While ransomware is about a decade old, hackers are becoming more sophisticated in their practices. Ransom attacks most often begin with an email attachment innocently opened by an employee. Security-enhancing technology may assist in keeping systems safe, including software that scans every incoming email. There may be ransomware victims who do not come forward due to the embarrassment of the situation (Conn, 2016). This situation prompted California Senator Bob Hertzberg to introduce legislation (Senate Bill 1137) that provided bigger penalties for ransomware extortion attacks and classified them as felonies. Ransomware perpetrators could be fined $10K and imprisoned for two to four years. An estimated $209 million was extorted from United States companies in the first quarter of 2016 using ransomware, compared to $25 million in 2015, validating the need for stricter penalties (HIPAA Journal, 2016). According to Young (2016), Senator Hertzberg's website was hit by ransomware one day after his bill for stricter penalties passed in the Senate.

Administrative and Personnel Issues

The final responsibility for creating and managing the infrastructure to protect client privacy and confidentiality lies with healthcare administrators who must develop a plan, policies, a designated implementation structure, user-access levels, and an adequate budget (Semel, 2016). Upper-level management must have security-awareness training and set a positive example for all stakeholders, including employees, students, consultants, and contractors because privacy and security is a responsibility shared by everyone in the organization. Administration must also work with IT personnel to establish the following centralized security functions:

- *A comprehensive security plan.* This plan needs to be developed with input from administrators, information services personnel, and clinical staff. It should define security responsibilities for each level of personnel, as well as a timeline for the development and implementation of policies, procedures, and physical infrastructure. Incorporation of computer forensics as a plan component helps to build and maintain a strong security readiness. Computer forensics refers to the collection of electronic evidence for purposes of formal litigation and simple internal investigations.

- *Accurate and complete information-security policies, procedures, and standards.* These should be published online for easy access, with notification of employees as new policies are released.

- *Information-asset ownership and sensitivity classifications.* Ownership in this context refers to who is responsible for the information, including its security. Sensitivity classification is a determination of how damaging an item of information might be if it were disclosed inappropriately. The level of sensitivity may be used to determine what information should be encrypted.

- *Identification of a comprehensive security program.* A well-defined security plan can avert or minimize threats. A key part of the plan is the identification of responsibility for information integrity, privacy, and confidentiality. A strong plan incorporates computer forensics.

- *Information-security training and user support.* Education is an important component in fostering proper system use. Most problems with information-system security are primarily related to the human factor, rather than the technical one.

- *An institution-wide information-security-awareness program.* Formal IS training and frequent suggestions are needed to remind users of the need to protect information.

For an information-security plan to be effective, responsibility must be shared by healthcare administrators, IT and healthcare professionals, and all system users. Involving users in system-security development fosters ownership of this responsibility and facilitates the ability to trace problems, limit damage, and make corrective changes. This involvement can occur on an individual level or through an institutional security committee. Security committees should consider routine maintenance, confidentiality clauses in vendor contracts, third-party payer needs, legal issues inclusive of monitoring, ongoing security needs as the institution and system evolve, and disaster planning. The IT department should address these areas when there is no security committee. Individual users are responsible for protecting their passwords, saving and backing up work files on a regular basis, securing removable storage media, adherence to safe-computing policies, and not leaving confidential information unattended on the computer screen or in paper form. They should also be responsible for reporting any observed unauthorized access. It may be necessary to outsource security if there are insufficient resources internally, but this decision needs to be carefully weighed. Collaboration is required for security to be truly effective in an organization.

Levels of Access

Access should be strictly granted on a need-to-know basis. This means no personnel, including IT staff, should have routine access to confidential information unless it is required by a particular event, at which time an audit trail should be established. Access should be based on job duties, and access for all personnel should be very limited. This should also be reviewed on an annual basis, or sooner if needed.

Access Limitations

Access should be determined by who needs a healthcare record, and under what conditions and locations. For example, direct-care providers require information about their clients under a wide range of conditions and locations. Access levels should be decided by defining roles for every level of personnel. Levels of personnel can be referred to as user classes. Each user class has a different set of privileges. Initial system access should be contingent on successful completion of system training and demonstration of competence. User training should address appropriate uses of information and the consequences of information misuse. User roles and audits must be incorporated into the design of information systems to best ensure security, privacy, accessibility, and confidentiality. A definition of each user role is instrumental in preventing unauthorized access to sensitive healthcare information. For example, nursing assistants are responsible for the documentation of hygiene, dietary intakes, vital signs, and fluid intake and output; however, this user should not be able to access diagnostic and patient history information. Access limitations can prevent any unauthorized access by employees. It is an added layer of security.

User Authentication

Access by authorized individuals can be verified through user authentication. User authentication can be based on (a) what you know, for example, passwords; (b) what you have, for example, smartcard; (c) what you are, for example, fingerprint; or (d) what you do, for example, voice recognition. Third-party authentication systems, such as Kerberos and Sesame, can be used. One common form of authentication is the appearance of the user's name or employee ID on the screen. In the event that other staff members discover a discrepancy, they have the responsibility to report it immediately. It is important to develop authentication policies jointly with IT personnel, business staff, and end users. It is also critical to factor in time to install and test drivers and hardware, as well as to consider the time and resources required to enroll and update users. Support costs and training times increase as the complexity of the authentication process increases. Unwieldy authentication systems can reduce staff productivity.

Personnel Issues

Clear policies and procedures must be established and communicated to all personnel who handle information. Staff education is a key element of information and system security. Education for information handling and system use should include an orientation, system training, and a discussion of what is acceptable and unacceptable behavior. Staff should also be informed of the consequences of unauthorized access and information misuse, the use of audit trails, and ongoing measures to heighten security awareness. Staff needs to know what constitutes an incident and how it should be handled. There should be periodic reminders that client information belongs to the client as well as what constitutes professional, legal, and ethical behavior. Yearly review of the ethical-computing statement is one way to emphasize the importance of ethical behavior. Education and monitoring activities show administrative commitment to ethical-information use. Explicit written policies and procedures provide the discipline to achieve information and system security. Policies and procedures should address information ethics, privacy and security, staff training for information and system security, access control, system monitoring, data entry, backup procedures, responsibilities for the use of information on mobile devices and at remote sites, and exchange of client information with other healthcare providers. Information-ethics policies should do the following:

- *Plan for audit trails.* **Audit trails** are a record of system activity. Users should know that their system access is monitored and that audit-trail records will be kept for a period of years.

- *Establish acceptable computer uses.* This includes authorized access and using only authorized and legal copies of software. One example of how this might be enforced is requiring licenses for all software used within the institution.

- *Collect only required data.* Limiting the collection of information to what is needed, and no more, eliminates the danger of inappropriate disclosure of unneeded information and may lessen the workload.

- *Encourage client review of files for accuracy and error correction.* Client inspection of records ensures information integrity.

- *Establish controls for the use of information after hours and off-site.* As many employees and clinicians work at home or complete projects on their own time, it is important to develop policies related to downloading files or carrying information off the premises. Both the types of information that may be carried on mobile devices and the responsibilities of the staff member to safeguard that information must be communicated to all employees.

For information security, integrity, confidentiality, accessibility, and privacy policies to be effective, they must meet the following criteria:

- Be disseminated
- Be reviewed
- Be understandable
- Be compliant
- Be enforceable and enforced.

Information-ethics policies are most credible when practiced by top administrators and IT personnel. After policies have been developed and implemented, a security education, training, and awareness program (SETA) must be implemented. A SETA program should consist of three elements: security education, security training, and security awareness.

System Security Management

System security involves protection against deliberate attacks, errors, omissions, and disasters. Good system management is a key component of a strong framework for security, because it encompasses the following tasks:

- Monitoring
- Maintenance
- Operations
- Traffic management
- Supervision
- Risk management.

Monitoring includes setting and enforcing standards, tracking changes, and observing all system activity in the operational environment. Monitoring also alerts managers to problems, such as intruders or the introduction of a virus. Maintenance encompasses all activity needed for proper operation of hardware, including preventive measures, such as testing, periodic applications of patches, and replacement of select components, to ensure that data are available when needed. Maintenance includes documentation of all configuration settings, server protocols, and network addresses, and any changes, so that records are available in the event that the system must be restored. Operations management includes all activities needed to provide, sustain, modify, or cease system usage and telecommunications. Traffic management permits rerouting of transmissions for better system performance. Supervision requires monitoring traffic, as well as system performance and taking measures to prevent system overload and crashes.

Risk management helps to identify and curtail high-risk problem areas in a timely fashion. Although software is available to facilitate system-management tasks, the lack of comprehensive commercial packages available for the management of systems across networks has forced institutions to develop in-house solutions or use outsourcing agents for customized applications. Many organizations have different staff members for network and systems management. Network staff traditionally focus on hardware—such as switches, routers, and connections—whereas IT personnel track information and software use. The security officer plays a pivotal role in tracking personnel information about system use. It is the security officer who should assign access codes and passwords to authorized users, who deletes codes for staff no longer with the organization, and changes access rights when personnel move from one department to another. Increased computing needs and limited budgets require greater staff efficiency. Effective use of system and network management tools will help provide staff efficiency, minimize the number of required support staff, reduce support costs, and improve information security.

Audit Trails

Audit trails record activity, both by system and application processes and by user activity of systems and applications. In conjunction with appropriate tools and procedures, audit trails can assist in detecting security violations, performance problems, and flaws in applications. Auditing software helps to maintain security by recording unauthorized access to certain programs, screens, or records. Audits show access to records by user or by password, and all access by an individual or level of employee, for example, user class. For this reason, all users should sign off after each use; if they encounter an active session that belongs to another user, they should log that user off and sign in under their own access credentials. Frequent review of audit trails for unusual activity quickly identifies inappropriate use. Poorly audited systems invite fraud and abuse. The level of control in many audit systems is not sufficient for HIPAA compliance. Optimally, audits should be able to track all access, creations, updates, and edits at the data-element level for each patient record. This ability supports a consumer's right to view logs of who has accessed his or her data, what was viewed, and when the data were accessed. Audit-trail records must now be available for longer periods of time. Before HIPAA, audit logs were usually kept for limited periods. Consideration must be given now to the retention period for audit logs. Department managers must be advised when audit trails indicate that members of their staff have accessed records without a justifiable need. Audit trails are essential, but may still fail to capture the full range of security issues. In the event that an audit trail identifies unauthorized access, it is important to enforce the written security policy. At a minimum, this should be a verbal reprimand, or possibly a notation on the employee's performance evaluation. In many institutions, however, employees are held to the statement they signed on receipt of their access code and password, acknowledging termination of employment as a possible consequence of inappropriate system use. When employees are terminated for this reason, they may be escorted off the premises by the security department to prevent any further opportunity for unauthorized access. Audit trails may also reveal unauthorized access from outside sources, although little legal recourse has been available to punish the guilty parties until recently. There is now increased legislative activity to prevent and punish cybercrime.

Handling and Disposal of Confidential Information

Although most people recognize the need to keep electronic health records confidential, many pay less attention to safeguarding information printed from the record or extracted from it electronically for reporting purposes. All client-record information should be treated as confidential and kept from unauthorized view regardless of its form or format. Computers, including workstations on wheels, should also be secured. These mobile computers are often a high risk because they are left in visible areas.

Computer Printouts

In the past, the primary sources of inadvertent disclosure of information were printouts of portions of client records and faxes. All papers containing PHI, such as prescriptions, laboratory-specimen labels, identification bracelets, meal descriptions, addressograph plates, and any other items that carry a patient's name, address, Social Security number, date of birth, or age must be destroyed. This may entail using shredders, or locked receptacles for later shredding and incineration. Shredding on-site may offer better control, as well as cost savings. Nurses may also be responsible for erasing from a computer's hard drive files containing calendars, surgery schedules, or other daily records that include PHI. Disposal policies for records must be clear and enforced. For tracking purposes, each page of output should have a serial number or other means of identification so that an audit trail is maintained that identifies what each paper record is, as well as the date and method for destruction and the identity of individuals witnessing the destruction. The person designated to oversee this destruction can vary, but it may be a secretary or staff from information services. Control must be established over the materials that users print or fax. Some institutions include a header on all printouts, such as lab results, which display the word *confidential* in capital letters. This reminds staff to dispose of materials appropriately. It is very important to maintain confidentiality and privacy at all times. This is especially important in high-visibility areas, such as nurses' stations. Any paper that is printed should be turned over while the user is away, and eventually destroyed when it is no longer needed.

Email, Social Media, and the Internet

Policy should dictate what types of information may be allowed in email and social media. Email is a good way of disseminating information, such as announcements, to large numbers of people quickly and inexpensively, but it should not be used for sensitive information unless it is encrypted. Nonencrypted messages can be read, and public email password protection of mailboxes can be hacked. When looking at encryption, ask whether email encrypts all messages between users, whether messages are encrypted both in transit and when stored in the mailbox, and whether messages remain encrypted when sent between different email programs. Unauthorized or dormant mail accounts should be destroyed, and firewalls should be used for additional protection. It is easy to inadvertently send out messages to the wrong party, attach the wrong document, or include persons who are not authorized to see the information. Software can be used to monitor network traffic for patterns that represent client information, such as lists or Social Security numbers. This same software can detect requests for files, and monitor web-based mail to determine if requests come from appropriate parties, or if there are problems with information being sent to unauthorized recipients.

If social media is used for professional purposes, its use should remain professional in context to provide information, educate patients, and empower consumers to engage in their healthcare. Piscotty, Martindell, and Karim (2016) concluded that social media can provide instant access to current evidence that may improve patient outcomes. Social media use will continue to grow in response to consumer demand and may serve as a robust outlet for providing present-day information. It is not an appropriate media for sharing protected health information. Understanding the tensions between privacy, audience, and information disclosure, as well as an environment that can balance all of these factors, is necessary for the future of these technologies (Vitak, Blasiola, Patil, & Litt, 2015). Healthcare providers need to use good judgment and safe computing practices when using social media.

HIPAA regulations affect email use and routing infrastructures. Private and confidential patient information should only be sent as encrypted email. Most email networks allow messages to travel through any available simple mail transfer protocol (SMTP) relay until it reaches its destination. Messages are stored at each relay and then forwarded. These relays can be hacked; encryption helps to ensure that intercepted mail cannot be read, but it does not keep it secure. Security lies with access and control of decryption keys. Central administration for encryption, key management, and disclosure should be addressed via policies and training. Another concern related to email and information-system security is spam, which is also discussed in this chapter.

Web-Based Applications for Healthcare

There is a high level of concern over the security of health information transmitted via the Internet. The debate over whether the Internet is safe enough to use for health information is likely to continue for some time. Patients often access websites that provide some healthcare information. Some use the information in the manner intended, while others use it to self-diagnose or self-treat. It is the responsibility of the healthcare professional to properly guide the patients in understanding their disease state and accessing credible websites.

Electronic Storage

Increased access to information through an ever-increasing number of interconnected storage devices and networks also creates additional concerns over security. Security threats to stored information mirror those that may affect any network. Unauthorized access to information is a major threat that can be curtailed through careful management of the interfaces between systems. It is crucial to ensure that authorized users can access information when they need it, but that sufficient security measures are in place to prevent unauthorized access. These measures include requirements for user identification and encrypted passwords to access the various components of the network. Confidential information may also be copied from the system in the form of electronic records. Administrators may download these records for report purposes. Once the records are no longer needed, electronic copies of sensitive data should be deleted or subjected to shredder software. **File-deletion software** overwrites files with meaningless information so that sensitive information cannot be accessed.

Special Considerations with Mobile Computing

Mobile computing has the potential to improve information access, enhance workflow, and promote evidence-based practice to make informed and effective decisions at the point of care. Handheld computers, tablets, and smartphones offer portable and unobtrusive access to clinical data and relevant information at the point of care. They also prove useful in areas of documentation and healthcare reference. For these reasons, mobile devices are used widely in healthcare-providers' practices, and the level of use continues to rise.

Staff who use mobile devices should work with the information-services department to help secure those devices from unauthorized view. Other problems identified with the adoption of mobile technology include usability and lack of technical and organizational support. Point of care devices, and the software that they use, must actually serve to facilitate, not hinder, the work of the bedside caregiver in order to realize the benefits associated with point of care technology. The mobility that provides an advantage can also pose problems because mobile devices may be left unattended in patient-care areas subject to unauthorized view or theft. Wi-Fi is vulnerable in a number of ways that wired networks are not. The main reason is because Wi-Fi signals are simultaneously broadcast in all directions. Therefore, special care must be taken to secure all mobile devices used by healthcare professionals. Some organizations even require employees to only use devices that have been secured by their IT department. This increases the security since the IT department maintains control of the security of the device. If it is lost, they can simply lock it or turn it off.

Security for Wearable Technology/ Implanted Devices/Bedside Technology

Wearable technology is technology that is worn on the body and uses sensors to connect to the person, while making use of a web connection to connect wirelessly to a device of the user's choice, like a smartphone (Skiba, 2014). Wearable technology includes, but is not limited to, physical activity monitors like FitBit, smart watches, smart shoes and clothes, and smart glasses that give the user the ability to connect to the Internet using voice commands. These devices can take pictures, record videos, and interface with online tools like Facebook and Twitter. Although wearable technology seems pretty innocuous in regards to privacy and security, as the wearer is using the technology to monitor their personal data and send that data to a device of their choice, most of the time, there are definite implications in regards to keeping the data secure.

Anytime data is sent from one device and received at another there is a security concern. As technology grows in the way it accesses and transmits little pieces of data about a person's health and behavior, there need to be security protocols that ensure confidentiality and prevent the device from being hacked directly. PHI can be sold on the black market for approximately ten times more than a stolen credit card number. The reason PHI is more valuable than a credit card is that a credit card can be cancelled; PHI never goes away. Even something seemingly minor, such as heart rate and fitness information, is finding its way to employers, insurance companies, and the black market, resulting in problems as diverse as higher insurance premiums and identify theft. The National Institute of Standards and Technology (NIST) states that encryption on a device that is not verified and validated by NIST provides no protection (Computer Security Division Computer Security Research Center, 2016). And it is rare to find consumer wearables that have deployed NIST-approved encryption in their product. The Health Insurance Portability and Accountability Act's (HIPAA's) security rule is concerned with protecting PHI. For covered entities, the rule defines 18 criteria that define PHI, like name, address, phone, fax, Social Security number, medical plan and account numbers, device identifiers and serial numbers, biometric identifiers, and more (Lee, 2015). Noncovered entities currently can do whatever they want with someone's data, including sharing and selling the data, as long as the actions are covered in the terms of service. Many of the wearables invoke terms of service by which the user essentially gives up the right to keep their information private. Regulations need to catch up to these many loopholes associated with new technologies. Until then, users of new technology need to be aware of what they are signing when registering for a new app or device. As for employers using wearable technology to promote employee well-being, transparency is needed about how that data will be used. Plans using wearable technology should only be run on an opt-in basis and not be compulsory to avoid the perception of coercion for the employee (Everett, 2015).

When a wearable device has the ability to interact with the outside world, an organization needs to address security concerns that arise with that functionality. Smart glasses that can record video and audio bring forth concerns that confidential information could be recorded and transferred outside the network, free from security measures. There is also concern that recorded data could be used to bring litigation against an organization. Smart watches have the ability to both store and transfer data. Although the data being stored may seem harmless, the watch does not discriminate between sensitive data and non-sensitive data and, therefore, presents another security concern. An organization must develop a security solution that addresses the capabilities of wearable technology so that it can develop acceptable-use policies for employees, clients, and visitors. The organization should also consider ensuring an advanced-network-security infrastructure that can analyze data flow, as well as identify the type of device sending and receiving data. Real-time identification of traffic out of the network, originating from a specific device, provides organizations with the ability to mitigate security threats. Even if the transfer of data cannot be blocked, the detection of a threat can notify administrators that an unacceptable device is being used on the network and trigger an alert to enforce policy (Martini, 2014).

Implanted Medical Devices

Implantable medical devices (IMDs) are devices that are surgically implanted to treat a medical condition, monitor the internal state or improve the functioning of a particular body part, or provide a patient with a capability not previously possessed (Camera, Peris-Lopez, & Tapiador, 2015). Some of the earlier devices were sent out without any type of encryption or defense mechanisms in place, or the ability to receive security updates without surgery. Limited battery power was also a problem (Song, et al., 2016). Some of the latest devices incorporate more sophisticated computing, communication, and networking functions. This gives the IMD more intelligence, and the patient more autonomy, because they need not be present at the medical center for medical personnel to access data and reconfigure the device, as it can be done remotely. Along with these benefits come numerous security and privacy risks for the patient. And, although these risks are common in computing scenarios, there have been more critical repercussions in the case of implanted devices. Direct attacks against an IMD can have serious consequences for the patient, sometimes fatal (Camara et al., 2015).

The wireless communication capabilities of IMDs, especially when the patient is in an open or non-medical environment, can lead to a major security risk. The presence of the IMD can be remotely detected, and eavesdroppers can hear the unsecured transmitted data.

Security for these devices must be based on the possible communication interactions between these devices. In one scenario, the communication is between the patient with the IMD and the medical programmer who receives the data. In this case some programmers want to introduce another device, which acts as a proxy, so that instead of a direct connection, in which an active or passive listener can kidnap the data, the middle device can authenticate the programmer and send the information forward.

Camara et al. (2015) discussed security needs in two potential modes: normal and emergency. In normal mode, the patient controls access and interaction with his or her IMD. Strong access control and protocols can be used to prevent unauthorized access, making the device undetectable to unauthenticated parties. In emergency mode, it may be necessary for unauthorized parties to access the IMD. An example of this may be the need for healthcare staff to deactivate the device during surgery when the patient is travelling. To do this they must be able to over-ride security protocols in place, thus leaving the device open to attackers. Balancing the conflicting needs between normal mode and emergency mode is difficult, and there is no answer acceptable to all. In the end, however, a majority agree that if there is doubt about a patient's safety, it is necessary to grant access to unauthorized users.

One solution that has been proposed is a wearable jammer (Cass, 2011). This device can be worn outside the body and stop unauthorized users from hacking into the medical device. However, medical personnel could remove the jammer in an emergency. Some security researchers feel that adequate security should be built into devices, but they do agree that this can help with medical devices already implanted with little security. In the end, it is up to manufacturers to strengthen the cybersecurity of IMDs. The patient can play a role as well by complying with change-out dates to ensure they have the device with the latest security.

An interesting twist to the issue of security and IMDs is that patients don't have access to the data being generated by their own medical device. Hugo Campos hacked into his implanted cardioverter defibrillator (ICD) to get his own medical information, data which his physician had access to on a 24/7 basis (Singer, 2011). When patients are expected to be an active participant in their own care it seems strange, at the very least, that they do not have access to the data being collected by their own medical device. The FDA needs to do more to encourage the manufacturers of IMDs to give the patient and healthcare providers the ability to authenticate to the device in real time, while devising improved protocols to prevent unauthorized access.

Wireless Radio Frequency Bedside Devices

Some devices at the bedside use radio frequency technology to connect one device to another. An example of this includes a mobile workstation that uses a Bluetooth device to connect the scanner to the computer. The nurse scans the patient identification band or a medication and verifies the right patient or the right medication with the right medical record.

Radio frequency (RF) wireless technology works by creating electromagnetic waves at the source with the ability to pick up the electromagnetic waves at a specified destination. Signals with longer wavelengths travel longer distances and can penetrate through objects better than signals with shorter wavelengths (Karygiannis, Eydt, Barber, Bunn, & Phillips, 2007). Such RF wireless technologies operate under a grant of certification and/or issuance of a license from the Federal Communications Commission (FCC) (2013).

To prevent unauthorized access of RF data, and to ensure that the data sent is received by the device it is intended for, security measures must be in place. As discussed previously, authentication and wireless encryption play important roles in an effective wireless security plan. The security scheme must also take into consideration that some wireless technologies can sense other like technologies and "pair," or make connections, to a network. Bluetooth devices use this type of technology. This could lead to safety and effectiveness concerns as it might allow unintended remote control of the medical device.

The US Food & Drug Administration (FDA) (2013) offers these guidelines for RF wireless devices

- Utilize data encryption methods at a level appropriate for the risks presented:
- For the medical device
- The environment of use
- Type and probability of threats to which it could be exposed
- Probable risks to the patient if a security breach should occur
- Use the most up-to-date wireless encryption in the design and build of all devices.

In summary, any device that sends data from one device to another is at risk for a security breach. Methods must be in place to mitigate those risks based on the environment, severity of the risk, the potential for harm, and the ways in which the information is being sent and received. Security concerns are not just concerns for healthcare organizations, but also for individuals using these devices.

Future Directions

The necessity of uninterrupted access to information makes it imperative that the systems that store, process, and transmit information are adequately secured. Information technology will continue to grow as will the need for qualified professionals including, but not limited to, the informatics nurse specialist (INS). Security of information and devices that store or transmit information falls within several functional areas of nursing informatics practice, with the most obvious areas being safety, security, and environmental health (American Nurses Association, 2015b). Security should also be considered when developing or designing HIT applications, which fall under the functional areas of development, as well as systems analysis and design. And the last functional area of nursing informatics practice with a major security concern is compliance and integrity management, where the INS employs legal and ethical safeguards to ensure the protection of information and information quality. In truth, one might argue that security is a consideration with each of the functional areas of nursing informatics practice.

Security has not received the attention that it deserves, as is evident from the number of high-profile cases of identity theft, loss, and accidental disclosure of personal and health information. Greater awareness, sufficient resources, and an organization-wide commitment to information security are needed, particularly as the amount of personal health information collected and stored increases. Healthcare institutions and providers have an ethical and legal obligation to consumers to secure health information. Present methods are not good enough. New technologies must be combined with existing measures and ongoing vigilance in a constant effort to ensure that health information is secure. The INS should tap into another functional area of nursing informatics practice—policy development and advocacy—to develop policies, lobby for legislation that creates harsher penalties for cybercriminals, and provide additional tools to aid in this effort.

Summary

- The primary goals of healthcare information-system security are the protection of client confidentiality and information availability and integrity.
- Privacy and confidentiality are important terms in healthcare-information management. With privacy one chooses to disclose personal information, while confidentiality assumes a relationship in which private information has been shared for the purpose of health treatment.
- Information privacy is the right to choose the conditions under which information is shared, and to ensure the accuracy of collected information.
- Threats to information and system security and confidentiality come from a variety of sources, including system penetration by thieves, hackers, unauthorized use, denial of service and terrorist attacks, cybercrime, errors and disasters, sabotage, viruses, and human error.
- Planning for security saves time and money, and is a form of insurance against downtime, breaches in confidentiality, and lost productivity.
- Security mechanisms combine physical and logical restrictions.

- If social media or email is used for work purposes, care should be taken to protect confidentiality and privacy.
- Examples of security measures include automatic sign-off, physical restriction of computer equipment, strong password protection, and firewalls.
- Ultimately, healthcare administrators are responsible for protecting client privacy and confidentiality through education, policy, and creating an ongoing awareness of security.
- One aspect of system-security management includes monitoring the system for unusual record-access patterns, as might be seen when a celebrity receives treatment.
- Health information on the Internet requires the same types of safeguards provided for information found in private offices and information systems.
- All chart printouts, forms, and computer files containing client information should be given the same consideration as the client record itself to safeguard confidentiality.
- More secure methods of authentication are needed, as even the best passwords can be compromised.
- Mobile computing supports point of care, but also introduces additional security issues related to theft of devices and vulnerabilities associated with wireless connectivity.
- Wearable technology, widely used for fitness tracking, collects and transmits personal health data, often without adequate security measures in place.
- The wireless-communication capabilities of implanted medical devices allow changes to settings without further surgery, but it also opens these devices to hacking.
- Several functional areas of nursing informatics practice encompass security, most notably the areas of safety, security, environmental health, and compliance and integrity management, although security is a pervasive concept throughout informatics practice.

Case Study

Your institution has a well-publicized policy against the use of unauthorized, unlicensed software copies. One of the nurse managers has noted during the course of conversation, that she loaded a copy of the spreadsheet program she uses on her home office PC onto one of the unit PCs so that she can work on projects at both locations. As a staff nurse, what should you do? Explain your response. Would you respond any differently if you were the informatics nurse specialist? If so, how?

About the Authors

Dr. Bhatt earned her BSN from Wayne State University and her MSN, MBA, and Informatics certificate from the University of Phoenix. Her DNP is from Oakland University in Rochester, Michigan, and she is enrolled in the DNP to PhD program at UNLV. Her passions include teaching, reading, and acquiring new knowledge. Dr. Bhatt created hospice software with IT partners that is now used by hospices across the United States, and currently teaches informatics courses. She believes that through dedication and hard work, all things are possible.

Ms. Mulberger MSN, RN-BC contributed the content, "Special considerations with mobile computing." Ms. Mulberger is the Clinical Informatics Quality Supervisor at Kalispell Regional Healthcare where she works with clinicians to build and support documentation and order pathways. An experienced presenter and author on nursing informatics topics, Pat is a member of Health Information Management Systems Society, and serves on the American Nursing Informatics Association Board of Directors.

References

American Nurses Association. (2015a). Code of ethics for nurses with interpretive statements. Retrieved from www.nursingworld.org

American Nurses Association. (2015b). *Nursing informatics: Scope and standards of practice* (2nd ed.). Silver Spring, MD: nursesbooks.org

Britton, K. (2016). Handling privacy and security in the Internet of things. *Journal of Internet Law, 19*(10), 3–7.

Brown, C. L. (2012). Health-care data protection and biometric authentication policies: Comparative culture and technology acceptance in China and in the United States. *Review of Policy Research, 29*(1), 141–159. doi:10.1111/j.1541-1338.2011.00546.x

Camera, C., Peris-Lopez, P., & Tapiador, J. (2015). Security and privacy issues in implantable medical devices: A comprehensive survey. *Journal of Biomedical Informatics, 55,* 272–289.

Camp, L. J. (2015). Respecting people and respecting privacy. *Communications of the ACM, 58*(7), 27–28. doi:10.1145/2770892

Cass, S. (2011). Personal security. Retrieved from www.technologyreview .com/s/425059/personal-security

CERT Insider Threat Center at Carnegie Mellon's Software Engineering Institute (SEI). (2016). CERT insider threat center. Retrieved from www.cert.org/insider-threat/cert-insider-threat-center.cfm

Chaudhary, R., & Ward, J. J. (2014). A practical approach to health care information security. *Journal of Health Care Compliance, 16*(3), 11–66.

Computer Security Division Computer Security Research Center. (2016). Retrieved from http://csrc.nist.gov/groups/STM/cmvp/index.html

Conn, J. (2016). Hospital pays hackers $17,000 to unlock EHR's frozen in "ransomware" attack. *Modern Healthcare.* Retrieved from www.modernhealthcare.com/article/20160217/NEWS/160219920

Department of Health and Human Services. (2007). HIPAA security series: 4 security standards technical safeguards. Retrieved from www.hhs.gov/sites/default/files/ocr/privacy/hipaa/administrative/securityrule/techsafeguards.pdf

Everett, C. (2015). Can wearable technology boost corporate wellbeing? *Occupational Health, 67*(8).

Federal Communications Commission. (2013). Radio frequency safety. Retrieved from www.fcc.gov/general/radio-frequency-safety-0

Grimm, J. (2016). PKI: Crumbling under the pressure. *Network Security, 2016*(5), 5–7. doi:10.1016/S1353-4858(16)30046-0

Hallman, S., Stahl, A., & Ahmadov, V. (2011). The causes, security issues, and preventive actions associated with data integrity. *Communications of the IIMA, 11*(1), 17–26.

HealthIT.gov. (2013). How can you protect and secure health information when using a mobile device? Retrieved from www.healthit.gov/providers-professionals/how-can-you-protect-and-secure-health-information-when-using-mobile-device

HIPAA Journal. (2016). California ransomware bill passed by state senate committee. Retrieved from www.hipaajournal.com/california-ransomware-bill-passed-state-senate-committee-3395/

Information Security Forum (ISF). (2016). Threat horizon 2018: Executive summary. Retrieved from www.securityforum.org/research/

Joint Commission on Accreditation of Healthcare Organizations. (1996). *Medical records process.* Chicago, IL: Accreditation Manual for Hospitals.

Karygiannis, T.T., Eydt, B., Barber, G., Bunn, L., & Phillips, T. (2007). *Guidelines for Securing Radio Frequency Identification (RFID) Systems.* NIST Special Publication 800-98. Retrieved from http://ws680.nist.gov/publication/get_pdf.cfm?pub_id=51156

Lee, K. (2015). Wearable health technology and HIPAA: What is and isn't covered. Retrieved from http://searchhealthit.techtarget.com/feature/Wearable-health-technology-and-HIPAA-What-is-and-isnt-covered

Martini, P. (2014). A secure approach to wearable technology. *Network Security*, 2014(10) 15–17.

MITRE Corporation. (2014). Electronic consent management: Landscape assessment, challenges, and technology. Retrieved from www.healthit.gov/sites/default/files/privacy-security/ecm_finalreport_forrelease62415.pdf

Murdock, L. E. (1980). The use and abuse of computerized information: Striking a balance between personal privacy interests and organizational information needs. *Albany Law Review*, 44(3), 589–619.

National Institute of Standards and Technology (NIST). (2012). Guide for conducting risk assessments. *National Institute of Standards and Technology Special Publication* 800-30 Revision 1. Retrieved from http://nvlpubs.nist.gov/nistpubs/Legacy/SP/nistspecialpublication800-30r1.pdf

Nazareth, D., & Choi, J. (2015). A system dynamics model for information security management. *Information & Management*, 52(1), 123–134.

Park, J. S., Chandramohan, P., Suresh, A. T., Giordano, J. V., & Kwiat, K. A. (2013). Component survivability at runtime for mission-critical distributed systems. *Journal of Supercomputing*, 66(3), 1390–1417.

Perkins, E. (2016). Top 10 security predictions through 2020. Retrieved from www.forbes.com/sites/gartnergroup/2016/08/18/top-10-security-predictions-through-2020/#1aa2bb1e3cbe

Piscotty, R., Martindell, E., & Karim, M. (2016). Nurses' self-reported use of social media and mobile devices in the work setting. *Online Journal of Nursing Informatics*, 20(1).

Rezaeibagha, F., Susilo, W, & Win, K.T. (2015). A systematic literature review on security and privacy of electronic health record systems: Technical perspectives. *Health Information Management Journal*, 44(3), 23–38. doi:10.12826/18333575.2015.0001.

RF Basics. (n.d.). Retrieved from www.digi.com/resources/standards-and-technologies/rfmodems/rf-basics

RSA. (2014). The current state of cybercrime 2014: An inside look at the changing threat landscape. Retrieved from www.emc.com/collateral/white-paper/rsa-cyber-crime-report-0414.pdf

Selvakumaraswamy, S., & Govindaswamy, U. (2016). Efficient transmission of PKI certificates using elliptic curve cryptography and its variants. *International Arab Journal of Information Technology*, 13(1), 38–43.

Semel, M. (2016). Why security and compliance are executive responsibilities. *Journal of Health Care Compliance*, 18(2), 17–51.

Shekokar, N. M., Shah, C., Mahajan, M., & Rachh, S. (2015). An ideal approach for detection and prevention of phishing attacks. *Procedia Computer Science*, 49, 82–91. http://doi.org/10.1016/j.procs.2015.04.230

Singer, E. (2011). Getting health data from inside your body. Retrieved from www.technologyreview.com/s/426171/getting-health-data-from-inside-your-body/

Skiba, D. J. (2014). The connected age and wearable technology. *Nursing Education Perspectives*, 35(5), 346–347. Retrieved from http://search.proquest.com/docview/1561005652?accountid=458

Song, K., Han, J. H., Lim, T., Kim, N., Shin, S., Kim, J., & ... Lee, J. (2016). Subdermal flexible solar cell arrays for powering medical electronic implants. *Advanced Healthcare Materials*, *5*(13), 1572–1580. doi:10.1002/adhm.201600222

Tajuddin, S., Olphert, W., & Doherty, N. (2015). Relationship between stakeholders' information value perception and information security behaviour. *AIP Conference Proceedings*, *1644*(1), 69–77. doi:10.1063/1.4907819

US Food & Drug Administration (FDA). (2013, August 14). Radio frequency wireless technology in medical devices - guidance for industry and food and drug administration staff. Retrieved from www.fda.gov/downloads/MedicalDevices/DeviceRegulationandGuidance/GuidanceDocuments/UCM077272.pdf

Vasalou, A., Joinson, A., & Houghton, D. (2015). Privacy as a fuzzy concept: A new conceptualization of privacy for practitioners. *Journal of the Association for Information Science & Technology*, *66*(5), 918–929. doi:10.1002/asi.23220

Vitak, J., Blasiola, S., Patil, S., & Litt, E. (2015). Balancing audience and privacy tensions on social network sites. *International Journal of Communication*, *9*, 1485–1504.

Winland-Brown, J., Lachman, V. D., & Swanson, E. O. (2015). The New 'Code o f Ethics for Nurses With Interpretive Statements' (2015): Practical Clinical Application, Part I. *MEDSURG Nursing*, *24*(4), 268–271.

Wójtowicz, A., & Joachimiak, K. (2016). Model for adaptable context-based biometric authentication for mobile devices. *Personal & Ubiquitous Computing*, *20*(2), 195–207. doi:10.1007/s00779-016-0905-0

Wulf, G. (2007). *HIPAA information and consent form*. Retrieved from www.wulfclinic.com/document/hipaaform.pdf

Yang, Z., Kankanhalli, A., Ng, B., & Lim, J. (2013). Analyzing the enabling factors for the organizational decision to adopt healthcare information systems. *Decision Support Systems*, *55*(13), 764–776.

Young, S. (2016). California senate website hit with ransomware. *Techwire*. Retrieved from www.govtech.com/security/California-Senate-Website-Hit-with-Ransomware.html

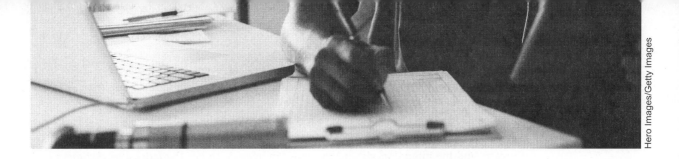

Chapter 14
Information Networks and Information Exchange

Jane M. Brokel, PhD, RN, FNI

Learning Objectives

After completing this chapter you should able to:

- Define the concept of health information networks.

- Compare and contrast the different models for their respective advantages and disadvantages.

- Differentiate between clinical-data networks and health information networks.

- Explain the value of interoperability for health information.

- Describe the current status of the nationwide health information network in the United States.

- Discuss the need for international standards for integration of information.

- Describe the implications of interoperability for healthcare professionals and impact on healthcare delivery.

- Describe the process and use cases for health information exchange (HIE).

- Discuss key factors in the infrastructure for HIE.

- Describe obstacles to network development and sustaining the operations for information exchange.

Introduction

Information networks for the healthcare industry are defined as states and entities meeting a set of standards, specifications, and policies that enable the secure exchange of health information over the Internet (Office of the National Coordinator for Health Information Technology, 2016a). Any social-networking society shares details to inform a select community interested in knowing the same information. Both individuals and families interact with

271

many providers for many reasons, such as physical and mental health; hearing, vision, and dental checkups; sports medicine and physical therapy for conditioning; occupational-health nurses for prevention; or school nurses for school health, nutrition, and more. Each professional provider must legally maintain a record—increasingly, an electronic record—for documenting healthcare problems, health risks, and health-promotion needs, along with a plan for care, and the interventions and therapies delivered. Today, the federal government has provided a foundation for the exchange of health information across these diverse private and public entities. Federal agencies that need to securely exchange electronic health information include the Centers for Disease Control and Prevention (CDC), Centers for Medicare and Medicaid Services (CMS), Department of Defense (DoD), Department of Veterans Affairs (VA), and the Social Security Administration (SSA). These agencies and private providers are accountable for the privacy and security of patient data, and must sign the Data Use and Reciprocal Support Agreement (DURSA), which outlines the roles and responsibilities among participants to have mechanisms in place to protect data. Many healthcare institutions and agencies are able to share more and more individual health information to make cost-effective, timely, and efficient decisions. The health information stored within comprehensive, longitudinal electronic health records within data warehouses and repositories hold allergy and medication profiles, problem lists, laboratory results, radiology images and interpretations, treatment plans for care, and more. Repositories of information are extracted and held within centralized infrastructures for information exchange by state or regional organizations, or within decentralized care-delivery systems.

Health Information Network Models

The preparations for an information network include organizing a governing body and establishing financial sustainability. Several options for operational and business models exist. The US Internal Revenue Service Code, Section 501, and its respective sub-sections, stipulate criteria for organizations to qualify as tax-exempt. Tax-exempt organizations include not-for-profit 501c(3) charitable organizations, 501c(4) social-welfare organizations, and 501c(6) mutual-benefit organizations, as well as virtual businesses linked contractually, but with no separate new entity form; quasi-governmental entities; state agencies; a partnership or limited-liability corporation (LLC) pass-through entity; a special joint-powers authority; or a cooperative (Internal Revenue Service, 2016). The tax-free status for a 501 organization applies to entities that reinvest in the development of services, but these models are not always sustainable due to the challenges of meeting evolving standards. University of Massachusetts Medical School Center for Health Policy and Research (2009) provided information on sustainable models for states to implement sustainable information networks.

Three of the conceptual public-governance models are described as sustainable models (Nolan, Campbell, Thomasian, & Sailors, 2009) and these models exist today. A government-led network with a direct government program, which provides services for the network infrastructure and oversight for the information network, has been used in ten states. In this model, the state government directly runs the health information network through an existing agency, such as the Iowa Department of Public Health with the Iowa Health Information Network (IHIN) and Illinois Health Information Exchange (ILHIE); the Nevada Department of Health and Human Services in their Office of Health Information Technology; and Medicaid Agency with the governor-appointed Alabama Health Information Exchange Advisory Commission (Milken Institute School of Public Health, 2013). These models are subject to government administrative rules and processes, which may limit and delay services associated with legislating changes.

The second type of sustainable model is a public-utility information network with government oversight, where a public sector serves an oversight role and regulates the private-provided services of the information network. Information networks that are a joint effort of a previously existing state agency and a newly created organization include the Health Care Authority Washington and the OneHealthPort, and CareAccord and the Oregon Health Information Exchange, with similar networks in Florida and Arizona. With this model, the state government creates an agency of the state in the form of a nonprofit authority with comprehensive and extensive powers to operate the state health information network in a businesslike manner. This type of model is accountable to the people of the state through audits, legal oversight, and financial disclosure. These models are foundations for states or regions to provide oversight with or without a level of regulatory control by state governments to exert over the information network's infrastructure.

The third type of sustainable model is an information network led by the private sector with government collaboration, where the government acts as a stakeholder and the private sector operates the services. In this model, the state government has contracted health information exchange capabilities to an existing organization. This model exists in 11 states: California, Montana, Texas, New Mexico, Louisiana, Georgia, Indiana, Wisconsin, Rhode Island, and New Jersey. Connecticut uses the Rhode Island information network. The Rhode Island Quality Institute and an Indiana collaborative were early research projects using this model, which were funded by the Agency for Healthcare Research and Quality. These networks are nimble and adaptable to changing service needs.

A fourth model, existing within 22 states, creates an organization to manage and operate the information network. One example of this model is seen within the Utah Clinical Health Information Exchange (cHIE), which was one of the early research-funded models. Another example is the Massachusetts eHealth Institute, which was developed prior to any 2009 Health Information Technology for Economic and Clinical Health (HITECH) federally funded networks. Two other structures for information networks without an organization exist. One in Nebraska, known as Nebraska Health Information Exchange (NeHIE), is a collaborative of the four largest Nebraska healthcare organizations. The Idaho Health Data Exchange, a nonprofit 501(c)(6) company with volunteers, launched its services in late 2015 to fulfill the federal agenda for all states to connect to a nationwide health information network.

Clinical Data Networks or Health Information Networks

Health information networks have been vendor, community-wide, regional, statewide, and global enterprises, such as at military operating sites (Adler-Milstein, Lin, & Jha, 2016), with a goal to exchange patient-level information. Integrated delivery networks (IDN) and health systems within multiple states are organizations that predate the proposed models for health information networks IDNs have been able to exchange standard content and identifiers adopted across all member hospitals, nursing homes, hospice, homecare, and clinics. All IDNs experienced the challenges of adopting common-information formats and learning new workflows for use cases.

Information network organizations are led by multiple representatives from professional groups and healthcare entities responsible for treatment, payment, and operations. Delaware was the first statewide-initiated health information network, while many before this were regional health information organizations. The Department of Defense and the Veterans

Administration healthcare settings have exchanged information between settings, and have collaborated to achieve the same externally with a private healthcare organization (Office of the National Coordinator for Health Information Technology, 2016a). These information networks are centered on patient-care services, and have personal-health records (PHRs) tethered to the hospital or physician office with web-based portals to allow the patient or parent to document symptoms or statuses as in a health-record bank. The two parties upload and download information to help the patient continue care.

In contrast, clinical-data networks were developed to support research on patient outcomes rather than the care delivered. The National Patient-Centered Clinical Research Network hosts a coordination of clinical-data-research networks (CDRNs) comprised of different types of health systems partnered to conduct research as a network (Timble et al., 2015). These data-research networks involve two or more healthcare systems, and include integrated delivery systems, academic medical centers, and safety-net clinics. Each CDRN will develop capacity to conduct randomized trials and observational comparative-effectiveness studies, using data from specific practices and their patient populations (Timble et al., 2015). Some examples of clinical-data research networks include: the Oregon Community Health Information Network (OCHIN), Greater Plans Collaborative (GPC), PEDSnet, Patient-Centered Network of Learning Health Systems (LHSNet), and Scalable Collaborative Infrastructure for a Learning Healthcare System (SCILHS).

Interoperability

Interoperability is the ability of two or more health information systems to exchange electronic clinical information with, and use electronic clinical information from, other systems (Office of the National Coordinator for Health Information Technology, 2016b). This ability is possible because health information systems are designed using common standards. When provided access to longitudinal information that follows consistent and shared ways of representing the meaning of clinical concepts and terms, healthcare providers quickly identify what the information is and understand the meaning (Office of the National Coordinator for Health Information Technology, 2016b). In 2016, only meaningful-use EHR users designated under the CMS Medicare and Medicaid EHR Incentive Programs and their exchange partners (i.e., behavioral health, long-term care, and post-acute care providers) were required to meet the need for interoperability exchange and use. The short-term goal for 2017 focuses on electronically sending, receiving, and finding queried and requested information; integrating the received information into a patient's medical record; and the subsequent use of that information (Office of the National Coordinator for Health Information Technology, 2016b). Public health, emergency-medical services, schools, social services, and research consortiums will be engaged after 2017 to exchange interoperable information.

The Medicare Access and CHIP Reauthorization Act of 2015 mandated, among other requirements, that Medicare providers report on how they are using EHRS technology, with an emphasis on interoperability and exchanging information. The Office of the National Coordinator for Health Information Technology (ONCHIT) published the required measures in 2016 and will be implemented by the end of 2018. If identified barriers exist to achieving this interoperability by December 2019, the federal government is asked to recommend actions to achieve interoperability. Nurses and nurse informaticians have a significant role in ensuring that interoperability is achieved. Nurses and other caregivers in all settings (e.g., clinics, homes, schools, community-based resident facilities, and work settings) where healthcare is managed long term need interoperable data to understand the electronic health information received from settings where the patient may have been. The near-term goals are availability of information (i.e., sending, receiving, finding, and using electronic health information) from outside sources (e.g., retail pharmacies, homecare services, long-term resident facilities, schools, and individuals), and use of information from outside sources in decision making and managing care (Office of National Coordinator for Health Information Technology, 2016b). The MACRA 106(b) mandate is for physicians and hospitals to use the outside sources of electronic health information. This goal for interoperability is necessary to augment safety and evidence-based care, as well as decrease inappropriate utilization and increase efficiency.

In 2015, the ONCHIT described three classifications for interoperable data: emerging, pilot, and national. Emerging technical standards and implementation specifications require additional specification by the standards-development community, have not been broadly tested, have no or low adoption, and/or have only been implemented within a local or controlled setting. Pilot technical standards and implementation specifications have reached a level of maturity, specification clarity, and adoption, where some entities use them to exchange health information either in a testing or production environment. National technical standards and implementation specifications have reached a high-level of maturity and adoption by different entities such that most entities are using them, or are readily able to adopt them for use, to exchange health information (Office of the National Coordinator of Health Information Technology, 2016c).

In 2016, the ONCHIT first published interoperability standards describing both standards and implementation specifications. Yearly updates to the interoperability standards are expected following healthcare-provider adoption and use in multiple settings among multiple systems. In Table 14-1, some international standards that impact the documentation of nurses, nurse practitioners, and other healthcare professionals are shared.

Table 14-1   Best Available Interoperability Standards and Implementation Specifications

Type of Need	Standard/Implementation Specifications	Adoption Level	Federally Required
Allergic reactions	SNOMED CT	Medium-High	No
Allergens: medications	Rx NORM	Medium-High	Yes
Allergens: medications	NDF-RT (value–substance reactant for tolerance)	Unknown	No
Allergens: food substances	SNOMED CT	Unknown	No
Allergens: environmental substances	SNOMED CT	Unknown	No
Care team member	National Provider Identifier (NPI) (not required for non-billable healthcare providers)	Low	No
Patient medical encounter diagnosis	SNOMED CT	Medium-High	Yes
Patient medical encounter diagnosis	ICD-10-CM	Medium-High	Yes
Patient dental encounter diagnosis	SNOMED CT	Medium-High	Yes
Patient race and ethnicity	OMB Standards for Maintaining, Collecting, and Presenting Federal Data on Race and Ethnicity, Statistical Policy Directive No. 15, Oct. 30, 1997	Medium-High	Yes
Patient family health history	SNOMED CT	Medium	No
Functional status/disability	Support varied and not included (ICF or SNOMED CT considered)		
Gender identity	SNOMED CT	Unknown	Yes

(Continued)

Table 14-1 *(Continued)*

Type of Need	Standard/Implementation Specifications	Adoption Level	Federally Required
Sex at birth	For Male and Female, HL7 Version 3 Value Set for Administrative Gender; For Unknown, HL7 Version 3 Null Flavor	Medium-High	Yes
Patient-identified sexual orientation	SNOMED CT	Unknown	Yes
Immunizations historical	HL7 Standard Code Set CVX—Clinical Vaccines Administered	High-Widespread	Yes
Immunizations historical	HL7 Standard Code Set MVX—Manufacturing Vaccine Formulation	Medium-High	No
Immunizations administered	HL7 Standard Code Set CVX—Clinical Vaccines Administered	High-Widespread	No
Immunizations administered	National Drug Code	High-Widespread	Yes
Patient industry and occupation	Varied support for National Institute for Occupational Safety and Health (NIOSH) list, which includes an Industry and Occupation Computerized Coding System (NIOCCS), US Department of Labor, Bureau of Labor Statistics, Standard Occupational Classification, and National Uniform Claim Committee Health Care Taxonomy (NUCC) codes standards		
Numerical laboratory test results	LOINC	Medium	Yes
Medications	RxNorm	High-Widespread	Yes
Medications	National Drug Code (NDC)	Medium	No
Medications	National Drug File—Reference Terminology (NDF-RT)	Medium	No
Units of measure (numerical references and values)	The Unified Code for Units of Measure	Low-Medium	Yes
Patient clinical problems and conditions	SNOMED CT	High-Widespread	Yes
Patient preferred language	RFC 5646	Unknown	Yes
Dental procedures performed	Code on Dental Procedures and Nomenclature CDT	Medium-High	Yes
Dental procedures performed	SNOMED CT	High-Widespread	Yes
Medical procedures performed	SNOMED CT	High-Widespread	Yes
Medical procedures performed	CPT-4/HCPCS	High-Widespread	Yes
Medical procedures performed	IDC-10-PCS	Medium-High	Yes
Imaging (diagnostic, interventions, procedures)	LOINC	Low-Medium	No
Tobacco use	SNOMED CT	High-Widespread	Yes
Unique implantable device identifiers	Unique device identifier as defined by the Food and Drug Administration at 21 CFR 830.3	Low	Yes
Patient vital signs	LOINC	High-Widespread	Yes
Notification of patients' admission, discharge, and transfer status to other providers	HL7 2.5.1	High-Widespread	No
Patient care plans—standard	HL7 Clinical Document Architecture (CDA), Release 2.0, Final Edition	High-Widespread	Yes
Patient care plans—implementation specifications	HL7 Implementation Guide for CDA Release 2: Consolidated CDA Templates for Clinical Notes (US Realm), Draft Standard for Trial Use, Release 2.1	Unknown	Yes

Type of Need	Standard/Implementation Specifications	Adoption Level	Federally Required
Shareable clinical decision support	HL7 Implementation Guide: Clinical Decision Support Knowledge Artifact Implementation Guide, Release 1.3, Draft Standard for Trial Use.	Unknown	No
Electronic prescribing—implementation specification	NCPDP SCRIPT Standard, Implementation Guide, Version 10.6	High-Widespread	Yes
Prescription refill request—implementation specification	NCPDP SCRIPT Standard, Implementation Guide, Version 10.6	Medium-High	Yes
Cancel a prescription—implementation specification	NCPDP SCRIPT Standard, Implementation Guide, Version 10.6	Unknown	Yes
Medical imaging formats for data exchange and distribution	Digitalized Imaging and Communications in Medicine (DICOM)	High-Widespread	No
Format for medical imaging reports for exchange and distribution—standards	DICOM	High-Widespread	No
Format for medical imaging reports for exchange and distribution—implementation	PS3.20 DICOM Standard-Part 20: Imaging Reports using HL7 Clinical Document Architecture	Low	No
Receive electronic laboratory reports—standard	HL7 2.5.1	High-Widespread	No
Receive electronic lab reports—implementation specifications	HL7 Version 2.5.1 Implementation Guide: S&I Framework Lab Results Interface, Release 1—US Realm [HL7 Version 2.5.1: ORU_R01] Draft Standard for Trial Use, July 2012	Medium-High	Yes
Ordering labs for a patient—standard	HL7 2.5.1	High-Widespread	No
Ordering labs—implementation specifications	HL7 Version 2.5.1 Implementation Guide: S&I Framework Laboratory Orders from EHR, Release 1 DSTU Release 2—US Realm	Low	No
Patient education materials—standard	HL7 3 standard: Context aware knowledge retrieval application (Infobutton). Knowledge Request Release 2	Medium-High	Yes
Patient education materials—implementation specifications	HL7 Implementation Guide: Service-Oriented Architecture Implementations of the Context-aware Knowledge Retrieval (Infobutton) Domain, Release 1.	Medium	Yes
Patient education materials—implementation specifications	HL7 Version 3 Implementation Guide: Context-Aware Knowledge Retrieval (Infobutton), Release 4.	Medium	Yes
Reporting antimicrobial and resistance information to public health agencies	HL7 Clinical Document Architecture (CDA), Release 2.0, Final Edition	High-Widespread	No
Reporting antimicrobial and resistance information to public health agencies	HL7 Implementation Guide for CDA Release 2—Level 3: Healthcare Associated Infection Reports, Release 1, US Realm.	Low	Yes
Reporting cancer cases to public health agencies	HL7 Clinical Document Architecture (CDA), Release 2.0, Final Edition	High-Widespread	Yes
Transition of care or referral to another healthcare provider—standard	HLT Clinical Document Architecture, (CDA), Release 2.0, Final Edition	High-Widespread	No
Transition of care or referral to another healthcare provider—implementation specifications	Consolidated CDA Release 1.1 (HL7 Implementation Guide for CDA Release 2: IHE Health Story Consolidation, DSTU Release 1.1—US Realm)	High-Widespread	Yes
Nursing assessments (observations)	LOINC or SNOMED CT	Unknown	No
Outcomes of nursing	LOINC	Unknown	No
Nursing diagnoses (problems, risks, needs)	SNOMED CT	Unknown	No
Nursing interventions (procedures)	SNOMED CT	Unknown	No

Reference: 2016 Interoperability Standards Advisory from Office of National Coordinator for Health IT.

International Standards

The harmonization of concepts and data normalization are both necessary to achieve a level of interoperability, allowing reuse of information for multiple purposes. This interoperability requires international standards, as noted in Table 14-1, to share patient health and care information, initially, for healthcare professionals to provide care and, subsequently, for public-health use and for researchers to generate new evidence. For example, the physicians' and nurses' documentation of patients' clinical problems and conditions uses SNOMED CT, an international standard terminology, in the problem list. The international standards work to communicate the patients' conditions among healthcare professionals, as well as for patients and families. Patients, family members, and even new healthcare professionals who do not understand what these problems and conditions represent can use knowledge databases to search, not only the definition of the condition, but also the knowledge context associated with the condition. Medical-knowledge databases and medical journals are frequently linked to electronic patient-record systems to support searching medical conditions. Drug databases may be purchased and linked to the electronic patient-record and pharmacy systems for searching. Nursing-knowledge databases and nursing journals for nursing diagnoses, nursing problems, problem risks, and needs for health enhancement and interventions may be linked as well; these sources are not linked as often as medical sources. Publishers have translated the knowledge databases into multiple languages to inform healthcare professionals, patients, and the general public. International standards are necessary to communicate information worldwide and, when linked to appropriate translated knowledge resources, provide meaning for intelligent or learned use of the information and knowledge when making decisions. Consequently, users not only need the terms, but also the knowledge context to support accurate meaning for decision making in managing care. Not all health information technology (HIT) meets the demands of a broad scope of healthcare professionals and patient users.

Not all standards are developed in a method that fully supports nurses' practices when coordinating nursing care across many settings, and helping patients and families continue healthcare. Extra steps are necessary for including details for treatment plans, health-enhancement plans, and risk-aversion interventions until the electronic health information systems meet the demands for decision making and managing care for all populations in all settings. Current electronic health information systems remain inadequate for vulnerable populations at home, such as infants and children with genetic disorders associated with developmental delays, congenital disorders, and unknown developmental and genetic disorders. The current standard for the plan of care constructed by the *HL7 Implementation Guide for CDA Release 2: Consolidated CDA Templates for Clinical Notes* lacks the nursing-process details that support this population (Lavin, Harper, Barr, 2015; Gonzalez, 2014). Therefore, nurses need to communicate the additional electronic information and not assume that the continuity of care document standards have achieved the communication intended for the next level of care, whether for homecare nursing services, school nurse, or other setting.

Using the consolidated CDA guide as an example, all healthcare professionals need to understand the intentions of interoperability and how these standards support healthcare professionals. The CDA templates of the future will incorporate and harmonize previous efforts from HL7: *Integrating the Healthcare Enterprise Patient Care Coordination (IHE)*, the *Continuity of Care Document*, and the *HITSP Summary Documents Using HL7 Continuity of Care Document (CCD) Component*.

The updates for clinical notes that could help support the CDA Release 2 for Patient Care Plan include the Home Health Plan of Care (HHPoC), Consultation Note, Continuity of Care Document (CCD), Diagnostic Imaging Reports (DIR), Discharge Summary, History, and Physical (H&P), Operative Note, Procedure Note, Progress Note, Referral Note, Transfer Summary, and Unstructured Document, and Patient Generated Document (US Realm Header).

Additionally, the Commission for Certification of Health Information Technology (CCHIT) (Heo et al., 2012) was a regulating body that certified HIT, using the American National Standards Institute (ANSI) standards and Health Information Technology Standards Committee (HITSC) standards. The technical standards for transport of health information to and from electronic destinations include industry-recognized transport types (e.g., Internet Protocol Version 6) and the recipient's technical capability (e.g., broadband, electronic, fax, and print). The Federal Communications Commission (FCC) collaborates with the Department of Health and Human Services (DHHS) to ensure the connectivity bandwidth for download and upload speed requirements—upload speeds greater than 200 kilobytes per second (kbps)—for broadband connections to support rural settings with HIT. At this time, a number of carriers are now offering download speeds of 1.5 Mbps and 3.0 Mbps, and an estimated 3,600 out of approximately 307,000 small providers face a broadband connectivity gap below required FCC recommendations (Federal Communications Commission, 2010).

Nationwide Health Information Network

Nationwide Health Information Network (NHIN) is broadly defined as the set of standards, specifications, and policies that support the secure exchange of health information over the Internet (Public Health Data Standards Consortium, 2018). The Office of the National Coordinator for Health Information Technology is responsible for the support and promotion of the adoption of information technology and health information exchange (HealthIT.gov, 2017). Working with the Health Information Technology Standards Committee (HITSC), the Office of the National Coordinator outlined a standards and interoperability framework with principles and processes for the NHIN. The framework for the NHIN identified standards and implementation guides for the use cases (e.g., practice and services). In 2016, the ONCHIT (2016b) published the best available interoperability standards and implementation specifications. The implementation specifications included programs of tools and services to guide the implementation of standards, allowing interoperable exchange of information. The interoperability standards, highlighted in Table 14-1, allow providers, organizations, and agencies to join the national network to exchange health information when participating in state or regional networks.

The NHIN is a set of standards, services, and policies that will bring together the state-level HIE and community health information organizations (HIOs) when all stakeholders are using the evolving information-exchange standards (Adler-Milstein et al., 2016). Kuperman and McGowan (2013) identified concerns with the completeness, accuracy, and timeliness in accessing and using the exchanged information during the provider's clinical workflow, and that the information presented for the physician may not be sufficient for the care coordinator's work, and could lead to unintended consequences when integrated into practice. This network has already connected a diverse set of federal agencies and private organizations that needed to securely share reliable electronic health-related information in the past five years (Department of Health and Human Services, 2016). The state-level HIE programs are responsible for organizing and facilitating the implementation of interoperability standards among stakeholders through state-wide operational planning. The state-wide information network ensures all stakeholders and communities are included, rather than excluded, and can legislate the standards to carry out functions through a single entity accountable to the citizens. The role of the state-level HIE program is to adapt to the state's needs and priorities, based on the characteristics of providers taken from an evaluation of current HIT use. The agencies, such as public health and Medicaid services within the state government, are stakeholders and will be involved with HIE services. The success for the NHIN is dependent on the information networks.

Implications of Interoperability

When the NHIN was first envisioned more than a decade ago, the issue for healthcare professionals was how to use the HIE; that is, how to query patient records and find providers to share and receive patient information. This is a process for bidirectional sharing of patient health-related information among primary providers (nurse practitioners, physicians, and physician assistants), consulting specialists, hospitals, ambulatory centers, nursing homes, post-acute providers, dentists, audiologists, optometrists, and occupational and school-health professionals. Each citizen contributes to the collection of health information when participating in interviews at healthcare settings, when applying for a job or position that requires physical and cognitive abilities to perform occupational tasks, or when participating in school activities.

The electronic health record (EHR) and personal health record (PHR) are tools that provide background information on individual abilities and disabilities (such as vision, hearing, and mobility). The records include common elements that support decisions, such as immunization status, allergies (foods, environment, and medications), values (preferences, and cultural and religious beliefs), social habits (alcohol or tobacco use), family history, advance directives, and insurance coverage or noncoverage. The health record is about health patterns and functioning, using information to keep persons safe and healthy, and not just for medical conditions or diseases. A visit to a primary-care practitioner or urgent clinic allows providers to access the information through a record-locator application to obtain the person's allergies or past history. This past health information, once validated by a clinician, helps ensure appropriate selection of interventions or medications for safe care.

Process and Use Cases for Health Information Exchange

A health information exchange (HIE) is defined as the electronic movement of health-related information or clinical data that follows patients across delivery settings, according to nationally recognized standards (Adler-Milstein et al., 2016). Adler-Milstein et al. (2016) found healthcare organizations were in agreement that broad-based HIE was needed to improve care and should support multiple approaches to HIE. The HIE processes have been developed to support a geographic region by a community of stakeholders or within a state health information network. A national survey identified 106 operational HIE network, community, and regional organizations providing services to over a third of all US providers in 2014 (Adler-Milstein et al., 2016). The organizations provide oversight in authorizing the infrastructure, location of health information, and the secure transfer and reuse of that health information electronically.

The HIE network sustains operations through a membership fee, where stakeholders pay to support shared services for all. The fees may be tiered toward size or volume of activity, or may be based on relative value to each type of participant. Another method to sustain operations is through a transaction fee where the regional or state-level network charges transaction fees for services or products on the basis of benefit to the participants. The fees could be for clinical results delivered, covered life per month, each hour of technical assistance, or monthly use of an HIE application. Additionally, a program and service fee is charged to stakeholders for participation in the HIE services, or for purchasing and implementing the HIE program. Some HIEs do not charge a fee to physicians and nurse practitioners for access to patient information, such as laboratory results, pathology reports, diagnostics reports, discharge summaries, and consultation reports. This is not a universal practice with all HIEs, and professional providers may be charged a fee for transactions when using the HIE. When the data are used for group-practice management, eprescribing, EHR-lite (i.e., basic components of EHR data), quality-measures monitoring, biomedical devices, and pharmaceutical manufacturers, fees are considered for use of the HIE. Only half of the 106 operational HIE networks and community-based organizations reported they were financially viable without government support in 2014 (Alder-Milstein et al., 2016). The secondary use of data for profit presents ethical concerns that consumers and participating providers will raise as HIPAA violations. The third-party payers have provided incentives for HIE participating providers by offering quicker reimbursements and payment for performance. CMS has offered meaningful-use incentives due to the HITECH Act, which encouraged adoption and implementation of electronic health records in eligible provider practices and hospitals. This practice resulted in disincentives for nonuse of EHRs and HIEs after 2014.

Key Factors

Health information exchanges are used for patient-care treatment, healthcare operations, and payment. The use of HIE to acquire lab results and patient summaries in primary care practices for individual patient care ranged from 55% in New Zealand to 14% in Canada, while the United States was around 31% with greater use seen in large integrated health systems (Schoen et al., 2012). Healthcare operations use included options for professional clinical decision making to diagnose, plan interventions and surveillance, coordinate care, and to evaluate patient outcomes through alerts, messages, or regular reports among health professionals. Healthcare payment includes managing operation and fiscal resources, monitoring processes for quality and continuous improvement, and reporting for accreditation and regulatory requirements within an agency or organization. Public-health related uses include processes for population health and safety, including disease surveillance and registries for births, deaths, immunizations, cancer, and trauma.

To accomplish exchanges for patient, professional, organizational, and public uses, a HIE infrastructure requires not only technology, but also an organizing structure for processes. The organizing structure establishes secure processes and rules of operation, technical and content standardization for interoperable exchanges among entities, and outlines the use cases and workflow to obtain meaningful information use. There are eleven key factors considered indispensable prerequisites for the HIE organizing infrastructure. These factors include:

- *Data storage.* Data storage is necessary to enable the ability to aggregate data from disparate sources. Large health systems are often well-positioned to store and share patient-protected information within secure structures with private access. This is not the case for many small clinics, community centers, schools, and occupational-health staff for small businesses who need data storage to allow access to their health-related information for sharing when the agency closes on evenings and weekends. A central repository can temporarily hold information from small providers as it is collected for electronic medical or health record applications. This **repository** may also store data to serve as a core component for public-health use of data registries for birth certificates, immunizations, work-related injuries, cancer, diabetes, and trauma, or for monitoring communicable illnesses. The infrastructure for data storage may be consolidated with a centralized cooperative data repository to push and pull data. The **infrastructure** may be decentralized or federated with access to information through multiple health systems. A hybrid infrastructure is a combination of the consolidated and federated models. A hybrid-infrastructure model enables the access and exchange of data stored in existing provider networks as well as through a central-data repository maintained for smaller providers who would not be able to maintain 24/7 services for HIE access.

- *A master person index.* A **master person index (MPI)** is a standard person-identifier code that uniquely identifies an individual and permits the correlation process to match the person's data from a variety of different sources of health providers (e.g., clinics, hospitals, pharmacies, and nursing homes). Health systems often use enterprise-wide MPI applications and processes to maintain only one electronic health record for a person across many organizations within the system. When the MPI is not used or is unknown for a patient, an algorithm of multiple identifiers (name, birth date, address, etc.) will need to be used to make a match with multiple external records. The risk in not matching records with a level of certainty, which can lead to either using information from another person's record or result in duplicate collection for the person whose identifier is not found.

- *Record-locator service.* A **record-locator service** used to access and find health information that matches the identified individual. Some describe the record-locator services as a map or pointer to search and locate the information. The record locator can point to specific types of information (e.g., laboratory results, medications from pharmacies, allergies, or continuity of care documents).

- *Methods of authentication.* **Authentication** is necessary to identify who is allowed to access health information through the HIE record-locator services. This individual will find important information for decision-making about patient care, and can download the information into the local record or simply document the original source of data used for local decisions. Valid users will include clinical professionals and public-health staff who use the healthcare data for patient populations and information-technology professionals who audit user access. Patients could potentially have access in the future.

- *Authorization for users.* The **authorization** process can occur through the healthcare organizations that already manage employment or through professional appointments. These organizations are positioned to facilitate role-based security for a clinician user to gain access to the record-locator service for health information exchange. This authorization process includes steps to train individuals to locate and obtain correct patient-level information during their daily workflow of care or for public reporting.

- *Security policies and procedures to ensure a person's privacy and confidentiality.* These procedures clarify when information requests and reuse require patient consent. The operating rules include establishing data agreements among organizations to retrieve and reuse patient information previously collected and managed within other healthcare organizations. Additionally, each state or regional HIE establishes procedures to allow persons either to opt-in (allow data to be shared) or to opt-out (data are not to be shared) from health information exchange. Networks and regional organizations may vary in their procedures. The Health Information Security and Privacy Collaborative (HISPC) provided a framework, toolkit, and templates for data agreements, patient consents, and requests for opt-in and opt-out; public-education materials; and interstate and intrastate policies and legislation. Regional and state organizations need to apply broad restrictions on access to specific health information to allow individual protections, while permitting exchanges for both public safety and statistics. In the future, after the development of common request standards, an individual may have the opportunity to specify access limits for specific health information (e.g., genetic code) or allow information to be shared (e.g., healthcare systems or clinical research). The HIPAA guidelines expand on meeting needs for exchange of PHI for continuous care, while requiring informed consent and tracking disclosure of other requests for information.

- *Audits and logs of HIE activity.* This includes both intentional and unintentional connections, and disconnections to network services. These networking activities allow improved configuration and generation of alerts and notifications during connection for users. The networks and organizations monitor and report on activity and response levels to track thresholds for technical stability and for any security violation.

- *Criteria-based standards.* **Criteria-based standards** are needed for data transport, messaging, transfer of care, and other use cases that specify content formats and workflows for use of health information. A referral for consultation, a discharge summary, and a continuity of care document are examples of using standardized formats for content exchange. HIT users must conform in order to exchange information within statewide networks. Requirements include data-storage configurations and processes (e.g., edge servers and web services), determining the frequency in which data is made available through the HIE, and disaster recovery. The previously mentioned standards for interoperability align with this factor.

- *Determination of scope of services.* The scope of services is determined by functionality that enables sets of standard types of data to be exchanged through the networks. These data are exchanged through HIE using a **push or pull function** that may be triggered by user-initiated events. An example could include a request for a continuity of care document being pulled in anticipation of receiving a patient in transfer from one facility to another. Push examples include a push of final pathology results to update previously sent preliminary results, a push of new prescriptions or the changes in medications prescribed to a pharmacy, or a push to notify a public-health department about the occurrence of communicable illness for a disease-surveillance registry.

- *Knowledge of workflow between providers and other users for patient- and public-health outcomes.* The Health Information Technology Standards Panel developed, harmonized, and integrated technical standards for facilitating widespread adoption and use of interoperability in healthcare. This panel was created by the ONCHIT and conducted its work from 2007 to 2010. A complete library of the panel's work products is available at the HITSP website: www.hitsp.org/default.aspx. Recent interest and efforts in workflow and HIE have focused on understanding the standard data needs for precision medicine and global sharing of accurate genotypic and phenotypic data for novel genes or variants (Ashley, 2016). Use cases for precision medicine will require a deeper knowledge about diseases such as cancer, and targeting interventions on cardiovascular and other body systems with greater therapeutic precision (Ashley, 2016).

- *A portal for access.* The **portal for access** enables authorized users to sign on to the HIE. Different portals may be necessary to support different types of information exchanges (or HIE services) required for continuous care delivery, public reporting, and quality monitoring. An example is a provider portal aligned within the EHR to query a patient record, and retrieve and download the continuity of care document and laboratory results, or make a referral to a physician or nurse specialist or therapists, with key data included. For a consumer and patient, the portal would allow going to a PHR to collect self-monitored blood-glucose levels, daily weight, responses to a pre-visit questionnaire, or logging respiratory symptoms with chronic diseases.

In summary, the constituents who set up regional or state health information exchange infrastructures need to engage consumers, providers, and public-health professionals from the community to design processes. Consumer focus groups and healthcare-professionals' feedback sessions are important methods to stimulate dialogue with providers and consumers, in order to test ideas and develop procedures for the HIE and privacy protections. The providers will likely store data captured about the patient within a repository that is external to the active electronic health record. This storage (e.g., cache with edge server) will allow others to find and pull data from healthcare providers on an as-needed basis without disrupting the clinicians' workflow. Statewide toolkits and communication plans help guide entities and consumers on how to work together to standardize content, as well as to find and use it with the exchange technology. The implication is to educate the population in the state to allow information to be stored and shared—and thus, be accessible. However, for the HIE processes to accomplish these goals, the adoption of EHRs must first be broadly implemented.

Driving Forces

The steps toward exchange began back in 1965, when Medicare and Medicaid programs required accurate and timely information for reimbursement procedures (Staggers, Thompson, & Snyder-Halpern, 2001), as well as with the 2003 Medicare Modernization Act, which supported the first electronic prescribing through HIE. The HITECH Act legislation in 2009 was the driving force for funding state HIE programs. Today, the level of centralization of the community or network decision making, the establishment for EHRs in all care settings, the diversity of EHR systems that need to be integrated into the exchange, and the vast number of patient records are all factors affecting the rate of adopting HIE; while meaningful-use requirements with incentive payments, and the need for information at transitions of care in order to reduce fragmentation drive HIE (Frankel, Chinitz, Salzberg, & Reichman, 2013). Since 2016, MACRA rules have initiated Medicare performance-incentive payments to eligible clinicians who electronically find, use, and share health information with external providers.

The impacts on HIE is that it reduces duplication by sharing information often and in many different settings (i.e., clinics, pharmacies, ambulatory services, nursing homes, hospitals, schools, occupational-health centers, and public-health centers). The costs of fragmentation in delivering healthcare have resulted in duplicated tests, quality gaps due to multiple records and discrepancies within those records, and increased costs to deliver. A person's complete longitudinal health record is important because a uniform holistic picture of the person's symptoms, conditions, and functional health patterns can impact the person's receipt of appropriate and timely care and treatment. HIE allows reuse of patient health information.

The methods to transfer information across settings vary widely in format (e.g., letter, report, or note) and method (e.g., mail, fax, or portal to HIE record locator). When the information is not easily obtained, providers are forced to recreate the information or take action with incomplete information because the person often does not remember. The primary goals of HIE are to facilitate access to and retrieval of clinical data to provide safe, timely, efficient, effective, equitable, and patient-centered care. The associated benefits of HIE are to save money, improve outcomes, and improve provider-patient relationships.

Current Status

In 2016, all states had an operational process for information networks to exchange health information. In 2014, within the United States, 82% of office-based physicians used an electronic health record system (EHRS), and 74.1% used systems certified by the CDC (2015). Six states exceeded adoption rates: Iowa (83.4%), North Carolina (84.8%), Oregon (85.0%), Vermont (85.0%), South Dakota (86.1%), and Minnesota (88.6%). In 2013, while nine states exceeded the national average for use of EHRSs in office-based clinics, the range in use of any part of an EHR ranged from 66% to 94%. The state-initiated HIEs and regional HIEs have supported 42% of all primary-care physicians to share data (Center for Disease Control and Prevention, 2015). Of the physicians with a certified EHRS, those offices electronically sharing patient health information with external providers ranged from 17.7% in New Jersey to 58.8% in North Dakota. In exchanging health information, Adler-Milstein et al. (2016) found the patient summary was shared most often (89%), followed by sharing of discharge summaries (78%), messages alerting providers of admission/discharge/transfers from the hospital (69%), medication lists and problem lists from ambulatory settings (66%), and lab results (63%). Acute-care hospitals were providing and receiving data in operational HIE with 81% to 82% effort in the nation, followed by ambulatory physician practices with 75% effort in providing data with 88% effort in receiving information (Adler-Milstein et al., 2016). Long-term facilities were providing information effort at 40%, while receiving data at 51%; while public-health departments were at 44% effort in providing information and receiving data at 56% effort (Adler-Milstein et al., 2016). Adler-Milstein et al. found laboratories, imaging services, and other healthcare professionals and providers at, or well below, 50% effort in providing information and receiving data from HIE.

Information networks continue to evolve and seek stakeholder buy-in to adopt use cases, while improving response to operation and technology issues. Early return-on-investment models suggest that federal and state governments may indeed benefit the most from HIE and NHIN exchanges by reducing duplicated tests and consultations, and by reducing readmissions for the same medical condition; thus, controlling Medicare costs and Medicaid reimbursements to providers. With this expectation, the employers or purchasers of health-insurance plans, the insurers themselves, and even consumers should see declines in cost over time with the reductions of duplicated services when moving the patient between multiple settings. Hospitals can benefit as well, with reduction of costs, fewer test supplies required to take care of a patient, having prospective payment plans, and shorter lengths of stay from better care coordination. Understanding this expected ROI forecast would mean those collecting information electronically will see an increase in burden and costs associated with documenting aspects of care in standard formats, or they may see an eventual decline in tests or in paperwork when fully automated. In this picture, the benefit to individual physicians, nurses, and pharmacists are minimal because the burden to collect and validate more data to ensure safety and prevention of error increases.

Obstacles

Developing a sustainable HIE business model was the greatest barrier to progressing the efforts of HIE in 2014, as reported by 33% of operational HIEs (Alder-Milstein et al., 2016). Another barrier that impacts adoption of technology solutions is the integration of the HIE process into the professionals' daily workflow. The lack of funding remains a barrier reported by those responding to the evaluation of HIE by Adler-Milstein and colleagues. Twenty-five %

of HIE respondents identified the limitations of interface standards and a lack of resources to implement interface standards as barriers for practices. Providers were asked to pay for costly interfaces to share documentation with the network's HIE in addition to the costs of EHR systems, which delayed the timely adoption of HIE processes.

Even successful state and regional information networks are struggling to engage ambulatory providers and community agencies outside the traditional healthcare system. Only 15% of office-based physicians with a certified EHRS electronically shared patient information with external providers. Among all specialist and primary-care physicians, sharing was far less with home health (11.8%), long-term care (10.6%), and behavioral-health providers (11.4%) (CDC, 2015). This lack of capability for healthcare operations and EHRSs to interface data across applications (e.g., EHR documentation systems, scheduling and staffing systems, and accounting systems) remains a barrier. This impacts the ease of extracting data for sharing health information with these external providers, and directly impacts continuous services for vulnerable populations, such as infants and children with disabilities and congenital conditions, geriatric people with disabilities and chronicity, and persons with mental and behavioral conditions who require multiple services.

For the community of providers, the challenge will be to ensure the additional adoption of new 2016 standards for EHRSs to exchange common data (see Table 14-1). The process for adoption of new standards includes the adoption of implementation specifications, new workflows, and new functions within EHRS technology. The education of end users on the use of clinical terminologies, information models, evidence-based content, and redesigned workflows must accompany the information technology to ensure the right clinical data is captured by the right persons, at the right time, in the right place, and is stored and retrievable for interpretation when needed. New skills are necessary to support these needs.

Future Directions

The need to generate greater value from sharing healthcare data may have to come through analytics, decision support, and patient engagement, to overcome the barriers of cost, which are passed onto providers, though this value is hindered without more providers using HIE services (Adler-Milstein et al., 2016). The era of accountable care models with bundled payment models could create more demand for HIE sharing of information. This is because hospital and primary-care providers need the information about their patients from other healthcare professionals who share in the care of their patients within homes, schools, workplaces, and community services, but are not part of their organization. There is room for the adoption of HIE services within primary-care practices and imaging services, but also across many of the community service professionals who serve patients. These professionals include optometrists; dentists; audiologists; chiropractors; physical and occupational therapists; dietitians; nurses in work, school, or home settings; and others providing healthcare outside of the traditional healthcare systems.

Critical implications for the future of health information networks are additional adoption of EHRSs by external providers, and the far-reaching adoption of the 2016 interoperable standards at all levels of providers (Office of the National Coordinator for Health Information Technology, 2016b). This chapter shares many of the standards and implementation specifications published within the final 2016 advisory. The 2016 interoperability standards include the transition of care to another healthcare provider and public-health reporting, but likely will expand to include standards relevant for all external providers. For instance, the standards and implementation specifications for nursing documentation were not explicitly outlined for nursing-process data elements—though shared within the standards, the standards are in need of further public comment and input from the greater nursing community, which represents a lot of external providers outside the traditional healthcare system. Any future standards and implementation specifications will include future public comments and HITSC recommendations for 2017 and future years. At this time, the advisory did not include within its scope administrative healthcare operations or payment-data needs, nor were the administrative-transaction requirements for HIPAA and CMS included. The ONCHIT advisory provided reference to the best available standards and implementation specifications, and therefore, the Secretary of Health and Human Services has not formally approved these interoperability standards.

The best-available published interoperability standards, shown in Table 14-1, have been studied and will require more research in trial sites for the Nationwide Health Information Network. The performance category of advancing care information (ACI) was recently added to the meaningful-use incentive program, with 11 meaningful-use indicators. Eligible clinicians will need to meet certain MACRA criteria for the advanced alternative payment model (APM) professionals. The administrative rules for MACRA requirements on sharing information would distribute incentive payments to eligible clinicians in 2019. CMS intends to have budget neutrality, where the negative adjustments for care delivered offset the positive adjustments to eligible clinicians. CMS expects this to drive quality improvement in care to Medicare beneficiaries and patients.

Summary

- The health information exchange (HIE) infrastructure is a process for bi-directional sharing of patient health-related information among primary providers (nurse practitioners, physicians, and physician assistants), consulting specialists, hospitals, ambulatory centers, nursing homes, dentists, audiologists, optometrists, and occupational- and school-health professionals.
- Shared information includes standard elements such as immunization status, allergies (foods, environment, and medications), values (preferences, cultural and religious beliefs), social habits (alcohol or tobacco use), family history, medication list, care plan, and insurance coverage or non-coverage that support decisions.
- HIE requires an organizing structure, in addition to technology, for exchange at individual, professional, organization, public-health, and national levels.
- Key factors for consideration in creating the HIE infrastructure include data storage, a master person index (MPI) or code that can be used to uniquely identify an individual and his or her information from different sources, a record-locator service used to access and find health information that matches the identified individual, authentication of allowed users, security policies and procedures to ensure privacy and confidentiality, audit trails of all activity, standards for transport and messaging, scope of services, knowledge of workflow, and a portal for access.
- Regional or state health information-exchange infrastructures need to engage consumers, providers, and public-health professionals from the community to design processes.
- The impetus for HIE began with the inception of the Medicare and Medicaid programs.
- HIE has the potential to reduce duplication and provide reuse of patient health information.

- Preparations for an HIE include organizing a governing body and establishing financial sustainability.
- There are several models for information networks including not-for-profit, public utility, mutual benefit, for-profit, government-led initiatives, and for-research, as well as permutations of these models.
- The public-authority HIE is accountable to the people of the individual state through audits and legal oversight and financial disclosure.
- Integrated delivery networks (IDNs) and health systems within multiple states predated the proposed models for HIE organizations.
- The Department of Defense and the Veterans Administration healthcare settings have HIE within these organizations and are working to achieve HIE with external enterprises.
- The challenge with information-network models is to be financially self-sustaining over time. Many were started with public funds, some charge for access to patient information, while others only charge for other services or generate revenue from the secondary use of data. Third-party incentives for HIE include quicker reimbursement payment for services.
- All states have implemented HIEs with the ONC-HIT oversight.
- The success of HIEs will be determined by the level of responsiveness to what stakeholders need and want for improving patient-centered healthcare and population health.
- Even successful HIEs have endured a variety of obstacles with policy, organizational structure, financial sustainability, legal procedures, technical designs and equipment, and operational processes.
- The NHIN is a structure that will bring together the state-level HIE and regional HIOs when the stakeholders are using the evolving information-exchange standards.
- Characteristics that greatly affect the state-wide HIE initiative are stakeholders driving the effort, the capabilities and availability of skilled human resources for the effort, ability to access sufficient financial resources, and the strength of leadership.

Case Study

Patient-Emergency Room

A widowed 85-year-old male is in transport to the emergency room for a fractured hip after being found dazed and semi-oriented at home by a visiting neighbor. The triage nurse receives the emergency medical service (EMS) phone call that the patient is 20-minutes out. The nurse uses the patient's name and other identifiers to search within the state's information-network record-locator service to access essential information. The nurse finds one unique patient, based on the EMS-reported patient name and address. After logging into the information network for HIE, the emergency-room nurse views information from the patient's primary-care physician and cardiologist, the patient's pharmacy, the public-health registry, the laboratory results on his last INR and chemistry, and hematology results. An old hospital record is located and used to help prepare for the patient. On his arrival, the nurse and the emergency physician find the patient unable to state allergies and some of his medications, so they use HIE information to verify past history. The nurse verifies the information with the patient and uses the provider-data repository to contact the pharmacy on recent dosing protocols for the patient's anticoagulant. They are able to complete assessments, determine the patient's current status, and route the patient to the radiology department for additional testing.

What is the standard healthcare information the nurse will be able to find through the health information exchange?

What types of services could the triage nurse and emergency physician use after accessing the HIE?

Case Study

Transfer from the Hospital to a Skilled-Nursing/Long-Term Care Facility

An 85-year-old male had a total-hip replacement, is stable, and agrees to complete his rehabilitation and strengthening at the local nursing home, which has skilled nursing services. The staff nurse prepares the patient for discharge and transfer. The assessments are completed prior to discharge within the hospital EHRS. New electronic prescriptions are sent to the patient's pharmacy for delivery to the nursing home. The nurse updates the patient's problem list and adds the problem of risk for falls, and ensures that interventions (e.g., fall prevention, pain management, and exercise promotion) and the current status on patient outcomes for pain and mobility level are up-to-date on the care plan. The nurse contacts the receiving setting and provides the name and other identifying information to the receiving manager or clinical nurse leader. While on the phone, the nurse at the nursing home accesses the state's information network through a web portal to use a record-locator service to search for the patient. The receiving nurse pulls in the advance directive, the plan of care, the problem list, new prescriptions, and continued medications. The last INR test result was posted this morning with the most recent dose for anticoagulation, which was administered in the morning. The two nurses discuss the plans for the anticoagulant protocol that was ordered by the cardiologist for the patient during the patient's rehabilitation.

Will the long-termcare setting be able to use the record-locator service to obtain the information if they do not have a full electronic health record system?

How does the nursing home access the patient's information before arrival?

Should the long-termcare facility wait to use the state's health information network after they implement the EHRS? How can the facility receive training?

Case Study

School Nurse Accessing Public-Health Immunization Registry

The parents of a four-year-old girl register her for preschool, but cannot remember the dates and types of immunizations that were administered at the local clinic and public-health office over the past three years. The parents are concerned about her food allergies and use the little girl's personal health record to keep her allergies and records up-to-date. The school nurse can use record-locator services to obtain the little girl's data and to determine if any immunization is missing. The nurse will provide teaching on immunizations and ask if there are any medications for the known allergies, and what type of reactions are possible. This information was partially complete in the state's health information network resources.

How does the school nurse update the information within the HIE?

About the Author

Dr. Brokel served on the executive committee and advisory council from 2009 to 2016 to guide the development, implementation, and operations for the Iowa Health Information Network. She teaches family-nurse-practitioner students online for Simmons College, and is an adjunct faculty for the University of Iowa College of Nursing. Dr. Brokel is an active practicing nurse clinician and advocate for identifying future information solutions to coordinate better care for pediatric clients at home and in schools.

References

Adler-Milstein, J., Lin, S. C., & Jha, A. K. (2016). The number of health information exchange efforts is declining, leaving the viability of broad clinical data exchange uncertain. *Health Affairs, 35*(7), 1278–1285.

Ashley, E. A. (2016). Towards precision medicine. *Nature Reviews Genetics, 17*(9), 507–522.

Center for Disease Control and Prevention (CDC). (2015). National ambulatory medical care survey (NAMCS) EHR survey. Retrieved from www.cdc.gov/nchs/data/ahcd/nehrs/2015_web_tables.pdf

Department of Health and Human Services (DHHS). (2016). Nationwide health information network exchange. Retrieved from www.healthit.gov/sites/default/files/pdf/fact-sheets/nationwide-health-information-network-exchange.pdf

Federal Communications Commission. (2010). Healthcare broadband in America: Early analysis and a path forward. OBI Technical Paper No. 5. Retrieved from www.healthit.gov/providers-professionals/faqs/what-recommended-bandwidth-different-types-health-care-providers

Frankel, M., Chinitz, D., Salzberg, C. A., & Reichman, K. (2013). Sustainable health information exchanges: The role of institutional factors. *Israel Journal of Health Policy Research, 2*(21), 1–11.

Gonzales, E. I. (2014). *Clinical documentation strategies for home health.* Danvers, MA: HCPro.

Heo, E. Y., Hwang, H., Kim, E. H., Cho, E. Y., Lee, K. H., Kim, T. H., ... Yoo, S. (2012). Comparing the certification criteria for CCHIT-certified ambulatory EHR with the SNUBH's EHR functionalities. *Healthcare Informatics Research, 18*(1), 57–64.

HealthIT.gov. (2017). About ONC. Retrieved from www.healthit.gov/newsroom/about-onc

Internal Revenue Service. (2016). Publication 557. Tax-exempt status for your organization. Department of the Treasury. Retrieved from www.irs.gov/publications/p557

Kuperman, G. J., & McGowan, J. J. (2013). Potential unintended consequences of health information exchange. *Journal of General Internal Medicine, 28*(12), 1663–1666.

Lavin, M., Harper, E., & Barr, N. (2015). Health information technology, patient safety, and professional nursing care documentation in acute care settings. *The Online Journal of Issues in Nursing, 20*(2) 6–6.

Milken Institute School of Public Health. (2013). Status of health information exchanges: 50 state comparison. *Health Information & the Law.* Washington, DC: George Washington University and The Robert Wood Johnson Foundation. Retrieved from www.healthinfolaw.org/comparative-analysis/status-health-information-exchanges-50-state-comparison

Nolan, K., Campbell, C., Thomasian, J., & Sailors, R. (2009). Preparing to implement HITECH: A state guide for electronic health information exchange. 2009 Report from the State Alliance for EHealth. National Governors Association. Retrieved from www.nga.org/files/live/sites/NGA/files/pdf/0908EHEALTHHITECH.PDF

Office of the National Coordinator for Health Information Technology. (2016a). Nationwide health information network exchange. Retrieved from www.healthit.gov/sites/default/files/pdf/fact-sheets/nationwide-health-information-network-exchange.pdf

Office of National Coordinator for Health Information Technology. (2016b). Connecting health and care for the nation. A shared nationwide interoperability roadmap — Final version. Retrieved from www.healthit.gov/sites/default/files/hie-interoperability/nationwide-interoperability-roadmap-final-version-1.0.pdf

Office of National Coordinator for Health Information Technology. (2016c). 2016 interoperability standards advisory: Best available standards and implementation specifications. Final version. Retrieved from www.healthit.gov/sites/default/files/2016-interoperability-standards-advisory-final-508.pdf

Patient-Centered Outcomes Research Institute. (2016). *Clinical data research network.* Retrieved from www.pcornet.org/clinical-data-research-networks/

Public Health Data Standards Consortium. (2018). Nationwide Health Information Network (NHIN, also NwHIN). Retrieved from www.phdsc.org/health_info/nationwide-health-architecture.asp

Schoen, C., Osborn, R., Squires, D., Doty, M., Rasmussen, P., Pierson, R., & Applebaum, S. (2012). A survey of primary care doctors in ten countries shows progress in use of health information technology, less in other areas. *Health Affairs, 31*(12), 2805–2816.

Timble, J. W., Ruden, R. S., Towe, V., Chen, E. K., Hunter, L. E., Case, S. R., et al. (2015). National patient-centered clinical research network (PCORnet) Phase I: Final evaluation report. Patient-Centered Outcomes Research Institute. Retrieved from www .rand.org/pubs/research_reports/RR1191.html.

University of Massachusetts Medical School Center for Health Policy and Research. (2009). Report to the state alliance for eHealth: Public governance models for a sustainable health information exchange industry. Retrieved from www.nga.org/files/live/sites/ NGA/files/pdf/0902EHEALTHHIEREPORT.PDF.

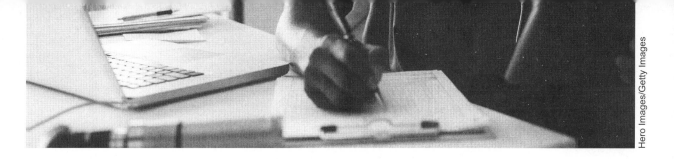

Chapter 15

The Role of Standardized Terminology and Language in Informatics

Susan Matney, PhD, RN-C, FAAN

 ## Learning Objectives

After completing this chapter, you should be able to:

- Explain standardized healthcare terminology and its importance to nursing.

- Describe the American Nurses Association (ANA) criteria established for recognizing standardized terminologies.

- Describe each of the ANA-recognized terminologies and the benefits of use when implemented within an electronic healthcare record system.

- Discuss standardized terminologies used for the different parts of the nursing process and their similarities and differences.

- Define the different types of terminology structures, such as a classification system (e.g., NANDA, NIC, or NOC) versus a reference terminology (ICNP, or SNOMED CT).

- Demonstrate how standard terminologies facilitate the use of evidence-based practice and decision-support rules.

- Illustrate how using standardized healthcare terminologies correlates to the US meaningful use criteria.

- Identify the benefits of using structured terminologies within electronic healthcare record systems.

Introduction to Terminology

Person-centered care requires treating patients in a variety of settings across the entire healthcare continuum, and necessitates the ability to share the most accurate and up-to-date information among a multitude of providers and care settings (Payne et al., 2015). The current state of information use in the healthcare community is evolving from paper-based to computerized records. The introduction of computerized information systems and their increasing use has amplified the need for structured and controlled vocabularies that can be used to represent care.

Standardized Terminology

Standardized terminologies have been developed for use within electronic health record systems (EHRSs). Standardized terminologies are structured and controlled languages developed according to terminology-development guidelines and approved by an authoritative body (Healthcare Information and Management Systems Society, 2013). These terminologies are often referred to as controlled terminologies.

Healthcare-terminology standards are designed to enable and support widespread interoperability among healthcare-software applications for the purpose of sharing information. The use of standardized terminology is a means of ensuring that the data collection is accurate and valid (Payne et al., 2015; Westra, Delaney, Konicek, & Keenan, 2008). The requirement for standardized-terminology development has increased tremendously to support the use of national and international health-information standards.

Standardized terminology is essential for successful development and implementation of an EHRS. Terminology is required to represent, communicate, exchange, manage, and report data, information, and knowledge. It enables safe, patient-centric, high-quality healthcare that optimizes data collection for the measurement of patient outcomes. EHRSs can no longer be developed or implemented without standardized terminologies. Data exchange between EHRS must take place without loss of meaning. Data sharing and reuse that address the effectiveness and efficiencies of care are greatly enhanced when data are defined using common terminologies (McCormick et al., 2015).

The implementation of standardized terminology within an EHRS is essential for healthcare organizations to meet the criteria of meaningful use. The American Recovery and Reinvestment Act of 2009 defined meaningful use as a certified EHRS used in a meaningful way. Meaningful use was one piece of a broader health information technology (HIT) infrastructure needed to reform the healthcare system and improve healthcare quality, efficiency, and patient safety (Health Information Technology, 2015). One of the primary criteria identified for meaningful use is the use of standardized terminologies. The goal of meaningful use is to exchange clinical structured data in a manner that is accurate and complete to improve patient care in a cost-efficient way.

TERMINOLOGY DEFINITIONS Before discussing specific terminologies, some basic elements need to be explained: concepts, codes, and the different types of terminologies. A concept is an expression of an idea with a single unambiguous meaning (International Organization for Standardization/International Electrotechnical Commission 17115, 2007). Clinical concepts are used to document ideas related to patient care or express orders, assessment, and outcomes within an EHRS. A concept can have one or more representations, called synonyms or terms. Concepts have unique identifiers known as codes. Codes are made up of letters or numbers, or a combination of both. Codes are used to designate concepts in a computer system (de Keizer, Abu-Hanna, & Zwetslook-Schonk, 2000). A concept with an assigned code is considered codified. Concept codes facilitate the development of evidence-based practice and decision-support rules; reporting of administrative and financial standards for diagnoses, procedures, and drugs; and the core quality measures. Codified data is used to track key clinical data such as disorders, nursing problems, allergies, procedures, and signs and symptoms. Providers use the collected data for activities such as care coordination, data mining, reporting of clinical-quality measures, and public-health information. Although many individuals working within the healthcare industry recognize coded data only as a source for determining reimbursement, health-information-management professionals have always understood the many uses of coded data.

Clinical terminology enables the capture of a patient's data at the level of detail necessary for patient-care documentation, and is used to describe health conditions and healthcare activities (International Organization for Standardization/International Electrotechnical Commission 17115, 2007). Clinical terminologies consist of concepts that support diagnostic studies, patient history, physical examinations, visit notes, ancillary-department information, nursing care, assessments, flow sheets, vital signs, and outcome measures. A clinical terminology can be mapped to a broader classification system for administrative, regulatory, and fiscal reporting requirements (Giannangelo, 2014).

TYPES OF TERMINOLOGIES Different types of clinical-terminology systems used in healthcare were described by de Keizer et al. (2000), and are still referenced and relevant today. Table 15-1 outlines the terminology types.

A classification system is used to categorize the details of a clinical encounter. It does not capture the level of detail necessary to document specific items at the point of care. Classifications consist of mutually exclusive categories that can be used for specific purposes. An example would be to group data to determine costs and outcomes of treatment. This kind of classification could provide data to consumers on costs and outcomes of treatment options. The International Classification of Diseases (ICD), which is a classification system, does not consist of definitions or definitional relationships between terms such as "has body location."

The term ontology is frequently used within the HIT world. Ontologies help to facilitate interoperability because concepts are organized by their meanings to describe the definitional structure-relationship. Ontologies contain machine-processable definitions in the form of relationships; for example, the concept of *finger* is a part of the concept of *hand*. Ontologies also organize concepts for storage and retrieval of consistent well-formed data. Using the previous example, the ontology can be queried to find the concepts that are defined as *a part of the hand*. The concepts returned would include "thumb," "pointer finger," and so on. The concepts in the ontologies have unique codes.

REFERENCE VERSUS INTERFACE TERMINOLOGY Terminologies are used two different ways within EHRSs: first, as a reference terminology, and second, as an interface (point of care) terminology. A reference terminology consists of a set of concepts with definitional relationships. A reference terminology is necessary to analyze data, develop evidence-based practice, and improve the quality of care. A reference terminology is frequently an ontology and can, therefore, be used to support data aggregation, disaggregation, and retrieval.

Table 15-1 Types of Standardized Healthcare Terminologies

Types of Terminology	Description	Example
Nomenclature	A set of terms composed according to pre-established rules	LOINC, NANDA-I
Terminology	A set of terms representing concepts in a particular field or domain; for example, nursing problems and nursing observations	
Vocabulary	A terminology accompanied by definitions or descriptions	NANDA-I
Classification	An arrangement of concepts based on essential characteristics and arranged in a single hierarchy	ICD, CPT, NIC, NOC
Ontology	A set of concepts formally organized by meaning	SNOMED CT, ICNP

A reference terminology is used to retrieve data across healthcare settings, domains, and specialties in a standardized manner. In a work that remains relevant through the present, Rosenbloom, Miller, Johnson, Elkin, and Brown (2006) stated that an **interface terminology** is what the clinicians see on the screen, and it consists of terms with which clinicians are familiar. It is usually made up of synonyms from the reference terminology and supports the entry of patient-related information into EHRSs. To illustrate: the reference term for a prothrombin-time blood test is "Coagulation tissue factor induced" and the interface term the providers see on their screens is "Protime."

TERMINOLOGY-DEVELOPMENT GUIDELINES Standard terminologies are developed according to terminology-development guidelines. These guidelines, or rules, were clearly articulated by Cimino (1998) and have been adopted as a gold standard in the healthcare industry for evaluating terminologies. Table 15-2 depicts these guidelines.

TERMINOLOGY AND NURSING For years, nurses have expressed nursing care using different terms to say the same thing. Standardized nursing language is a common language, readily understood by computers and nurses, that is used to describe care (Thede & Schwirian, 2014). A uniform representation of nursing care supports a complete and unambiguous description of how nursing problems, interventions, and outcomes are documented. The use of coded standardized terminology for nurses is vital to bedside nursing and to the nursing profession. It is essential because it enables consistent use of terminologies across clinical settings and specialties. The use of standardized nursing terminology will result in better communication to the interdisciplinary team, an increase in the visibility of nursing interventions, enhanced data collection used to evaluate and analyze patient-care outcomes, and

Table 15-2 Cimino's 12 Terminology Development Guidelines

Guideline	Explanation
1. Content	Healthcare terminologies should be rich in content.
2. Concept orientation	Healthcare terminologies should be based on concepts, rather than on terms. Terms must correspond to at least one meaning (nonvagueness) with no more than one meaning (nonambiguity). The meanings correspond to no more than one term (nonredundancy).
3. Concept permanence	Once a concept enters a terminology, it should not be deleted or reused.
4. Nonsemantic concept identifier	Concept identifiers are the codes that identify concepts in a terminology. The code must have no meaning, and each concept must have a unique identifier.
5. Polyhierarchy	A strict hierarchy consists of a root concept used for traversing the hierarchies.
6. Formal definition	Formal definitions add semantic exactness to a terminology by making the relationship between concepts explicit.
7. Reject "not elsewhere classified"	The problem with such terms is that they can never have formal definition other than one of exclusion.
8. Multiple granularities	Terminologies should not restrict users or applications to terms at some particular level of granularity.
9. Multiple consistent views	It should be possible to view the concept hierarchies in multiple consistent ways.
10. Beyond healthcare concepts representing context	Terminologies should not specify how different pieces on clinical information are related.
11. Evolve gracefully	The terminology should allow for long-term growth.
12. Recognize redundancy	Redundancy is the condition in which the same information can be stated in two different ways.

greater support of adherence to the standards of care. Furthermore, the use of standardized nursing terminology can be used to assess nursing competency.

The need for standardization in nursing documentation is critical to support interoperability—the ability to share comparable data with other healthcare organizations via electronic transmission. The collection of standardized nursing-care documentation can enable a comparison of different terminologies that can be used to research patient-care outcomes nationally and worldwide. Given the federal requirements to EHRSs, there is a need to establish standards for the implementation of terminologies within an EHRS. Healthcare terminology needs to be universally understood across all healthcare providers and organizations in order for healthcare systems to be interoperable and to uniformly exchange data. To accomplish interoperability, standardized clinical terminologies must be implemented within EHRs (McCormick et al., 2015).

Languages and Classification

Billing Codes

Healthcare encounters are coded for billing by code sets mandated by the Health Insurance Portability and Accountability Act (HIPAA). HIPAA mandates that all electronic transactions include only HIPAA-compliant codes (Giannangelo, 2014). The code sets described here are the ICD, Current Procedural Terminology (CPR) codes, and the Alternative Billing Codes (ABC). These codes are used to classify and catalog diseases and procedures. These code sets are reviewed and subject to modification annually. Use of billing codes at the point of care is discouraged, but some systems use them to build problem and procedure lists. This chapter will give only a brief overview of the code sets and is not intended for training of health-information-management professionals.

INTERNATIONAL CLASSIFICATION OF DISEASES The International Classification of Diseases (ICD-10), developed by the World Health Organization (World Health Organization, 2016) is the international standard diagnostic classification for health-management purposes, and clinical use. The ICD diagnoses are used to classify mortality and morbidity data from inpatient and outpatient records. They are used to classify diseases and other health problems recorded on many types of health- and vital-statistics records, including death certificates. In addition to enabling the storage and retrieval of diagnostic information for clinical, epidemiological, and quality purposes, these records also provide the basis for the compilation of national mortality and morbidity statistics used throughout the world.

The original intent of ICD was the creation of diagnostic and procedural coding for statistics and research. Since 1983, ICD has also been used for reimbursement. In October 2015, the United States transitioned to a US-specific version known as ICD-10-CM/PCS. ICD-10 contains two different code sets: *International Classification of Diseases, 10th Revision: Clinical Modification (ICD-10-CM)*, and *International Classification of Diseases, 10th Revision: Procedure Coding System (ICD-10-PCS)*.

ICD-10-CM replaces ICD-9-CM volumes 1 and 2. ICD-10-CM is the version used in the United States to identify diagnosis reimbursement codes in all healthcare settings. Two departments within the Department of Health and Human Services (DHHS)—the Centers for Medicare and Medicaid Services (CMS) and the National Center for Health Statistics (NCHS)—develop and maintain the ICD-10-CM official Guidelines for Coding and Reporting. The guidelines should be used as a companion document to the official version of ICD-10-CM. WHO requires that mortality data be submitted as ICD-10. ICD-10-CM contains more than 69,000 codes, whereas ICD-9 contained more than 14,000 codes. The official ICD-10-CM is currently comprised of the following three volumes:

Volume 1: Tabular List—contains an alphanumeric list of ICD-10 codes arranged by chapter

Volume 2: Instruction Manual—contains instructional materials as to how to use volumes 1 and 3

Volume 3: Alphabetical Index—contains alphabetical index to diseases, disorders, injuries, and other conditions found in volume 1.

ICD-10-PCS replaces ICD-9 Volume 3 Procedure Codes. ICD-10-PCS is used by facilities to report procedures in the hospital inpatient setting. The PCS codes are not required for outpatient settings.

The ICD classification system consists of a monohierarchy, which means that the concepts are classified by a disease header with the disease variations underneath. The monohierarchy provides a means of data collection against one point of view. The collection of the ICD data does not support the specificity necessary for clinical description of patients, research, quality analysis, and health-policy development. The structure of ICD-10-CM codes has increased from three to seven characters. Table 15-3 provides some examples of ICD-10-CM codes and one example of an ICD-10-PCS code.

CURRENT PROCEDURAL TERMINOLOGY CODES The American Medical Association (AMA)   is a classification system used for billing and reimbursement of outpatient procedures and interventions. CPT is the most widely accepted medical nomenclature used to report medical procedures and services under public and private health-insurance programs. CPT codes are used to code all medical procedures performed in healthcare, except for alternative medicine. CPT code sets are copyrighted by the AMA and are released once each year.

Table 15-3   Examples of ICD-10-CM Codes (Version: 2016)

ICD-10-CM	Diagnosis
P00-P96	Chapter XVI—Certain conditions originating in the perinatal period
P00-P04	Fetus and newborn affected by maternal factors and by complications of pregnancy, labor, and delivery
P02	Fetus and newborn affected by complications of placenta, cord, and membranes
P02.7	Fetus and newborn affected by chorioamnionitis
E00-E90	Chapter IV Endocrine, nutritional, and metabolic diseases
249-259.99	Diseases of other endocrine glands
E10	Type 1 diabetes mellitus
E10.1	Type 1 diabetes mellitus with ketoacidosis
ICD-10-PCS	**Procedure**
	Resection of Gallbladder, Percutaneous Endoscopic Approach
1 = Section	B = Medical and Surgical
2 = Body System	F = Hepatobiliary System and Pancreas
3 = Root Operation	0 = Resection (Cutting out or off, without replacement, all of a body part)
4 = Body Part	3 = Gallbladder
5 = Approach	Y = Percutaneous Endoscopic
6 = Device	Z = No Device
7 = Qualifier 3	Z = Qualifier

Source: From International Statistical Classification of Diseases and Related Health Problems 10th Revision (ICD-10)-WHO Version for; 2016. Published by WHO.

Table 15-4 Examples of CPT Codes

CPT Code	Description
Level 1: 80000–89398	Pathology and laboratory tests
Level 2: 81000–81099	Urinalysis procedures
81015	Urinalysis; microscopic only
81005	Urinalysis; qualitative or semiquantitative, except immunoassays
Level 2: 80100–80103	Drug testing
80100	Drug screen, qualitative; multiple drug classes, chromatographic method, each procedure

Source: From CPT Code.Published by AMA.

The CPT listings have divisions including: evaluation and management, anesthesia, surgery, radiology, pathology, and laboratory and medicine. Within these divisions are subsections that include section headings, subsections, categories and subcategories, guidelines, symbols, colons, semicolons, modifiers, appendices, indices, and examples. For example, CPT codes that fall under the pathology and laboratory category range in number from 80048 to 89356. If a urinalysis was done under this category, the code would range from 81000 to 81099, and is classified according to the specific type of urinalysis performed, for example: urinalysis microscopic. The range's specific details or procedures dictates the precise number. When trying to locate a surgery code (10000 to 69999), locate that section's heading and find the corresponding subheading to classify what type of procedure was conducted and where on the body it was performed. For example, if a procedure took place within the patient's integumentary system (10040 to 19499), and an excision was done on a benign lesion (11400 to 11471), detail should be coded regarding where the incision was made and how big it was. Table 15-4 displays some examples of CPT codes.

Clinical Terminologies

Clinical terminologies are those used for documenting patient care within an EHRS. This section will give a brief overview of two categories of clinical terminologies: multidisciplinary and nursing specific.

Most of the terminologies discussed here are listed as source vocabularies within the **Unified Medical Language System (UMLS)** developed by the National Library of Medicine (NLM). The UMLS is a large metathesaurus that contains more than a hundred source vocabularies (National Library of Medicine, 2016a). The NLM provides a web-based application to the UMLS with which users can do multiple types of searches, such as finding synonymous terms from two or more sources and the association between concepts (NLM, 2016b).

The American Nurses Association (ANA) recognizes terminologies appropriate for use by nursing (American Nurses Association, 2014). Terminologies must meet defined criteria for approval. The criteria specify that terminologies must be used to support nursing practice that reflects the nursing process. The nursing-process data elements include assessment, diagnosis, outcome identification (goal), planning, implementation (interventions), and evaluation. The terminologies have to contain concepts that are clear and unambiguous, with a unique identifier. The terminology developer should have outlined processes for maintenance and growth. The Nursing Management Minimum Data Set (NMMDS), Nursing Minimum Data Set (NMDS), and ABC are data sets approved by the ANA, but will not be discussed in this chapter. All of the approved terminologies are outlined in Table 15-5. The ANA-released a position statement supporting documentation using the

Table 15-5 ANA-Recognized Languages that Support Nursing Practice

Terminology	Website	Diagnosis/ Problem	Intervention	Outcome	Other
Alternative Billing Concepts (ABC Codes)	www.abccodes.com				Billing Codes
Clinical Care Classification (CCC)	www.sabacare.com	X	X	X	
International Classification of Nursing Practice (ICNP)	www.icn.ch/icnp.htm	X	X	X	Assessment
Logical Identifiers Names and Codes (LOINC)	http://loinc.org/			X	Assessment
North American Nursing Diagnosis International (NANDA-I)	www.nanda.org	X			
Nursing Interventions Classification (NIC)	www.nursing.uiowa.edu/cncce/nursing-interventions-classification-overview		X		
Nursing Outcomes Classification (NOC)	www.nursing.uiowa.edu/cncce/nursing-outcomes-classification-overview			X	
Nursing Management Minimum Data Set	www.nursing.umn.edu/ICNP/USANMMDS/home.html				Nursing Management Codes
Nursing Minimum Data Set	www.nursing.umn.edu/ICNP/				
Omaha System	www.con.ufl.edu/omaha	X	X	X	
Perioperative Nursing Data Set (PNDS)	www.aorn.org	X	X	X	
SNOMED CT	www.ihtsdo.org/SNOMED CT	X	X	X	

ANA-recognized terminologies, but for comparison across health systems and/or transmission, the ANA-recognized terminologies should be mapped to LOINC and SNOMED CT (American Nurses Association, 2015).

In 2015, the NLM developed a new web resource entitled *Nursing Resources for Standards and Interoperability* (Warren, Matney, Foster, Auld, & Roy, 2015). This resource provides detailed information about why particular standards are pertinent and necessary for use in nursing and nursing-care documentation. The new web page supports synonymous mappings between SNOMED CT, LOINC, and other ANA-recognized terminologies, thus providing a valuable resource for nurses.

The Office of the National Coordinator (ONC) identifies the best-available standard vocabularies, messaging structures, and implementation specifications for the healthcare industry, and outlines them in the Interoperability Standards Advisory (ISA) (Office of the National Coordinator for Health IT. 2015). The ISA functions as a roadmap to interoperability and includes standard-terminology specifications. The ISA is not a ruling in itself, but a reference, illustrating a single public list of the best-available standards and implementation specifications available for clinical health-information-interoperability needs. The most recent roadmap includes draft-terminology recommendations for nursing. The ISA endorses encoding data, collected by nurses, with LOINC and SNOMED CT.

Multidisciplinary Terminologies

SNOMED CLINICAL TERMS SNOMED Clinical Terms (SNOMED CT) is a globally recognized, controlled-healthcare vocabulary that provides a common language for electronic health applications. SNOMED CT enables a consistent way of capturing, sharing, and aggregating health data across specialties and sites of care. The use of SNOMED CT within EHRSs facilitates interoperable data collection, which can be analyzed and used in the implementation of evidence-based practice, decision-support rules, reporting of quality measures, and administrative billing.

SNOMED CT is in conformance with federal regulatory standards and the Consolidated Health Informatics Initiative (Department of Health and Human Services, 2005). In 2007, the College of American Pathologists transferred the SNOMED CT intellectual property to the International Health Terminology Standards Development Organization (IHTSDO) to support the development of an international effort to produce and enhance a global clinical terminology standard (IHTSDO, 2016). The IHTSDO has developed a set of principles that guide decision making for the SNOMED CT. The IHTSDO initially consisted of nine founding-country members; this number recently increased to over 20 member-countries. Each member country has a SNOMED CT release center responsible for managing concept requests and distributing SNOMED CT. SNOMED CT is continually updated to meet the needs of users around the world. Revisions to the international version of SNOMED CT are released twice a year, once at the end of January and again at the end of July. Each release includes the core of the terminology (concepts, descriptions, and relationships), together with works to support the implementation of SNOMED CT.

SNOMED CT updates are driven by users of the terminology, who can request new concepts and submit them through the IHTSDO. Examples include refinements to descriptions, remodeling of new concepts to place them into the correct hierarchy, or the addition of new concepts. Prior to a release, SNOMED CT undergoes a clinical-quality-review process to ensure that concepts have been defined accurately.

SNOMED CT is recognized by the ANA as one of the standardized terminologies for supporting nursing practice. It is a clinical terminology comprised of codes, concepts, and relationships used in recording and representing clinical information across the scope of healthcare. It is concept-based, meaning that each concept has a distinct definition with a unique code identifier. SNOMED CT consists of 19 top-level hierarchies: procedures (medical and surgical procedures, laboratory and radiology procedures, interventions, education, and management procedures), clinical findings (nursing diagnoses, disorders, diseases that are necessarily abnormal, and signs and symptoms also known as assessments), body structures, observable entity (questions being asked during an assessment), devices, substances, and medications.

SNOMED CT hierarchies are created through defining relationships linking one concept to another concept for the purpose of defining each concept down to its specific meaning. Defining concepts by using a parent-child relationship begins to build vertical hierarchies within SNOMED CT. Concepts lower in the hierarchy are more specific in meaning than those higher up in the hierarchy, creating multiple levels of granularity. Specifying the attributes (characteristics) of each relationship further defines a given concept's meaning by connecting all the necessary and sufficient relationships between concepts required to fully represent a given concept's definition. An example of how the concept of *ineffective breathing* is mapped within SNOMED CT is illustrated in Table 15-6.

SNOMED CT is used to document care by clinicians, specialists, and practice domains using an interdisciplinary approach. It is used to document patient care across all sites of care and healthcare facilities (acute care, home care, hospice care, spiritual health, long-term care, and healthcare-clinic visits, as well as community and public health). The documentation of assessments, flow sheets, care plans, task lists, order sets, education plans, problem lists, allergies and allergic reactions, task lists, and medication-administration records can be encoded to SNOMED CT.

Table 15-6   SNOMED CT Example: Ineffective Breathing

SNOMED CT: Ineffective breathing pattern (finding)
SNOMED Concept ID: 20573003
Is_A Clinical finding
Is_A Finding related to ability to perform breathing functions (finding)
Is_A Respiration alteration (finding)
Finding Site: Structure of respiratory system (body structure)
Interprets: Ability to perform breathing functions (observable entity)

Source: Copyright by SNOMED International.

SNOMED CT updates are driven by users of the terminology, who can request new concepts and submit them through the IHTSDO. Examples include refinements to descriptions, remodeling of new concepts to place them into the correct hierarchy, or the addition of new concepts. Prior to a release, SNOMED CT undergoes a clinical-quality-review process to ensure that concepts have been defined accurately.

In March 2010, a collaboration agreement was signed between the International Council of Nurses (ICN) and IHTSDO to establish a harmonization board with the objective of future integration between ICNP and SNOMED CT (eHealthNews, 2010).

LOGICAL OBSERVATION IDENTIFIERS NAMES AND CODES The Logical Observation Identifiers, Names, and Codes (LOINC) is a terminology that includes laboratory and clinical observations. The laboratory portion of the LOINC database contains the usual laboratory categories such as chemistry, hematology, and microbiology. The domain and scope of clinical LOINC is extremely broad. Some of the sections of terms include vital signs, obstetric measurements, clinical-assessment scales, outcomes from standardized-nursing terminologies, and research instruments (Matney et al., 2016a). LOINC is also used for document and section names (Hyun, 2006; Richesson & Chute, 2015).

Terminology content used to document nursing assessments are contained within clinical LOINC (Matney et al., 2016a; Matney, 2003). In 2002, LOINC was recognized by the ANA. The ANA determined that both laboratory and clinical LOINC are appropriate for use by nursing. Because of their breadth and the early focus on laboratory testing, nursing-assessment observations are not yet well represented.

LOINC provides identifiers and names for observations, not values. Each LOINC record corresponds to a single observation, measurement, or test result. The record includes the axis fields specified in Table 15-7.

Nursing Terminologies

CLINICAL CARE CLASSIFICATION The Clinical Care Classification (CCC) System is a nursing classification designed to document the six steps of the nursing process across the care continuum (Saba, 2012). It facilitates patient-care documentation at the point of care. CCC was developed in 1991 and was last revised in 2012. The CCC consists of two interconnected terminologies, the CCC of nursing diagnosis and outcomes and the CCC of nursing interventions. The two taxonomies are tools that support the documentation of nursing care. Both terminologies are classified by 21 care components that represent the functional, health, behavioral, physiological, and psychological patterns of a patient.

CCC nursing diagnoses consist of 182 diagnostic concepts classified into 59 major categories and 123 subcategories. Outcomes are assigned by expanding the nursing diagnosis concepts with one of three qualifiers: improved, stabilized, or deteriorated.

Table 15-7 LOINC Axes with Examples

Axis	Description of the Axis	Sample Values
Component (analyte)	The substance or entity measured, evaluated, or observed	Systolic blood pressure, pain onset, and sodium
Kind of property	The characteristic or attribute of the component measured, evaluated, or observed	Length, volume, time stamp, mass, ratio, number, and temperature
Time aspect	The interval of time over which the observation or measurement was made	Point in time, and over an 8-hour period
System	The system (context) or specimen type with which the observation was made	Urine, serum, fetus, patient (person), and family
Type of scale	The scale of measure	Quantitative (a true measurement), ordinal (a ranked set of options), nominal, or narrative
Type of method	The procedure used to make the measurement or observation. Method is the only axis that is optional and is only included when different methodologies would significantly change the interpretation of the result.	Patient reported, measured

CCC uses a five-character code to codify the terminology. Each code can be decomposed to determine the meaning. The syntax of the code categorization is as follows:

Code 1 = care component

Codes 2 and 3 = major category (followed by a decimal point)

Code 4 = one digit code for a subcategory (followed by a decimal point)

Code 5 = one of three expected outcomes, *or* one of four nursing intervention types.

CCC nursing interventions consist of 198 categories classified into 72 major categories and 126 subcategories that represent interventions, procedures, treatments, and activities. The interventions can be modified by one of four intervention types: (1) assess or monitor; (2) care, direct, or perform; (3) teach or instruct; or (4) manage or refer.

CCC is an open-source terminology with no license fees. The terminology tables can be freely downloaded from www.sabacare.com. CCC is copyrighted, and its use within an EHRS requires written permission.

CCC has mappings to SNOMED CT. CCC codes can be obtained from the CCC terminology developer. CCC outcomes are mapped to LOINC and are freely downloadable from the LOINC database.

INTERNATIONAL CLASSIFICATION OF NURSING PRACTICE The International Classification of Nursing Practice (ICNP) is a unified nursing language system developed by the ICN in Geneva, Switzerland (International Council of Nurses, 2015). ICN is responsible for ensuring that the content reflects the domain of nursing. ICNP Version 2.0 was released in 2009. ICNP is a compositional terminology for nursing practice that facilitates the development of, and the cross-mapping among, local terms and existing terminologies. ICNP has been implemented as both an interface (ICNP Catalogues) and reference terminology.

ICNP contains nursing phenomena (diagnoses), nursing actions, and nursing outcomes (International Council of Nursing, 2015). ICNP is represented using a seven-axis model. The ICNP has developed specific guidelines for using the seven-axis model to develop nursing diagnosis, outcome, and intervention statements. The seven axes and a short description of each are listed here:

- *Focus.* The problem area or concern. Examples could include, but not be limited to, self-care abilities, pain, or knowledge deficits.
- *Judgment.* The assignment of priority to the area of concern by the nurse.

- *Means.* The method by which an intervention to address the problem area or concern is accomplished. For example, the patient with mobility issues can use a cane, crutch or walker to enhance mobility.
- *Action.* The intentional process to accomplish an intervention. With the above mobility example, the action would be to teach the patient how to use the mobility aid.
- *Time.* The relevant period or duration of the problem area or concern, whether that might be upon admission, post-operatively, or discharge. The patient with mobility issues after an injury would require instruction on crutch-walking prior to discharge.
- *Location.* The anatomical or spatial designation for a problem area or concern. As an example, the location could designate where a patient experiences pain or that the patient was sent to the physical therapy department for rehabilitation after a right total-knee replacement.
- *Client.* The individual, family, or community recipient of focus and interventions.

ICNP DIAGNOSIS

- A term from the focus axis is required.
- A term from the judgment axis is required.
- Additional terms from the focus, judgment, and other axes are included as needed.

INTERNATIONAL CLASSIFICATION OF NURSING PRACTICE

- A term from the action axis is required.
- At least one target term is required. Target terms come from all of the other seven axes except for judgment.

ICN recognized early that the terminology would need to be organized so it could be used at the point of care (Coenen & Bartz, 2010). In an ongoing process, ICNP catalogues are developed by interested parties to address specific health concerns or healthcare needs. ICNP catalogues are designed to support clinical documentation in an EHRS. The first two catalogues published by ICN were "Partnering with Individuals and Families to Promote Adherence to Treatment" and "Palliative Care for Dignified Dying." More catalogues are in development and testing. These catalogues will generate more content that nurses can use to document care.

NORTH AMERICAN NURSING DIAGNOSIS INTERNATIONAL North American Nursing Diagnosis International (NANDA-I) dates back to 1970 and was the first terminology to be recognized by the ANA (Gordon, 1994). A nursing diagnosis is a clinical judgment about individual, family, or community experiences and responses to actual or potential health problems and life processes.

NANDA-I diagnoses are used to identify human responses to health promotion, risk, and disease (Herdman, & Kamitsuru, 2014). Each nursing diagnosis has a description, a definition, and defining characteristics. The defining characteristics are manifestations, signs, and symptoms that assist the nurse in determining the correct diagnosis to assign.

NANDA-I is classified into 13 domains. Within each domain are two or more classes. The domains and classes have formal definitions. The following is a list of the domains. For each domain, up to two examples of the classes are shown:

Domain 1: Health Promotion—Health Awareness and Health Management

Domain 2: Nutrition—Ingestion and Digestion

Domain 3: Elimination/Exchange—Urinary Function and Gastrointestinal Function

Domain 4: Activity/Rest—Sleep and Rest

Domain 5: Perception/Cognition—Attention and Orientation

Domain 6: Self-Perception—Self-Concept and Body Image

Domain 7: Role Relationship—Caregiving Roles and Role Performance

Domain 8: Sexuality—Sexual Identity and Sexual Function

Domain 9: Coping/Stress Tolerance—Post-Trauma Responses and Coping Responses

Domain 10: Life Principles—Values and Beliefs

Domain 11: Safety/Protection—Infection and Physical Injury

Domain 12: Comfort—Physical Comfort and Environmental Comfort

Domain 13: Growth/Development—Growth

The first NANDA-I taxonomy was an alphabetical listing of the nursing diagnosis. In 2001, NANDA-I released NANDA-I Taxonomy II in which the nursing diagnoses were formatted using a multiaxial structure. The seven axes of the taxonomy are dimensions of the human response (Herdman, 2011). Table 15-8 depicts the NANDA-I axes with examples.

NANDA-I is used to document nursing diagnoses within all settings and across the care continuum. The coding system can be used within an EHRS. NANDA-I has been linked to the NIC interventions and NOC outcomes. The NANDA-I coding system can be used within an EHRS either by mapping the nursing problems that nurses document directly, or by mapping to the NANDA-I, NIC, and NOC linkages. The linkages can be loaded into an EHRS and can be used together to document the elements of the nursing process within the care plan.

NURSING INTERVENTIONS CLASSIFICATION The Nursing Interventions Classification (NIC) is a standardized classification of interventions that describes the activities that nurses perform. NIC is used in all care settings. An intervention is described as, "any treatment, based upon clinical judgment and knowledge that a nurse performs to enhance patient/client outcomes" (The University of Iowa, 2016a). The current NIC edition has 542 interventions (Butcher, Bulechek, McCloskey Dochterman, & Wagner, 2013). The interventions are grouped together by 30 classes and 7 domains. Each intervention includes a label name, a definition, a unique code, and associated nursing activities. There are more than 1,200 activities. Below is a list of the NIC domains:

Domain 1: Physiological: Basic

Domain 2: Physiological: Complex

Domain 3: Behavioral

Domain 4: Safety

Table 15-8 NANDA-I Axes with Examples

Axis	Description of the Axis	Sample Values
Axis 1: The diagnostic concept	The principle element or root of the diagnostic statement. May consist of one or more nouns.	Activity intolerance Fatigue Fear Pain Sorrow
Axis 2: Time	Duration of a period or interval.	Acute, chronic, short-term, long-term
Axis 3: Unit of care	Person or population for which the nursing diagnosis is determined.	Individual, family, community
Axis 4: Age	Physical development stage.	Fetus, adolescent, young adult, old, old adult
Axis 5: Health status	State of health or illness.	Wellness, actual, risk for
Axis 6: Descriptor	A modifier that limits or defines the nursing diagnosis meaning.	Ability, decrease, delayed, excessive, impaired
Axis 7: Topology	Parts or regions of the body.	Auditory, bowel, urinary, skin

Domain 5: Family

Domain 6: Health System

Domain 7: Community

The NIC coding system can be used within an EHRS either by mapping the nursing interventions and activities that nurses perform directly, or by mapping to the NANDA-I, NIC, and NOC linkages. The linkages can be loaded into an EHRS. They were developed to be used together to document the elements of the nursing process within the care plan.

NURSING OUTCOMES CLASSIFICATION The Nursing Outcomes Classification (NOC) is a classification system that describes patient outcomes sensitive to nursing interventions. The NOC is a system to evaluate the effects of nursing care as a part of healthcare. NOC consists of outcomes for individual patients, families, and communities. An outcome is, "a measurable individual, family, or community state, behavior, or perception that is measured along a continuum and is responsive to nursing interventions" (The University of Iowa, 2016b). NOC can be used across all clinical settings and specialties. The NOC classification is structured using three levels: domains, classes, and outcomes. The outcomes are organized into 31 classes and 7 domains (Moorhead, Johnson, Maas, & Swanson, 2013). Each outcome concept consists of a definition, a measurement scale, a list of associated indicators, and supporting references. The following is a list of the NOC domains:

Domain 1: Functional Health

Domain 2: Physiological Health

Domain 3: Psychosocial Health

Domain 4: Health Knowledge and Behavior

Domain 5: Perceived Health

Domain 6: Family Health

Domain 7: Community Health.

Each outcome, associated indicators, and measurement scale(s) are coded for use in EHRSs.

The NOC coding system can be used within an EHRS either by mapping the nursing outcomes directly, or by mapping to the NANDA-I, NIC, and NOC linkages. The linkages can be loaded into an EHRS. They were developed to be used together to document the elements of the nursing process within the care plan.

THE OMAHA SYSTEM The Omaha System is a taxonomy that provides a framework for integrating and sharing clinical data. As noted by Martin (2005), and still true today, it is widely used in settings such as home care, hospice, public health, school health, and prisons. ANA initially recognized the Omaha System in 1992 as a standardized terminology to support nursing practice.

The Omaha System consists of three relational components: an assessment component (problem classification scheme), an intervention component (intervention scheme), and an outcomes component (problem rating scale for outcomes) (Topaz, Golfenshtein, & Bowles, 2014). The three components are designed to be used together and create a comprehensive problem-solving model for practice, education, and research. Concepts from the components can be assigned to an individual, family or group, or community (Correll & Martin, 2009). Table 15-9 provides an overview of the Omaha System.

PERIOPERATIVE NURSING DATA SET The Perioperative Nursing Data Set (PNDS) language, developed by the Association of periOperative Registered Nurses (AORN), is a standardized perioperative-nursing vocabulary that provides nurses with a clear, precise, and universal language for clinical problems and surgical treatments. PNDS provides wording

Table 15-9 Omaha System Overview

Component	Terms	Purpose
Problem Classification Scheme	• Four domains • Forty-two problems • Two sets of modifiers • Clusters of problem-specific signs or symptoms	Organize assessment (needs and strengths) for individuals, families, and communities
Intervention Scheme	• Four categories • Seventy-five targets and one "other" • Client-specific information	Organize multidisciplinary practitioners' care plans and the services they deliver
Problem Rating Scale for Outcomes	• Three concepts • Five-point Likert-type scale	Individual, family, and community

A full description of the components is available online at www.omahasystem.org.

and definitions for nursing problems, interventions, and outcomes, thus, furnishing clinicians with the same terms to describe patient care in the perioperative setting. The AORN's initial goal was to develop a unified language for nursing care that could be systematically quantified, coded, and easily captured in a computerized format in the perioperative setting (Morton, Petersen, Chard, & Kleiner, 2013). The PNDS provides a systematic approach to define and recognize the contributions of the perioperative nurse in healthcare.

The second edition of the *Perioperative Nursing Data Set* (PNDS) was superseded by the third edition (PNDS 3) in 2011 and the PNDS fourth edition (PNDS 4) in 2016. The PNDS 4 terminology is only distributed through AORN and AORN Syntegrity licensed vendors (Hunt, Howard, Hill, & Hillanbrand, 2015). The PNDS language is mapped to SNOMED CT, meaning that terms in the PNDS correlate with the terms and coding in SNOMED CT, and allow the PNDS to provide data that can be exchanged (Maxwell-Downing, 2013).

The PNDS vocabulary is structured using four domains. Three of the four domains are patient-centric and the other represents the perioperative settings administrative or performance concepts that affect patient care. Each domain has three levels: patient outcomes or performance measures, actual or potential nursing problems or measurement/analytical reporting, and nursing interventions or standardized data elements. Each patient-outcome concept consists of a unique identifier, a definition, an interpretive statement, and a domain. Below is a list of the PNDS domains:

Domain 1–Safety: 0-199
Domain 2–Physiological Response: 200-499
Domain 3A–Behavioral Responses-Individual & Family Knowledge: 500-699
Domain 3B–Behavioral Responses-Individual & Family Rights/Ethics
& Competency: 700-899
Domain 4–Health System: 900-1100
Interventions:
      Assessment–**A.xx** (e.g., A.30)
      Implementation–**Im.xx** (e.g., Im.240)
      Evaluation–**E.xx** (e.g., E.550)
Outcomes–O.xx
PNDS Nursing Problems–NP.xx (SNOMED CT Nursing Problem List)

SOURCE: Janice Kelly.

In summary, this section has described the terminologies used within an EHRS. The ANA-recognized nursing classifications codify data used during the nursing process such as assessments, nurse-sensitive problems, interventions, and outcomes. One or more terminologies can be used for nursing documentation. The next section will illustrate a use case showing how the nursing terminologies can be used for documenting nursing care.

Storyboard Illustrating Terminology Use

The following storyboard illustrates the use of SNOMED CT, LOINC, CCC, ICNP, NANDA, NIC, and NOC. Examples show encoding concepts used in the nursing process, and not everything can be encoded within the storyboard (e.g., gender = male):

> Joe is a 24-year-old male paraplegic admitted to an inpatient unit from his home with right lower-lobe pneumonia. During his admission assessment, the nurse notes that he has no sensation from the shoulders down. He is confined to a wheelchair and requires two-person assistance with movement. He could move himself with his upper body before this illness. His oxygen saturation is 85% on room air by pulse oxymetry. Evaluation of his vitals shows a temperature of 101°F. His skin is moist and clammy.

ASSESSMENT The process of nursing assessment includes items such as vital signs, physiological signs, and patient symptoms within the realm of nursing practice (Matney et al., 2016b). Assessments are observations documented as a name-value or question-and-answer pair. Assessment name-value pairs depicted in the storyboard are oxygen saturation = 85%, temperature = 101°F, skin type = moist and clammy, and skin temperature = cold. SNOMED CT and LOINC both include content that supports the encoding of point of-care assessments. Table 15-10 illustrates how the assessments can be encoded.

Table 15-10 Nursing Assessment Coding Examples

Assessment Measure	SNOMED CT	LOINC	Assessment Value
Oxygen saturation	**Fully Specified Name:** Hemoglobin saturation with oxygen (observable entity) **Concept Code:** 103228002 **Defined as:** Is A: hematologic function	**Name:** Oxygen saturation in capillary blood **Code:** 2709-4 **Fully Specified Name:** Oxygen saturation:MFr:PT:BldC:QN:: Component = Oxygen Property = Mass fraction Time = Point in time System = Blood mixed venous Scale = Quantitative	**Numeric value = 85** **Units of measure = Percent**
Temperature	**Fully Specified Name:** Body temperature (observable entity) **Concept Code:** 386725007 **Defined as:** Is A: body temperature measure Is A: vital signs	**Name:** Body temperature **Code:** 8310-5 **Fully Specified Name:** Body Temperature:Temp:PT: ^Patient:QN:: Component = Body temperature Property = Temperature Time = Point in time System = Patient Scale = Quantitative	**Numeric value = 85** **Units of measure = Degrees Fahrenheit**
Skin moisture	**Fully Specified Name:** Moistness of skin (observable entity) **Concept Code:** 364532007 **Defined as:** Is A: skin observable	**Name:** Moisture of Skin **Code:** 39129-2 **Fully Specified Name:** Moisture:Type:PT:Skin:Nom:: Component = Moisture Property = Type Time = Point in time System = Skin Scale = Nominal	**Coded Value** **SNOMED CT Code = Fully Specified Name:** Clammy skin (finding) **Concept Code:** 102598000 **Defined as:** Is A: Finding of moistness of skin

NURSING DIAGNOSIS/PROBLEM AND ICD-10 CODING After the patient has been assessed, a nursing diagnosis or problem is determined. Even though Joe is a paraplegic, he has impaired mobility because he could move himself with his upper body before his pneumonia. Other nursing diagnoses for Joe include impaired gas exchange and hypothermia. Table 15-11 illustrates NANDA, ICNP, and CCC coding examples. It should also be noted that Omaha System, PNDS, and SNOMED CT contain nursing diagnoses.

Joe will be assigned an ICD-10-CM billing code for his pneumonia by the medical coders of the hospital after discharge. The ICD-10-CM code for "Pneumonia, organism unspecified" is "J18.9."

NURSING INTERVENTIONS Nursing interventions are acts planned by the nurse and performed by the nurse for the client, by the client, or by the nurse and client acting together. Nursing interventions include acts such as assess, evaluate, educate, and monitor. Using the example of Joe, the interventions on his care plan included: assist with transfer, oxygen therapy, and monitor temperature. Table 15-12 shows NIC, ICNP, and CCC examples. It should also be noted that the Omaha System, PNDS, and SNOMED CT contain nursing interventions.

GOALS AND POTENTIAL NURSING OUTCOMES A goal is the desired outcome for the future. It is a scheduled observation in the future. Based on Joe's diagnoses, the nurse sets measurable goals that include improved mobility, improved gas exchange, and normothermia. The assessment data, diagnoses, and goals are written in the care plan for other care providers to access. When the goal is evaluated and given an outcome-measurement value, such as improved, it is then considered an outcome. Table 15-13 shows NOC, ICNP, and CCC examples. It should also be noted that the Omaha System, PNDS, and SNOMED CT contain nursing outcomes.

Benefits of Implementing Standardized Terminologies

Implementing standardized terminology has many benefits to multiple beneficiaries. Beneficiaries include the patient, the provider, the organization, and the healthcare industry in general. Using standardized terminologies ensures compliance with standards coming forth

Table 15-11 Nursing Diagnosis/Problem Coding Examples

Diagnosis/Problem	NANDA-I	ICNP	CCC
Impaired mobility	Impaired physical mobility **Axes:** **The diagnostic concept** = Physical mobility **Descriptor** = Impaired	Impaired mobility **Concept Code:** 10001219 **Axes:** **Focus** = Ability to mobilize **Judgment** = Impaired	Physical mobility impairment **Concept Code:** A01.5 **Concept Categorization:** Component 'A' = Activity Major category '01' = Alteration
Impaired gas exchange	Impaired gas exchange **Axes:** **The diagnostic concept** = Gas exchange **Descriptor** = Impaired **Defining Characteristic:** Hypoxia	Impaired gas exchange **Concept Code:** 10001177 **Axes:** **Focus** = Gaseous exchange **Judgment** = Impaired	Gas exchange Impairment **Concept Code:** L26.3 **Concept Categorization:** Component 'L' = Respiratory **Major Category** '26' = Alteration
Hyperthermia	Hyperthermia **Axes:** **The diagnostic concept** = **Descriptor** = **Defining Characteristic:** Body temp above normal range	Hyperthermia **Concept Code:** 10000757 **Axes:** **Focus** = Hyperthermia **Judgment** = Negative	Hyperthermia **Concept Code:** K25.2 **Concept Categorization:** Component 'K' = Physical regulation Major category '25' = Alteration

TABLE 15-12 Nursing Intervention Coding Examples

Nursing Intervention	NIC	ICNP	CCC
Assist with transfers	Transfer **Domain:** Physiological domain: Basic **Class:** Immobility management **Definition:** Moving a patient from one location to another	Transferring act **Concept Code:** 10020030 **Axes:** **Action:** Transferring **Description:** Positioning: Moving somebody or something from one place to another	Transfer care **Concept Code:** A03.3 **Categorization:** **Component:** 'A' = Activity **Concept:** '03.3' = Transfer care **Definition:** Actions performed to assist in moving from one place to another
Oxygen therapy	Oxygen therapy **Domain:** Physiological domain: Complex **Class:** Respiratory management **Definition:** Administration of oxygen and monitoring of its effectiveness	Oxygen therapy **Concept Code:** 10013921 **Axes:** **Action:** Therapy **Description:** Therapy	Oxygen therapy care **Concept Code:** L.35 **Categorization:** **Component:** 'L' = Respiratory **Concept:** 35 Oxygen therapy care **Definition:** Actions performed to support the administration of oxygen treatment
Monitor temperature	Temperature Regulation: Fever treatment **Domain:** Physiological domain: Complex **Class:** Thermoregulation **Definition:** Attaining and/or maintaining body temperature within normal range	Monitoring body temperature **Concept Code:** 10012165 **Axes:** **Focus:** Body temperature **Action** = Monitoring **Description:** Monitoring	Temperature **Concept Code:** K33.2 **Categorization:** **Component:** 'K' = Physical regulation **Concept:** '33.2' = Temperature **Definition:** Actions performed to measure body temperature

TABLE 15-13 Nursing Goal/Potential Outcome Coding Examples

Nursing Goal/Outcome	NOC	ICNP	CCC
Improved mobility	Immobility consequences: Physiological **Domain:** Functional health **Class:** Mobility **Definition:** Severity of compromise in physiological functioning due to impaired physical mobility	Effective mobility **Concept Code:** 10028461 **Axes:** **Focus** = Ability to mobilize **Judgment** = Positive	Physical mobility impairment improved **Concept Code:** A01.5.1 **Concept Categorization:** Improved = Fifth digit. '1' added to the diagnosis
Improved gas exchange	Respiratory status: Gas exchange **Domain:** Physiologic health **Class:** Cardiopulmonary **Definition:** Alveolar exchange of carbon dioxide and oxygen to maintain arterial blood gas exchange	Effective gas exchange **Concept Code:** 10027993 **Axes:** **Focus** = Gaseous exchange **Judgment** = Positive	Gas exchange impairment improved **Concept Code:** L26.3.1 **Concept Categorization:** Improved = Fifth digit. '1' added to the diagnosis
Normothermia	Thermoregulation: Vital sign status **Domain:** Physiologic health **Class:** Metabolic regulation **Definition:** Balance among heat production, heat gain, and heat loss	Thermoregulation **Concept Code:** 10014973 **Axes:** **Focus** = Thermoregulation **Judgment** = Positive	Hyperthermia improved **Concept Code:** K25.2.1 **Concept Categorization:** Improved = Fifth digit. "1" added to the diagnosis

for meaningful use, quality measures, and interoperability. Terminology facilitates the monitoring of trends and problems in the health of populations, developing clinical-decision support, and expanding our knowledge of diseases, treatments, and outcomes through research and clinical data mining.

Patient-Specific Benefits

Patient-care benefits include decreased costs, increased quality across the continuum of care, improved outcomes, and improved safety. Standard terminologies provide a means of sharing chart data electronically between other departments, facilities, and settings. The use of collected interoperable data can be analyzed to identify ways to reduce errors of omission via reminders and alerts (clinical-decision support), which are developed within an EHRS. Costs can be reduced by eliminating redundant testing and diagnostic investigation. Value is derived by maintaining continuity of care. With standardized clinical terminology, patient data will be available across the full spectrum of healthcare settings: Family history, medications, allergies, diseases, treatments, and interventions can be coded and shared among clinicians, sites of care, and even across national and international geographic boundaries, which improves communication, resulting in improved patient safety and outcomes. The ability to track a patient's health maintenance, follow-up activity, compliance, and progress will provide important information regarding quality of care outcomes.

Provider and Nursing Benefits

Providers and nurses will benefit by having access to complete data along the continuum of care. Healthcare organizations around the world are working to integrate EHRSs. Using structured vocabularies within and between systems will provide access to complete and accurate healthcare data. Lack of complete and accurate data is currently a frustration to providers who want to give the best patient care. This frustration occurs when important clinical information for the patient is unavailable at the point of care. These systems will provide access to healthcare records that will gain better control over healthcare information quickly, and when the information is needed most—at the point of care.

Nurses will benefit from using a standardized nursing language due to enhanced efficiency, accuracy, and effectiveness, resulting in a significant improvement in patient care. McCormick et al. (2015) described three examples in which the implementation of a standardized nursing terminology made a significant impact on patient outcomes. The study reported how standardized nursing terminology is structured and incorporated into the electronic nursing-documentation tools.

Organizational Benefits

The organization can benefit by cost savings, decision-support rules, outcomes measurement, and the ability to use the data for data mining. Using standardized-clinical terminology allows sharing of accurate health information across departments and facilities. The necessity of streamlining care processes to capture efficient gains that require fewer provider and staff hours devoted to administrative care will result in reduced hospital costs. Organizations that implement EHRSs using standard terminologies will observe benefits, such as the ability to measure an improvement in patient-care outcomes and cost efficiency. For example, healthcare organizations will experience a reduction in transcription errors and reduced coding and billing errors, resulting in reduced healthcare-claim denials. The ability to track a patient's health maintenance, follow-up activity, compliance, and progress will provide important information regarding the quality of patient-care outcomes.

Standardized terminologies support the development of **decision-support software (DSS)**. Decision support is the alerts and reminders used within an EHRS. The ability to collect codified data provides vital information that can be used for decision support (Lopez, Febretti, Stifter, Johnson, Wilkie, & Keenan, 2017). Clinical decision-support software is highly dependent on clinical information to function. To be useful, the clinical information must contain sufficient detail with respect to the right variables, the right wording and codes, and the right information modeling, and must, thus, be structured in a way that the decision-support software can use. DSS is used to prevent negative outcomes and support positive outcomes of patient care.

Documentation of healthcare using a standardized terminology is vital to support data mining. Data mining is the process of analyzing healthcare data from different perspectives and summarizing it into useful information that can be used to improve patient safety and quality of care and cut costs. It is becoming an important tool to transform data into information. Data mining is a key component in the analysis of workflow in complex healthcare organizations. It is also used for research (Salanterä, 2015). The data-mining process is carried out by the collection of standardized data with their associated codes from EHRSs. Analyzed results from data mining can identify patterns or trends in patient care and outcomes. The use of data mining by organizations can provide analysis for the identification of important questions that are directly related to increased errors, causing a reduction in patient safety and resulting in high healthcare costs. For example, a hospital organization may want to analyze questions, such as how many patients are at risk for falls and how many actually fall while in the hospital resulting in injury. The data collected and mined for these important questions can provide important information regarding patient falls and identify an improvement in the interventions provided for patients who are at risk for falls, and education that can lead to a reduction in the occurrence of falls.

National Healthcare Reporting Requirements

The Health Information Technology for Economic and Clinical Health (HITECH) Act seeks to improve American healthcare delivery and patient care through the adoption of interoperable EHRSs. The provisions of the HITECH Act are specifically designed to work together to provide the necessary assistance and technical support to providers, enable coordination and alignment within and among states, establish connectivity to the public health community in case of emergencies, and ensure that the workforce is properly trained and equipped to be meaningful users of EHRs (Health Information Technology, 2015).

Medicare is leading several eHealth initiatives to facilitate the triple goals of improving the health of populations, reducing the cost of healthcare, and improving the quality of care. CMS is collaborating with public agencies and private organizations, including the National Quality Forum (NQF), The Joint Commission, the National Committee for Quality Assurance, and the Agency for Health Care Research and Quality, to improve the quality of care (Centers for Medicare and Medicaid Services, 2013). The use of standardized terminology is mandatory for data collection and reporting of established quality measures for CMS-eligible hospitals and physicians (Centers for Medicare and Medicaid Services, 2014). For example, smoking status and venous-thrombosis prophylaxis are required to be tracked and collected. Also, the Health IT Standards Committee has established that hospitals are required to maintain an active-problem list mapped to SNOMED CT (Centers for Medicare and Medicaid Services, 2014). HL7 is a standards-development organization (SDO) accredited by the American National Standards Institute (ANSI) and dedicated to providing a comprehensive framework and related standards for the exchange, integration, sharing, and retrieval of electronic health information (Health Level Seven, 2016a). Healthcare organizations are required to send HL7-formatted messages containing patient demographic and clinical data. Messages sent containing laboratory-test names and results are required to be sent using

LOINC codes. Messages sent containing allergies should use SNOMED CT and RxNorm, a standardized nomenclature for clinical drugs and drug-delivery devices, developed by the NLM (Health Information Technology, 2009). In summary, to meet the CMS incentives, as well as provide safer patient care with improved quality, the implementation of standardized terminology is required.

Issues and Concerns

It is not easy to use standardized terminology within systems. Rector (1999), in his foundational article, described why "terminology is hard"; the issues he described still stand true today. He discussed challenges related to the implementation and maintenance of standardized terminologies, and we will address three high-level issues next in this chapter. First, there are numerous systems in use today with locally defined concepts; these will need to be mapped or linked to standardized terminology. Second, determining which terminology or terminologies to use is still a challenge. Third, data entry, presentation, and retrieval for clinical tasks must be considered. The mandate for the use of standardized terminologies in EHRSs for meaningful use has increased the need for systems to use standardized terminologies. Many systems in use today, both home grown and vended, have been created without using standard terminologies. The applications will have to be rewritten to use standardized terminologies. Methods will need to be developed to convert stored data, or retrieve data from the old system, so that patients' data will not be lost. Developers will need to determine how terminologies will be maintained and updated when new versions are released.

Specific terminologies have been mandated for laboratory and clinical systems, but the only nursing mandate is that SNOMED CT be used to message nursing data between systems. This causes two challenges: First, nurses need to determine which nursing terminologies they want to use to support the nursing process. Second, the terminology they choose will have to include a mapping to SNOMED CT to send patient data to other systems, such as a nursing home.

Finally, interface terms and synonyms for data entry, presentation, and retrieval for clinical tasks must be locally developed. Clinicians use different terms for the same concept across specialties and even between nursing units and settings. For example, a pediatrician or advanced nurse practitioner in an office setting will want to know that a newborn experienced transient tachypnea of the newborn. The screen display should specify this phrase for them, but providers in the NICU would rather see this information as TTN. Both of these are synonyms of the same concept and should be created based on context of use. The terms for medical and common items are different from country to country. For example, the American word, diaper, is called a nappy in the United Kingdom. Operational resources will be required for the development of the synonyms.

Future Directions

HIT allows comprehensive management of clinical information and its secure exchange between healthcare providers. Broad use of HIT has the potential to improve quality, prevent healthcare errors, increase administrative efficiencies, decrease paperwork, expand access to affordable care, and improve population and community health. The HITECH Act of 2009 sets forth a plan for the advancement of the Meaningful Use of HIT to improve the quality of care and to establish the foundation of the US health reform. The Office of the National Coordinator for Health Information Technology (ONCHIT) is at the forefront of the administration's

HIT efforts and is a source that supports the adoption of HIT and the promotion of a nation-wide health-information exchange to improve healthcare (Health Information Technology, 2015). To meet the standards defined by the HITECH Act, an EHRS will need to provide complete, accurate, and searchable health information available at the point of diagnosis and care, permitting more informed decision making to enhance the quality and reliability of the healthcare delivery. Other HITECH Act requirements needed to meet the standards include the need to develop a more efficient and convenient functionality, without waiting for the exchange of records or requiring unnecessary or repetitive tests or procedures. EHRSs are required in order to support reduction in adverse events through a stronger understanding of a patient's health history and potential for drug-drug interactions, providing an improvement in patient safety. Finally, healthcare information systems are required to support more efficient administrative duties, allowing for more interactions with, and the transfer of information to, patients, caregivers, clinical-case managers, and the monitoring of patient care.

To have good semantic interoperability, patient data needs to be encoded using standard terminologies and structures using pre-defined syntax (Matney, Dolin, Buhl, & Sheide, 2016b). Structured data facilitates computer processing by making data identifiable for tracking, trending-decision support, quality measures, data mining, and analytics (Dolin & Alschuler, 2011). The C-CDA (mentioned previously) and an emerging HL7 standard, called Fast Health Interoperability Resources (FHIR), are two examples of structured data syntax. CDA defines reusable patterns, called templates, using extensible mark-up language (XML) and standard terminologies (Dolin, Alschuler, & Boyer, 2006). Resources simulate paper forms by replicating different types of clinical and administrative information, and are the most important parts of the FHIR specification (Health Level Seven, 2016b). The FHIR resource specification defines a generic form template for types of clinical information such as observations, health conditions, and procedures.

Significant advances in the development and adoption of clinical terminologies and terminology standards has been illustrated in this chapter. In the last decade, and with the requirement to build EHRSs that meet the 2009 Meaningful Use criteria, the use of coded data has expanded to include pay for performance initiatives, care coordination, patient-safety monitoring, and public-health surveillance. Many benefits have yet to be realized from point of care to research and the development of evidence-based practice. There are still hurdles that need to be jumped in order for health-information systems to fully use terminologies. We will know we have succeeded when clinical terminologies are used and reused to capture healthcare data in a standardized format that has global meaning, and can be applied at both the individual and aggregate levels.

Summary

- Standardized terminologies have been developed for use within electronic health record systems (EHRS) as a means to ensure accurate, consistent meaning of data that is collected and shared across the healthcare-delivery system.
- The implementation of standardized terminology within an EHRS is essential for healthcare organizations to meet the criteria of Meaningful Use.
- Concept codes, used to designate concepts in a computer system, facilitate the development of evidence-based practice, decision support, and reporting.
- Clinical terminology enables the capture of data at the level of detail necessary for patient care documentation. Clinical terminologies consist of concepts that support diagnostic studies, history, physical examinations, visit notes, ancillary-department information, nursing notes, assessments, flow sheets, vital signs, and outcome measures.

- Standardization in nursing documentation supports research across settings on patient outcomes and interoperability.
- Healthcare encounters are coded for billing by code sets mandated by the Health Insurance Portability and Accountability Act (HIPAA). HIPAA mandates that all electronic transactions include only HIPAA-compliant codes. These include the ICD, CPT codes, and the ABC.
- Reference terminology supports data aggregation, analysis, and retrieval. Interface terminology represents what clinicians see on the screen.
- The American Nurses Association (ANA) Committee for Nursing Practice Information Infrastructure (CNPII) recognizes terminologies appropriate for use by nursing.
- Nursing terminologies include:
  - Clinical Care Classification (CCC)
  - International Classification of Nursing Practice (ICNP)
  - North American Nursing Diagnosis International (NANDA-I)
  - Nursing Interventions Classification (NIC)
  - Nursing Outcomes Classification (NOC)
  - The Omaha System
  - Perioperative Nursing Data Set (PNDS)
- Standardized-terminology beneficiaries include the patient, the provider, the organization, and the healthcare industry. The use of standardized terminologies provides access to complete and accurate healthcare data and ensures compliance with standards coming forth for Meaningful Use, quality measures, and interoperability.
- Documentation of healthcare using a standardized terminology supports data mining, a process of analyzing healthcare data from different perspectives, and summarizing it into useful information that can be used to improve patient safety and quality of care, as well as cut costs.
- Issues associated with the implementation of standardized terminology within systems include mapping considerations, determination of the most suitable terminologies, and retrofitting standardized terminologies into existing systems.
- Multidisciplinary terminologies include SNOMED CT, a comprehensive clinical terminology covering nursing, medicine, and allied health, and the Logical Observation Identifiers, Names, and Codes (LOINC), a terminology that includes laboratory and clinical observations.

Case Study

As the only informatics nurse at your small community hospital, your chief nursing officer heavily relies upon you to translate major developments in policy and reimbursement that have direct implications for the department and facility. How would you go about explaining the relationship between standardized terminologies and financial rewards related to Meaningful Use?

About the Author

Susan Matney, PhD, RN-C, FAAN is a Senior Medical Informaticist, Intermountain Healthcare, Murray, Utah. She develops clinical-information models bound to standard terminologies. She has represented Intermountain at international and national conferences and organizations, including SNOMED Clinical Terminology (SNOMED CT), Health Level 7

(HL7), Logical Observation Identifiers Names and Codes (LOINC), and American Academy of Nursing (ANA). She chairs the LOINC nursing subcommittee, is current vocabulary facilitator of the HL7 CIMI Working Group, and was the past chair of the SNOMED CT nursing special interest group.

References

American Nurses Association (ANA). (2014). *ANA recognized terminologies that support nursing practice.* Retrieved from www.nursingworld.org/MainMenuCategories/Tools/Recognized-Nursing-Practice-Terminologies.pdf.

American Nurses Association (ANA). (2015). *Inclusion of recognized terminologies within EHRs and other health information technology solutions.* Retrieved from www.nursingworld.org/MainMenuCategories/Policy-Advocacy/Positionsand-Resolutions/ANAPositionStatements/Position-Statements-Alphabetically/Inclusion-of-Recognized-Terminologies-within-EHRs.html

Butcher, H. K., Bulechek, G. M., McCloskey Dochterman, J. M., & Wagner, C. (2013). *Nursing intervention classification* (6th ed.). St. Louis, MO: Mosby/Elsevier.

Centers for Medicare and Medicaid Services (CMS). (2013). *ICD-10 and CMS eHealth: What's the connection?.* Retrieved from www.cms.gov/Medicare/Coding/ICD10/Downloads/ICD-10andCMSeHealth-WhatstheConnection_071813remediated%5B1%5D.pdf

Centers for Medicare and Medicaid Services (CMS). (2014). *CMS implementation guide for quality reporting document architecture category I and III?* Retrieved from www.cms.gov/regulations-and-guidance/legislation/ehrincentiveprograms/downloads/qrda_ep_hqr_guide_2015.pdf

Cimino, J. J. (1998). Desiderata for controlled medical vocabularies in the twenty-first century. *Methods of Information in Medicine, 37*(4–5), 394-403.

Coenen, A., & Bartz, C. (2010). ICNP: Nursing terminology to improve healthcare worldwide. In C. A. Weaver, C. Delaney, P. Weber, & R. L. Carr (Eds.), *Nursing and informatics for the 21st century: An international look at practice, education and EHR trends* (2nd ed., pp. 207–218), Chicago, IL: Healthcare Information and Management Systems Society.

Correll, P. J., & Martin, K. S. (2009). The Omaha system helps a public health nursing organization find its voice. *Computer, Informatics, Nursing, 27*(1), 12–16.

de Keizer, N. F., Abu-Hanna, A., & Zwetslook-Schonk, J. H. M. (2000). Understanding terminological systems I: Terminology and typology. *Methods of Information in Medicine, 39,* 16–21.

Department of Health and Human Services. (2005). Consolidated health informatics (CHI) initiative; health care and vocabulary standards for use in federal health information technology systems. *Federal Register.* Retrieved from www.gpo.gov/fdsys/pkg/FR-2005-12-23/pdf/05-24289.pdf.

Dolin, R. H., & Alschuler, L. (2011). Approaching semantic interoperability in Health Level Seven. *Journal of the American Medical Informatics Association, 18*(1), 99–103.

Dolin, R. H., Alschuler, L., Boyer, S., et al. (2006). HL7 clinical document architecture, release 2. *Journal of the American Medical Informatics Association, 13*(1), 30–39.

eHealthNews. (2010). *ICN and IHTSDO team-up to ensure a common health terminology.* Retrieved from www.ehealthnews.eu/research/1980-icn-and-ihtsdo-team-up-to-ensure-a-common-health-terminology

Giannangelo, K. (2014). *Healthcare code sets, clinical terminologies, and classification systems* (3rd ed.). Chicago, IL: American Health Information Management Association.

Gordon, M. (1994). *Nursing diagnosis: Process and application* (3rd ed.). St. Louis, MO: Mosby.

Health Information Technology (HIT). (2009). *HIT standards committee—joint working groups on quality and operations. Meaningful use measure grid*—data elements mapped to HITEP datatypes. Retrieved from www.healthit.gov/sites/default/files/standards-certification/MU_Grid_Data_Element_Standards_08202009.pdf

Health Information Technology (HIT). (2015). *Meaningful use definition & objectives.* Retrieved from www.healthit.gov/providers-professionals/meaningful-use-definition-objectives

Health Level Seven (HL7). (2016a). *About HL7.* Retrieved from www.hl7.org/about/index.cfm

Health Level Seven (HL7). (2016b). *Welcome to FHIR.* Retrieved from: http://hl7.org/fhir/index.html

Herdman, T. H. (2011). *Nursing diagnoses 2012–14: Definitions and classification.* New Jersey (NJ): John Wiley & Sons.

Herdman, T.H. & Kamitsuru, S. (Eds.). (2014). NANDA International Nursing Diagnoses: Definitions & Classification, 2015– 2017. Oxford: Wiley Blackwell.

Healthcare Information and Management Systems Society. (2013). *Terminology in heath informatics.* Retrieved from www.himss.org/terminology-heath-informatics

Hunt, P. S., Howard, C., Hill, B., & Hillanbrand, M. A. (2015). AORN surgical conference & expo 2015 speaker interviews. *AORN Journal, 101*(2), 183–187.

Hyun, S. (2006). *Toward the creation of an ontology for nursing document sections: Mapping section names to the LOINC semantic model.* Paper presented at the AMIA, Washington, DC.

IHTSDO. (2016). *International health terminology standards development organisation.* Retrieved from www.ihtsdo.org/

International Council of Nurses. (2015). *International classification for nursing practice (ICNP).* Retrieved from www.icn.ch/what-we-do/international-classification-for-nursing-practice-icnpr/

International Organization for Standardization/International Electrotechnical Commission 17115. (2007). *Health informatics—Vocabulary for terminological systems.* Geneva, Switzerland.

Lopez, K. D., Febretti, A., Stifter, J., Johnson, A., Wilkie, D. J., & Keenan, G. (2017). Toward a more robust and efficient usability testing method of clinical decision support for nurses derived from nursing electronic health record data. *International Journal of Nursing Knowledge, 28*(4), 211-218. doi:10.1111/2047-3095.12146

Martin, K. S. (2005). *The Omaha system: A key to practice, documentation, and information management.* (2nd ed.). St. Louis, MO: Elsevier.

Matney, S. (2003). Logical observation identifier names and codes (LOINC) ANA recognition commentary. *Online Journal of Nursing Informatics, 7*(3).

Matney, S. A., Dolin, G., Buhl, L., & Sheide, A. (2016a). Communicating nursing care using the Health Level Seven consolidated clinical document architecture release 2 care plan. *CIN: Computers, Informatics, Nursing, 34*(3), 128–136.

Matney, S. A., Settergren, T., Carrington, J. M., Richesson, R. L., Sheide, A., & Westra, B. L. (2016b). Standardizing physiologic assessment data to enable big data analytics. *Western Journal of Nursing Research, 39*(1), 63–77. doi: 10.1177/0193945916659471

Maxwell-Downing, D. (2013). Clinical issues. *AORN Journal, 97*(1), 140–147.

McCormick, K., Sensmeier, J., Dykes, P., Grace, E., Matney, S. A., Schwartz, K., & Weston, M. (2015). Exemplars for advancing standardized terminology in nursing to achieve sharable, comparable quality data based upon evidence. *Online Journal of Nursing Informatics (OJNI)*, *19*(2). Retrieved from www.himss.org/ojni

Moorhead, S., Johnson, M., Maas, M., & Swanson, E. (2013). *Nursing outcomes classification* (NOC) (5th ed.). St. Louis, MO: Mosby.

Morton, P., Petersen, C., Chard, R., & Kleiner, C. (2013). Validation of the data elements for the health system domain of the PNDS. *AORN Journal*, *98*(1), 39–48.

National Library of Medicine (NLM). (2016a). *UMLS metathesaurus vocabulary documentation.* Retrieved from www.nlm.nih.gov/research/umls/sourcereleasedocs/

National Library of Medicine (NLM). (2016b). *UMLS knowledge source server (UMLSKS).* Retrieved from https://login.nlm.nih.gov/cas/login?service=http://umlsks.nlm.nih.gov/uPortal/Login

Office of the National Coordinator for Health Information Technology. (2015). *2015 interoperability standards advisory.* Retrieved from www.healthit.gov/sites/default/files/2016-interoperability-standards-advisory-final-508.pdf

Payne, T. H., Corley, S., Cullen, T. A., Gandhi, T. K., Harrington, L., Kuperman, G. J., et al. (2015). Report of the AMIA EHR-2020 task force on the status and future direction of EHRs. *Journal of the American Medical Informatics Association*, *22*(5), 1102–1110. doi:10.1093/jamia/ocv066

Rector, A. L. (1999). Clinical terminology: Why is it so hard? *Methods of Information in Medicine*, *38*(4–5), 239–252.

Richesson, R. L., & Chute, C. G. (2015). Health information technology data standards get down to business: Maturation within domains and the emergence of interoperability. *Journal of the American Medical Informatics Association*, *22*(3):492–4. doi:10.1093/jamia/ocv039

Rosenbloom, S. T., Miller, R. A., Johnson, K. B., Elkin, P. L., & Brown, S. H. (2006). Interface terminologies: Facilitating direct entry of clinical data into electronic health record systems. *Journal of American Medical Informatics Association*, *13*(3), 277–288.

Saba, V. K. (2012). *Clinical care classification (CCC) system manual version 2.5, 2nd edition.* New York: Springer.

Salanterä, S. (2015). Advanced use of electronic health records: The depth of nursing notes. *Nursing Research*, *64*(6), 411–412.

Thede, L., & Schwirian, P. (2014). Informatics: The standardized nursing terminologies: A national survey of nurses' experience and attitudes—SURVEY II: Participants' perception of the helpfulness of standardized nursing terminologies in clinical care. *OJIN: The Online Journal of Issues in Nursing*, *20*(1). Retrieved from www.nursingworld.org/MainMenuCategories/ANAMarketplace/ANAPeriodicals/OJIN/Columns/Informatics/Perception-of-the-Helpfulness-of-Standardized-Nursing-Terminologies.html

The University of Iowa. (2016a). *CNC—Overview: Nursing interventions classification (NIC)*, © 2016. Retrieved from www.nursing.uiowa.edu/cncce/nursing-interventions-classification-overview

The University of Iowa. (2016b). *CNC—Overview: Nursing outcomes classification (NOC)*, © 2016. Retrieved from www.nursing.uiowa.edu/cncce/nursing-outcomes-classification-overview

Topaz, M., Golfenshtein, N., & Bowles, K. H. (2014). The Omaha system: A systematic review of the recent literature. *Journal of American Medical Informatics Association*, *21*(1), 163–170.

Department of Health and Human Services (DHHS). (2011). *The office of the national coordinator for health information technology.* Retrieved from http://healthit.hhs.gov/portal/server.pt?open=512&objID=1487&mode=2

Warren, J. J., Matney, S. A., Foster, E. D., Auld, V. A., & Roy, S. L. (2015). Toward interoperability: A new resource to support nursing terminology standards. *Computers, Informatics, Nursing, 33*(12), 515–519.

Westra, B. L., Delaney, C. W., Konicek, D., & Keenan, G. (2008). Nursing standards to support the electronic health record. *Nursing Outlook, 56*(5), 258–266, e251.

World Health Organization (WHO). (2016). *International classification of diseases (ICD) information sheet.* Retrieved from www.who.int/classifications/icd/factsheet/en/

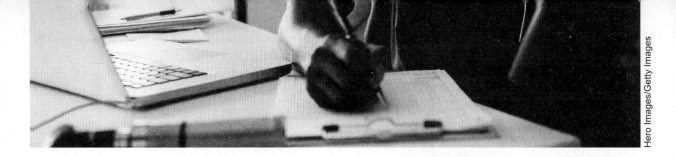

Chapter 16

Continuity Planning and Management (Disaster Recovery)

Carolyn S. Harmon, DNP, RN-BC

 ## Learning Objectives

After completing this chapter, you should be able to:

- Examine the continuity life cycle.

- Evaluate the importance of continuity planning.

- Explain the rationale for developing a business-continuity plan (BCP).

- Discuss the relationship between continuity planning and disaster recovery.

- Outline the steps of the continuity-planning process.

- Review the advantages associated with continuity planning.

- Identify events that can threaten business operation and information systems (IS).

- Discuss how information obtained from a mock or an actual disaster can be used to improve responses and revise continuity plans.

- Discuss legal and accreditation requirements for continuity plans.

Introduction and Background

In the past, disaster-recovery planning focused primarily on the recovery and restoration of data. However, as reliance on timely access to data has grown, the importance of continuity planning for all organizations that rely on continued operations for timely access to, and the processing of, information also has grown. This is especially true for healthcare organizations, with respect to their information systems, networks, freestanding personal computers (PCs), laptops, and hand-held devices. Lost or corrupted data, as well as a data breaches, have a negative impact on business processes, impede the delivery of operations, reduce productivity, and undermine public confidence in the organization (Brown, 2016). Lost or corrupted data are costly to recreate and threaten the survival of a business or healthcare-delivery system in a highly competitive environment.

Since the primary focus of healthcare delivery is the care and well-being of the clients, it is essential to protect the information technology (IT) and data that support client care. IT and its associated data must be viewed as critical resources to support daily operations. Healthcare providers have an obligation to determine how a disaster may affect the delivery of services and identify strategies and related procedures to ensure the availability of information and the continuity of care on a 24/7 basis. Disasters can be manmade or natural. Natural disasters include floods, hurricanes, tsunamis, extreme heat, landslides, winter storms, tornadoes, earthquakes, volcanoes, wildfires, thunderstorms, and lightning strikes (Medina, 2016). Man-made disasters can include cyber-attacks, terrorist attacks, bio-threats, acts of war, riots, explosions, train wrecks, chemical and toxic-waste spills, mining accidents, and shipwrecks. Blackouts, brownouts, and pandemics are also disasters that can occur. The effect of any of these disasters on a healthcare-delivery system could potentially be disastrous. During Hurricane Sandy in New York, patients were moved after the threat had occurred, but a hospital should plan for moving patients before the event, or be self-sustaining during and after such an event. The United States has suffered events such as mass shootings, devastating hurricanes, and horrific tornados—confirming that critical emergency-management capabilities must be increased from minimum disaster-management levels. When a catastrophic disaster occurs, significantly more business-continuity management capabilities, in relation to quantity and quality, are needed. **Business-continuity management (BCM)** is broadly defined as the process that seeks to ensure organizations are capable of withstanding any disruption to normal functioning (Snedaker & Rima, 2014).

Healthcare facilities have become increasingly dependent on IT services, which renders these facilities vulnerable to technology-related failure. Whenever a business is heavily dependent on IT, all risks and threats need to be considered when preparing for recovery. If a disaster occurs and the organization cannot recover fast enough, the consequences can be devastating. Unfortunately, IT also has to consider disgruntled employees and social unrest as threats; therefore, these must be added to the list of man-made disasters.

What Is Continuity Planning?

Continuity planning, usually called **business-continuity planning (BCP)**, is the creation and validation of a practiced logistical plan for how an organization will recover and restore partially or completely interrupted critical functions within a predetermined time after a disaster or extended disruption. The logistical plan is called a business-continuity plan. Continuity planning and **disaster recovery** are processes that help organizations prepare for disruptive events, whether the event is a hurricane or simply a power outage. Continuity planning is the process of ensuring the uninterrupted operation of critical services regardless of any event that may occur. This includes all critical applications and resident data, as well as hypertext transfer protocol (HTTP) data communications on the World Wide Web, databases, networks, and file servers utilized by an organization. A continuity plan is a critical aspect of an organization's risk-management strategy and is instrumental to its survival should a disaster occur (Bailey, 2015).

Historically, BCP began as disaster recovery, but as dependence on automation has increased for nearly all daily operations, this dependence has created a need for more detailed planning to maintain daily operations under a wide array of potential disruptive events.

Continuity planning is typically referred to as BCP or contingency planning. Risk analysis, contingency planning, disaster recovery, data backup, and emergency mode or crisis management are encompassed within BCP (Dooling, 2013). Continuity planning and disaster recovery are processes by which an organization resumes business after a disruptive event. The event might be a disaster such as a huge earthquake or a terrorist attack, or a smaller disruptive event like malfunctioning software caused by a computer virus.

Business-continuity planning suggests a comprehensive approach to making sure an organization can keep operating, not only after a natural calamity, but also in the event of smaller disruptions, including the illness or departure of key staffers, supply-chain problems, or other challenges that businesses are likely to face at some point in time. Disaster planning and recovery is primarily focused on the risks to IT and the data that they utilize. IT staff members are primarily responsible for this area of business-continuity. Data recovery and protection are required for healthcare providers because rapid access to usable data is essential and can literally become a life and death situation. BCP has evolved into its own specialty, resulting in the formation of the Disaster Recovery Institute International with a certification process for its experts. The development of a continuity plan is the most difficult aspect of business-continuity. The widening scope of continuity planning requires expertise from many different disciplines. The ultimate success of continuity planning requires the involvement of key persons across the organization, since they are in the best position to know its policies, standards, functions, data, clients, personnel, and operations (Snedaker & Rima, 2014). Developing continuity into the design of the organizational infrastructure helps prevent local events from disrupting the entire organization.

The BCP for IT needs to include servers, storage devices and media, networking equipment, connectivity links, vendors, suppliers, partners, and IT personnel, as well as air-conditioning and power supplies. The plan should ensure continued availability, reliability, and recoverability of all IT resources, including data, equipment, supplies, processes, personnel, and lines of communication. It should balance the costs of risk management with the opportunity cost of not taking action in preparing for disasters. The continuity plan should provide an enterprise-wide, risk-based approach, covering people, processes, technology, and the extended enterprise to ensure continued availability of operational support systems and minimize disruption risks. Disasters and system downtime can affect all aspects of a business, including facilities, workers, communications, clients, suppliers, partners, logistics, and data. Continuity of business is a backup plan to ensure business as usual in the event of a natural or man-made disaster. Hospitals and other healthcare-delivery organizations are businesses; the only difference is that the product is healthcare.

The processes and procedures a healthcare provider puts into place to avoid mission-critical business interruption or data loss during any type of disaster are essential to ensure that the right mechanisms or backup operational modes are in place to continue operations. These backup systems are often in geographically dispersed locations, so that data access can continue uninterrupted if one location is disabled. Systems, data, and applications that can be impacted include electronic health records, order entry, patient accounting, imaging services, reports, and distribution workflow. Other areas to be considered are emergency care, care management, patient monitoring, clinical profiles, laboratories, dictation equipment, practitioners' portals, healthcare supplies, and a variety of other applications.

IT performance is an area to be considered when establishing a continuity of business plan. Questions to be considered are:

- How will applications perform over a WAN or the Internet?
- What is the impact of distance on existing applications?
- How will the remote data center be managed?

- What are critical business-continuity and disaster-recovery applications?
- Should a separate business-continuity and disaster-recovery capability be devised for each application?
- If one application fails, how will it impact other applications?
- What are the points of potential or expected failure?
- Will the plan scale to fit future requirements?
- What are the potential security threats created by the business-continuity and disaster-recovery plans that are in place?
- How can the integrity and privacy of the data be preserved?

The National Disaster Life Support Foundation defines a disaster as: "an event and its consequences that result in a serious disruption of the functioning of a community, and cause widespread human, material, economic, or environmental losses that exceed the capacity of the affected area to respond without external assistance to save lives, preserve property, and maintain the stability and integrity of the affected area" (Medina, 2016, p. 282). Disasters may strike without warning and require immediate action. For this reason, every organization needs to develop a plan that anticipates potential technology and data-related problems, and provides implementation steps to avoid these problems by instituting policies and procedures to maintain the availability and security of client information under adverse or unexpected conditions. Continuity plans also address alternative means to support the retrieval and processing of information in the event that systems fail.

Disaster-recovery plans enable the retrieval of critical business records from backup storage, restoration of lost data, and resumption of system operations. Plans should ensure uninterrupted operation or expedite resumption of operation after a disaster, while maintaining data access, integrity, and security. Business-continuity plans must identify the plan's objectives—including multiple vendor platforms found in most organizations, and address the implications for other agencies when a system becomes inoperable (Cook, 2015). For example, if a healthcare IS is unavailable for a lengthy period of time, treatment of patients may be slowed, and information will not be available to third-party payers and suppliers. A comprehensive plan consists of separate plans for each of the following areas:

- *Risk analysis.* A risk assessment is performed to include essential functions on systems inside and outside the organization's walls (Dooling, 21013).
- *Downtime and contingency.* Downtime planning focuses on short periods of operational disruptions, with core processes documented during contingency planning (Dooling, 2013).
- *Emergency mode or crisis management.* This plan provides direction during, and immediately after, an incident. This may include a provision to switch to duplicate hardware and networks as a means to minimize disruption of services. This plan also includes the declaration of a disaster (Dooling, 2013).
- *Data backup.* This plan outlines the availability, integrity, and protection of health data (Dooling, 2013).
- *Disaster recovery.* Disaster-recovery planning restores full operational IS capabilities. This plan includes training, testing of mock drills, and evaluation of identified gaps (Dooling, 2013).

Consideration of each of these areas as separate plans may provide for better division of responsibility and increased awareness of the significance for each area. An organization's security officer should have a key role in continuity and disaster planning, starting with a basic understanding of the plan-development process to help direct the effort. Part of the security role is the protection of information. Data security is particularly important in order to comply with federal mandates and accreditation requirements.

Steps in Developing a Preparedness Program

Healthcare businesses can prepare for hazards and disasters by developing a preparedness program. This program plans for events that may occur today or in the future. A preparedness program protects patient safety, secures health information, ensures access and stability for continuity of care, and provides information recovery (Dooling, 2013). The US Department of Homeland Security (n.d.) has devised a five-stage process in developing a preparedness program (see Figure 16-1). These stages include:

1. Program management
2. Planning
3. Implementation
4. Testing and exercise
5. Program improvement.

Program Management

Program management is at the center of developing a preparedness program. The foundation of a preparedness program includes management leadership, commitment, and financial support (Snedaker & Rima, 2014). Management leadership develops and disseminates a detailed policy that is consistent with the organization's mission and vision. The policy defines the program's goals and objectives, as well as employee roles and responsibilities. Most often, program goals include protection of human safety, minimization of operational

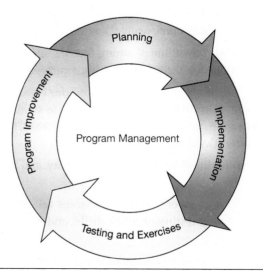

Figure 16-1 • Preparedness Program Planning Stages

SOURCE: From Program Management.Published by US Department of Homeland Security.

disruptions, facility preservation, and prevention of environmental contamination. The program objectives consider both short and long-term objectives, entailing all aspects of the program.

The program policy developed by leadership will authorize key employee positions to develop and manage the preparedness program (Cook, 2015). One employee position is assigned the role of program leader or coordinator. The designated coordinator is accountable to the organization's leadership team for achieving program goals. The responsibilities of the program coordinator entail developing a preparedness policy, program goals and objectives, program scope, regulations, priorities, budget, schedule, resources, program evaluation, and records management. The program coordinator guides program development and leads all essential communications regarding the preparedness-program plan to the organization's leaders, all employees, and a program committee, which is established by the program coordinator. This committee assists in the design, implementation, and management of the preparedness program, while all employees are expected to participate in some effort of the preparedness program. The program committee should encompass employees with all aspects of organizational knowledge and may include: management, human resources, risk, nursing, laboratories, respiratory, security, quality, IT, engineering, maintenance, environmental services, and so on.

After a program coordinator is selected, and the program committee is created, the program scope is established. The scope of the program is determined by a variety of factors, such as the complexity of the healthcare organization. The program scope is also determined by the risk assessment and business-impact analysis (Department of Homeland Security, n.d.). After the development of the program scope, the program budget and development schedule are established. The program schedule identifies milestones for achieving program goals and objectives.

Planning

Any community or organization may be impacted by a hazard or threat. The planning stage of the program utilizes an overall risk-management strategy (Cook, 2015). Strategies to prevent, deter, and mitigate risk are a part of the planning process. During this stage, threats and hazards are identified, and organizational vulnerabilities are assessed with their potential impact analyzed. Figure 16-2 depicts the Risk Assessment Process.

RISK ASSESSMENT A risk assessment identifies vulnerabilities. The risk assessment can be completed by using the Threat and Hazard Identification and Risk Assessment (THIRA)

Table 16-1 All-Hazards

All-Hazards	Examples
Natural	Hurricane or typhoon, flood, wildfire, winter storm, earthquake, tsunami, storm surge
Technological	Nuclear power-plant meltdown, dam failure, presence of hazardous materials, industrial accidents, plane crashes
Civil or political	Terrorism, civil war, conflicts
Hybrid	Train derailment or truck accident containing hazardous chemical materials, causing environmental hazard; tsunami causing electrical power failure, resulting in nuclear power-plant meltdown
Humanitarian or complex	Migration of refugees from war and poverty-stricken countries
Emerging infectious disease	Pandemic flu, Ebola epidemic, use of infection as a new technology that can be used against the population

Source: 'Types of disasters', Center for Domestic Preparedness, Healthcare Leadership for Mass Casualty Incidents, pp. 9–10. Participant/Student Manual, Department of Homeland Security/Federal Emergency Management Agency (FEMA), HCL PM 09.0,The Federal Emergency Management Agency (FEMA) website: Healthcare Leadership for Mass casualty Incidents Training, available at: www.fema.gov/medialibrary/assests/images/106224 (last accessed 30th November, 2015).

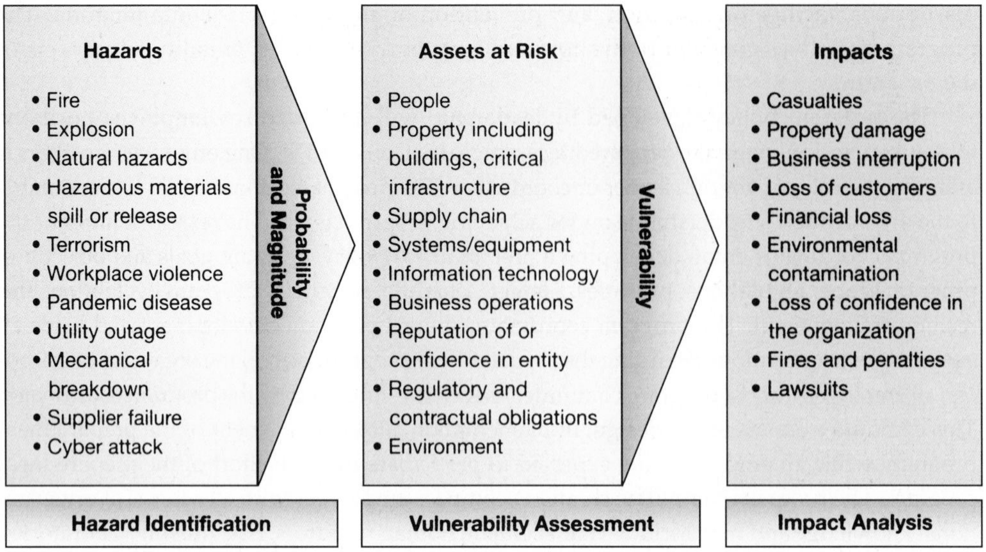

Figure 16-2 • Risk Assessment Process Diagram

SOURCE: From Risk Assessment.Published by US Department of Homeland Security.

process (Department of Homeland Security, 2013). THIRA includes a four-step process, outlined in Table 16-2. Potential loss scenarios are recognized during the risk assessment, resulting in documentation of resources needed. Some potential loss scenarios may consist of historical events that have previously interfered with business operations such as power failure, building damage, terror attacks, or natural disasters. Scenario development and documentation may involve business disruptions, threats, and an analysis of the possible impact to business operations.

A business-impact analysis (BIA) identifies the impact from disruption of time-sensitive or critical processes to a business (Snedaker & Rima, 2014). The BIA also identifies which processes are vital to continue business operations. In healthcare, the consequences of disruption may include patient harm or death, financial or patient-care-data loss, and increased expenses such as overtime or loss of supplies. The timing of disruption may be short- or long-term. Under long-term circumstances, supply replenishment and workforce replacement need to be considered.

During the conduction of a BIA, a BIA questionnaire is used to survey organizational managers (Snedaker & Rima, 2014; Department of Homeland Security n.d.). The program coordinator selects managers with detailed knowledge of day-to-day operations. The analysis recognizes critical operations, the maintenance of critical operations, and the support of data

Table 16-2 THIRA Process

Process Step	Description
Step 1. Identify the threats and hazards of concern	List community threats and hazards identified via experience, forecasting, subject matter experts, and other sources
Step 2. Give the threats and hazards context	Describe concerns with possible effects to community
Step 3. Establish capability targets	Assess threats and hazards utilizing capability concepts (prevention, protection, mitigation, response, and recovery)
Step 4. Apply the results	Estimate resource requirements

Source: From Threat and Hazard Identification and Risk Assessment Guide. Published by US Department of Homeland Security.

and information integrity. After the BIA identifies the critical needs of the organization, these needs are ranked in order of prioritization utilizing the following categorical methodology:

- Category 1: Mission-critical—recovery window 0 to 12 hours
- Category 2: Vital—recovery window 13 to 24 hours
- Category 3: Important—recovery window 1 to 3 days
- Category 4: Minor—recovery window more than 3 days (Snedaker & Rima, 2014).

The BIA leads to the documentation of the emergency-response plan, communications plan, IT plan, and the business-continuity plan (see Figure 16-3).

Implementation

The implementation of a preparedness program consists of resource management, employee training, and executing plans such as the emergency-response plan, crisis-communications plan, business-continuity plan, and IT plan (Snedaker & Rima, 2014). Resource management during the implementation stage entails the resources required for implementing the preparedness program such as people, technology, facilities, and funding. A needs assessment is conducted to determine the organization's specific resource needs. This needs assessment will include an exploration of the internal and external environment.

In addition to resource management, the implementation stage executes the emergency-response plan (ERP), crisis-communications plan (CCP), business-continuity plan, and IT plan (ITP). The ERP protects people, property, and the environment (Department of Homeland Security, n.d.). This plan includes evacuation and lockdown procedures. A CCP establishes the communication needs between the organization and employees, patients, families, and the media. Most often in healthcare, a spokesperson is appointed. The ITP outlines data-recovery strategies and data-backup plans. Data recovery may be internal or vendor supported. The BCP is a process of restoring and recovering an organization's day-to-day operations.

An incident-management system is developed during the implementation stage to manage operational disruptions by utilizing a combination of facilities, equipment, personnel, procedures, and communications (Jensen & Thompson, 2016). Incident-management systems utilize incident-command systems to define responsibilities, and coordinate activities (Jenson & Thompson, 2016). The incident-command system provides organization and structure to a crisis situation with clearly defined roles for each position. The next step in the implementation stage

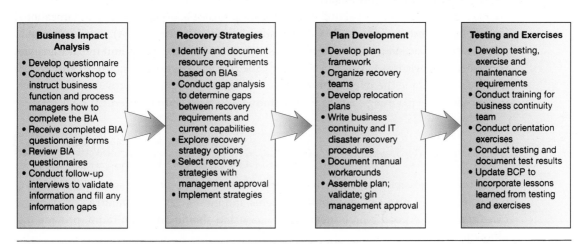

Figure 16-3 • Business Impact Analysis Process

SOURCE: From Risk Assessment.Published by US Department of Homeland Security.

Table 16-3 Training

Who Needs Training?	What Training Should Be Provided?
All employees	• Protective actions for life safety (evacuation, shelter, shelter-in-place, and lockdown) • Safety, security, and loss-prevention programs
Emergency-response team (evacuation, shelter, shelter-in-place)	• Roles and responsibilities as defined in the plan • Training to comply with regulations or maintain certifications (if employees administer first aid, CPR, or AED, or use fire extinguishers or clean up spills of hazardous chemicals) • Additional training for leaders, including incident management
Business-continuity team	• Roles and responsibilities as defined in the plan • Additional training for leaders, including incident management
Crisis-communications team	• Roles and responsibilities as defined in the plan • Additional training for leaders, including incident management • Training for spokespersons

Source: From Training. Published by US Department of Homeland Security.

is training. Training informs employees of their role during a disruption in routine operations. Members of emergency response, business-continuity, and crisis-communication teams should be familiar with their defined plans (Snedaker & Rima, 2014). Training information and content is utilized during the development or testing of scenarios, drills, and exercises. Table 16-3 describes who needs training and what training needs to be provided for that role or person.

Testing and Exercises

A schedule of training drills and exercises are developed and executed during the testing and exercises stage. The execution of disruption scenarios provides return demonstrations that validate users' comprehension of roles and responsibilities. Thus, the testing and exercises stage is used to evaluate training, as well as the overall-preparedness program (Snedaker & Rima, 2014). The advantages to testing and exercising a preparedness program include knowledge reinforcement and gap identification. Therefore, this stage is of utmost importance in determining the success of the organization's ability to prevent, deter, mitigate, and withstand risks.

Program Improvement

Program improvement may occur from the evaluation of the program test results or analyzing the program after an actual event has occurred. Quality-assurance techniques may include both internal review and external audits (Snedaker & Rima, 2014). Lessons learned, resolutions, and action plans are documented. These documented gaps and deficiencies are addressed via the corrective-action program. The corrective-action program is compiled of meetings to critique the overall-preparedness program. Program-improvement activities move back to the planning stage to recycle through the program-management stages.

Advantages of Continuity Planning

It is not always possible to avoid a disaster or to provide 100% protection against every threat, but a satisfactory plan can anticipate problems and minimize losses incurred by damage (Medina, 2016). A good plan is clear and concise and should, at a minimum, provide the following (Dooling, 2013):

• Identifies strategies for correction of vulnerabilities within the organization

- Provides a reasonable amount of protection against interruption in services, downtime, and data loss
- Ensures continuity of the client record and delivery of care
- Expedites reporting of diagnostic tests
- Captures charges and supports billing and processing of reimbursement claims in a timely fashion
- Ensures open communication with employees and ensures customers of availability of services or interim arrangements
- Provides a mechanism to capture information needed for regulatory and accrediting bodies
- Helps to ensure compliance with HIPAA legislation and requirements of The Joint Commission (TJC)
- Establishes backup and restoration procedures for systems, databases, and important files
- Allows time for restoration of equipment, the facility, and services.

Basically, an effective disaster plan saves patients from unnecessary delays in treatment and avoids redundant procedures. It also saves money upfront and over time by limiting loss of data, equipment, and services. Any organization that requires a high level of information integrity and availability cannot afford to be without a continuity plan that provides for disaster recovery. A good plan can make the difference between an organization's survival and demise.

Disasters versus System Failure

Hazards come from many sources, including environmental disasters, human error, sabotage, acts of terrorism and bioterrorism, high-tech crime, operating-system or application-software bugs or viruses, overtaxed infrastructure, power fluctuations and outages, and equipment failure (Medina, 2016).

A thorough appraisal by IT personnel can minimize the risk of damage from various hazard situations. The impact scenarios provide a means to understand the impact of a disaster versus a system failure. An annual review of the impact scenarios should be performed and the scenarios updated, because not only does the organization change, but also the IT and the environment in which it operates. Typically, an IT failure is something for which staff members are prepared, having resources already in place; for example, redundant equipment and data backups. A disaster, however, affects an entire organization: all its systems, equipment, processes, personnel, clients, partners, and information in all media and formats.

Continuity and Recovery Options

The 24/7 operations of healthcare providers make continuity of services essential. Although continuity planning must encompass all aspects of daily operations, the focus on information should guide the selection of computer services, hardware, and software for day-to-day operations, backup, and recovery. Problems are magnified by the fact that an estimated 60% of critical business data resides at remote sites away from IT staff, with backups and testing of backups frequently hampered by limited and busy staff, slow WAN connections, and constantly increasing data-storage requirements (Snedaker & Rima, 2014).

Hardware redundancy is the first line of defense in providing continuous system operations, because redundancy allows operations to continue even when individual components fail. This redundancy may be accomplished via redundant processors and disk arrays at one location, at two separate locations of the same organization, or at another facility. An increasing number of organizations now split their IT infrastructure between two locations for added protection. A second data-processing site requires sufficient space for equipment and staff, especially if it may double as a backup data center.

Functional requirements include mainframe and/or server capacity, printers, storage devices, network and communication equipment and services, sufficient cabling, an uninterrupted power source, and air conditioning, as well as space for a help desk, an operations center, and test room. Online replication of data is an integral part of business-continuity, providing data availability, averting disaster, and reducing costs and recovery time. Redundant network storage provides multiple data paths, preventing damage and loss. Advances in IT in recent years have helped organizations be better prepared in the event of a major disaster. These advances include improvements in data-replication hardware, servers, and other equipment that require less electricity and have better battery-backup systems for small businesses. Improved software and equipment options for emergency notification make it easier and quicker to contact key administrators, employees, vendors, and suppliers (Snedaker & Rima, 2014). Automated emergency-notification applications expedite the traditional calling tree to contact personnel within a span of minutes, using methods that range from interactive voice-response phone calls to email, freeing personnel for other tasks in the process. Managed-hosting services with Internet access also provide an option for a secondary site for backup and recovery. Communications management is essential in controlling rumors and contacting the media (Snedaker & Rima, 2014).

A managed-hosting site eliminates the need to perform backups; rent space; purchase antivirus and firewall software; and purchase server and networking equipment, disk and tape-storage hardware and media, and telecommunications lines; and is available wherever there is an Internet connection using Remote Desktop software or Virtual Private Network software. The latest versions of most database-management systems, such as SQL Server or Oracle, provide for database replication across a network, as well as incremental and full backup capabilities. Using replication across a network, a secondary-site database can be kept current with the production database in the organization's main site because each transaction that takes place for the production database also occurs at the replicated-database site. The connection between the primary site and the replication site can be either leased lines or the Internet. Redundancy of communication capabilities is important for replication.

Backup and Storage

Data availability, recovery time, disaster avoidance, retention requirements, and costs determine the best backup and storage options for a given organization (Dooling, 2013). Continuous delivery of services is the goal, but solutions to achieve zero downtime are expensive and not always possible. For these reasons, organizations must determine data-storage requirements and acceptable recovery time on a system-by-system basis.

These decisions help determine media choices for storage. Media choices include magnetic tape, hard disk, optical disc (CD and DVD), and solid-state storage (flash memory, thumb drives), as well as remote backup services. CDs, DVDs, and solid-state storage devices are convenient for backing up stand-alone PCs.

Common anti-disaster protection methods include the following: automated backups, off-site media storage, data mirroring, server replication, remote-data replication, a virtual tape library that emulates multiple tape drives (by backing up data to disks with later conversion to physical tapes for off-site vaulting), and snapshots of data at prescribed intervals (Sewell, 2016). Virtual-disaster recovery pools IT resources, masking boundaries between hardware to increase capacity. Data mirroring is the creation of a duplicate online copy. This technique eliminates wait time, but may also replicate corrupted data.

Best practices for long-term data retention include the selection of standardized file formats, good management of metadata, the selection of media intended for long-term storage and proper housing, and regular inspection and maintenance of stored media. Metadata is a set of data that provides information about how, when, and by whom data are collected, formatted, and stored (Kendall & Kendall, 2014). File metadata describes each file's permissions, owner, group, access control lists (ACLs), size, and so forth. System metadata is configuration information, and each operating system has a different way of storing such information. Metadata is essential to the creation and use of data repositories.

Backup allows restoration of data if, or when, they are lost. Losses may occur with disk or CPU crashes, file deletion, and file corruption due to power or application problems, or overwritten files. Fast data recovery minimizes the worst consequences of downtime, including a tarnished image and financial losses. Storage-area networks with electronic vaulting provides the type of protection needed to ensure business-continuity.

Server replication is recommended for the most widely used applications, because it ensures continuity by providing a reliable secondary infrastructure. Electronic vaulting sends backups over telecommunication links to secure storage facilities. This approach eliminates labor costs and the need to physically transport tapes. It also improves data integrity and shortens recovery efforts. Electronic vaulting may be provided by commercial enterprises that provide backup services for customers. Customers receive backup software at their site and at a central, remote file server. The customer connects to the remote server to back up data. Each customer has a separate account, and file access is limited to authorized persons.

Remote backup service (RBS) protects both data and data integrity. Data retrieval, when needed, is limited only by the speed of the communication link. RBSs also provide reports to show which files have been backed up. Tape and other older media do not support fast data-recovery efforts. Backups may fail because of faulty software, bad network connections, worn tapes, or poor storage conditions. For this reason, backups should be verified and periodically tested. Advancements in IT and changes in the costs of backup options and storage media provide more options to maintain business-continuity, backup, and storage. Newer tape drives have well-developed error correction, eliminating the need to verify backup copies, but not the need to test stored media.

Storage media differ, but should permit permanent or semipermanent record keeping. Magnetic tape is still used as a relatively inexpensive storage medium. Optical disks are another storage option with a longer shelf life, but a higher cost. Electronic transfer over high-speed telephone lines to another site is a faster, more reliable means of backup that eliminates transportation concerns. When electronic transmission is not an option, a second set of backup media should be made and transported separately to ensure against accidental loss or destruction. Archived data must be inspected regularly to ensure they can be processed, and that the medium has not deteriorated or become outdated in light of current backup systems. Cloud storage is an additional option for remote-backup and file-retrieval tools. The cloud is a model of networked storage with data in virtualized pools of storage (Lackey et al., 2014). The criteria for good backup systems include the following four points:

- Backups must contain the requested data
- Backups must complete within the prescribed time frame

- Backups must occur as scheduled—full backup on some days and incremental on others
- Backups must be set to expire at the correct time.

PERSONAL AND NOTEBOOK COMPUTERS Although the primary focus of an IT continuity/disaster-recovery plan is on the major systems in an organization, large amounts of information that is important for daily operations are also found on PCs, notebook computers, and smart phones. Most breaches involve individuals, removable or portable electronic devices or media, paper, and laptops, with theft and loss accounting for the major types of breaches encountered (Wikina, 2014). Mobile workers spend at least 50% of their time at locations outside of the main organization's site, using notebooks or PDAs. Homecare personnel exemplify one such group of mobile workers. Other healthcare professionals telecommute using the Internet and remote connections to access and transmit information. Telecommuters face IT threats that do not affect internal employees, such as firewall maintenance, denial-of-service attacks, and lost productivity when network connections are not available. For these reasons, IT-disaster plans need to include remote users and the devices they use. Routine maintenance prevents many problems faced by mobile users. Box 16-1 lists maintenance tasks recommended for personal computing devices (PCD).

Organizations should not assume that users know how to perform these tasks, or that they will perform them regularly. Instruction and assistance should be provided for PCD users. For example, computer-support personnel should perform periodic backups using standardized backup procedures and media.

Manual versus Automated Alternatives

The decision to use manual alternatives when a system has failed or is otherwise unavailable has implications for the delivery of care, the cost-of-care provided, records management, and employee IT system training. A backup alternative is a different means to accomplish a common task than what is ordinarily used. An example of a manual backup alternative is the completion of paper requests for laboratory tests that are then delivered to the laboratory, instead of selecting ordered tests from menus on computer screens. Implementation of a backup alternative may delay delivery of services for several reasons. First, personnel are less familiar with the alternative procedure and will take longer to accomplish their work, thereby delaying results reporting and processing requests for services. Second, manual forms may no longer exist or may not be current in terms of displaying the newest available tests or test names. Third, because automation eliminated personnel who supported the manual process, there may be few people available who know the manual alternative.

Automated backup alternatives may also be available. For example, staff may be able to access information through a different screen than the one they generally use. Despite these potential problems, implementation of backup alternatives permits ongoing delivery of care, even if it is somewhat slower. Calculation of backup costs goes beyond initial setup costs and ongoing expenditures. Recovery costs can be high for several reasons :

- The personnel cost for hiring and training staff to use backup alternatives
- Additional costs for dual entry of data
- Costs for cleanup, repair, or replacement of computer equipment
- Payment for backup computing or recovery services.

Another cost is the impact on the quality of services rendered during the time an information system is not available. The expense for manual versus automated alternatives varies according to the length of time that the system is unavailable, the type of backup alternatives

---

Box 16-1   Recommended PCD Maintenance

- Establish a secure place for backup media away from the PCD, preferably in a fire-proof safe or file cabinet. Backup media stored under poor conditions or kept in the same area as the device are vulnerable to the same threats. Another backup option is online backup. This may be accomplished through the information-services department or a vendor.

- Do an incremental backup daily, a full backup weekly, and a full system backup monthly; backup/store files on network drives whenever possible. This is particularly important for remote sites not covered by IT staff.

- Test backup media to ensure that the media are operational. Establish a policy for routine replacement of backup media.

- Periodically delete no-longer-needed files from the hard drive.

- Defragment all hard drives monthly.

- Maintain air flow around the PCD to allow cooling.

- Keep storage media away from magnetic fields, including electronic devices.

- Periodically clean PCDs.

- Run virus-protection software regularly and obtain updated versions as available.

---

employed, and the resources required. Because implementing a backup alternative is costly, administrators must decide if the anticipated time a system is not available merits initiating the alternative. Extremely short periods of system unavailability are usually not worth the additional time and trouble.

Costs for a manual alternative include additional labor for IT staff and other personnel, increased potential for error, and space requirements. Data entry into the system after a manual backup requires additional personnel and a place for them to work. For example, laboratory tests that were requested, but not completed before the system became unavailable must be requested again through the manual alternative. During the time a system is down, laboratory staff must try to match manual requisitions against those that were entered but not processed before the system failed. When the system is restored (goes live), laboratory tests that were ordered and completed during the time the system was down, along with test results, must be entered so that the client record is not fragmented.

Staff Training

The successful implementation of a manual alternative plan hinges on the cooperation and support of everyone in the organization. One way to ensure this success is through training (Wikina, 2014). Detailed instructions on every aspect of the system, the plan, and the implementation of manual alternatives should be incorporated into initial computer training. However, this approach requires a longer training period, and refresher training periodically. Recall of manual procedures is often poor when long periods elapse between instruction and execution. A more effective strategy entails posting plans in conspicuous places, yearly review of continuity plans, mock disasters, and the provision of step-by-step reference guides to help staff implement manual alternatives. Other measures to increase disaster awareness and ensure successful recovery efforts are listed in Box 16-2.

When it is not possible to maintain IT continuity, recovery is the next option. Recovery is not a simple undertaking and requires detailed and tested procedures. Few organizations have

---

Box 16-2 Ways to Ensure Business-Continuity and Successful Recovery

- Display continuity plans in conspicuous places and post revised versions as soon as they are available.
- List key contact people responsible for implementing continuity and recovery plans.
- Review staff responsibilities periodically.
- Provide clear step-by-step reference aids for staff to guide them through continuity and recovery options including manual alternatives.
- Emphasize the importance of disaster preparedness by incorporating mock-disaster situations into annual training for all employees.
- Review the continuity and recovery plans at least twice each year.
- Schedule at least two mock disasters per year—one of which is community-wide.
- Test backups periodically.
- Label backup materials and include explicit directions with them.
- Provide up-to-date, hot and cold site information to persons responsible for recovery.
- Test the emergency notification plan periodically. This may include a calling tree, but more likely it will rely upon special software that provides almost instant, simultaneous notification of all key persons.
- Emphasize the need for emergency-care arrangements for dependents and pets to personnel involved in disaster and recovery plan implementation.

---

actually reconstructed IS from their backups, and few IT staff are equipped to deal with data recovery (Poelker, 2012). Even when it would appear that equipment and storage media are damaged, assumptions should not be made that data are permanently lost, nor should persons unacquainted with salvage recovery techniques attempt to restore equipment or storage media (Snedaker & Rima, 2014). For these reasons, it is best to call in recovery specialists when significant data loss has occurred. Successful recovery requires stabilization of the affected system and good problem-solving skills, staff preparedness, and good backups. Recovery is complicated when backups are not verified, delaying the detection of problems until restoration is attempted. Also, large organizations typically have data stored in many locations, on many different devices, on many different media, and in several different formats.

Most organizations use a combination of backup formats and software programs. Restoration of system operation may result from one of several approaches. First, materials stored at a cold site can be shipped back to the organization and reloaded onto the information system. Second, information may be restored from RBSs or electronic vaulting. A third option is the use of hot sites such as a commercial managed-hosting site. Commercial hot sites are fully equipped with uninterrupted power supplies, computers, telecommunication capabilities, security, and environmental equipment. Hot sites may accept transmission of backup copies of computer data, allowing restoration of operations using backup media. This restoration is accomplished at another location served by a different power grid and central telephone office to avoid the effects of the disaster that affected the healthcare enterprise. The organization may develop its own hot site or outsource for services. When possible, hot sites should be close enough for practical employee travel, with sufficient space, power, cabling, parking, and satellite-dish accommodations to support IT function. A dedicated hot site usually sits idle when not needed, but is available in the event of an emergency and is compatible with the agency's systems for ease of system restoration and updates. The creation of redundant-computer capabilities and the acquisition of a dedicated hot site is costly. At one time, it was common to share the center with other healthcare alliance partners. In this arrangement, tenants agree to relinquish the site in the event of a disaster. Sharing a site presumes that it is unlikely that two or more partners at separate locations would have a disaster at the same time. Shared arrangements are no longer practical because most organizations' systems now have extensive online processing. Hot sites may not be adequate to process critical applications or be able to provide for special equipment needs, such as unique laser printers and forms-handling equipment.

Another option is the creation of a backup facility on-site in another building owned by the organization. This option reduces real-estate costs, but still requires system redundancy. Internal hot sites can continue to provide processing for critical business functions; although, typically, this occurs at a reduced level of service. When not in use as a hot site, it can be used for other processing activities, thereby eliminating certain types of fees. Commercial hot-site services or managed-hosting services charge monthly reservation fees in addition to restoration charges, but are less costly than establishing an independent site. Unfortunately, the uniqueness of most client–server environments made commercial recovery services unprofitable and unavailable until recently, forcing institutions to develop their own internal-recovery options. Although clinical staff have no involvement in the establishment of hot and cold sites, it may have relevance for them in terms of possible delays in information access.

Vendor Equipment

Vendors may offer processing capability through their equipment either at their location or at the location of the disaster. This solution may work for a select few applications but does not address the needs of an entire organization. There are also issues related to costs, software versions and customizations, availability, and testing. Sending equipment from other locations can take days before the equipment arrives, the software is loaded, and the data are recovered from backup media. An alternative to system restoration is distributed processing. Distributed processing uses a group of independent processors that contain the same information, but these may be at different sites. In the event that one processor is knocked out, information is not lost because remaining processors can continue IT operation with little or no interruption. Distributed processing is more expensive up front, but eliminates the time a system is not available. Rapid replacement of equipment is yet another recovery strategy, but it is not always feasible because it is costly to maintain extra hardware. An additional option is an online-data-backup service (ODBS). ODBS automatically backs up data at an offsite location (Lackey et al., 2014). Data can be retrieved via the Internet when using ODBS. Two popular ODBS options are Backblaze and Carbonite.

Salvaging Damaged Equipment and Records

Once alternative arrangements have been made to maintain business options, restoration of the equipment and required data records becomes the focus. Few IT personnel possess the skills necessary to salvage damaged records and equipment, but internal personnel should know how to act quickly and effectively to limit damage and to obtain outside help. Quick action, and a basic knowledge of recovery techniques, can expedite the return to full operation and minimize loss of equipment and records, as well as costs. Whether the information center was without climate control, or was physically damaged by an event that exposed it to heat, humidity, and/or smoke damage, there are guidelines to follow to salvage materials. Some of these guidelines are provided in Box 16-3.

> ## Box 16-3 General Salvage Rules
>
> - Stabilize the site.
> - Pump out water to minimize mold and mildew growth and damage.
> - Vent the area.
> - Do not restore power to wet equipment.
> - Open cabinet doors, remove side panels and covers, and pull out chassis to permit water to exit equipment.
> - Call in professional decontamination specialists when hazardous chemicals or wastes are present.
> - Initiate salvage options within 48 hours.

The first rule is to stabilize the site. In most scenarios, internal staff do not participate in the actual recovery process. Many processes require the use of hazardous knowledge of detailed salvage methods. Disaster-recovery experts can best ensure data recovery from damaged media, particularly from magnetic media. Fires, heat, and floods leave residues that damage electronic equipment and storage media. Additional damage may occur when media are improperly stored and handled after the disaster, and with the passage of time. Degradation of media also impedes recovery efforts. Data integrity is compromised when storage media are damaged. Recovery specialists must verify data on a bit-by-bit basis and reconstruct files before data can be recorded onto new media. It is important to have written agreements with restoration companies in times of widespread disasters, such as earthquakes or floods, when many organizations will be seeking help at the same time.

Recovery Costs

The cost for recovery is frequently overlooked in developing the continuity and disaster-recovery plan. Recovery costs should be determined as part of the continuity plan because unanticipated expenses during recovery are never well received, and it can be an extremely expensive process, involving the following cost factors:

- Lost consumer confidence
- Financial loss
- Temporary computer services, including space rental, equipment, furniture, extra telephone lines, and temporary personnel
- Shipping and installation costs
- Post-disaster replacement of equipment, repairs, and costs associated with bringing the building up to new codes
- Recovery and possible decontamination
- Overtime hours for staff during the disaster for the implementation of manual alternatives, as well as after the disaster, for entering data into the system that was generated during system downtime
- Reconstruction of lost data.

Insurance coverage is recommended as a means to help pay for information-system disasters. It is recommended to compile a list of assets to determine insurable values (Department of Homeland Security, n.d.).

One person should be designated to interact with the insurance company, and a mechanism should be identified for how disaster-related costs will be documented. Insurance will normally reimburse only for expenses associated with repair or replacement of a damaged building, but not additional costs associated with building-code changes implemented since the building was built.

Planning Pitfalls

Continuity plans are subject to the following pitfalls:

- *Inadequate commitment and involvement of leadership.* Senior management is too busy to oversee the continuity plan; therefore, the plan is delegated to a mid-level manager, and the plan visibility is reduced (Lingeswara, 2012).

- *Insufficient IT budgets.* Few IT budgets have sufficient funding for business-continuity efforts. Continuity-plan budgets need to be spread across the organization.

- *Lack of access to the plan.* If the plan is available online, measures must be taken to ensure that the computers that house the plan are accessible. All employees responsible for implementing any part of the plan should have a copy at home, at work, and in their briefcases. These copies may be on paper, PCDs, CD-ROM, or DVD; thumb drives may also be acceptable distribution methods. Everyone should be aware of their roles and responsibilities (Snedaker & Rima, 2014).

- *Failure to include all information and devices in the plan.* Businesses evolve and institute new processes. Many plans lag behind the information technology that is being used. An increasing amount of important information is found on laptops, desktop PCs, smart phones, and even in paper format. Many plans fail to consider the importance of email, enterprise resource-planning systems, and web-based transactions to daily operations. Many healthcare providers also have separate databases for various populations. Information services may not be aware of these separate databases until problems arise. There are also applications supported by application-service providers. One such example might include a renal database for dialysis patients. Continuity plans must consider how services will be provided in the event that the vendor's database is unavailable due to failure on the vendor's end, or because of an inability to access the database due to inoperable Internet or telephone connections (Lucci & Walsh, 2015). Another example might be the failure to consider the multivendor environment seen in most healthcare systems today. Data are frequently housed on several computers.

- *Failure to incorporate data growth into the plan.* Unprecedented data growth is a threat to recovery plans. Organizations need to focus on critical data to ensure business-continuity and reduce recovery time. Failure can occur during data recovery when a lack of thorough understanding of data dynamics exists among recovery personnel (Lingeswara, 2012).

- *Failure to update the plan.* The continuity plan is a dynamic document that is subject to change as operations and personnel change, and as determinations are made that some portions of the plan do not work well. The BCP workgroup should control the change process and should print review and revision dates on each page. A change manual can be used to note changes, including the date and reason for each change.

- *Failure to test the plan.* A significant percentage of organizations that have continuity and disaster-recovery plans have never tested them, do not know if they have been tested, or have not tested them within the past year (Snedaker & Rima, 2014).

- *Failure to consider the human component* (Lucci & Walsh, 2015). Preservation of human life is the top priority in any disaster, followed by preservation of critical business functions. In any disaster, the loss of personnel is a distinct possibility. In times of disaster, the organization should be prepared to assist employees and their families, including communication links to check on employees, and provide such amenities as transportation to work and possibly temporary housing. Restoration of peace of mind for employees and families is just as important as recovering data from a computer system and maintaining business-continuity. This includes reestablishing user confidence once normal operations are restored and addressing the emotional impact that the disaster has had on employees.

Using Post-Disaster Feedback to Improve Planning

Post-disaster feedback is invaluable in revising disaster plans for future use and should be an integral part of continuity planning (Medina, 2016). Personnel input after mock disasters or prolonged downtime should be used to identify what worked and what did not. Information systems, IT, society, and organizations change over time. Plans that looked adequate before a disaster may not prove adequate after a disaster has occurred. Recovery expenses usually exceed anticipated costs, leading to a change in recovery strategies for future use.

Another option for the development, revision, and management of continuity plans for organizations with limited resources is the use of a third-party data-management system. Managed-hosting-service providers offer continuous data backup, safeguarding against data loss while allowing for immediate recovery and restoration of services in the event of a disaster. Organizations using managed-hosting-service providers retain control of data-processing operations, while the managed-hosting-service provides the resources. Customers can manage their data processing through a personalized web-management interface that allows them to initiate recovery from any location. Challenges for the future include:

- Finding ways to protect the growing amount of information, no matter where it is stored or used

- Finding ways to make sure people can stay connected to their data, no matter what the disruption

Without addressing and linking these two elements, a plan may fall far short of its goals.

Legal and Accreditation Requirements

The Health Insurance Portability and Accountability Act security rule requires continuity planning and disaster-recovery processes (Snedaker & Rima, 2014). All healthcare organizations must have a data-backup plan, a recovery plan, an emergency mode of operation plan, and testing and evaluation procedures. Although HIPAA does not specify the exact processes or procedures for compliance, it does demand safeguards for the security of protected healthcare information while operating in both normal and emergency modes. These safeguards encompass the creation, access, storage, and destruction of manual records. The final continuity-planning component of the HIPAA regulations required compliance by April 2006.

The Pandemic and All-Hazards Preparedness Act (PAHPA) was enacted in 2006 at the end of the 109th Congressional session and reauthorized in March 2013 (Public Health Emergency, 2016). The purpose of this law was to improve the nation's public health and medical preparedness and response capabilities for emergencies, whether deliberate, accidental, or natural. This law authorized development of a national, near-real-time information network to coordinate federal and state response to public-health emergencies within two years of enactment. The Secretary of Health and Human Services was charged with leading the federal response to these types of emergencies, usurping the role previously accorded to the Department of Homeland Security. Similar legislation focused upon hospital readiness to deal with disasters.

The Joint Commission (TJC) requires disaster-preparedness standards for hospital accreditation. Until 2000, standards focused on disasters and accidents, such as power-plant failures and chemical spills. In 2001, TJC introduced new emergency-management standards for hospitals, long-term-care facilities, and behavioral health and ambulatory care that focused on the concept of community involvement in the management process. These guidelines address information security, disaster preparedness, and recovery planning. TJC recommends collaboration with essential community partners for staff training and exercises (Snedaker & Rima, 2014).

TJC suggests that organizations conduct at least two emergency drills per year with one community-wide drill. Accreditation standards mandate that healthcare organizations have an emergency plan that identifies potential hazards, their impact on services, and measures to handle and recover from emergencies. Accredited organizations must demonstrate a command structure, emergency-preparedness training for staff, and a mechanism to enact an emergency plan, and they must identify their role in community-wide emergencies. Hospitals respond more effectively when emergency-management standards are assigned to a high-level leadership position.

Together, TJC and HIPAA require that healthcare providers perform a BIA and crisis-management analysis, conduct employee training, implement ongoing continuity-plan reviews, plan for information-technology disasters and recovery, and audit their continuity-plan processes (Snedaker & Rima, 2014). Several other accrediting bodies require disaster plans, though their focus is personnel safety rather than information safety. There are other groups that demonstrate varying levels of interest in BCM including: the Food and Drug Administration, the Federal Emergency Management Agency (FEMA), the National Institute of Standards and Technology, the Disaster Recovery Institute International, the Bioterrorism Task Force of the Association for Professionals in Infection Control and Epidemiology, and the Bioterrorism Working Group of the Centers for Disease Control and Prevention. Recommendations from these other groups provide voluntary guidelines for better BCM that help continuity planners to achieve HIPAA and compliance with TJC.

There has been a move toward voluntary compliance with the Sarbanes-Oxley Act by not-for-profit healthcare organizations in recent years (Snedaker & Rima, 2014). The Sarbanes-Oxley Act of 2002 was enacted by the federal government as a means to legislate corporate accountability and responsibility. While it applied only to publicly traded corporations, Sarbanes-Oxley impacts the healthcare industry by increasing the demand for fiscal responsibility, accountability, and accurate financial reporting and disclosure. Voluntary compliance with Sarbanes-Oxley is widely seen as a part of enterprise-risk management and an opportunity to demonstrate good governance to the community. It requires the creation of audit functions and the presence of an expert in accounting on a corporate audit committee. Auditors must clearly see that a plan exists to protect and recover financial data. Voluntary compliance with Sarbanes-Oxley helps not-for-profit entities justify their not-for-profit status and maintain their reputation in the community. Compliance with Sarbanes-Oxley requires continuity of records.

Future Directions

Continuity planning in healthcare organizations will continue to receive greater attention for a variety of reasons as follows:

- Consumers have come to expect a level of service that requires immediate access to data.
- Wait time decreases satisfaction and can diminish quality of care.
- Healthcare organizations are catching up with other industries in understanding the business case for continuity of operations.
- Compliance will become a larger issue, particularly as more legislation and regulatory bodies require the presence of a workable continuity plan.
- More professional organizations are now focused upon various aspects of continuity planning and response to disasters.
- The creation of a national network that will allow improved monitoring of the population's health for suspicious symptoms or early onset of epidemics will make it more imperative to maintain all links in the process.

It is only a matter of time before another disaster occurs. The preparation provided by an effective business and continuity plan can minimize loss of life and data, and can support ongoing operations. Healthcare organizations must be able to effectively deal with crises. The availability of disaster-preparedness programs at schools of higher education, such as those at Penn State University and the University of North Carolina, along with certification programs by private and public organizations, such as the Association of Public Treasures of the United States and Canada, indicate the growing importance—as well as the rigors—of disaster preparedness and recovery, and business-continuity.

Summary

- Business-continuity planning is the process of ensuring the continuation of critical business services regardless of any event that may occur. It includes IT disaster planning. Continuity planning consists of several steps that are best defined as life cycle stages.
- The Department of Homeland Security recommends investing in a preparedness program. This program is built on the foundations of program management via leadership, commitment, and financial support.
- The planning stage for developing a preparedness program includes an all-hazards risk assessment and business-impact analysis. Strategies are developed to prevent, deter, and mitigate risk during the planning process.
- The implementation stage consists of resource assessments, plan writings, incident management, and employee training. The following plans are established during this stage: crisis-communications plan, business-continuity plan, and IT plan.
- The testing and exercises stage clarifies roles, reinforces knowledge, improves performance, reveals gaps, and evaluates policies, plans, and procedures.
- The program-improvement stage critiques the overall-preparedness program. Lessons learned with corrective action are documented during the program-improvement stage.
- Disasters that threaten IT operation may be natural or human-made. Continuity plans help to ensure uninterrupted operation or speedy resumption of services when

a catastrophic event occurs. The identification of information vital to daily operation is best determined through interviewing system users. The purpose, flow, recipients, need for timeliness, and implications of information unavailability must be considered in this process. Not all information used in daily operations is automated. A vital-records inventory should be conducted to identify additional information that requires protection.

- Documentation is essential to the development and successful implementation of a disaster plan. Plans must be detailed, current, and readily available to be useful.

- Careful attention to backup and storage helps ensure that information can be retrieved or restored later. Backup may be handled internally or outsourced. Commercial backup services provide transport or electronic transmission of backup media and special storage conditions until materials are needed.

- Manual alternatives to IT ensure ongoing delivery of services, although at a slower rate. Staff must receive instruction and support as they resort to manual methods.

- Restoration of information services post-disaster is not simple because backup media may be faulty and some information kept on other media is lost forever. System restoration may reload backup media stored at cold sites or resort to RBS or hot sites. Distributed processing and rapid replacement of equipment are other alternatives.

- Restoration is costly because it generally requires outside professional services, additional equipment, and extra hours from support staff. Expenses may be partially recouped through insurance coverage. Salvage of damaged records is an important aspect of recovery that is best handled by experts.

- System restarts require planning to avoid system overload as users try to catch up on work. Administrators must consider what functions should be restored first and how to integrate backup paper records with automated records. Post-disaster feedback is a major factor for the design and implementation of a better plan for future use.

- Continuity planning also needs to consider legal and regulatory requirements.

Case Study

As the clinical representative for your unit on the Disaster Planning Committee, you are charged with identifying all forms in your area that require completion of a physical vital-records inventory sheet. What forms would you list and why?

About the Author

Carolyn S. Harmon, DNP, RN-BC, is clinical assistant professor and program director for the Masters of Nursing Informatics and the Masters of Nursing Administration at University of South Carolina. Dr. Harmon received her DNP in Executive Leadership with a nursing-informatics research focus from the University of Alabama at Birmingham (2014), Masters in Nursing with a Health Systems Management specialty from Queens University of Charlotte (2003), and a Bachelor of Science in Nursing from Bluefield State College (1995). Dr. Harmon is a Board Certified Informatics Nurse, as well as a Certified Six Sigma Green Belt. She currently serves as the President-elect for the American Nurses Informatics Association.

References

Bailey, D. (2015). Business-continuity management into operational risk management: Assimilation is imminent . . . resistance is futile! *Journal of Business-Continuity & Emergency Planning, 8*(4), 290–294.

Brown, H. S. (2016). After the data breach: Managing the crisis and mitigating the impact. *Journal of Business-Continuity & Emergency Planning, 9*(4), 317–328.

Cook, J. (2015). A six-stage business-continuity and disaster recovery planning cycle. *SAM Advanced Management Journal,* 23–33, 68.

Department of Homeland Security. (n.d.). Ready, prepare, plan, stay informed. Retrieved from www.ready.gov

Department of Homeland Security. (2013). Threat and hazard identification and risk assessment guide (2nd ed.). *Comprehensive Preparedness Guide (CPG). 201,* 1–28. Retrieved from www.fema.gov/media-library-data/8ca0a9e54dc8b037a55b402b2a269e94/CPG201_htirag_2nd_edition.pdf

Dooling, J. A. (2013). It is always time to prepare for disaster. *Journal of Health Care Compliance, 15*(6), 55–56.

Jensen, J., & Thompson, S. (2016). The incident command system: A literature review. *Disasters, 40*(1), 158–182.

Kendall, K. E., & Kendall, J. E. (2014). *Systems analysis and design* (9th ed.). Boston, MA: Pearson.

Lackey, A. E., Pandey, T., Moshiri, M., Lalwani, N., Lall, C., & Bhargava, P. (2014). Productivity, part 2: Cloud storage, remote meeting tools, screencasting, speech recognition software, password managers, and online data backup. *Journal of the American College of Radiology, 11*(6), 580–588.

Lingeswara, R. (2012). Key issues, challenges and resolutions in implementing business-continuity projects. *ISACA Journal, 1,* 1–4.

Lucci, S. M., & Walsh, T. (2015). The changing face of disaster recovery. *For the Record (Great Valley Publishing Company, Inc.27*(10), 14–17.

Medina, A. (2016). Promoting a culture of disaster preparedness. *Journal of Business-Continuity & Emergency Planning, 9(3),* 281–290. Published by Henry Stewart Publications, © 2015.

Poelker, C. (2012). Don't roll the dice on data loss . . . Implement smart recovery to reduce disaster recovery costs in health care. *Health Management Technology, 33*(3), 14–15.

Public Health Emergency. (2016). Pandemic and all-hazards preparedness reauthorization act. Retrieved from www.phe.gov/Preparedness/legal/pahpa/Pages/pahpra.aspx

Sewell, J. (2016). *Informatics and nursing opportunities and challenges* (5th ed.). Philadelphia, PA: Wolters Kluwer.

Snedaker, S., & Rima, C. (2014). *Business-continuity and disaster recovery planning for IT professionals* (2nd ed.). Boston, MA: Elsevier.

Wikina, S. B. (2014). What caused the breach? An examination of use of information technology and health data breaches. *Perspectives in Health Information Management,* 1–16.

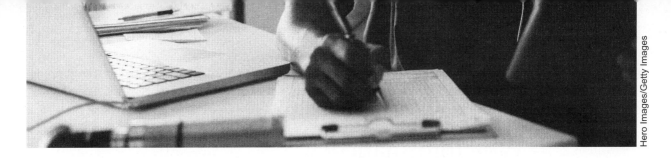

Chapter 17
Using Informatics to Educate

Diane A. Anderson, DNP, MSN, RN, CNE
Julie McAfooes, MS, RN-BC, CNE, ANEF, FAAN
Rebecca J. Sisk, PhD, RN, CNE

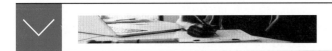

Upon completing this chapter, readers should be able to:

- Identify a variety of appropriate information-technology resources for educators.

- Discuss ways that informatics may be used to support and improve nursing education in academic and clinical locations.

- Promote learning through research, innovative strategies, and development, with a focus on student learning, supported by information technology.

- Discover new methods to meet the various educational needs of learners through the use of information technology in nursing education.

- Evaluate the impact of information technology on student engagement and teaching effectiveness.

The world of the nurse educator, just as with healthcare in general, has changed dramatically over the past few decades, from the chalkboard, overhead projector, hand-graded exams and assignments, face-to-face classrooms and phone calls, to text messages, Tweets, Snapchats, emails, online and virtual learning, and a host of other information-technology tools. Healthcare, along with nursing education, has changed dramatically. Information technology (IT) has the ability to enhance the concepts of teaching and learning. The use of IT has truly influenced the way nurses learn and care for patients safely. It has created the opportunity for nursing students to practice in virtual or simulated environments to learn and improve skills without causing harm to patients. Transforming the traditional classroom model is necessary to meet the educational needs of the next generation of nursing students. IT, in one way or another, has become a large part of our lives. As it continues to evolve, educators are challenged to integrate it into the curriculum in ways that support best teaching practices, meet quality standards, and, above all, enable the student to achieve learning and program outcomes.

In this chapter, two terms are used interchangeably: information technology (IT) and education technology (ET). Education technology refers to "resources, artifacts, tools, concepts and innovations associated with digital, that have a disruptive potential to transform or generate changes in the [educational] processes where they are used, regardless of whether these are new or old technologies" (Sosa Neira, Salinas, & de Benito Crosetti, 2017, p. 129).

Why Informatics?

What does this have to do with informatics? The Health Information Technology for Economic and Clinical Health Act (HITECH Act) strongly recommended that hospitals and healthcare providers increase the meaningful use of health information technology (HIT). Why? For one thing, it is necessary to decrease overall healthcare costs and to improve population health outcomes. In order for this to take place, healthcare personnel must be properly prepared to utilize HIT efficiently. This preparation begins with nursing education. For example, electronic health record systems (EHRS) are paramount in the healthcare environment today for data collection, collaboration, and communication. Significant errors impacting patient outcomes have long plagued the healthcare community, and IT, such as EHRS, has made strides to improve patient outcomes, assure safe delivery of care, and reduce healthcare errors (Herbert & Connors, 2016). Nursing faculty must prepare students for this environment. It is paramount that faculty are committed to the integration of informatics as well as EHRS throughout the academic process, in order to adequately prepare nursing students for clinical practice. According to Tellez (2012), major nursing, healthcare services, and national health policy organizations all recommend that "BSN curricular revisions are required to prepare nurses to meet the challenges of the 21st-century healthcare system" (p. 232). The healthcare industry has recognized the need for improved communication between IT personnel and healthcare practitioners, in order to address the issues of patient care through the creation of informatics nurse-specialist positions (Cassano, 2017). To meet the needs of nursing students today, it is essential to provide learning experiences with IT that replicates, as closely as possible, what the student will encounter in the actual clinical environment. The Institute of Medicine (IOM) suggested that integrating EHRS into nursing education can also pave the way for evidence-based nursing practice (Wyatt, Li, Indranoi, & Bell, 2012).

Preparing the Learner

Organizations, such as the American Association of Colleges of Nursing (AACN), IOM, and Quality and Safety Education of Nurses (QSEN, 2013), have encouraged schools of nursing to increase patient safety through the use of IT in nursing education. Tools can be as simple as a PowerPoint presentation, or as complex as a high-fidelity simulation. The question is, how does one utilize IT in education, when the age of learners today could conceivably range from the baby boomer to the so-called net generation? The immediate answer to this is not a simple one and is the reason that exploration of a variety of IT uses should be a priority consideration that can appeal to a wide range of learners. The students of today expect to utilize IT in all areas of their life, and this includes education as well. Let's begin by examining some of the benefits and barriers to the use of technology in nursing education.

Educational Software Sources

Educational software can provide learners with interactive experiences that may be viewed anytime and anywhere. The purpose of these tools may be to tutor learners in an endless range of topics, or to test them to determine attainment of outcomes and level of proficiency.

A software application may be sold in a variety of ways. It may be acquired as a stand-alone product, or it can come bundled with other resources as part of a learning package. Vendors may offer organizations a comprehensive solution that includes, not only the educational titles, but also the system software that can store, deliver, and track user performance.

The National League for Nursing Simulation Innovation Resource Center (NLN SIRC), at sirc.nln.org, is an excellent source of information regarding simulation products that are marketed for nursing education. Everything from injection pads to human patient simulators is listed.

Publishers are excellent places to search for software on topics that match their textbooks. Users may purchase an access code that allows them to view the software remotely, using a browser connected to the Internet.

An increasing number of vendors will provide educators with analytics that inform them of the status and progress of their learners. These diagnostic features can alert educators about which learners may have problems, allowing for early intervention that will encourage success.

A key factor to using much of today's educational software is access to the Internet. Software that streams from a remote server to the learner's device requires a reliable and sustained connection to operate smoothly. Learners who live in technologically underserved areas may find it difficult to engage in these experiences at home, and may need to seek locations such as libraries, workplaces, and businesses that offer access to the Internet.

Barriers and Benefits

Some of the challenges of utilizing IT in nursing education are the compatibilities or incompatibilities of certain products, as well as the phasing out of other products due to ever-evolving competition by IT companies. Sometimes products become outdated. Faculty may have concerns that the technology adds to their workload, contributes to alterations in faculty roles, leads to reduction in overall course quality, is not compatible with their teaching styles and values, or consumes time and resources for learning its use (Fiedler, Giddens, & North, 2014; Pereira & Wahi, 2017).

Conversely, the benefits of utilizing IT in education are many. Students who require a different type of inspiration to learn, or students who struggle with traditional education teaching methodologies, may benefit from some form of elearning. Flexibility of when and where one wishes to participate in class is an attractive benefit for many students, who can attend class via mobile phone applications, laptops, and tablet computers. Students are individuals who bring unique learning styles, life experiences, and needs to the classroom, whether it is a virtual or a traditional bricks-and-mortar location. Educational technology has the capability of bringing forth relevant and modern learning activities and opportunities for the diverse learner of today.

In an effort to facilitate student learning, educators need to develop the skills to use technology to support successful teaching and learning experiences. Additionally, choosing among various educational technologies, and applying them in a manner that results in a successful learning environment, promotes interactive collaboration, and can set the stage for lifelong learning. Integration of IT should not serve as a replacement for faculty, but rather complement a course, enhancing the faculty member's teaching style, and curriculum.

Necessary Tools

What is different about teaching with IT, rather than the traditional style that many of us grew up with? Using educational IT, along with an instructionally sound curriculum, can be a powerful synthesis of tools to aid in the engagement and successful graduation rates of online students. When faculty utilize a systematic design process to develop their online courses, learning outcomes and retention rates are at least equal to traditional or face-to-face (F2F) classroom learning environments. For nontraditional students, online courses may provide courses not otherwise available (James, Swan, & Daston, 2016). Manning-Ouelette and Black (2017) discovered that students in online courses are more engaged in deep learning than students in traditional learning settings.

Development of an online course is similar to that of a F2F classroom course, beginning with the course description, development of course objectives or outcomes, alignment with program outcomes and regulatory agencies, teaching strategies, course content development, and methods of evaluation. There is no hard and fast rule for getting started, but in general, it is essential to consider the many types of resources available. This may include support for the technology (fiscal as well as technical), student levels and learning styles compatibility with the current learning platform, and ease of integration. Other important points to ponder consist of faculty teaching preferences and limitations, pedagogical reliability, and the ability to achieve and assess outcomes. It is important to consider that it may be prudent to start out slowly: adding too many forms of IT at once in one course could end up being disastrous, as well as overwhelming for students and faculty alike. IT should complement the course, not overpower it.

Information Technology in the Classroom

Face-to-face classrooms, with the reputation of having a one-way direction of communication through lectures, can be greatly enhanced through the addition of IT (Sawang, O'Connor, & Ali, 2017). Though lecture is still an efficient way of delivering information to a larger group, going a step further—perhaps by adding an audience response system (ARS), a video, a writeable tablet device with an outline provided, or a PowerPoint presentation—may benefit students. The classroom, as well as the student, of today is very different than those from 20 or even 10 years ago, but so is healthcare, and nurse educators must rise to the challenge. Realistically, not all nurse educators are likely to pursue the use of new technologies in their classrooms. There is, now more than ever, a need for nurse educators who are creative, innovative, and who welcome the challenges of trying new technological teaching methods. Every nurse educator can use teaching methods that not only encourage learning, but also give the student the unique opportunity to be able to generate personal learning, rather than to simply sit and absorb content from faculty. The integration of information technology into the realm of nursing education allows the student the opportunity to hypothesize, problem-solve, learn the art of collaboration and respectful debate, associate the integration of nursing theory with professional nursing practice, and become an active participant in the way they learn (Oermann, 2015).

Web-Based Environments

In a 2017 systematic review of the literature, the software type of ET most frequently mentioned (52.9%) was Web 2.0 (Sosa Neira, Salinas, & de Benito Crosetti, 2017). Web 2.0 is best defined as the second generation in the development of the World Wide Web that focuses more on user collaboration, or communication, through the sharing of content, along with social networking. In other words, these web applications go beyond the display of privately viewed, individual pages, and enables a community of users to interact with the site—allowing each individual to add or update information. Facebook and Twitter are examples of web-based social-networking sites, where individuals post, update, or add to information seen by large groups of people. Web applications, such as Gmail, hosted services (Google Docs), video-sharing websites (YouTube), and wikis, such as Wikipedia, are other examples of Web 2.0 or networking technologies.

On Web 2.0's heels, is Web 3.0, also referred to as the semantic or data-driven web. In this evolution, the data is retrieved from an individual's unique web searches—the web intuitively adjusts to meet the needs of each user. In other words, if a user does a lot of searching for clothing or shoes, for example, that user will receive more advertisements related to the most frequent search parameters or combinations of items searched for most frequently. Note that a hard and fast definition of Web 3.0 is not possible, since elements and ideas are emerging continuously.

Some benefits of Web 3.0 have become reality largely due to the increasing use of smart phones and cloud applications, paving the way for the ability to access data from almost anywhere. These days, information access is not limited to the home only but wherever someone happens to be. Web 3.0 abilities continue to expand, including allowing televisions to collect user data and enabling smartphones to access data on users' computers.

Learning Management System

A learning management system (LMS) is the heart and soul of the online education system or classroom that focuses on structured partnerships between students and faculty, which typically include discussion forums and areas for submitting assignments electronically. Some of the other core components of a LMS include the ability to track and manage students, course materials, exams, announcements, email, and grading communication tools. In this LMS environment, faculty have control of what students view, the format in which they see information presented, when content becomes visible to students, and the ability to set timeframes for exams, where applicable. Having control within the LMS permits teaching faculty to be more organized and efficient in how they choose to manage or add to the course content.

Learning is most often asynchronous, requiring the learner to be diligent, self-directed, motivated, and organized, but can also be used where programs are hybrid (a mix of online and face-to-face classes) or in a F2F classroom. Offering courses in online and web-enhanced formats expands the opportunity and flexibility for those students who have either limited, or perhaps no, access to the F2F classroom, where there are specific class meeting times. The LMS (Moodle, Canvas, Schoology, and Blackboard for example) combines a collaborative style learning environment, along with additional learning tools that empower the teaching and learning process. This may include videos, voice-over PowerPoint presentations, or additional educational tools capable of bringing the course to life and adding items of interest to the content, making traditional online learning much more engaging and multidimensional.

Massive Online Open Courses

Massive online open courses (MOOC) are best defined as online courses intended to accommodate, with open and free access, an unlimited number of participants. It is thought that the role of the MOOC is to support lifelong or networked types of learning and to reach large groups of like-minded individuals. Having access to the Internet is the only prerequisite for someone to be able to sign-up and participate. Spring (2016) stated that MOOCs are often used as an opening to attract students to a school or a university, by offering some insight into what the school's tuition-based courses would have to offer them. At the very least, MOOCs do have the ability to connect large groups of people with large amounts of information. One of the benefits of a MOOC is that it has the capability of providing education to new groups of learners that include the working parent, international students who may have no access or only limited access to higher education, retired individuals, or those seeking lifelong learning. MOOCs have become a part of the regular course offerings of many universities. The concept of building a sense of community, and feeling connected, is thought to be an essential aspect of, as well as motivation for, the student's journey to success.

Multimedia and Presentation Software

Before the explosion of computers and IT, lectures may have included an easel with posters or hand-drawn diagrams for adding a visual effect for the audience. Others used manually operated projectors (a.k.a., an overhead projector) and transparent sheets overlaid with text or images to illustrate a specific concept or point they wished to emphasize. Today, PowerPoint is one of the most common presentation tools faculty use for lectures or other educational purposes. Also known as productivity software, PowerPoint runs on a computer, and assists the user in the development and enhancement of presentations. This has been a long-utilized teaching companion to a lecture, for displaying content including text, graphs, charts, videos, images, or photographs. Slides offer a visual aid for students, and faculty can make slides available either before or after the lecture as an aid for note-taking and review or for study-guide purposes. Additionally, the faculty is able to keep lectures on track, meet class time constraints, and ensure that no key points are left out of the presentation. PowerPoint is considered to have a straight-forward or linear format, as slides are displayed one after the other, and large quantities of information must be consolidated into brief bullet-point statements. Thus, PowerPoint is not the optimal modality for presentation of more complex material. Contemporary versions of PowerPoint allow presentations to be stored in the Cloud and are accessible from any location with Internet access and via any compatible devices. PowerPoint is compatible with both Mac- and Windows-based computer systems.

If Not PowerPoint, Then What?

Other presentation software includes Keynote, which is compatible with iOS or Apple products, such as iPad, iPhone, or Mac, and like PowerPoint, has a linear or slide type of format. Unfortunately, it is not currently available for Windows-based computers, but is extremely user-friendly, and, if one happens to be a die-hard Mac user, it works well with iCloud, allowing access to the information stored there from anywhere and has many intuitive, built-in animation features.

Prezi is an alternative type of presentation software that uses a map-style background and allows the presenter to tell a story by zooming in on specific components of the map, then back out again, and on to the next point of information on the map. Prezi is also Cloud-based software, allowing for better collaboration among multiple presenters, as well as easy access from any computer. Visually appealing, Prezi can be a welcome change from the traditional linear slideshow flow of a PowerPoint presentation, but it should be noted that the presentation's movement can cause queasiness for some audience members.

There are some different options in using presentation software for educational purposes. Screencasts, or video screen captures, are an excellent option when there is a need for a quick tutorial or lesson. Usually accompanied by audio, the screencast is essentially a movie, or recording, of what is happening on a faculty member's computer screen along with voice enhancement, which is then viewed by students on their devices. This is not to be confused with a screenshot, which is a single image of computer screen content. Screencasts can be viewed at a student's convenience and started, stopped, or repeated as often as desired. Other benefits include the ability to present material visually, such as key points, images, or a step-by-step process. Screencasts are one way to appeal to the visual learner, or to explain a complex concept. Numerous products exist for creating screencasts, and range from free downloads (such as Screencast-O-Matic and Jing) that offer the product with restricted capabilities, to full-version products that must be purchased. Screencasts can provide educators and students the opportunity to extend teaching and learning well beyond traditional limitations and embrace the opportunity to transform the way the information is taught, as well as how students learn.

Social Media

Communication is an important tool in any educational environment, but when used as a teaching tool, social media can be a powerful method of relaying information to a group of individuals. There are many different types of social media, with Facebook being one of the most utilized and well known. Clark (2017) explained that Facebook can be a valuable educational tool because it has the potential to inspire users to collaborate and share knowledge and experiences in a social media group setting, while targeting a specific population. For example, similar to the healthcare professional who has a Facebook group dedicated to reaching Type 1 diabetics, the nurse educator can utilize social media as a tool to get information out to nursing students, or utilize this media to deliver announcements or resources with just a click.

Social media has become an essential part of online daily activity, as social media websites and similar applications multiply. Facebook allows an individual to create a profile; choose privacy options; and upload and share photos, videos, and life events, along with a plethora of other opportunities for staying connected to a specific group or community of individuals. From a business perspective, social media can be utilized to educate, communicate, market, and promote businesses or products, and attract new, as well as stay connected to current, customers. In healthcare, social media can be an inexpensive and far-reaching tool to promote education for patients, for example, by distributing pertinent information related to a specific health condition. This provides the individual with a casual forum where they are able to ask questions, learn, share experiences and tips, or develop and build a support system with others that have similar health difficulties.

Can one Tweet contain a meaningful or powerful message in 280 characters or less? Twitter allows an individual to create a personal Twitter handle; then, using a smartphone, iPad, or computer, the person may send out messages to those who are followers, and retweet or forward messages from those the user is following. Twitter users can also follow specific sites or content, using a hashtag (#) before a keyword (#DiabetesSux or #lovemydog). A study by Waldrop and Wink (2016) found support for the use of Twitter in nursing education, and the authors suggested that, in some respects, it may not yet be utilized to its full potential. Using this technology to send out course-related information, announcements, links to current events, or additional activities for learning has been received well by students. The potential for Twitter use to send out follow-up information to the class to encourage dialog, and after-hours connection and learning from one another, are also positive considerations, which, again, reinforces the sense of community and belonging.

Other commonly used forms of social media include Instagram, a visual sharing application, where photos and videos may be shared by using a smartphone, allowing viewers to like their activity, tag others in specific photos, or leave comments. Interaction on Instagram is the same as other social networking where individual profiles are set up, and photographs posted from those followed are viewed in the follower's newsfeed and vice versa.

If social networking interests are strictly professional, LinkedIn may be the answer. Individuals interested in growing their professional network or thinking of making a job or career move, often look to LinkedIn because human resource professionals, as well as recruiters, are on LinkedIn. Professionals may collaborate with like-minded individuals who may be able to add value to their line of work, whether locally, nationally, or internationally. LinkedIn allows members to conduct polls on various topics. LinkedIn provides the opportunity for its users to blog, network, post a resume, apply for jobs, and follow specific businesses or specific interests. In other words, it is Facebook for business professionals.

Should social media be used in education? The advantages are numerous, and the opportunity for students to collaborate is a great way for the shy student to open up and post in an online forum, building confidence and encouraging participation. Students may ask a question regarding an assignment or lecture or for assistance by posting to the wall where all group members can see it, permitting all students to review the follow up responses; or they may view an announcement from faculty.

With every positive, there are also negative considerations. In a F2F classroom, the use of social media may prove to be more of a distraction to students, who use it during class time. Additionally, there is always the possibility of untrue or inappropriate information being added to the site, necessitating careful monitoring by the group administrator. There are also issues with privacy being potentially compromised; and, even with the adjustment of privacy settings, there is the possibility of reputation damage if incorrect or outdated information is posted or shared. This can be avoided if the user profile is regularly updated, relevant, and accurate.

Social media users continually connect with one another, sharing information day in and day out, linking students and educators to wonderful resources through the simple click of a mouse, or a touch screen tap. It is far more likely that faculty are the ones that need to be convinced of the value of using technology in the world of education; students have already been won over, so it makes sense to engage students in the online world where they are already very involved!

Web Conferencing

Web conferencing gives attendees an opportunity to attend online or virtual meetings over the Internet. With a computer's speakers and microphone, a connection to a meeting can be made—even while one is "on the go"—simply by making a telephone call and using a specific phone number and meeting identification code. This can be very advantageous, as individuals from multiple time zones can be connected all at once, without requiring either travel, or the need to find and book a meeting room. Attendees can also easily log into or out of the call with minimal disturbance to other meeting participants, particularly if the meeting room host has the capability of muting all in attendance, to prevent background noises and outside conversations from being audible. Some web-conferencing technology includes video conferencing capability, ideal for presenting difficult concepts, or lecturing to students, giving them a feeling of connection to faculty or peers that—particularly in an online class—makes for a stronger feeling of classroom community, as well as appealing to the visual learner. Just as there are advantages, some of the disadvantages are related to connectivity, audio or video quality, system errors, and virtual conference-room size limitations.

Web conferencing is an excellent tool for the nurse educator, allowing either synchronous or asynchronous access to classroom activities, and adding an interactive element that is appealing to different student learning styles, particularly in distance education. There are times when simply reading assigned materials is insufficient for certain types of content, making it difficult for learners to easily comprehend or keep them engaged. In the F2F classroom, a presenter can lecture to students all over the country with the use of web conferencing, allowing these students the opportunity to virtually attend a presentation that they otherwise would not have been able to. Web conferencing will no doubt continue to evolve and create new opportunities for the way that we can use it to educate our students.

Audience Response Systems

The audience response system (ARS), also referred to as student response systems, or clickers, are utilized in the classroom by using a radio frequency receiver connected to the presenter's computer, along with individual radio transmitters, which are given to every member of the audience, each with its own identifier. Typically, a PowerPoint presentation is projected, which allows the audience to view the results. Once everyone has had the opportunity to respond or "vote" on a question or poll, the ARS system then collects the audience responses, and presents a graph or aggregated data based upon the results. Some educators may consider this technology antiquated, however. Gousseau, Sommerfeld, and Gooi (2016) suggested that learners may now be engaged via their smartphones, laptops, and/or tablet technology, rather than through traditional clickers.

Issues to consider with the ARS technology include cost, safety and security, training, equipment, updates, and technical support. Additional considerations may include the anticipated types of questions that would be utilized for the ARS system, along with whether or not it would be used simply for question and answers, or individually graded questions. Either way, an ARS can enhance and promote an active and engaged learning environment, and provide quick and meaningful feedback for questions asked of learners.

Academic Electronic Health Record

Nursing education professional organizations have recognized the need for an integration of informatics in nursing programs. The AACN and the QSEN are examples of such organizations that have developed competencies, and strongly recommend that nursing students be well-prepared to access and evaluate patient information using the electronic health record systems (EHRS) used in healthcare facilities (Titzer & Swenty, 2014). School of nursing program and course objectives should be tailored to meet the Essential IV of the AACN *Essentials of Baccalaureate Education*, which addresses information management and application of patient care technology (American Association of Colleges of Nursing, 2008). The addition of technology-teaching strategies throughout the curriculum also supports the QSEN competencies, which have emphasized the importance of informatics as an area of focus.

Incentive programs have played a large part in the push to bring healthcare into the digital age. The Health Information Technology for Economic and Clinical Health (HITECH) Act of 2009 requires health care providers and organizations to implement an EHRS, demonstrate meaningful use, and validate improvements made in healthcare safety through the use of health IT (HealthIT.gov, 2016). Clearly, information technology should also be recognized as an important component in the education process, and, along with other innovative strategies, make the education process dynamic and complete.

Videos, Podcasts, and Mobile Applications

Videos have been a part of nursing education since the advent of film. Videos were typically outdated, did not always demonstrate evidence-based practice clearly, and the original intent of the video was often lost due to how distracting, outdated, and egregious the nursing techniques, errors, and behaviors were. Schools of today, however, are more apt to use a laptop and click on YouTube, or an educational website, loaded with demonstration style videos. Almost anything imaginable is available in video format, but the concern is always the authenticity and validity of the information being presented. Particularly with YouTube, faculty must review all content in that it is comprised of content that is uploaded by anyone with video capability. Today anyone with a smartphone can create and upload a video to YouTube. On the other hand, YouTube also offers some privacy settings, which limit the viewing audience and protects copyrighted material from being uploaded to other websites (YouTube help, 2017). However, copyright protection is limited and, eventually, become public domain once works lose their copyright protection. It is paramount to verify whether the material one wishes to use is indeed public domain before uploading it to a personal or educational website, or to YouTube.

YouTube, and sites of its kind, can be a beneficial and engaging learning tool for students of all generations. Options are limitless, and creativity and imagination will only continue to propel the use of this technology even further for the benefit of nursing education.

Podcasts provide another option to enhance the learning experience because the student can access and listen to recordings using an iPod, tablet, computer, smartphone, or MP3 player. A study by Marrocco, Wallace-Kazer, and Neal-Boylan (2014) concluded that "faculty and students appreciated the many positive aspects of podcasting; including the ability to create a venue for hesitant students to participate in class discussion and provide asynchronous education that spanned learning and geographic barriers" (p. 52). The video podcast is also a consideration, when an audio file is insufficient for presenting a topic that would be better explained using video in addition to the audio. These files are shared via the Internet in the form of a recorded lecture (with or without video), or an informational discussion, and students are then able to access them using their smartphones, computers, or tablets. Video podcasting is very similar to what is found on YouTube, which includes both audio and video. Podcasts alone are also an excellent way for faculty to notify students of emergency situations necessitating class cancellation, or learning-management system outages. Either way, this technology is one way to engage learners who prefer to listen to a lecture, whether F2F or online. Many of the application downloads are free and easy to use, even for the beginning podcaster. Audacity, Auphonic, and Camtasia are some examples of podcast and video podcast products that are available. It is always advisable to research compatibilities, security, and support prior to use of any downloaded app. Table 17-1 provides some technology examples used for instruction.

Table 17-1   Classroom Information-Technology Resource Examples

Commonly Utilized Technology	Examples	Website
Online learning platforms/ learning management systems	Blackboard, Canvas, Schoology, Moodle	www.blackboard.com/ https://canvas.instructure.com/ register_from_website www.schoology.com/ https://moodle.org/
Massive online open courses (MOOCs)	edX, NovoEd, Khan Academy	www.edx.org/ http://novoed.com/ www.khanacademy.org/
Multimedia and presentation software	PowerPoint, KeyNote, Prezi, Jing, Screencastomatic,	www.microsoftstore.com https://support.apple.com/keynote# https://prezi.com www.techsmith.com/jing.html https://screencast-o-matic.com/
Social media	Facebook, Twitter, Instagram, LinkedIn	https://facebook.com https://twitter.com www.instagram.com www.linkedin.com
Web/Video conferencing	WebEx, Adobe Connect, GoToMeeting, BlueJeans, Skype	www.webex.com www.adobe.com/products/adobeconnect .html www.gotomeeting.com www.bluejeans.com www.skype.com/en/
Audience response system (Clickers)	Meridia, Vistacom, Qwizdom, Polleverywhere	www.meridiaars.com/ http://vistacomusa.com/ http://qwizdom.com/us/ www.polleverywhere.com/
Academic EHR	SimChart	https://evolve.elsevier.com/education/nursing/ simchart-for-nursing/
Videos	YouTube, F.A. Davis	www.youtube.com/ http://davisplus.fadavis.com/
Podcasts	Auphonic, Audacity, Camtasia, Adobe Audition	https://auphonic.com/ https://audacity.en.softonic.com/ http://discover.techsmith.com/ camtasia-brand-desktop/ www.adobe.com/products/audition.html
Simulation	Simulation Innovation Resource Center (SIRC) Laerdal	http://sirc.nln.org/ www.laerdal.com/us/
Mobile applications	Epocrates, Skyscape Medical Resources, Pocket Lab Values, Symptomia	https://online.epocrates.com/ www.skyscape.com/ https://play.google.com/store/ apps/details?id=com.medplusapps. pocketlabvalues&hl=en http://appcircus.com/apps/symptomia
Test banks/test analysis	Examsoft, Scantron	http://learn.examsoft.com/ www.scantron.com/
Virtual learning environment	Shadow Health, Second Life, The Neighborhood	https://shadowhealth.com/ http://secondlife.com/ www.pearsonhighered.com/products-and- services/course-content-and-digital-resources/ interactive-learning-and-assessment/neighbor- hood.html
Telehealth, telepresence robots	eVisit, Doctor on Demand, TelaDoc	https://evisit.com/ www.doctorondemand.com/ www.teladoc.com/

(Continued)

Table 17-1 *(Continued)*

Commonly Utilized Technology	Examples	Website
Infographics	VisMe, Venngage, Piktochart	www.visme.co/ https://venngage.com/ https://piktochart.com/
Augmented reality	ZygoteBody, BioDigital, Anatomy4D	https://zygotebody.com/ www.biodigital.com/ http://anatomy4d.daqri.com/
Exam proctoring software	ProctorU, ProctorCam, B Virtual	www.proctoru.com/ https://home.pearsonvue.com/test-owner.aspx http://bvirtualinc.com/
Apple software/applications	Podcasts	www.apple.com/
Cloud services	Box, Sharepoint, Dropbox	www.box.com/home https://products.office.com/en-us/SharePoint/ www.dropbox.com/

Simulation and Virtual Learning Environments

The topics of simulation and virtual learning environments are covered more extensively later, but it is worth mentioning that simulations today are the descendants of the first simulation manikin, Mrs. Chase, used in schools of nursing in the early 1900s. Figure 17-1 depicts Mrs. Chase, as well as a few of the simulation manikins available today. Considered by today's standards to be a low-fidelity manikin, Mrs. Chase was utilized to teach basic nursing tasks, such as making an occupied bed, bathing, dressing, bandaging, and patient-transfer techniques. Fast forward 100 plus years to Sim Man 3G, which is capable of breathing, showing signs of arrhythmias, bleeding, and seizures, as well as exhibiting a host of neurological, cardiovascular, trauma, and wound-care symptoms. Nearly any emergency situation can be replicated in a realistic manner through the magic of simulation. The method of experiential

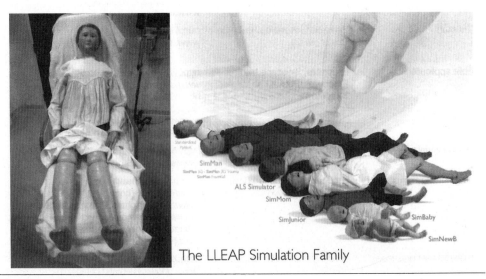

Figure 17-1 • Mrs. Chase 1911 (Hartford Courant) and Laerdal Simulation Manikins today.

SOURCE: Hartford Courant (Left); Laerdal Medical Corporation (Right)

learning is a method that allows the student to practice skills, through a hands-on style of learning, without causing harm to any patient in the process.

3-D Virtual Learning Environment

The term, virtual learning environment (VLE), has been defined broadly as "a system for delivering learning materials to students via the web" (Oxford University Press, 2016, para. 1). However, for the purpose of this chapter, virtual learning environments will refer to learning that occurs in three-dimensional (3-D) VLEs such as Second Life (SL). Ahem and Wink (2010) described SL as an "Internet-based, multiplayer virtual world designed by its residents, called avatars" (p. 225).

A virtual learning environment consists of multiple strategies that can include a computer- or Internet-based platform. It may be found with an online classroom, or interactive, asynchronous learning environments, such as Second Life or Shadow Health, which are an enhancement to the computer- and Internet-based platforms. Students using avatars are immersed in role-playing, or situational learning activities, that bring to life a circumstance that requires a response from the student. Students can role-play "in world" with Second Life, where a personal avatar is created and is capable of interacting with specific areas of the environment or other avatars. Shadow Health, creator of Digital Clinical Experiences, includes a natural language conversation engine with both speech-to-text and typing options through which the Digital Standardized Patient responds verbally to key questions that are asked by the student. At this point in time, these avatars have the capability of responding to more than 300,000 questions. Technologies such as this afford students the opportunity to interview and conduct a physical assessment of a virtual patient, while learning to formulate and organize assessment questions, respond empathetically, and provide patient education (Foronda, et.al, 2017). Figure 17-2 depicts a Shadow Health standardized patient.

3-D virtual learning environments are a form of multiuser virtual environments (MUVEs), and are especially useful when a teacher needs to design safe learning experiences that meet specific objectives (Calandra & Puvirajah, 2014). As with other forms of simulations, students can make mistakes, receive formative feedback, and improve their decision making without risking a patient's health or life.

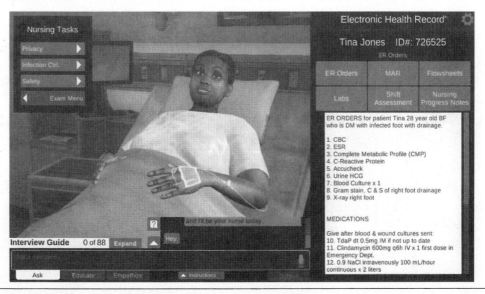

Figure 17-2 • Shadow Health Digital Clinical Experience for Health History with Digital Standardized Patient Tina Jones

Getting Started in 3-D VLE

Joining SL and designing an avatar are free, but real estate and fixtures are not. In addition to the cost of real estate, the cost of designers, programmers, and technical help staff must be considered when using 3-D VLEs. Information and advice about how educators can access resources are available on the "Second Life Wiki Education/Resources" page (2017a).

To provide a safe environment for learning, educational institutions buy SL islands and make those islands private to protect students and staff members from pesky and inappropriate "griefers" (SL users who harass other users). While selected SL public sites are available, the uninterrupted learning and the psychological safety of students should be considered. Educational and nonprofit organizations can purchase islands at a discount from Linden Labs (Second Life Wiki, 2017b) and make them private or public. For example, public islands, such as the HealthInfo Island, provide information on a variety of health issues; the American Cancer Society has a public island on SL; and a few public islands owned by colleges of nursing are also available. Getting started in SL requires patience while becoming accustomed to its features; consultation and programming by experts, and funds for purchasing private assets comprise other considerations.

Theories Applicable to 3-D VLE

UNDERLYING THEORIES

SOCIAL PRESENCE AND IMMERSION. The theories related to the 3-D VLE concern the experience participants have within the environment. Acting through avatars, participants and facilitators alike experience a sense of social presence due to immersion into the 3-D VLE (Esteve-González, Cervera, & Martínez, 2016). This immersion sets the stage for educational activities, such as group meetings or simulations, where interactions among participants and facilitators feel real. Figure 17-3 depicts a nursing student providing patient care in Second Life. Reality, or fidelity, is important in simulation design (Jeffries, Rodgers, & Adamson, 2016), but in 3-D VLEs, the reality is related to the perception of being an actual person interacting with others within the virtual environment. Beck, Fishwick, Kamhawi, Coffey, and Henderson (2011) describe a phenomenon called sentient presence, which means that

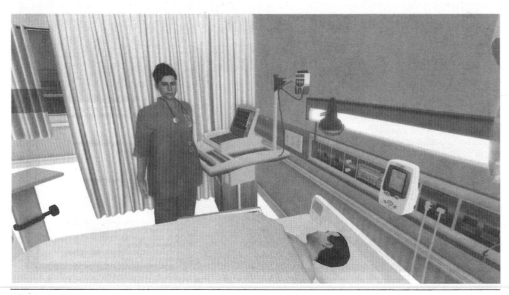

Figure 17-3 • Nursing Students Caring for a Patient in SL.
SOURCE: Prof. Rebecca J Sisk

avatars are present in the physical environment while thoughtfully interacting in a virtual society. The physical environment is enhanced by the ability of avatars to communicate and express their public personalities. This collaborative interaction results in learning, according to social constructivists (Beck et al., 2011).

SOCIAL CONSTRUCTIVISM. Since learning occurs in the interactions and tasks available in the 3-D VLE, social constructivism explains the learning that results as students work together. According to Vygotsky's social constructivist theory (1980), learning is developed by individuals as they interact with each other in a socially-constructed environment, such as Second Life. For example, Salmon, Nie, and Edirisingha (2010) investigated the learning activities of students in archeology, media and communications, and digital photography. They described a five-stage model that illustrates the process of social constructivism in their study. When this process was applied, students entered the environment and learned how to log on, name their avatars, and practice communicating and moving around. They then began interacting with each other, exploring, communicating, and working together in various activities, getting to know each other as they learned. As they began to know other students, they shared information, sought ways to network, and helped each other meet their goals. Finally, they began to understand not only what they learned, but also how they learned through their efforts to learn together. Nursing students in SL, in addition to participating in clinical simulation, can also practice various graduate-level roles in 3-D VLEs, such as in an educator, executive, or informatics role.

DESIGNING SIMULATIONS—THE NLN/JEFFRIES THEORY The NLN/Jeffries theory was designed to guide simulation experiences (Forneris & Fey, 2016). It features several concepts: the context, or place and purpose of a simulation; the background, such as goals for student learning and place in the curriculum; the design of the simulation, including its content and problem-solving elements; the experience itself; the facilitator; the educational strategies included; the participants; and the expected outcomes. Thus, within a given context, and assuming given goals for a simulation, educators ask themselves, "What content and problem-solving activities can we design, and what types of facilitation and educational strategies could we use to help students achieve the expected learning outcomes of the simulation?"

Though the literature focuses on applying this theory in bricks-and-mortar simulation labs, the same concepts and relationships can be applied in 3-D VLEs. For example, in a mental-health nursing course, students can perform a needs assessment in the home for an avatar-patient, and practice therapeutic communication. The context is the home setting, and the student goals would be to conduct a needs assessment and to speak to the patient-avatar therapeutically. In designing the simulation, one student could play the part of the patient, with a scripted set of challenges to present to another student playing the part of the nurse. The educator would give feedback to the students and lead a debriefing session to evaluate the outcomes of the simulation. The NLN/Jeffries theory provides an evidence-based tool for designing 3-D VLE simulations that is useful for planning.

Instructional Methods Used in 3-D VLEs

The literature on learning activities that can be used in 3-D VLEs is extensive. They have been categorized into four broad categories: communicating/collaborating, building/creating, exploring/processing, and role play/simulation.

COMMUNICATING/COLLABORATING A major advantage of SL is the ability to meet together, communicate, and collaborate (Ludlow & Hartley, 2016). Communication can take place through SL speakers or on telephone conference lines. Additionally, teachers and students can get together and participate in written chats, producing transcripts that can be saved, analyzed, and discussed. Avatars can instant message (IM) each other, locate each other, and teleport throughout a SL island. Organizational meetings can be conducted in SL, with avatars representing each member sitting in a virtual room together, and includes notecards for agendas, and web pages accessible through SL browsers.

Students can also participate in networking sessions or even celebrate their accomplishments. Some documented examples of communicating/collaborating include (1) a perioperative continuing education conference sponsored by the University of Texas at Arlington College of Nursing site in SL, which was designed by nursing informatics students (Baker & Brusco, 2011); (2) a journal club conducted across seven different health organizations and conducted in SL (Billingsley, Rice, Bennett, & Thibeau, 2013); and (3) nursing students practicing communication with each other to collect health histories that included potentially embarrassing content (Sweigart & Hodson-Carlton, 2013).

BUILDING/CREATING The 3-D VLE environment would be quite sterile without buildings, furniture, and various fixtures. These can be designed in place for students, or students can learn to program and set up environments that match the teaching that is anticipated. An example of this type of activity was described by Cook (2012), in a virtual pediatric primary-care clinic designed by family nurse-practitioner students. They applied a model by de Freitas and Oliver (2006) that considered the situation or context to be displayed, the pedagogy or learning activities that would be used, the characteristics of the learner, and the design needed to build such a clinic. Note that building a clinic in SL often requires staff help to build and furnish structures with required equipment. Otherwise, there is a steep learning curve for the instructor in SL.

Students can also build business plans, models, posters, and other artifacts in SL for future learners. For example, students in a teacher-education study in Second Life designed a professional development plan (Hartley, Ludlow, & Duff, 2015), and nursing students in a care-coordination simulation in SL successfully designed a patient-teaching plan for their virtual patients (Holland, Tiffany, Tilton, & Kleve, 2017). Many examples of posters designed for learning can be found through exploration of various university or nonprofit organizations, such as the University of Texas at Arlington Second Life poster exhibit, where nursing students' research posters are displayed. The exhibit can be accessed by going to this Second Life URL and signing in: http://maps.secondlife.com/secondlife/UTArlington%20III/196/197/23). Any learning objects students can create in this world, such as images, artwork, or photographs, can be left as artifacts for future learners to view or experience.

EXPLORING/EXPERIENCING SL field trips are commonly described in the literature. For example, as part of the orientation for a research course designed for graduate students in psychology, students were assigned to explore the UCLA library and other sites (Fitzsimons & Farren, 2016). Students took pictures in-world during their tours as they worked individually and in groups. Finally, they proposed research hypotheses and survey questions, thus gaining authentic experiences as researchers. Some of the advantages described by Fizsimons and Farren were the ability to help students work in groups as well as on individual assignments, and improve students' negotiation skills as they worked in groups.

Likewise, Koivisto, Multisilta, Niemi, Katajisto, and Eriksson (2016) studied the efficacy of using an experiential game in a 3-D VLE in which students applied the nursing process in caring for virtual patients. Students reported that they learned most when interviewing virtual patients and implementing interventions, providing some confirmation that clinical reasoning can be developed within 3-D VLEs. Another example of student exploration in SL was designed for community-health nursing students at the University of Wisconsin-Oshkosh (Schmidt & Stewart, 2010). Although an older study, the idea can still be applied today. The faculty used a public health department in SL to display a description of public health, its purpose, and its services. This display demonstrated various public-health activities, such as the Women, Infants, and Children (WIC) program and sanitation, as well as links to support groups in SL. Yet another example is an experience described by Reinsmith-Jones, Kibbe, Crayton, and Campbell (2015), who assigned an exploration of a model of the United States Holocaust Museum in Washington, DC, to educate social work students about the experiences of German Jews in World War II. Thinking creatively, real-world attractions can be replicated "in world" in various academic fields.

ROLE PLAY AND SIMULATION. Clinical simulations in SL are challenging because actual hands-on skills are not possible. However, students can set priorities, interview patients, and care for patient avatars based on history and physical data. Students can also try out new roles and solve problems "in world" (Esteve-González, Cervera, & Martínez, 2016) through various learning activities. This type of simulation should be carefully structured around expected learning outcomes to assure authenticity. For example, Kidd, Knisley, and Morgan (2012) used a 3-D VLE to teach undergraduate students to complete mental-status tests in a mental health course. Students successfully completed mental health assessments and health histories on virtual patients played by their instructors.

Students can also practice communication and assessment skills in a safe environment in SL. For example, Schaffer, Tiffany, Kantack, and Anderson (2016) used three scenarios in SL to provide clinical experiences in an undergraduate community-health nursing course: an airplane crash, a family health situation, and a home safety assessment. Finally, Rose (2013) described a 3-D VLE simulation in which students received a report on a patient who needed pain medication and a dressing change. After the script was played, two students worked together to develop a care plan for the patient and reflected on the simulation and what they learned.

DEVELOPING LEARNING ACTIVITIES IN 3-D VLEs Many examples of communicating/collaborating, building resources, exploring/experiencing, and role-play and simulation are described in the literature outlined previously. Other learning activities can be designed within each category, based on expected learning outcomes, by brainstorming or adapting real world assignments into "in world" activities. Some specific ideas for implementing each category of learning activity are displayed in Figure 17-4.

Communicating/ Collaborating	Building resources	Exploring/Experiencing	Role play & simulation
☐ Continuing education	☐ Research posters	☐ Virtual heart tours	☐ Scripted simulation
☐ Journal clubs	☐ Clinics	☐ Heart and lung sounds	☐ Unscripted simulation
☐ Lectures/discussions	☐ Business plans	☐ Community assessment	☐ Communications practice
☐ Faculty office hours	☐ Emergency staffing plans	☐ Disaster drill	☐ Job interviewing practice
☐ Study sessions	☐ Marketing campaigns	☐ Scavenger hunt	☐ Marketing communications practice
☐ Organizational meetings	☐ Anatomy/physiology models	☐ Observational research	

Figure 17-4 • Examples of Learning Activities Possible in 3-D VLEs

Assessment of Learning in 3-D VLEs

CHALLENGES Though younger, traditional students have been exposed to technology-based learning methods, not all students embrace applications such as SL. Their resistance is not entirely baseless—new skills need to be learned, the technology is sometimes unreliable, and some of the student computer systems may be inadequate for the task at hand. Additionally, students need to be oriented to the skills needed in SL, which takes valuable class time. Therefore, faculty members need to plan ahead and make clear expectations for their students (Hartley, Ludlow, & Duff, 2015).

STUDENT SATISFACTION VERSUS LEARNING OUTCOMES Most research conducted on teaching in SL or other 3-D VLEs has focused on student satisfaction. By far, the greatest negative feedback from students is on difficulties with the technology, including getting in and operating it, and having trouble walking or talking. However, other types of satisfaction have been measured. For example, Foronda, Lippincott, and Gattamorta (2014) found that, although students reported anxiety at the beginning of learning in SL as well as technical difficulties, they also expressed appreciation with the support provided by the instructors, and appreciation for the experience and skill-development.

Though student satisfaction is important, a satisfied student is not necessarily an educationally successful student. Whether students have actually met learning outcomes also needs to be assessed. Learning-outcome measurement in 3-D VLEs is similar to assessment in other contexts. When a 3-D VLE is used within a course, examinations, projects, and student papers can be used to assess whether students meet course or unit objectives, and to compare 3-D VLE versus onsite sections of a course. Likewise, rubrics can be used to evaluate how well students meet learning outcomes when they complete a simulation, whether live or videotaped. Other outcomes that have been used in 3-D VLE research include learning self-efficacy (Cheong, 2010; Xu, Park, & Back, 2011), student engagement (Pellas & Ioannis, 2015; Schaffer, Tiffany, Kantack, & Anderson, 2016), reflective journaling (Tandy, Vernon, & Lynch, 2016), and debriefing.

DEBRIEFING Several debriefing tools have been used for high-fidelity clinical simulation, but little has been published on debriefing specifically in SL. Some of the most common tools for debriefing in high-fidelity simulations include Debriefing Assessment for Simulation in Health-Care (DASH) ©, a tool developed by the Center for Medical Simulation (Brett-Fleegler, Rudolph, Eppich, Monuteaux, Fleegler, Cheng, & Simon, 2012), debriefing with good judgement (Rudolph, Simon, Raemer, & Eppich, 2008), debriefing for meaningful learning (DML) (Dreifuerst, 2015), and plus-delta (Decker, Lopreiato, & Patterson, 2013). Most of these models involve students reflecting upon what went well in a simulation, what did not go well, and what could be improved, while being respectful of students and other participants, and promoting critical-thinking skills through effective questioning. Since existing debriefing tools focus on high-fidelity clinical simulation, research is needed on developing debriefing tools uniquely suited to 3-D VLEs.

High-Fidelity Simulation

As the fidelity of a simulation increases, the quality of the experience increases along with the resources required to offer it. Decisions regarding the level of fidelity to offer should consider whether the return on investment of time, money, and effort are necessary. In general, the lowest level of fidelity should be chosen that will satisfy the objectives for the simulation.

When is high-fidelity simulation warranted? The National Council of State Boards of Nursing published the results of a study on the use of simulation to replace clinical experiences in 2014, and found that up to half of the clinical hours in a prelicensure program could be substituted with high-quality simulation (Hayden, Smiley, Alexander, Kardong-Edgren, & Jeffries, 2014).

Students with all types of learning styles value high-fidelity simulated experience (Tutticci, Coyer, Lewis, & Ryan, 2016). A well-designed and managed simulation can prepare them adequately for professional practice.

The complex technologies needed to conduct high-fidelity simulation are major barriers to its implementation (Al-Ghareeb & Cooper, 2016). Faculty training to increase the skill level of those managing simulated experiences, along with technical support, can reduce this problem (Doolen et al., 2016).

The design of high-fidelity simulation varies widely. Further research is needed to determine best practices for creating these experiences to achieve an optimal level of learning.

Lack of time is another frequently cited reason for the avoidance of high-fidelity simulation (Al-Ghareeb & Cooper, 2016). Strategies to address this include hiring dedicated simulation staff, which requires administrative support.

Even when there are knowledgeable and skilled staff and sound educational designs, lack of funding may limit the level of fidelity that can be realistically offered (Doolen et al., 2016). One approach to managing cost is to create regional simulation centers that serve several organizations, including colleges and healthcare institutions. Education and practice partners may collaborate on funding and operating a regional center, or outside users may pay a fee to utilize the services of the center.

Student Evaluation

Students engaged in high-fidelity simulation may be evaluated in a number of ways. One is through the use of video capture of the simulation. Video lets educators review student performance multiple times and make more accurate assessments, especially during high-stakes scenarios. Students may review their actions on video to promote self-critique. The benefits of video-assisted debriefing over standard oral debriefing when comparing performance and stress have yet to be proven (Rossignol, 2017). The extra cost and complexity of videotaping simulation should be weighed when pursuing this option.

Debriefing after Simulation

Debriefing following a simulation is a key activity that helps educators elaborate on lessons to be learned, and lets students express their understanding of the experience. Although debriefing can encompass elements of student assessment, it is not the same (Dreifuerst & Decker, 2012). Debriefing is appropriate following all types of simulation, including those that incorporate high-fidelity simulations, that may include formal evaluation along with assessment, critique, and grading. In this instance, debriefing is an opportunity to review the findings of the evaluation.

The INACSL Standards Committee has published standards of best practice regarding debriefing that describe criteria and required elements (INACSL Standards Committee, 2016). Debriefing must be conducted in a supportive learning environment by a competent person who was attentive during the simulation. The information shared during the debriefing should be based on a theoretical framework and align with the simulation's objectives and outcomes.

Technical Support for Simulation

When microcomputers first emerged in the early 1980s as teaching tools for nursing students, many educators purchased hardware and software for their new computer centers with the belief that this would revolutionize nursing education. But they were disappointed when computer-based learning was not immediately embraced. Kathleen Mikan (1980), an early pioneer in IT for nursing education, was one of the first nurse educators to notice that much of the material purchased was underutilized, explaining that the mere availability of a computer does not ensure its use. And the same holds true for each new generation of IT that has followed, including simulation, where the mere availability of simulators, trainers, manikins, and virtual environments does not ensure that educators and students will intuitively understand how to learn from them.

The role of the educator in simulation varies. Some are solely responsible for every aspect of the simulated experience, including creating the physical space, designing the instructional approach, and teaching the learners. This may be a necessity in a small school or institution where there are few staff. Most educators are supported by others who assume roles such as programming and maintenance. This allows the educator more time to focus on the pedagogical aspects of simulation, from assessing ways to integrate simulation into the curriculum, to evaluation of its effectiveness in achieving educational outcomes. Job titles for support personnel include simulation technologist, simulation coordinator, and simulation specialist. Informatics nurse specialists (INSs) often fill these roles.

Vendors who sell products may provide education and training for clients as part of the purchase agreement, or as a separate contract. Another arrangement is to sign a service agreement where the vendor will provide the clients with ongoing support via phone, email, or on-site visits to install, repair, troubleshoot, or maintain simulation products.

A review of current practices regarding simulation may reveal gaps where support is needed. Whether to have internal staff provide support, or to contract for this service, requires careful consideration of the knowledge and skills of personnel, and how best to utilize their time and efforts to learn and carry out support functions.

Certification in Simulation

Certification in healthcare simulation is still relatively new. The Society for Simulation in Healthcare (SSH) offered the first certification for healthcare simulation experts in 2011 (Rutherford-Hemming & Lioce, 2015). There is an increasing demand for verification of competency prior to employment in positions where significant resources are allocated to the design and development of simulated-learning experiences. On-the-job training is giving way to formal programs and educational degrees where simulation specialists learn industry standards for best practice, and receive external validation of their knowledge, skills, and attributes (Decker, Lopreiato, & Patterson, 2015).

Reasons to become certified include gaining professional recognition and demonstrating knowledge and skill to employers, peers, and the public. Advantages include increased networking among colleagues that will nurture the sharing of insight and experience. SSH offers three certifications: the Certified Healthcare Simulation Educator (CHSE), the Certified Healthcare Simulation Educator-Advanced (CHSE-A), and the Certified Healthcare Operations Specialist (CHSOS). The CHSE must have a minimum of a bachelor's degree and two years of continuous use of simulation in the education role (Society for Simulation in Healthcare, 2017a). The CHSE-A certification is for advanced leaders in healthcare simulation who have a master's degree and five years of experience in simulation in the education role (Society for Simulation in Healthcare, 2017b). The third certification, CHSOS, has similar requirements to the CHSE, but is also focused on the simulation operations role. All candidates must successfully pass an examination to earn any SSH certification (Society for Simulation in Healthcare, 2017c).

The workforce encompasses a growing number of simulation technicians. Training may result in awarding a certificate of attendance, but more associate degree programs are educating graduates in healthcare simulation technology to prepare them for the field (Escobar-Castillejos, Noguez, Neri, Magana, & Benes, 2016).

Future Directions

Where will informatics in education go from here? It is quite clear that the information age mindset of students today has led educators to seriously evaluate and change the ways that the teaching and learning process is delivered, and the ways in which students will learn. As information technologies evolve, they will continue to have a lasting impact on the way that the curriculum is delivered, how nursing students are taught, and how the nurses of tomorrow will begin their professional practices in a rapidly paced and continually evolving world of healthcare. Traditional methods of nursing education must also move into the twenty-first century to meet these challenges and to adequately prepare the next generation of nurses for the increasingly complex challenges they will face. The world of nursing education must keep up with technological trends and advances to enhance the curriculum and educational process as healthcare continues to rapidly change and evolve.

Summary

- Information technology can enhance teaching and learning.
- Information technology and education technology are terms used to refer to tools or resources that have the potential to transform educational processes.
- Informatics provides a means to prepare nurses for the workforce, primarily through the use of academic EHRS.
- Information technology in nursing education can be used to heighten awareness of patient safety through interactive technology and simulation.
- Technology offers tools for educators to track learning.
- Barriers to technology adoption and use in nursing education include inability to keep up with innovation, concerns over workload, and achieving a fit with the curriculum.
- Benefits to incorporating technology in education include flexibility and addressing the needs of a diverse learner population.
- Information technology should complement, not replace, instruction.
- Information technology should be part of the instructional design process.
- Web-based environments foster collaborative learning.
- Learning management systems provide a platform for online instruction.
- Massive online open courses (MOOCs) are online courses intended to accommodate—with open and free access—an unlimited number of participants.
- Presentation software goes beyond basic slide preparation to incorporate different computing platforms, nonlinear formats, collaboration, and audio.
- Social media can be used successfully to relay education, although there are risks that include distraction and inappropriate use, as well as concerns related to privacy.
- Web conferencing provides opportunities to attend online or virtual meetings over the Internet.
- Audience response systems use radio frequency receivers to engage learners in classroom activities.
- Academic electronic health records provide students with competencies needed in the workplace, including information management.
- Online tools increase the available options to produce, share, and view videos; listen to podcasts; and locate mobile applications that can enhance learning.

- Simulation and virtual learning environments provide opportunities for experiential learning in a safe environment.
- Virtual learning environments are a mechanism to deliver learning materials to students via the web, including environments such as Second Life and Shadow Health.
- Second Life is free to join, and designing an avatar is free, but real estate and fixtures are not.
- In order to ensure a safe learning environment, schools using Second Life purchase real estate that can be kept private or made public.
- Optimal use of instructional technology, including virtual reality and 3-D environments, require comprehension of underpinning theories.
- Sentient presence refers to the situation when avatars are present in the physical environment while thoughtfully interacting in a virtual society.
- Social constructivism explains the learning that results as students work together in a virtual environment.
- The NLN/Jeffries theory was designed to guide simulation experiences. Central concepts of the theory include: context, background, design, the experience itself, the facilitator, the educational strategies, participants, and expected outcomes.
- Learning activities that can be used in 3-D VLEs are extensive, but may be grouped into the following categories: Communicating/collaborating, building/creating, exploring/processing, and role play/simulation.
- Challenges to virtual learning include concerns over learning new skills, discomfort with technology, and inadequate student technology to host virtual learning.
- Debriefing, while heavily discussed in traditional simulation, has not been covered well with virtual environments.
- High-fidelity simulation can increase the quality of the experience and replace traditional clinical hours, but it is resource-intensive and requires complex technologies.
- Further research is needed to determine the best design for optimal high-fidelity simulation.
- Certification in healthcare simulation is offered by the Society for Simulation in Healthcare (SSH) and serves to demonstrate competencies to employers, peers, and the public.
- Information technology will continue to evolve and impact how nursing students are taught and prepared for the workforce.

Case Study

As a nurse educator in a prelicensure BSN nursing program, you have been asked to create a new eight-week long Complex Adult Health course using at least three different forms of educational technologies.

What might be some ways that you would accomplish this?

1. Map out course content by week and assign learning objectives for each week's content. How would the use of information technology enhance these topics?
2. With course lectures, how might information technology be integrated in order to enhance this material for optimal and straightforward learning?
3. For course assignments, how will the guidelines and rubrics be developed, and where does technology fit in?
4. Would online exams be a consideration? Reflect upon the risks and benefits of this.

Your Course Outcomes are as follows:

Upon completion of this course, the student will be able to:

1. Demonstrate the ability to aptly respond to the physiological, psychological, and spiritual needs of the adult patient with multifaceted care needs.
2. Apply assessment data obtained to plan, implement, and evaluate evidence based interventions specific to the complex health problems of the adult patient.
3. Analyze pathophysiological and pharmacological characteristics related to the nursing care of the adult patient, and design an appropriate plan of care.
4. Maximize growing confidence and independence in providing nursing care for the adult patient with complex health needs.

About the Authors

Ms Diane Anderson has been a nurse for nearly 40 years starting as a LPN, then earned her diploma from Shadyside Hospital School of Nursing, Pittsburgh, Pennsylvania, and her BSN, MSN, and DNP, from Chatham University, Pittsburgh, Pennsylvania. She has taught at diploma, RN to BSN, pre-licensure BSN, and MSN levels and now teaches in the Chamberlain College of Nursing graduate program.

Ms. Julie McAfooes is a curriculum technology manager for the online RN-to-BSN Option at the Chamberlain College of Nursing. Ms. McAfooes has been a nurse educator teaching in all types of programs. Her special interest is in uses of educational technology for interactive learning, in particular, simulation.

Dr. Rebecca Sisk has been a nurse educator for more than 35 years and has spent the last four years developing a Second Life practicum for graduate students in nursing education. Together with her students and colleagues, she has developed several simulation experiences focused on communicating and collaborating, creating various learning activities, exploring possibilities, and role playing. She teaches in the Chamberlain College of Nursing graduate programs and serves as a mentor in Second Life.

References

Ahem, N., & Wink, D. M. (2010). Virtual learning environments: Second Life. *Nurse Educator, 35*(6), 225–227.

Al-Ghareeb, A. Z., & Cooper, S. J. (2016). Review: Barriers and enablers to the use of high-fidelity patient simulation manikins in nurse education: An integrative review. *Nurse Education Today, 36,* 281–286. doi:10.1016/j.nedt.2015.08.005

American Association of Colleges of Nurses. (2008). *The essentials of baccalaureate education for professional nursing practice.* Retrieved from www.aacnnursing.org/Education-Resources/AACN-Essentials

Baker, J. D., & Brusco, J. M. (2011). Nursing education gets a Second Life. *AORN Journal, 94*(6), 499–605. doi: 10.1016/j.aorn.2011.09.004

Beck, D., Fishwick, P., Kamhawi, R., Coffey, A. J., & Henderson, J. (2011). Synthesizing presence: A multidisciplinary review of the literature. *Journal of Virtual Worlds Research, 3*(3), 3–35. https://doi.org/10.4101/jvwr.v3i3.1999

Billingsley, L., Rice, K., Bennett, M., & Thibeau, S. (2013). Using a multiuser virtual environment to facilitate nursing journal clubs. *Clinical Nurse Specialist, 27*(3), 146–154. doi: 10.1097/NUR.0b013e31828c8408

Brett-Fleegler, M., Rudolph, J., Eppich, W., Monuteaux, M., Fleegler, E., Cheng, A., & Simon, R. (2012). Debriefing assessment for simulation in healthcare: development and psychometric properties. *Simulation In Healthcare: Journal Of The Society For Simulation In Healthcare, 7*(5), 288-294. doi:10.1097/SIH.0b013e3182620228

Calandra, B., & Puvirajah, A. (2014). Teacher practice in multi user virtual environments: A fourth space. *Techtrends: Linking Research & Practice to Improve Learning, 58*(6), 29–35. doi:10.1007/s11528-014-0800-3

Cassano, C. (2017). *The right balance—Technology and patient care.* Retrieved from www.himss.org/online-journal-nursing-informatics-volume-18-number-3

Center for Medical Simulation. (2017). *Debriefing assessment for simulation in healthcare (DASH).* Retrieved from https://harvardmedsim.org/debriefing-assessment-for-simulation-in-healthcare-dash/

Cheong, D. (2010). The effects of practice teaching sessions in Second Life on the change in pre-service teachers' teaching efficacy. *Computers & Education, 55,* 868–880. doi:10.1016/j.compedu.2010.03.018

Clark, K. R. (2017). Managing multiple generations in the workplace. *Radiologic Technology, 88*(4), 379–396.

Cook, M. J. (2012). Design and initial evaluation of a virtual pediatric primary care clinic in Second Life. *Journal of the American Academy of Nurse Practitioners, 24,* 521–527. doi: 10.1111/j.1745-7599.2012.00729.x

Decker, S. I., Lopreiato, J. O., & Patterson, M. D. (2015). Certification in clinical simulations: The process, purpose, and value added. In P. R. Jeffries (Ed.). *Clinical simulations in nursing education: Advanced concepts, trends, and opportunities* (pp. 191–205). Philadelphia, PA: Wolters Kluwer Health.

de Freitas, S., & Oliver, M. (2006). How can exploratory learning with games and simulations within the curriculum be most effectively evaluated? *Computers & Education, 46*(3), 249–264. doi:10.1016/j.compedu.2005.11.007

Decker, S., Fey, M., Sideras, S., Caballero, S., Rockstraw, L., Boese, T., & Borum, J. C. (2013). Standards of best practice: Simulation standard VI: The debriefing process. *Clinical Simulation in Nursing, 9*(6), S26–S29. https://doi.org/10.1016/j.ecns.2013.04.008

Doolen, J., Mariani, B., Atz, T., Horsley, T. L., Rourke, J. O., McAfee, K., & Cross, C. L. (2016). High-fidelity simulation in undergraduate nursing education: A review of simulation reviews. *Clinical Simulation in Nursing, 12,* 290–302. doi:10.1016/j.ecns.2016.01.009

Dreifuerst, K. T., & Decker, S. I. (2012). Debriefing: An essential component for learning in simulation pedagogy. In P. R. Jeffries (Ed.). *Simulation in nursing education: From conceptualization to evaluation* (2nd ed.), (pp. 105–130). New York: National League for Nursing.

Dreifuerst, K. T. (2015). Getting Started With Debriefing for Meaningful Learning. *Clinical Simulation In Nursing, 11*(5), 268–275. doi:10.1016/j.ecns.2015.01.005

Escobar-Castillejos, D., Noguez, J., Neri, L., Magana, A., & Benes, B. (2016). A review of simulators with haptic devices for medical training. *Journal of Medical Systems, 40*(4), 1-22. doi: 10.1007/s10916-016-0459-8.

Esteve-González, V., Cervera, M. G., & Martínez, J. G. (2016). Exploring the social presence in 3D virtual learning environments. *Proceedings of the European Conference on Games Based Learning,* 977–980.

Fiedler, R., Giddens, J., & North, S. (2014). Faculty experience of a technological innovation in nursing education. *Nursing Education Perspectives, 35*(6), 387–391. doi: 10.5480/13-1188

Fitzsimons, S., & Farren, M. (2016). A brave new world: Considering the pedagogic potential of virtual world field trips (VWFTS) in initial teacher education. *International Journal for Transformative Research, 3*(1), 9–15. doi:10.1515/ijtr-2016-0002

Forneris, S. G., & Fey, M. (2016). NLN vision: Teaching with simulation. In P. Jeffries (Ed.). *The NLN Jeffries simulation theory,* (pp. 43–49). Philadelphia, PA: Wolters Kluwer.

Foronda, C. L., Alfes, C. M., Dev, P., Kleinheksel, A. J., Nelson, D. A., O'Donnell, J. M., & Samosky, J. T. (2017). Virtually nursing: Emerging technologies in nursing education. *Nurse Educator, 42*(1), 14–17. doi:10.1097/NNE.0000000000000295

Gousseau, M., Sommerfeld, C., & Gooi, A. (2016). Tips for using mobile audience response systems in medical education. *Advances in Medical Education and Practice, 7,* 647–652. doi:10.2147/AMEP.S96320

Hartley, M. D., Ludlow, B. L., & Duff, M. C. (2015). Second Life: A 3D virtual immersive environment for teacher preparation courses in a distance education program. *Rural Special Education Quarterly, 34*(3), 21–25. https://doi.org/10.1177/875687051503400305

Hayden, J. K., Smiley, R. A., Alexander, M., Kardong-Edgren, S., & Jeffries, P. R. (2014). The NCSBN national simulation study: A longitudinal, randomized, controlled study replacing clinical hours with simulation in prelicensure nursing education. *Journal of Nursing Regulation, 5*(2), supplement.

HealthIT.gov. (2016). Health IT legislation and regulations. Retrieved from www .healthit.gov/policy-researchers-implementers/meaningful-use-regulations

Herbert, V. M., & Connors, H. (2016). Integrating an academic electronic health record: Challenges and success strategies. *CIN: Computers, Informatics, Nursing, 34*(8), 345–354. doi:10.1097/CIN.0000000000000264

Holland, A. E., Tiffany, J., Tilton, K., & Kleve, M. (2017). Influence of a patient-centered care coordination clinical module on student learning: A multimethod study. *Journal of Nursing Education, 56*(1), 6–11. doi:10.3928/01484834-20161219-03

INACSL Standards Committee. (2016). INACSL standards of best practice: Simulation debriefing. *Clinical Simulation in Nursing, 12*(s), S21–S25. dx.doi.org/10.1016/j.ecns.2016.09.008

James, S., Swan, K., & Daston, C. (2016). Retention, progression and the taking of online courses. *Online Learning, 20*(2), 189–210.

Jeffries, P., Rodgers, B., & Adamson, K. A. (2015). NLN Jeffries Simulation Theory: Brief narrative description. *Nursing Education Perspectives, 36*(5), 292–293.

Kidd, L. I., Knisley, S. J., & Morgan, K. I. (2012). Effectiveness of a Second Life simulation as a teaching strategy for undergraduate mental health nursing students. *Journal of Psychosocial Nursing, 50,* 28–37. doi:10.3928/02793695-20120605-04

Koivisto, J. M., Multisilta, J., Niemi, H., Katajisto, J., & Eriksson, E. (2016). Learning by playing: A cross-sectional descriptive study of nursing students' experiences of learning clinical reasoning. *Nurse Education Today, 45,* 22–28. doi:10.1016/j.nedt.2016.06.009

Ludlow, B. L., & Hartley, M. D. (2016). Using Second Life for situated and active learning in teacher education. In D. H. Choi, A. Diley-Hebert, & J. S. Estes (Eds.), *Emerging Tools and Applications of Virtual Reality in Education,* pp. 96–120. Morgantown, WV: West Virginia University Press.

Manning-Ouellette, A., & Black, K. M. (2017). Learning leadership: A qualitative study on the differences of student learning in online versus traditional courses in a leadership studies program. *Journal of Leadership Education, 16*(2), 59. doi:10.12806/V16/I2/R4

Marrocco, G. F., Wallace-Kazer, M., & Neal-Boylan, L. (2014). Transformational learning in graduate nurse education through podcasting. *Nursing Education Perspectives, 35*(1), 49–53 Published by National League for Nursing, Inc., © 2014. doi:10.5480/10-421.1

Mikan, K. (1980). Learning Resources Center Conference: Proceedings and evaluation. Bethesda, MD: National Library of Medicine.

Oermann, M. (2015). Technology and teaching innovations in nursing education: Engaging the student. *Nurse Educator, 40*(2), 55–56. doi:10.1097/NNE.0000000000000139

Oxford University Press. (2016). *Learn about virtual learning environment/Course management system content* © 2014. Retrieved from http://global.oup.com/uk/orc/learnvle

Pellas, N., & Ioannis, K. On (2015) the value of Second Life for students' engagement in blended and online courses: A comparative study from the higher education in Greece. *Education and Information Technologies, 20*(3), 445–466. doi:10.1007/s10639-013-9294-4

Pereira, A. S., & Wahi, M. M. (2017). Course management system's compatibility with teaching style influences willingness to complete training. *Online Learning, 21*(1), 36–59. doi: 10.24059/olj.v21i1.763

Quality and Safety Education for Nurses (QSEN). (2013). Pre-licensure knowledge, skills and attitudes. Retrieved from http://qsen.org/ competencies/pre-licensure-ksas/#informatics

Reinsmith-Jones, K., Kibbe, S., Crayton, T., & Campbell, E. (2015). Use of Second Life in social work education: Virtual world experiences and their effect on students. *Journal of Social Work Education, 51*, 90–108. doi: 10.1080/10437797.2015.977167

Rose, D. (2013). I've heard report, now what do I do? Avatars prepare novice students for patient handoffs. *Nurse Educator, 38*(2), 54–55. doi:10.1097/NNE.0b013e31828299d1

Rossignol, M. (2017). Effects of video-assisted debriefing compared with standard oral debriefing. *Clinical Simulation in Nursing, 13*(4), 145–153. https://doi.org/10.1016/j.ecns.2016.12.001

Rudolph, J., Simon, R., Raemer, D., & Eppich, W. (2008). Debriefing as formative assessment: Closing performance gaps in medical education. *Academic Emergency Medicine, 15*(11), 1010–1016. doi: 10.111/j.1553-2712.2008.00248.x

Rutherford-Hemming, T., & Lioce, L. (2015). Certified simulation healthcare educators: Descriptive exploratory analysis using survey research. *Clinical Simulation in Nursing, 11*, 222–227. https://doi.org/10.1016/j.ecns.2015.02.001

Salmon, G., Nie, M., & Edirisingha, P. (2010). Developing a five-stage model of learning in Second Life. *Educational Research, 52*(2), 169–182. https://doi.org/10.1080/00131881.2010.482744

Sawang, S., O'Connor, P., & Ali, M. (2017). Using technology to enhance students' engagement in a large classroom. *Journal of Learning Design, 10*(1), 11–19.

Schaffer, M. A., Tiffany, J. M., Kantack, K., & Anderson, L. J. (2016). Second Life® virtual learning in public health nursing. *Journal of Nursing Education, 55*(9), 536–540. doi: 10.3928/01484834-20160816-09.

Schmidt, B., & Stewart, S. (2010). Implementing the virtual world of Second Life into community nursing theory and clinical courses. *Nurse Educator, 35*(2), 74–78. doi: 10.1097/NNE.0b013e3181ced999

Second Life Wiki. (2017a). Linden Lab Official: Education and nonprofit discount terms and conditions. Retrieved from http://wiki.secondlife.com/w/index.php?title=Linden_Lab_Official:Education_and_Non-Profit_Discount_Terms_and_Conditions&printable=yes

Second Life Wiki. (2017b). Second Life Education/Resources. Retrieved from http://wiki.secondlife.com/wiki/Second_Life_Education/Resources

Society for Simulation in Healthcare. (2017a). CHSE. Retrieved from www.ssih.org/
Certification/CHSE

Society for Simulation in Healthcare. (2017b). CHSE-A. Retrieved from www.ssih
.org/Certification/CHSE-A

Society for Simulation in Healthcare. (2017c). CHSOS. Retrieved from www.ssih
.org/Certification/CHSOS

Sosa Neira, E. A., Salinas, J., & de Benito Crosetti, B. (2017). Emerging technologies
(ETs) in education: A systematic review of the literature published between 2006 and
2016. *International Journal of Emerging Technologies in Learning, 12*(5), 128–149 © 2017.
doi:10.3991/ijet.v12i05.6939

Spring, H. (2016). Online learning: The brave new world of massive open online courses
and the role of the health librarian. *Health Information & Libraries Journal, 33*, 84–88.
doi: 10.1111/hir.12134

Sweigart, L., & Hodson-Carlton, K. (2013). Improving student interview skills. The virtual
avatar as client. *Nurse Educator, 8*(1), 11–15. doi: 10.1097/NNE.0b013e318276df2d

Tandy, C., Vernon, R., & Lynch, D. (2016). Teaching note—Teaching student interviewing
competencies through Second Life. *Journal of Social Work Education, 53*(1), 66–71.

Tellez, M. (2012). Nursing informatics education: Past, present, and future. *Computers,
Informatics, Nursing*, 229–233. doi:10.1097/NXN.0b013e3182569f42

Titzer, J., & Swenty, C. (2014). Integrating an academic electronic health record in a nursing
program creating a sense of urgency and sustaining change. *Nurse Educator, 39*(5), 212–213.
doi: 10.1097/NNE.0000000000000064

Tutticci, N., Coyer, F., Lewis, P. A., & Ryan, M. (2016). High-fidelity simulation: Descriptive
analysis of student learning styles. *Clinical Simulation in Nursing, 12*, 511–521.
doi:10.1016/j.ecns.2016.07.008

Vygotsky, L. S. (1980). *Mind in society: The development of higher psychological processes.*
Cambridge, MA: Harvard University Press.

Waldrop, J., & Wink, D. (2016). Twitter: An application to encourage information
seeking among nursing students. *Nurse Educator, 41*(3), 160–163. doi:0.1097/
NNE.0000000000000235

Wyatt, T. H., Li, X., Indranoi, C., & Bell, M. (2012). Developing iCare v. 1.0: An academic
electronic health record. *Computers, Informatics, Nursing, 30*(6), 321–329. doi: 10.1097/
NXN.0b013e31824af81f

YouTube help. (2017). Frequently asked copyright information. Retrieved from YouTube
https://support.google.com/youtube/answer/2797449

Xu, Y., Park, H., & Back, Y. (2011). A new approach toward digital storytelling: An activity
focused on writing self-efficacy in a virtual learning environment. *Educational Technology
& Society, 14*(4), 181–191.

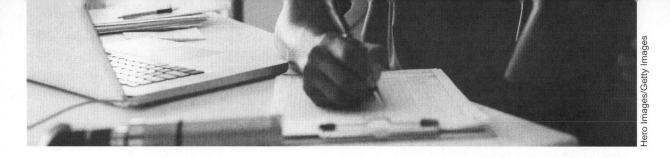

Chapter 18
Consumer Health Informatics

Melody Rose, DNP, RN
Toni Hebda, PhD, RN-BC, MSIS, CNE

 ## Learning Objectives

After completing this chapter, you should be able to:

- Distinguish between consumer health informatics and other subspecialties of healthcare informatics.

- Recognize driving factors behind the development of consumer health informatics.

- Discuss issues associated with consumer health informatics that can negatively impact access to care or ability to self-manage care.

- Examine ways that consumer health informatics is changing how health advice and care are sought and delivered.

- Distinguish key features, advantages, and disadvantages of various consumer health informatics applications.

- Provide recommendations for consumer evaluation of online information.

- Examine the informaticist role in the design, adoption, and use of consumer health informatics applications.

- Explore future directions for consumer health informatics.

Consumer health informatics (CHI) is a field within health informatics devoted to the consumer, or patient, view. According to the American Medical Informatics Association (2017, Para. 1), CHI concentrates on the "information structures and processes that empower consumers to manage their own health" citing health information literacy, easy-to-understand language, personal health records, and Internet-based strategies and resources as examples of those structures and processes. **eHealth**, which delivers health information and services through information technology (IT), falls under CHI (Hogan et al., 2014). In the current model of health informatics, the focus has shifted from provider to consumer (Wiesner, Griebel, Becker, & Pobiruchin, 2016). In comparison, the patient is emphasized within clinical informatics, and the community in public health informatics (Mancuso & Myneni, 2016). The emphasis upon the consumer differentiates CHI from its parent discipline and other branches of health informatics.

Edelstein noted that healthcare reform cannot be fully achieved without an expanded view of who is responsible for health and healthcare and that "dramatic and sustainable improvement in the quality and cost efficiency of our healthcare" is contingent upon a significant percentage of the population accepting ownership or responsibility for their own health (2016, p. 10). CHI plays a role in reform because it can empower patients, and improve patient engagement and shared decision making (SDM). Patient engagement is associated with improved outcomes, satisfaction, and compliance with treatment regimens. Engagement is contingent upon consumers' ability to access, understand, and manage personal health information (Hogan et al., 2014; Institute of Medicine, 2013; Demiris, 2016) This chapter examines the evolution of CHI, associated issues, the relationship between patient engagement and CHI, exemplars of CHI, the role of the informatics nurse with CHI, and future applications.

Evolution

CHI emerged 20 years ago as a way to assess the quality and validity of written health information, and then grew to encompass the online world inclusive of social media and SDM (Demiris, 2016; Flaherty, Hoffman-Goetz, & Arocha, 2015). According to CHI pioneer Gunther Eysenbach (2000), consumerism, evidence-based medicine, and a paradigm shift from clinical medicine in the Industrial Age toward public health in the Information Age influenced the development of CHI. Today, online health information quality is even more important because the Internet serves as a major information source for consumers, as well as a means to communicate with their providers and each other (Mancuso & Myneni, 2016). Yet, not all online information is created equal in terms of quality, and not all consumers possess the skills to identify quality information. Both situations are cause for concern because healthcare decisions based upon inaccurate or outdated materials are flawed. Attributes associated with quality information are listed in Box 18-1.

Box 18-1   Attributes of Quality Information

- **Timely:** Available when it is needed.
- **Precise:** Each detail is complete and clear.
- **Accurate:** Without error.
- **Numerically quantifiable:** Can be measured.
- **Verifiable by independent means:** More than one source provides the same or similar information.
- **Rapidly and easily available:** Can be located in a reasonable amount of time.
- **Free from bias or modifications with the intent to influence:** Information is not posted to generate profits.
- **Comprehensive:** Required details are present.
- **Appropriate to the user's needs:** Different users have different data needs. The appropriate data must be available for each user.
- **Clear:** Free from ambiguity, reducing the likelihood of misinterpretation, and at a level that can be understood.
- **Reliable:** Comes from a trusted source or can be independently replicated.
- **Current:** Most recent, prevalent, and/or accepted.
- **Convenient form for interpretation and use:** The user must be able to access and use the data without difficulty.

CHI is also transforming the dynamics of the consumer-provider relationship and healthcare culture from a paternalistic relationship—where the physician dispensed advice—to a situation where consumers come informed to appointments and expect to actively participate in the treatment plan (Borycki et al., 2011). A systematic review of research on patients' online health information seeking, covering the period between 2000 and 2015, and the impact on the provider-patient relationship, suggested that online health information-seeking behaviors could improve the provider-patient relationship, assuming that patients discussed the information with their provider (Tan & Goonawardene, 2017). Discussion provides the opportunity to determine the source and overall quality of information that consumers find, and provides an opportunity to direct consumers to better sources when indicated.

Driving Forces

A series of reports from the Institute of Medicine, including *Best Care at Lower Cost* (Institute of Medicine, 2013), called for patient engagement as key to US healthcare system reform. Engaged consumers are a critical factor in achieving successful healthcare outcomes (Mancuso & Myneni, 2016). Engaged consumers collaborate with providers, receive information related to the management of their health and conditions, and share in decisions related to their care (Singh et al., 2016).

Federal initiatives within the United States, such as meaningful use and patient-centered medical homes, provide incentives for the development of electronic patient portals to improve data sharing and communication with healthcare consumers, with the idea that access will help to educate and empower consumers (Ancker, Miller, Patel, & Kaushal, 2014; Demiris, 2016). In addition to government initiatives and rising consumerism, the push for healthcare consumer empowerment comes from groups, such as eHealth Initiative, which draws membership from executives across the healthcare-delivery industry committed to reforming the system (eHealth Initiative, 2017; Smith, 2016).

CHI continues to grow and evolve as emerging trends, such precision medicine and a sharing society, introduce both new opportunities and challenges (Demiris, 2016). A shift to care in the community with a need for increased self-management with the use of remote monitoring systems, personal health records (PHRs), decision support, and online health communities comprise some of the many other factors driving the further development of CHI (Valdez, Holden, Novack, & Veinot, 2015).

Issues

Several impediments to the full adoption and best use of CHI have been identified. These include a lack of consensus on what comprises CHI, literacy issues, inequities with access to online applications, varying levels of patient engagement, and persistent societal attitudes when it comes to healthcare delivery.

Unclear CHI Expectations

Despite the 2017 definition provided by the American Medical Informatics Association (AMIA), a systematic review of published definitions prior to that definition found no widely accepted definition for CHI (Flaherty et al., 2015). This situation, and the relative newness of CHI, has made it difficult to identify or develop core competencies for healthcare professionals needed to understand their roles.

Literacy and Information: Computer, Health, and eHealth Literacy

When discussing CHI, it is important to discuss literacy, as well as information, computer, health, and eHealth literacy. **Literacy** is the ability to read and write, but it is more than the mechanics of being able to sound out words or reproduce script. Central to the concept of literacy is the ability to process and critique meaning using reading, writing, and oral language within a specific context (Frankel, Becker, Rowe, & Pearson, 2016). An individual may be highly educated, but not literate in the dominant language of a setting, as may be seen when travelling abroad. Another example is seen with the individual who exhibits either cognitive limitations or is unable to read and write. Both situations require special measures to assure meaningful communication, whether that entails the services of a translator, printed materials in the consumer's native language, or reliance upon diagrams and demonstrations instead of printed materials.

Closely aligned to the concept of literacy is **information literacy**, which is the process of knowing when specific information is needed, why it is important, and then being able to locate it, evaluate it, and apply it (Sonya, 2014; Saranto & Hovenga, 2004). This definition remains in common use, although the Association of College and Research Libraries (ACRL) in its publication, *Framework for Information Literacy for Higher Education* (2016, p. 3), updated the definition to "the set of integrated abilities encompassing the reflective discovery of information, the understanding of how information is produced and valued, and the use of information in creating new knowledge and participating ethically in communities of learning." The ACRL definition presumes the creation of new knowledge in using information, and the application of ethics over previous definitions.

Definitions for **computer literacy** vary from the simple ability to use a computer for an express purpose, such as information retrieval, communication, or solving a problem, to definitions that require comprehension of the economic, psychological, and social effects of computers on the individual and society (Gürdaş Topkaya & Kaya, 2015). As may be inferred, computer literacy supports information literacy. The term **digital literacy** may be used interchangeably with computer literacy, although it refers to the use of computer technology and smartphones to read and interpret media, reproduce data and images, and evaluate and apply knowledge gained through exploration of the digital world (US Digital Literacy, 2016).

Health literacy enables consumers to directly interact with a complex health system to better manage their own health. In a definition still used today, the *National Action Plan to Improve Health Literacy* stated that health literacy is "the degree to which individuals have the capacity to obtain, process, and understand basic health information and services needed to make appropriate health decisions" (Department of Health and Human Services, Office of Disease Prevention and Health Promotion, 2010). Language in Title V of the Patient Protection and Affordable Care Act (P.L. 111148) of 2010 amended the definition to read, "the degree to which an individual has the capacity to obtain, communicate, process, and understand basic health information and services in order to make appropriate health decisions" noting that consumers must also be able to express their needs and preferences, and respond to information and services provided to them (Centers for Disease Control and Prevention, 2016). High levels of health literacy can enable informed decision-making, but motivation and willingness to change behavior must also be present (Valdez, Holden, Novak, & Veinot, 2015). Low levels of health literacy are associated with decreased compliance with prescribed treatment and poorer health outcomes (Jacobs, Caballero, Ownby, & Kane, 2014; Zuzelo, 2016). This presents a major concern with populations, such as the elderly, who are most impacted by chronic diseases. Using data from the Health and Retirement Study—a longitudinal survey of a nationally representative sample of older Americans—found that only 9.7% of persons 65 years of age and older with low health literacy used health information obtained online, compared to 31.9% of those with adequate health literacy (Levy, Janke, & Langa, 2015).

eHealth literacy is the ability to use electronic sources to search for, find, comprehend, and evaluate information and images found online, and apply knowledge acquired to address or solve a health issue (Hayat, Brainin, & Neeter, 2017). eHealth literacy brings with it an increased awareness of risks associated with unreliable online information, as well as the capability to make better decisions (Hayat et al., 2017; Vâjâean & Băban, 2015). The eHealth Literacy Scale (eHEALS) is a tool that measures eHealth literacy (Sudbury-Rile, FitzPatrick, & Schultz, 2017). eHEALS has an important place, particularly among populations that are not digital natives. The ability to find, comprehend, create, evaluate, and use images is known as visual literacy (Emanuel & Challons-Lipton, 2013; Yan, 2015).

Although distinct, the concepts of information, computer, and health literacy have become intertwined over time, largely because we rely upon computer and IT processes to locate information. By definition, eHealth requires elements from both computer and health literacy.

Locating and evaluating healthcare information has become more complex with the exponential growth in the volume and availability of information. Consumers can access a wide range of resources that have the potential to inform their healthcare decisions and promote a greater responsibility for self-care. While there is agreement that the Internet provides easier access to information, clinicians express concern that poor quality information can undermine informed decision-making (Usher, Gudes, & Parekh, 2016). Mounting concerns about quality, timeliness, and potential misinterpretation of online information have driven the development of a national and international quality standards agenda to help professionals and consumers alike access and evaluate online health information that is accurate, current, valid, appropriate, intelligible, and free of bias. One organization that emerged to address these concerns was the Health on the Net (HON) Foundation. HON (2016) is a nonprofit, nongovernmental organization, accredited by the Economic and Social Council of the United Nations that provides a process for approval of websites. HON provides a set of rules to hold web developers to basic, ethical standards in the presentation of material, and to help readers know the source and purpose of the data they are reading. Certified sites display a seal to indicate adherence with established principles, but HON does not rate the quality of information displayed. The HON seal contains the date of certification or indication that the site is either under reexamination, or was once certified but is no longer in compliance with HON principles. HON also provides downloads for Chrome, Internet Explorer, and Firefox browser toolbars that automatically check the certification of the site viewed, displaying the seal for compliant websites. Other initiatives include application of codes of conduct from sponsoring organizations, user guides, external certification, and quality filters (Nădăşan, 2016).

Discriminating between evidence-based and commercial information can be difficult. Many reputable Internet-based healthcare resources and websites, including commercial and other privately developed websites, meet the HON and other quality standards such as those put forth by the American Medical Association (AMA) (Nădăşan, 2016).

Statistics vary on how many individuals seek health information online, as well as the search methods used and whether information was verified with providers. Results from the 2011 National Health Interview Study reported that approximately one-half of the participants used chat rooms or Internet searches to locate health information online

(Amante, Hogan, Pagoto, English, & Lapane, 2015). A national survey in 2012 by the Pew Institute reported that 72% of adult Internet users searched for health information online (Fox & Duggan, 2013). Cheng and Dunn (2015) found that almost 80% of Internet users in Australia sought health information online. Another study found 98% of the parents surveyed reported using the Internet to search for information about their child's health, with 80% starting with a public search engine, and less than 20% starting their search on university or hospital websites (Pehora et al., 2015). Only one-half of those respondents verified the information they found with a provider, despite the fact that only 24% thought that public search engines provided safe, reliable information.

In summary, the widespread availability and use of online healthcare resources by consumers have both benefits and disadvantages. Standards must be in place to prevent the propagation of inaccurate or outdated online health information. Improving eHealth literacy among consumers can also help them to make decisions using quality information.

Bridging the Digital Divide

The disparity in access to IT tools and electronic healthcare resources is commonly referred to as the "digital divide" (van Deursen & van Dijk, 2015). In recent years, researchers have come to recognize that, in addition to whether a population has, or does not have, access to the Internet, there are other issues that contribute to the divide, including inequities in skills and usage. The digital divide becomes more critical as the amount and variety of online health resources increase, and as consumers need more sophisticated skills to use them and the information contained in their electronic health record (EHR). Equitably distributed online healthcare resources, skill in using these resources, and a robust telecommunications infrastructure can help close the digital divide and meet the overarching goal first set by *Healthy People 2010* to eliminate health disparities that remains relevant today (*Healthy People*, n.d.). *Healthy People* is a US initiative that establishes and monitors attainment of science-based population health goals and objectives with ten-year target dates (Centers for Disease Control and Prevention, 2017). *Healthy People* objectives are developed with input from the public.

To understand the importance of closing this divide, consider the impact of widespread access to interactive multimedia healthcare resources. The merging of media (computers, telephones, television, radio, video, print, and audio) and the evolution of the Internet have created a nearly universally networked telecommunication infrastructure. This infrastructure facilitates access to an expanse of health information and health-related services by extending the reach of health communication delivery. Rapidly rising smartphone ownership contributes to Internet access (Poushter, 2016). The Internet increases communication choices available for health practitioners to reach consumers, and for consumers to interact with providers and each other via online discussion groups. Yet, in a 2011 European study, the number of individuals impacted by chronic diseases over the age of 50 with Internet access varied from less than 20 to 53% in some regions, negatively impacting the ability to disseminate information and monitor health status (Romano et al., 2015). A 2016 Pew Research Center survey found that 42% of adults aged 65 and older owned smartphones, 67% used the Internet, and slightly more than one-half had broadband access, but fewer senior citizens were confident with their digital skills, and approximately one-fourth reported physical issues that could negatively impact their ability to get online (Anderson & Perrin, 2017).

Despite a rise in access to these technologies, their availability is not ubiquitous. Often, individuals who are the most vulnerable have the least access to information, communication technologies, healthcare, and supporting social services. For example, a 2016 survey found that more than 90% of lower income American families had Internet access, but only via mobile devices or older computers with slower connection speeds that negatively impacted their access to information (Rideout & Katz, 2016). A review of 31 studies conducted between 2005 and 2012 concluded that health information computer kiosks placed in clinical and community settings could help address these access problems (Joshi & Trout, 2014). The digital divide and poor health literacy limit the ability to achieve the potential of CHI (Demris, 2016).

Patient Engagement

Patient engagement is a concept that everyone agrees is important, although its definitions have varied over the years, as was noted in the National eHealth Collaborative's 2012 NeHC Stakeholder Survey (Patient Engagement, 2012). Some survey participants felt that the term referred to patients taking a more active role in planning their care while others thought that it referred to improved access to health information and education. Stage 2 of the Centers for Medicare and Medicaid Services' Meaningful Use EHR Incentive Program helped to put patient engagement in the spotlight with its introduction of patient-centric initiatives, which included online record access, the ability to communicate with providers via portals, and increased exposure to personalized health education (Esposito, 2016). In keeping with that focus, the Healthcare Information and Management Systems Society (HIMSS) (2017, Para. 1) stated that patient engagement is the ongoing, constructive communication "between patient and practitioner" that, within health IT, is driven by patient portals, secure messaging, mobile applications, and consumer-generated health data.

Patient engagement is associated with a better overall healthcare experience, increased satisfaction with care and quality of life, better medical adherence, and potentially lower costs (Hogan et al., 2014; IOM, 2013; Singh et al., 2016). In their review of literature, Singh et al. (2016) noted that self-management of chronic disease and promotion of patient engagement were key to successful care management for populations with high needs and high costs, and also served to decrease hospital use. Engagement requires the ability to access and manage one's personal health information, but is not in of itself a guarantee of participation in SDM. Engagement and self-management do not just happen; active efforts to educate and provide interventions that enhance consumer ability to monitor/manage their information and their health are needed, and consumers must assume accountability for their health and healthcare decisions (Edelstein, 2016). Healthcare providers can use evidence-based tools, such as the Patient Activation Measure (PAM), to measure engagement and allocate staff, money, and time resources accordingly (Edelstein, 2016). PAM is a 13-question validated survey-style tool that has been used in more than 20 countries and in different languages that places respondents into one of four levels:

- Disengaged and overwhelmed.
- Increasing awareness but struggling.
- Taking charge.
- Maintaining behaviors and pushing further.

Engaged healthcare consumers demonstrate a greater level of high-value behaviors to promote and maintain health, such as seeking information and services and practicing a healthy lifestyle, with the benefit for providers of improved outcomes at lower cost. On the other end of the scale, limited health literacy and the digital divide negatively impact engagement and SDM (Demiris, 2016).

SDM is an active process that requires comprehension of treatment options, the ability to evaluate potential benefits and harms, and mutual respect between patients and providers. SDM is associated with increased patient satisfaction and, sometimes, improved health outcomes (Qing et al., 2016). Tools, known as decision aids, have been developed to provide balanced information and facilitate SDM (Institute of Medicine, 2013). Decision aids can improve knowledge of treatment options, value-based decision making, accuracy of healthcare consumer perception of risks and benefits, increase participation, and reduce decision conflict (Hoffman et al., 2014). Qing et al. (2016) detailed efforts to develop a prototype tool called "Hearts Like Mine" (HLM), using electronic health record system (EHRS) data to personalize information on potential treatment outcomes for patients. The sample size was small, but participants reported a high level of confidence with their decisions. In another example, Kukafka et al. (2015) designed a web-based decision aid, RealRisks, to improve preference-based decision making for breast cancer prevention in women with low numeracy. Significant improvement in the accuracy of perceived breast cancer risk was found after exposure to the decision aid.

Changing Healthcare Delivery Models

Successful attainment of healthcare reform with patient-centered care requires SDM where consumers and healthcare providers collaborate to make treatment decisions and manage care (Institute of Medicine, 2013; Borycki et al., 2011). With SDM, patients bring their past experiences, preferences, and perspectives on healthcare, while healthcare providers bring research evidence and clinical expertise to the equation, resulting in an exchange of information, further communication, and treatment decisions. In order for consumers to engage in SDM, they must feel empowered. CHI not only provides important changes in the way that both providers and patients obtain information and communicate to support decision making, but it is also necessary to create a healthcare delivery system that supports cooperation, because self-care management requires cooperation with providers (Jung, 2016).

Consumer Health Informatics Applications

CHI provides structures and processes that allow consumers to track their health status and participate in treatment and prevention activities (Flaherty et al., 2015; Laxman, Banu Krishnan, & Dhillon, 2015; Nădăşan, 2016). Common applications include education, health games, telehealth, mHealth, personal health records or portals, and social media. Some examples of targeted applications have included smoking cessation, suicide prevention, and provision of cancer information (Flaherty et al., 2015). Barriers to the use of these applications can be grouped into system- and individual-level barriers. System-level barriers include technology-related issues, such as a lack of compatibility with legacy computer systems, usability, workflow, security, and reimbursement, while individual-level barriers may involve either the consumer or healthcare provider and will be discussed further under each application. The sheer number of CHI applications is overwhelming. The HealthIT. gov website (2016) provides information for consumers on personal wellness devices, wellness applications or apps, and other resources for wellness information, along with some exemplars.

Education

The Internet provides widespread access to information surpassing reliance upon print, television and radio in terms of influence and approaching the influence of physician advice for health decisions (Smith, 2016). Online health information is often seen as more up-to-date, quicker, and easier to access than other media; offers anonymity; and may be trusted and used more often in lieu of an intervention with a healthcare provider (Walsh, Hamilton, White, & Hyde, 2015). According to the Pew Research Center, 59% of American adults have looked online to find health information (Nădăşan, 2016). Bratucu et al. (2014) noted that consumers found online information helpful in understanding their symptoms and treatments, so that they could more readily engage in medical decision making—although, information alone does not guarantee that healthy behaviors will result. Using a nationally representative dataset, Shneyderman et al. (2016) found that people who sought health and cancer information on the Internet were more likely to follow cancer screening guidelines. Research has shown differences in health information seeking behaviors by educational level, age, and economic status. In their review of data from the Program for the International Assessment of Adult Competencies (PIACC) Feinberg et al. (2016) noted that adults without high school diplomas tended to rely upon advice from others, while adults with high school diplomas used more text-based sources, and Internet users were more likely to report a good to excellent health status. Usher, Gudes, and Parekh (2016) found extensive use of technology for health information, along with positive changes in behaviors in their study of Australian university students. In a systematic review of the literature, Sayakhot and Carolan-Olah (2016) examined how pregnant women used the Internet for information. One paper they reviewed reported that women with higher education levels were three times more likely to seek advice than women with less than a high school education, and most women did not discuss the information with their providers, so there was no way to determine if they had found accurate information. Perez et al. (2015, 2016) suggested that search patterns and use of credible information to make decisions may differ by level of socioeconomic status, education, and prior healthcare experiences, possibly placing individuals with limited resources at a disadvantage. While a comprehensive search of all information available about conditions and treatment options is most likely to result in a high-quality decision and desired outcome, not everyone searches systematically. Perez et al. (2015) found 27 unique search patterns with four organizing themes characterized by number of steps, and whether a hypothesis was formed and symptoms explored before or after searching interventions. The Perez study population was a small, convenience sample not representative of the general population in terms of age, gender, race, or insurance status, but a significant number of the participants ended their search after finding an acceptable solution, rather than the best solution, leading Perez et al. (2015) to suggest additional education of consumers by healthcare providers on search methods. Regretfully, a meta-analysis of 37 articles conducted by Hallows (2013) found that the Internet does not have the same impact upon the ability of senior citizens to make informed health decisions.

Another approach to search for health information online is the web-based question-and-answer (Q&A) forum found within many online communities. A disadvantage of this approach is that consumers often repeat questions that have been asked (Luo, Zhang, Wentz, Cui, & Xu, 2015). It is not only healthcare consumers who seek health information. Nguyen et al. (2017) studied surrogates of septic patients hospitalized in 19 ICUs and found that most of the surrogates indicated that they would like to receive a list of selected websites relative to the diagnoses. Another issue that impacts information search results is the use of filters imposed by search engines and social media in an attempt to meet individual preferences.

This practice is often not known by the public who should have the option to perform unfiltered searches (Holone, 2016).

Healthcare organizations have been working to meet consumer demands inclusive of wait lists, and information on services and disease management (Borycki et al., 2011). Despite these efforts, an assessment of health system websites for accessibility, content, marketing, and technology found many performed poorly, evoking concern because websites may provide the first impression of the organization (Ford, Huerta, Schilhavy, & Menachemi, 2012). This study considered accessibility on the basis of educational level for posted material and ease of navigation from page to page using embedded links, and found this to be the area most in need of improvement. On the technology side, Ford et al. (2012) found that many websites lacked clear descriptions of links needed to enable search engines to collect information. Standardization of information quality, and measures to ensure accessibility and compliance, as well as the provision of tailored disease-management information to prevent information overload, confusion, and inappropriate decisions represent improvements that organizations can make.

Health Games

Health games (gamification) provide a means to educate. The Internet can be accessed by various means—computer, smartphones, and kiosks—and provides many opportunities for health education. Kaufman, Sauve, and Renaud (2011) listed useful feedback, innovative learning methods, technology integration, and active engagement in real world problems as relevant and meaningful criteria for health games. Barriers related to health games include lack of expertise in design as well as by participants, a lack of interest and/or understanding of content by consumers, limited acceptance, usability issues, and costs associated with design and production (Laxman et al., 2015). Despite these issues, the popularity and promise of gamification in health has been growing, as evidenced by the number of available apps, and gamification is being embraced as a means to encourage healthier lifestyles and manage chronic diseases (AlMarshedi, Wills, & Ranchhod, 2016; Gamification Leads, 2013; Lister, West, Cannon, Sax, & Brodegard, 2014).

Telehealth

Telehealth is an important consumer health application because it allows consumers the option to remain in place for care, yet it still faces barriers that include professional licensure, legislative issues, reimbursement, lack of supportive infrastructure, and protection of storage and devices (Laxman et al., 2015). Telehealth is discussed at length in Chapter 19.

mHealth

mHealth is the use of wireless devices and sensor networks to access healthcare information or services from the community, or to transmit healthcare information to healthcare professionals (HCPs) (Laxman et al., 2015). The ubiquity of the smartphone makes it a convenient tool for mHealth. Hartzler and Wetter (2014) concluded that mobile phones showed great promise to leverage mHealth for consumer empowerment from their review of literature describing services for education, reminders, peer support, epidemiologic reporting, and case management. And like telehealth monitoring, smartphones move healthcare from a provider focus to a patient-focus. According to a Pew Institute survey, "62% of smartphone owners have used their phone in the past year to look up information about a health condition" (Smith & Page, 2015, p. 5). Young adults rely upon their phones for Internet use.

Examples of mHealth applications include real-time monitoring of vital signs, and tracking metrics, such as glucose, weight, or calories.

Wearable technologies can provide personalized health data that aid diagnosis and behavior change. One in six consumers in the United States has used some form of wearable technology, such as a smartwatch or fitness tracker, and the number of fitness devices is expected to grow to 110 million in 2018 (Piwek, Ellis, Andrews, & Joinson, 2016). The line between consumer wearables and medical devices has blurred as devices for fitness tracking are now being used by HCPs. Typically, persons who purchase wearables already demonstrate a healthy lifestyle. Advances in technology now make implantable medical devices to manage chronic diseases a viable alternative for many individuals (Amar, Kouki, & Hung, 2015).

mHealth technology is ideal for healthcare consumers and HCPs who are accustomed to using technology while on the go. It is particularly well-suited for adolescents and teens with chronic illness such as asthma. Smartphone technology can support:

- Personalized diaries
- Medical regimen information on schedules
- Automated system reminders and tailored messages (Perret, Bonevski, McDonald, & Abramson, 2016; Perri-Moore et al., 2016)
- Action plans
- Summary and detailed patient data
- Web portal access
- Exception reports on noncompliant patients (for the provider).

Barriers to mHealth include lack of physician support, concerns over regulation, efficacy, data integrity, security, and usability, particularly for the less technologically savvy or disabled. mHealth may also be perceived as less personal, and occasionally there are connectivity issues, or even safety concerns, with wearables (Piwek et al., 2016).

Personal Health Records and Patient Portals

Many of today's healthcare consumers are accustomed to having ready access to computerized personal information in their daily lives, so the ability to access and manage health information online would be a logical extension of that capability. Unlike the electronic health record, which is built upon healthcare provider input, the PHR allows users to electronically collect, track, and share past and current information about their health or someone in their care (Laxman et al., 2015; Genitsaridi, Kondylakis, Koumakis, Marias, & Tsiknakis, 2015). A PHR can be as simple as a paper document or thumb drive, but in recent years it has evolved to include online access. PHRs can stand alone or be tethered to a health plan or EHRS portal. The consumer enters and maintains all information with the stand alone PHR. This is in contrast with the tethered PHR, where portions are populated by the healthcare plan or healthcare delivery system EHRS that supports it. Microsoft's HealthVault (2017) is an example of a PHR that might be considered standalone, although healthcare consumers can now direct providers, pharmacies, and tracking applications to send data to their HealthVault PHR. The PHR continues to evolve to support data from self-monitoring devices and personal wellness applications, with findings from big data, genomics, and translational research expected to follow to support personalized healthcare (Pinciroli & Pagliari, 2015).

Despite the potential of PHRs, adoption rates have been low (Laxman et al., 2015; Vydra, Cuaresma, Kretovics, & Bose-Brill, 2015; Watters, Bergstrom, & Sandefer, 2016). Box 18-2 lists barriers to PHR adoption.

Box 18-2   Barriers to PHR Adoption

Barriers to PHR adoption for Consumers
- Concerns about privacy and security
- Lack of perceived benefit
- Usability
- Access issues
  - No Internet-capable device or Internet service
  - Physical or cognitive disabilities
  - Literacy issues (basic literacy, computer literacy, health literacy)

Barriers to Adoption by Providers
- Low levels of awareness
- Need for new workflow demands associated with PHR use
- Resistance to change
- Concerns related to confidentiality
- Limited technological literacy

Physician endorsement and engagement is key to increased adoption of PHRs. Today, the line between PHR and portal has blurred. Tethered PHRs are also known as portals (Vydra et al., 2015). Patient portals provide patients with a 24/7 path to their records from any Internet-accessible location, and have been shown to improve outcomes for individuals with chronic conditions (Elkind, 2017). Portals are password-protected websites that bring information together from different sources for a uniform look (Coughlin et al., 2017). Portals began to appear in the United States in the 1990s in response to the Health Insurance Portability and Accountability Act of 1996 requirement that patients have the right to see and obtain copies of their records. In subsequent years, the American Recovery and Reinvestment Act (ARRA) extended these rights through modifications to HIPAA, requiring providers using EHRSs to give patients electronic copies of their records. Stage I meaningful use requirements also called for providers to provide record access (Murphy-Abdouch, 2015). Meaningful use requires that patients receive a clinical summary after each visit, the ability to securely message providers, patient-specific education, patient reminders for preventative care, and medication reconciliation—features that lend themselves readily to incorporation into a portal (Centers for Medicare and Medicaid Services, 2016; Coughlin et al., 2017; Cronin et al., 2015). By 2015, approximately one-half of US hospitals and HCPs had secure portals in place. Box 18-3 describes common portal features.

Box 18-3   Common Portal Features

- Record access
- Ability to view test results
- Secure messaging capability
- The ability to schedule appointments
- Bill management
- Medication reconciliation
- Reminders for preventive services
- Delivery of personalized health information

Portals are expected to dramatically change care as use expands and consumers complete screenings and forms prior to appointments, thereby giving HCPs an opportunity to review records prior to seeing patients, enabling them to collaborate during the appointment (Smith, 2016). Optimal portal use requires good design and management, engaging features, and organization-wide support to meet patient needs (HealthIT.gov, 2013; Osborn et al., 2011; Otte-Trojel et al., 2015).

The number of patient portals continues to increase, affording record access and communication with healthcare providers; yet, overall portal adoption remains low with no agreement on how or where to best encourage adoption (Fix et al., 2016). However, a retrospective study conducted at Vanderbilt University Medical Center found that patient-initiated, secure-message use rapidly followed portal deployment with messaging interactions, sometimes exceeding face-to-face clinic visits (Cronin et al., 2015).

Social Media

Social media (SM), or social networking, encompasses a variety of forms from sites such as Facebook, Twitter, YouTube, blogs, to Internet-based support groups (Prybutok, Koh, & Prybutok, 2014). SM can share the wisdom of many (Bratucu et al., 2014), and over the years, SM sites such as Facebook have expanded to include use by individuals seeking information and support for healthcare issues. SM tools have gained prominence for self-management of chronic conditions. Two popular SM sites are patientslikeme.com and inspire.com. Both sites have similar features. PatientsLikeMe is briefly described here.

PatientsLikeMe (patientslikeme.com, 2017) provides a platform for individuals who have a specific health condition in common to share information about treatments, symptoms, and other issues. Health consumers use discussion boards and access other users' health profiles. Graphs and other visual displays provide rapid access to information regarding medications, symptoms, and other data. PatientsLikeMe was initially developed for individuals with amyotrophic lateral sclerosis (ALS) to share information and provide support to families and each other. The site currently provides communities for individuals with ALS, as well as a number of other chronic health conditions. Users create a profile that contains:

- A summary representation of their current health status.
- A diagram that maps functional impairment to areas of the body.
- A personal photo.
- An autobiographical statement.
- Their diagnosis history.
- A series of charts.

Members can locate others with the same condition with shared medical experiences for discussion of profiles and reports. Data entered by users are aggregated to create graphs and charts to show how one is progressing compared to others with similar conditions. Analysis of patient use of the site revealed three categories of comments posted by users: targeted questions, advice and recommendations, and building support relationships.

PatientsLikeMe (2017) bills itself as a clinical research platform that provides real-time insights into various diseases and conditions. PatientsLikeMe has partnered extensively with government, academic, nonprofit, and private organizations to support research, and is a well-known example of stakeholder involvement in research. The importance of stakeholder involvement in research has been recognized by funding agencies and researchers. One exemplar study of PatientsLikeMe members with diabetes examined patient perceptions of diabetes, and was used to help set research priorities (Schroeder et al., 2015).

HCPs are also turning to SM to market services and to ask consumers to provide feedback and ratings of their services. Glover et al. (2015) did a comparative analysis of Facebook ratings with the Hospital Compare metric, specifically 30-day all-cause unplanned hospital readmission rates, and found a correlation between higher hospital ratings on Facebook and lower 30-day readmission rates, than for facilities with lower Facebook ratings. This led the researchers to conclude that aggregate measures of consumer satisfaction on SM correlated with traditionally used measures of hospital quality.

Health Tracking and Disease Management

As the demand for healthcare increases due to an increase in the aging population, information technology may provide an alternative for some Americans in health tracking and simple disease management. Ancker et al. (2015) estimated over 90 million people in the United States have more than one chronic disease, and that this number will continue to grow. Common multiple chronic conditions (MCC) include such conditions as: chronic obstructive pulmonary disorder, heart failure, chronic pain, depression, diabetes, asthma, arthritis, obesity, HIV, as well as a number of mental illnesses. Patients that have MCC typically see more than one health provider.

Health-IT offers the consumer the ability to track their own health information, putting the consumer in control of shared data. In many instances, the consumer makes sure all information is shared between providers. There is a risk of lack of engagement by consumers, or intentional suppression of information (Ancker et al., 2015).

Stage one meaningful use guidelines opened the door for consumers to gain access to their EHR. Through the use of information technology, consumers can now access their EHRs, maintain their (PHR), communicate with their provider(s), schedule appointments, find educational materials, and be a full contributing member of their healthcare team. LeRouge, Van Slyke, Seale, and Wright (2014) reported that the Baby Boomer generation (birth years 1946 to 1964) had similar technology use compared to younger generations, but were less likely to use podcasts, kiosks, smartphones, blogs, and wikis for healthcare information. Generations older than Baby Boomers (Silent Generation and GI Generation) were considered less likely to utilize healthcare technology.

Typical barriers exist for health tracking and disease management. The consumer has to have available technology to connect and maintain connectivity to Internet websites. For patients/consumers that live in rural or remote areas, Internet access has to be available to gain access to appropriate websites. Because of the private and confidential nature of the information available, the consumer must be able to successfully log in and log out of personal accounts. Also, not all providers fully participate in patient portal websites. What this means is, if a provider does not place a patient's health information on the patient portal website, the patient will not have access to the information. This is a choice made by the provider, and becomes a choice by the consumer whether or not to stay with a provider that does not fully participate in a complete patient portal.

Home Monitoring

The concept of home monitoring is part of connected health—the blending of healthcare with technology at the level of the home. The American Telemedicine Association (2016) defines telehealth as a general term describing remote healthcare services, but not always involving clinical services. The types of home monitoring options are on the rise. In addition to monitoring chronic conditions, such as congestive heart failure, cardiac arrhythmias, high blood pressure, diabetes, and sleep disorders, there is a growing focus upon devices that support aging in place.

Technology that supports aging in place may stand-alone or be part of a larger unit such as a smart home. One stand-alone exemplar is an electronic pillbox that reminds the consumer to take their medication, which may also communicate compliance to a monitor. Smart homes combine several technologies that communicate and monitor through cameras and sensors (Ye, Stevenson, & Dobson, 2016). A smart home can be adapted for healthcare needs allowing older adults and persons with disabilities the independence of living at home while being monitored. Monitoring can be done by concerned family members or through contracted services. Smart home technology commonly measures activities of daily living, cognitive function, safety—including fall detection—and social connectedness (Czaja, 2015; Liu et al., 2016). Evolving smart home technology can integrate artificial intelligence and mobile phone technology to allow users to control conditions within their homes from any location, and increase the use of robots. Robots can serve as a coach, provide instructions and reminders, augment movement, and assist with domestic chores.

The technology that supports telehealth has the typical barriers of supporting hardware, software, and infrastructure. Cost, insurance coverage, and acceptability to the consumer may present other barriers. Chapter 19 provides an in-depth discussion of multiple facets of home monitoring.

Personalized Healthcare Medicine/Genomics

Perhaps the most wide-sweeping change in CHI will be that of personalized healthcare. The Department of Health and Human Services (DHHS) defines personalized healthcare as:

> Medical practices that are targeted to individuals based on their specific genetic code in order to provide a tailored approach. These practices use preventive, diagnostic, and therapeutic interventions that are based on genetic tests and family history information. The goal of personalized healthcare is to improve health outcomes and the healthcare delivery system, as well as the quality of life of patients elsewhere (Department of Health and Human Services, 2010, paragraph 7).

Genomic medicine customizes the practice of medicine specifically to the unique genetic makeup of a person. Genetics and genomics examine detailed information about genetic disorders, the background on genetic and genomic science, pharmacogenomics, along with family health history (National Human Genome Research Institute, 2016). According to Abrahams and Silver (2009), personalized medicine has the potential to shift the focus of medicine from reaction toward prevention, help providers select optimal therapy to make drugs safer, improve clinical trials, rescue drugs that are failing in clinical trials, and reduce the cost of healthcare.

Consider the advantage to patients and healthcare teams with the integration of cancer genomic data into health records. Warner, Jain, and Levy (2016) indicated that genomic data will help guide decision making in cancer treatment and improve patient care. With much of this data online, the patient can be an active participant in their own care through CHI tools, such as personal health records, telemedicine, telehome health monitoring, social networking, and smartphone applications.

Over the last several years, the market for direct-to-consumer (DTC) genetic testing has grown. In April 2017, the Food and Drug Administration announced that the DTC company 23andMe had been granted permission to test for ten disease conditions through their Personal Genome Service Genetic Health Risk (GHR) (US Food and Drug Administration, 2017). This decision was granted based on 23andMe's statistical track record for consistency and accuracy in their product results, and their ability to disseminate information to their clients in a professional, meaningful manner.

As this field grows, there will be bumps along the road regarding the ethics of genetic and genomic testing and attempts to predict the future based on today's limited knowledge. Technology will help with the aggregation of raw data which may shift the focus of care from treating chronic conditions to proactively preventing diseases. These tools will proliferate and have the potential to significantly impact consumer satisfaction with healthcare, as well as health outcomes.

The Role of the Informatics Nurse with CHI

The informatics nurse has several roles within CHI—guide, educator, designer, advocate, and researcher, are just a few of these roles. Sands and Wald (2014) stated that adapted healthcare systems that serve consumer needs require data streams to better support self-management, SDM, and provide increased virtual care options. Smith (2016) noted that ongoing barriers to the health information exchanges, needed for facilitating patient-centered care, included incomplete information, exchange access issues, and ineffective organization of data.

Informatics Specialist as Guide

Smith (2016) noted the need for HCPs to direct patients to the best available online resources. But, realistically, HCPs may require some help so that informatics nurses can educate patients on recommended examples, as well as guiding principles to use in order to guide consumers to appropriate sources, especially given the fact that there are thousands of resources to evaluate. There are resources available to assist the informatics professional with the development and promotion of consumer health informatics applications. The Department of Health and Human Services (DHHS) Office of Disease Prevention and Health Promotion (ODPHP) (2016) first developed the research-based guide, *Health Literacy Online: A Guide for Simplifying the User Experience*, in 2010, which has since been updated and is in its second edition. This guide is consistent with President Obama's Digital Government Strategy, an initiative that calls for providing online information to enhance transparency and support decision-making.

Amante et al. (2015) noted that individuals experiencing difficulties accessing healthcare services for reasons other than insurance coverage were more inclined to use the Internet to search for health information, and that improving the quality of online health information could help this population. The informatics nurse specialist can help guide the computer and technology literate consumer to the best resources for their needed services. de-Luque and Staccini (2016) suggested that consumers with chronic illnesses should be encouraged and trained to actively seek online information, noting that it significantly decreases anxiety. They also concluded that a trusted, connected healthcare environment can be created when patients, HCPs, and the healthcare industry all come together to build a shared model of health-data management.

Informatics Specialist as Educator

Technology has provided the infrastructure by which consumers can now have two-way communication with their HCPs. And efforts are being made to use normalized words and phrases to help consumers understand medical terminology and intent (Mowery et al., 2016). Some experts call this a "vocabulary gap," which is a barrier that forms when consumers try to use technology to access or send health information, but cannot due to language (Zeng & Tse, 2006). One approach to eliminating this health communication barrier is the development of consumer health vocabularies (CHVs).

Experts (Keselman et al., 2008; Zeng & Tse, 2006) noted that the use of CHVs has the potential to benefit not only human understanding, but also machine processing. Specifically, the use of CHVs has the potential to help practitioners use terms that are easily understood and recognizable by the consumer. Conversely, computer systems that may not recognize lay health terms not included in a controlled vocabulary, such as the unified medical language system (UMLS), would be able to process searches and retrieve information better if consumers used standard recognized terms.

The informatics specialist as educator can assist in these efforts by contributing to the design of consumer-friendly information retrieval tools, by designing electronic education that is readable at a sixth-grade level, and by providing consumers with helpful hints about vocabulary translations. Additionally, the informatics specialist as educator can assist in these efforts by including techniques from marketing, entertainment, and news media that will enhance the attractiveness or aesthetics of these healthcare communications.

Another lesser-known issue that impacts information search results is the use of filters imposed by search engines and social media in an attempt to meet individual preferences. This practice is often not known by the public, who should have the opportunity to perform unfiltered searches (Holone, 2016). Educating the consumer regarding search engine filters is one method of working around this barrier. Another method is educating consumers on trusted websites and relying on certified HON websites. The best education comes with full disclosure of information gained from Internet searches with healthcare providers for complete discussion.

Informatics Specialist as Designer

The informatics specialist as a designer of health information is in a distinctive position to create and promote the development of effective consumer health digital resources. The design of consumer applications needs to consider ease of use, appeal to all literacy levels and socioeconomic backgrounds, privacy and security concerns, and costs, particularly as interaction with the online healthcare system continues to increase via the use of portals and telehealth applications (Crotty & Slack, 2016; Laxman et al., 2015). In their study of Australian online health information, Cheng and Dunn (2015) found the readability of health websites to be above average reading levels, suggesting guidelines to ensure that readability levels are addressed in order to facilitate health literacy.

Perhaps the most important concept to consider when designing patient-centered CHI applications is that the developer must understand and align with consumer and family member activities, otherwise known as "patient work." Patient work considers human factors, principles, context, skills, and behaviors (Valdez et al., 2015). The World Health Organization has designated Nova Southeastern University's Center for Consumer Health Informatics (CCHIR) as a collaborating center in the patient-centric branch of CHI (PR Newswire, 2013).

A challenge to designing applications is trying to anticipate how they will be used, which suggests the need for more research in this area (Novak, Simpson, Slagle, & Mulvaney, 2015). Prybutok, Koh, and Prybutok (2014) found content relevance essential to effective message communication when the goal is behavior change in their study to identify factors most highly correlated with content relevance for online health information for 18 to 30-year-old college students. The designer of consumer health information needs to be mindful of end-users' needs, and the context in which information is used. Today's technology can change within moments. The informatics specialist must be able to adapt and translate these changes to the CHI setting.

Informatics Specialist as Advocate

In order to advocate for CHI, the INS needs to not only be aware of issues and barriers to its use, but also of viable solutions. Begany (2014) noted that the cost for Internet access in the US was twice what counterparts in other developed countries pay. Van Deursen and van Dijk (2015) found significant differences in the numbers and types of Internet-accessible devices in their study in the Netherlands. Working to ensure both access and affordability through policy and legislative efforts, provides a path to begin to address the issue of eHealth literacy (van Deursen & van Dijk, 2015). Increased connectivity and access to a higher quality of health-information resources is an important goal for fostering eHealth literacy and closing the digital divide.

As CHI applications become more pervasive across the care continuum, the INS must consider whether the tools are appropriate to serve populations diverse in culture, socioeconomic status, levels of education and literacy, disability, types of illnesses related to ethnicity (Chaet, Morshedi, Wells, Barnes, & Valdez, 2016), and physical or mental illnesses (Crangle & Kart, 2015). Ancker et al. (2014) found barriers to the use of technology related to patient data access via technical changes, rapid changes within organizations, and cultural issues. They concluded there was no simple solution, and progress requires continued policy development. Guynn (2016) noted that many health information websites were not accessible to screen reader software, thereby negatively impacting the visually impaired consumer.

The healthcare informatics specialist can play an important advocacy role through the engagement of consumers to use IT that supports informed healthcare decision making. As the role of CHI has evolved, so have plans to promote its use. There is a growing body of scholarly knowledge that is helping to delineate factors for success and proposals, such as the eHealth initiative that identifies best practices. Both efforts support CHI use and adoption.

eHEALTH INITIATIVE The eHealth Initiative (eHI) is an organization that brings together executives from multiple stakeholder groups in order to identify the best methods to transform healthcare through the use of IT and innovation (eHealth Initiative, 2017). eHI achieves this mission through its support of research, and education and advocacy activities. Since its inception approximately two decades ago, eHI has widely shared its vision and spearheaded several initiatives. In 2007, it released *eHealth Initiative Blueprint: Building Consensus for Common Action*, which represented the consensus of the group's shared vision and provided a set of principles, strategies, and actions for improving health and healthcare.

Believing that consumers can be engaged in their healthcare by using information and tools that facilitate consumer action and informed decision making, the *eHealth Initiative Blueprint and eHealth Toolkit* was designed to provide helpful information to healthcare leaders in their pursuit of health IT, and health information exchange adoption. Successful adoption includes a partnership between healthcare providers and consumers based on the following guiding principles.

- *Consumer engagement in healthcare.* Engaging consumers to use health IT and health information exchange practices to communicate with providers is critical to supporting informed decision making and improving healthcare.

- *Consumer access and control of personal health information.* Controlling access to his or her personal health information is the right of every consumer. Consumers have the right not only to access their personal health information, but to also annotate and request corrections.

- *Consumer access to electronic health information tools and services.* Having access to tools that engage consumers through the mobilization of electronic health information should be universal. These tools should also be designed explicitly to meet the needs of diverse consumer groups, including those who are poor, rural, older, physically disabled, or do not speak English.

- *Consumer privacy.* Having the privacy of their personal health information consistent with all applicable federal, state, and local laws is the right of every consumer.
- *Consumer trust.* Making public the policies surrounding the privacy and information use of personal health information is critical. Consumers want assurance that their personal electronic health information is gathered with appropriate consent, and is stored and used in a secure and auditable way.
- *Consumer participation and transparency.* The functioning of all governing bodies or individuals that oversee, implement, and/or develop policy for the electronic exchange of health information should be made transparent and open.

In subsequent years, eHI created the *2020 Roadmap in 2014,* which provided a framework for much of its work through the present. And in more recent efforts, eHI has begun to examine the status of genomics and precision medicine, and has launched the Electronic Medication Adherence Collaborative with the intention to improve outcomes and contain costs (eHealth Initiative, 2017).

Informatics Specialist as Researcher

As the rates of portal and secure messaging use increase, research is needed to understand the impact upon provider workload and its impact upon patient care (Cronin et al., 2015; Fix et al., 2016). Flaherty et al. (2015) identified five assessment criteria for CHI that include: citation—providing cited sources for represented materials; multidisciplinary—referencing necessary fields; impact—scholarly prestige of the journal the material is published in; comprehensibility—the material is understandable by the lay public; and simplicity/readability—terms are written with good definitions that are understandable. Although we typically think of a researcher as someone that conducts statistical research, in the instance of CHI research, the informatics specialist is researching information that meets these criteria.

The informatics specialist researcher is also aware of current technology trends and advancements that bring changes to patient care. Mobile health (mHealth) is a rapidly growing market to consumers that include devices from personally purchased fitness monitoring devices to provider prescribed monitors. In a study completed by Rai, Chen, Pye, and Baird (2013) consumers indicated favorable usage of mHealth as a compliment to in-person provider visits, but consumers that preferred mHealth to in-person visits also reported stronger use of mHealth devices. As this trend evolves, the informatics specialist will need to study the technology further.

EVIDENCE-BASED STUDIES Traditional research remains a role for the informatics specialist. CHI can impact consumers' health only if CHI is accepted and used. As healthcare informatics specialists consider factors that will enhance the successful adoption of CHI, research is beginning to identify attributes that facilitate or hinder CHI acceptance.

The Future of CHI

The future of CHI is exciting. Consumers now have more frequent opportunities to utilize CHI to find information, communicate with the healthcare team, share health-related data, participate in virtual communities, receive advice tailored to them, and learn more about their health conditions than anytime in previous history. Federal regulations provide consumers with access to their health records, and technology provides the means to gain access. CHI enables consumers to partner with providers in their care. Even so, more must be done to remove inequities in technology access, generational knowledge, and address literacy issues to enable consumers that hunger to be a part of their own healthcare team realize that capability.

As technology continues to evolve, consumers will have even more options for managing their healthcare. More healthcare information will be available online, and opportunities for health-related interactive social networking and communication with providers will become the norm. Technology applications, such as the use of sensorized garments that include unobtrusive sensors and monitors that provide real-time feedback regarding vital signs, gait, activity levels, and other information, will become commonplace. And the use of emerging technology in "smart homes," where unobtrusive sensors can allow monitoring of safety issues (falls, poor eating, and changes in sleep habits) in the home setting, will afford greater independence for older adults.

As CHI grows in its popularity, the role of the informatics expert as consumer health especialist will also advance. CHI truly has the potential to transform healthcare delivery.

Summary

- Consumer health informatics (CHI) is a field devoted to the consumer, or patient, view.
- eHealth delivers health information and services through information technology (IT) and falls under CHI.
- Quality information is critical to inform decisions.
- Quality information attributes include: timely, precise, accurate, quantifiable, verifiable by independent sources, easily available, complete, appropriate to user needs and level of understanding, unambiguous, reliable, current, and convenient.
- CHI is changing the provider-patient relationship.
- The development of CHI has been driven by the need for consumers to be accountable for their own health, and as a means to improve the healthcare system.
- Issues that impact CHI include: unclear expectations, literacy issues, and inequalities in Internet and technology access.
- Patient engagement is critical to consumers assuming responsibility for their own healthcare.
- Patient engagement is the ongoing, constructive communication between patient and practitioner that is driven by patient portals, secure messaging, mobile applications, and consumer-generated health data.
- Engaged consumers are more likely to share in their healthcare decisions and lead a healthier life.
- Shared decision making (SDM) is the process that occurs between provider and consumer that requires comprehension of treatment options, and the ability to evaluate potential benefits and harms in order to make treatment determinations.
- CHI applications include: education, health games, telehealth, mHealth, personal health records and portals, and social media.
- The Internet is widely used to search for health information online, surpassing reliance on other media. There are differences in the use of the Internet for online searches by levels of education, age, and economic levels.
- Health games are used to educate and motivate consumers and are gaining in popularity.

- Telehealth services allow consumers to stay in place to receive services.
- mHealth is the use of wireless devices and sensor networks to access healthcare information or services from the community, or to transmit healthcare information to HCPs.
- Personal health records (PHRs) and portals afford consumer control over their health information, and increasingly support other services, such as messaging providers and, sometimes, wellness and tracking applications.
- Social media (SM), or social networking, has gained prominence for sharing health information and self-management of chronic conditions.
- Health tracking and disease management provide additional options for consumers to be involved in their health.
- Home monitoring allows consumers to monitor chronic conditions from their homes.
- Personalized healthcare based upon one's genetic makeup provides a way for targeted treatment that is more effective for the individual.
- The informatics professional, including the informatics nurse, has multiple roles within CHI that include guide, educator, designer, advocate, and researcher.
- The future of CHI continues to evolve before our eyes bringing with it new possibilities.

Case Study

You have oversight for the design of your hospital's web portal. What factors must you consider from a consumer health informatics perspective and why? Select two factors for an in-depth analysis.

About the Authors

Dr. Rose is a 2014 graduate of Duke University School of Nursing DNP program, 2011 graduate of Walden University School of Nursing MSN—Informatics Specialty, 1986 graduate of Illinois Central College, Associate Degree of Nursing program. Dr. Rose lives in Murfreesboro, Tennessee, and is an Assistant Professor of Nursing at Cumberland University Jeanette C. Rudy School of Nursing, a Visiting Professor of Nursing at Chamberlain College of Nursing, and works PRN as a Nursing Supervisor at Southern Hills Medical Center in Nashville, Tennessee.

Dr. Hebda, graduated from Washington Hospital School of Nursing, and then earned her BSN at Duquesne University. She earned her MNEd, PhD, and MSIS from the University of Pittsburgh. She has had a long-standing interest in nursing informatics and teaches nursing informatics classes in the Chamberlain College MSN nursing informatics track.

References

Abrahams, E., & Silver, M. (2009). The case for personalized medicine. *Journal of Diabetes Science and Technology*, 3(4), 680–684.

AlMarshedi, A., Wills, G., & Ranchhod, A. (2016). Gamifying self-management of chronic illnesses: A mixed-methods study. *JMIR Serious Games*, 4(2), e14. doi:10.2196/games.5943

Amante, D. J., Hogan, T. P., Pagoto, S. L., English, T. M., & Lapane, K. L. (2015). Access to care and use of the Internet to search for health information: Results from the US national health interview survey. *Journal of Medical Internet Research*, 17(4), e106. doi:10.2196/jmir.4126

Amar, A. B., Kouki, A. B., & Hung, C. (2015). Power approaches for implantable medical devices. *Sensors (14248220)*, *15*(11), 28889. doi:10.3390/s151128889.

American Medical Informatics Association (AMIA). (2017). Consumer Health Informatics © 2017. Retrieved from www.amia.org/applications-informatics/consumer-health-informatics

American Telemedicine Association. (2016). *Telemedicine Nomenclature*. Retrieved from American Telemedicine Association (ATA) www.americantelemed.org/resources/nomenclature#.V1oYzSDD_IU

Ancker, J. S., Miller, M. C., Patel, V., & Kaushal, R. (2014). Sociotechnical challenges to developing technologies for patient access to health information exchange data. *Journal of the American Medical Informatics Association*, *21*(4), 664–670. doi:10.1136/amiajnl-2013-002073

Ancker, J. S., Osorio, S. N., Cheriff, A., Cole, C. L., Silver, M., & Kaushal, R. (2015). Patient activation and use of an electronic patient portal. *Informatics for Health & Social Care*, *40*(3), 254–266. doi:10.3109/17538157.2014.908200

Anderson, M., & Perrin, A. (2017). Tech adoption climbs among older adults. *Pew Research Center*. Retrieved from http://assets.pewresearch.org/wp-content/uploads/sites/14/2017/05/16170850/PI_2017.05.17_Older-Americans-Tech_FINAL.pdf

Association of College and Research Libraries. (2016). Framework for information literacy for higher education Published by American Library Association, © 2016. Retrieved from www.ala.org/acrl/standards/ilframework

Begany, G. (2014). Addressing eHealth literacy and the digital divide: Access, affordability and awareness. *Bulletin of the Association for Information Science & Technology*, *41*(1), 29–32.

Borycki, E. M., Bartle-Clar, J. A., Househ, M. S., Kuziemsky, C. E., Schraa, E. G., & Reid, P. (2011). Emergence of a new consumer health informatics framework: Introducing the healthcare organization. *Studies in Health Technology & Informatics*, *164*, 353.

Bratucu, R., Gheorghe, I. R., Purcarea, R. M., Gheorghe, C. M., Popa Velea, O., & Purcarea, V. L. (2014). Cause and effect: The linkage between the health information seeking behavior and the online environment—A review. *Journal of Medicine and Life*, *7*(3), 310–316.

Centers for Disease Control and Prevention. (2016). What is health literacy? Retrieved from www.cdc.gov/healthliteracy/learn/index.html

Centers for Disease Control and Prevention. (2017). National center for health statistics: Healthy people. Retrieved from www.cdc.gov/nchs/healthy_people/index.htm. From Healthy People 2020. Published by Office of Disease Prevention and Health Promotion.

Centers for Medicare and Medicaid Services (CMS). (2016). Eligible hospitals, critical access hospitals and dual-eligible hospitals attesting to CMS EHR incentive program stage 3 objectives and measures objective 3 of 6. Retrieved from www.cms.gov/Regulations-and-Guidance/Legislation/EHRIncentivePrograms/Downloads/MedicareEHStage3_Obj3.pdf

Chaet, A. V., Morshedi, B., Wells, K. J., Barnes, L. E., & Valdez, R. (2016). Spanish-language consumer health information technology interventions: A systematic review. *Journal of Medical Internet Research*, *18*(8), e214. doi:10.2196/jmir.5794

Cheng, C., & Dunn, M. (2015). Health literacy and the internet: A study on the readability of Australian online health information. *Australian & New Zealand Journal of Public Health*, *39*(4), 309–314. doi:10.1111/1753-6405.12341

Coughlin, S. S., Prochaska, J. J., Williams, L. B., Besenyi, G. M., Heboyan, V., Goggans, D. S., et al. (2017). Patient web portals, disease management, and primary prevention. *Risk Management & Healthcare Policy, 10*, 33–40. doi:10.2147/RMHP.S130431

Crangle, C. E., & Kart, J. B. (2015). A questions-based investigation of consumer mental-health information. *Peerj, 3e867*. doi:10.7717/peerj.867

Cronin, R. M., Davis, S. E., Shenson, J. A., Chen, Q., Rosenbloom, S. T., & Jackson, G. P. (2015). Growth of secure messaging through a patient portal as a form of outpatient interaction across clinical specialties. *Applied Clinical Informatics, 6*(2), 288–304. doi:10.4338/ACI-2014-12-RA-0117

Crotty, B. H., & Slack, W. V. (2016). Designing online health services for patients. *Israel Journal of Health Policy Research, 522*. doi:10.1186/s13584-016-0082-7

Czaja, S. J. (2015). Can technology empower older adults to manage their health? *Generations, 39*(1), 46–51.

Demiris, G. (2016). Consumer health informatics: Past, present, and future of a rapidly evolving domain. *Yearbook of Medical Informatics, Suppl 1*, S42–S47. doi:10.15265/IYS-2016-s005

Department of Health and Human Services, Office of Disease Prevention and Health Promotion. (2010). National action plan to improve health literacy. Washington, DC.

Edelstein, P. (2016). Correcting critical misperceptions about patient engagement. *Health Management Technology, 37*(1), 10–11. Published by NP Communications, © 2016

eHealth Initiative. (2017). Our vision. Retrieved from www.ehidc.org/

Elkind, E. (2017). The patient portal: Considerations for NPs. *The Nurse Practitioner, 42*(3), 1–4.

Emanuel, R., & Challons-Lipton, S. (2013). Visual literacy and the digital native: Another look. *Journal of Visual Literacy, 32*(1), 7–26.

Eysenbach, G. (2000). Consumer health informatics. *British Medical Journal (Clinical Research Ed.), 320*(7251), 1713–1716.

de-Luque, L., & Staccini, P. (2016). All that glitters is not gold: Consumer health informatics and education in the era of social media and health apps. Findings from the yearbook 2016 section on consumer health informatics. *Yearbook of Medical Informatics*, (1), 188–193.

Esposito, E. M. (2016). Ambulatory care nurse-sensitive indicators series: Patient engagement as a nurse-sensitive indicator in ambulatory care. *Nursing Economics, 34*(6), 303–306.

Feinberg, I., Frijters, J., Johnson-Lawrence, V., Greenberg, D., Nightingale, E., & Moodie, C. (2016). Examining associations between health information seeking behavior and adult education status in the US: An analysis of the 2012 PIAAC data. *Plos ONE, 11*(2), 1–20. doi:10.1371/journal.pone.0148751

Fix, G. M., Hogan, T. P., Amante, D. J., McInnes, D. K., Nazi, K. M., & Simon, S. R. (2016). Encouraging patient portal use in the patient-centered medical home: Three stakeholder perspectives. *Journal of Medical Internet Research, 18*(11), 9. doi:10.2196/jmir.6488

Flaherty, D., Hoffman-Goetz, L., & Arocha, J. F. (2015). What is consumer health informatics? A systematic review of published definitions. *Informatics for Health & Social Care, 40*(2), 91–112. doi:10.3109/17538157.2014.907804

Ford, E. W., Huerta, T. R., Schilhavy, R. M., & Menachemi, N. (2012). Effective US health system websites: Establishing benchmarks and standards for effective consumer engagement. *Journal of Healthcare Management/American College of Healthcare Executives, 57*(1), 47–64.

Fox, S., & Duggan, M. (2013). Tracking for health. Retrieved from www.pewinternet.org

Frankel, K.K., Becker, B.L.C., Rowe, M,W., & Pearson, P.D. (2016). From "What is reading?" to what Is literacy? *Journal of Education, 196*(3), 7–17.

Gamification leads tech health engagement surge. (2013). *Corporate Adviser*, 7.

Genitsaridi, I., Kondylakis, H., Koumakis, L., Marias, K., & Tsiknakis, M. (2015). Evaluation of personal health record systems through the lenses of EC research projects. *Computers in Biology and Medicine, 59*, 175–185. doi:10.1016/j.compbiomed.2013.11.004

Glover, M., Khalilzadeh, O., Choy, G., Prabhakar, A. M., Pandharipande, P. V., & Gazelle, G. S. (2015). Hospital evaluations by social media: A comparative analysis of Facebook ratings among performance outliers. *Journal of General Internal Medicine, 30*(10), 1440–1446. doi:10.1007/s11606-015-3236-3

Gürdaş Topkaya, S., & Kaya, N. (2015). Nurses' computer literacy and attitudes towards the use of computers in health care. *International Journal of Nursing Practice, 21*, 141–149. doi:10.1111/ijn.123

Guynn, J. (2016, March 24). For people with disabilities, surfing the web a daily struggle. *USA Today*.

Hallows, K. M. (2013). Health information literacy and the elderly: Has the Internet had an impact? *Serials Librarian, 65*(1), 39–55. doi:10.1080/0361526X.2013.781978

Hartzler, A., & Wetter, T. (2014). Engaging patients through mobile phones: Demonstrator success factors, and future opportunities in low and middle-income countries. *Yearbook of Medical Informatics, 9*, 182–194. doi:10.15265/IY-2014-0022

Hayat, T. Z., Brainin, E., & Neter, E. (2017). With some help from my network: Supplementing ehealth literacy with social ties. *Journal of Medical Internet Research, 19*(3), e98. doi:10.2196/jmir.6472

Health on the Net (HON). (2016, June 9). Health on the net celebrates its 20th anniversary. Retrieved from www.healthonnet.org/

Healthcare Information and Management Systems Society (HIMSS). (2017). Patient Engagement. Retrieved from www.himss.org

HealthIT.gov. (2013). National learning consortium: How to optimize patient portals for patient engagement and meet meaningful use requirement. Retrieved from www.healthit.gov/sites/default/files/nlc_how_to_optimizepatientportals_for_patientengagement.pdf

HealthIT.gov. (2016). eHealth: Stay well. Retrieved from www.healthit.gov/patients-families/stay-well

Healthy People. (n.d.). What are its goals? Retrieved from www.healthypeople.gov/2010/About/goals.htm

Hogan, T. P., Nazi, K. M., Luger, T. M., Amante, D. J., Smith, B. M., Barker, A., et al. (2014). Technology-assisted patient access to clinical information: An evaluation framework for blue button. *Journal of Medical Internet Research, 16*(3), 1. doi:10.2196/resprot.3290

Hoffman, A. S., Llewellyn-Thomas, H. A., Tosteson, A. A., O'Connor, A. M., Volk, R. J., Tomek, I. M., et al. (2014). Launching a virtual decision lab: Development and field-testing of a web-based patient decision support research platform. *BMC Medical Informatics & Decision Making, 14*(1), 1–27. doi:10.1186/s12911-014-0112-8

Holone, H. (2016). The filter bubble and its effect on online personal health information. *Croatian Medical Journal, 57*(3), 298–301. doi:10.3325/cmj.2016.57.298

Institute of Medicine. (2013). *Best care at lower cost: The path to continuously learning health care in America*. Washington, DC: The National Academies Press.

Jacobs, R. J., Caballero, J., Ownby, R. L., & Kane, M. N. (2014). Development of a culturally appropriate computer-delivered tailored internet-based health literacy intervention for Spanish-dominant Hispanics living with HIV. *BMC Medical Informatics & Decision Making, 14*(1), 103–112. doi:10.1186/s12911-014-0103-9

Joshi, A., & Trout, K. (2014). The role of health information kiosks in diverse settings: A systematic review. *Health Information & Libraries Journal, 31*(4), 254-273. doi:10.1111/hir.12081

Jung, M. (2016). Consumer health informatics: Promoting patient self-care management of illnesses and health. *The Health Care Manager, 35*(4), 312–320.

Kaufman, D., Sauve, L., & Renaud, L., (2011). Enhancing learning through an online secondary school educational game. *Journal of Educational Computing Research, 44*(4), 409–428.

Keselman, A., Logan, R., Smith, C. A., Leroy, G., & Zeng-Treitler, Q. (2008). Developing informatics tools and strategies for consumer-centered health communication. *Journal of the American Medical Informatics Association, 15*(4), 473–483. doi:10.1197/jamia.M2744

Kukafka, R., Yi, H., Xiao, T., Thomas, P., Aguirre, A., Smalletz, C., et al. (2015). Why breast cancer risk by the numbers is not enough: Evaluation of a decision aid in multi-ethnic, low-numerate women. *Journal of Medical Internet Research, 17*(7), e165. doi:10.2196/jmir.4028

Laxman, K., Banu Krishnan, S., & Dhillon, J. S. (2015). Barriers to adoption of consumer health informatics applications for health self management. *Health Science Journal, 9*(5), 1–7.

LeRouge, C., Van Slyke, C., Seale, D., & Wright, K. (2014). Baby boomers' adoption of consumer health technologies: Survey on readiness and barriers. *Journal of Medical Internet Research, 16*(9), 1438–8871.

Levy, H., Janke, A., & Langa, K. (2015). Health literacy and the digital divide among older Americans. *Journal of General Internal Medicine, 30*(3), 284. doi:10.1007/s11606-014-3069-5

Lister, C., West, J. H., Cannon, B., Sax, T., & Brodegard, D. (2014). Just a fad? Gamification in health and fitness apps. *JMIR Serious Games, 2*(2), e9. doi:10.2196/games.3413

Liu, L., Stroulia, E., Nikolaidis, I., Miguel-Cruz, A., & Rios Rincon, A. (2016). Review article: Smart homes and home health monitoring technologies for older adults: A systematic review. *International Journal of Medical Informatics, 91,* 44–59. doi:10.1016/j.ijmedinf.2016.04.007

Luo, J., Zhang, G., Wentz, S., Cui, L., & Xu, R. (2015). SimQ: Real-time retrieval of similar consumer health questions. *Journal of Medical Internet Research, 17*(2), e43. doi:10.2196/jmir.3388

Mancuso, P. J., & Myneni, S. (2016). Empowered consumers and the health care team. *Advances in Nursing Science, 39*(1), 26. doi:10.1097/ANS.0000000000000101

Microsoft. (2017). HealthVault. Retrieved from https://international.healthvault.com/

Mowery, D. L., South, B. R., Christensen, L., Jianwei, L., Peltonen, L., Salanterä, S., & ... Chapman, W. W. (2016). Normalizing acronyms and abbreviations to aid patient understanding of clinical texts: ShARe/CLEF eHealth Challenge 2013, Task 2. Journal Of Biomedical Semantics, 71-13. doi:10.1186/s13326-016-0084-y

Murphy-Abdouch, K. (2015). Patient access to personal health information: Regulation vs. reality. *Perspectives in Health Information Management, 12,* 1–10.

Nădășan, V. (2016). The quality of online health-related information—An emergent consumer health issue. *Acta Medica Marisiensis, 62*(4), 408–421. doi:10.1515/amma-2016-0048

National Human Genome Research Institute. (2016). Genomic medicine for patients and the public. Retrieved from www.genome.gov/19016903/genomic-medicine-for-patients-and-the-public/

Novak, L. L., Simpson, C. L., Slagle, J., & Mulvaney, S. A. (2015). Technology and the ecology of chronic illness in everyday life. *Studies in Health Technology and Informatics, 215,* 145–156.

Nguyen, Y., Porcher, R., Argaud, L., Piquilloud, L., Guitton, C., Tamion, F., et al. (2017). "RéaNet," the internet utilization among surrogates of critically ill patients with sepsis. *Plos ONE, 12*(3), 1–12. doi:10.1371/journal.pone.0174292

The Office of Disease Prevention and Health Promotion (ODPHP). (2016). *Health literacy online: A guide for simplifying the user experience.* Retrieved from https://health.gov/healthliteracyonline/

Osborn, C. Y., Rosenbloom, S. T., Stenner, S. P., Anders, S., Muse, S., Johnson, K. B., et al. (2011). MyHealthAtVanderbilt: Policies and procedures governing patient portal functionality. *Journal of the American Medical Informatics Association, 18 Suppl 1*, i18–i23. doi:10.1136/amiajnl-2011-000184

Otte-Trojel, T., Rundall, T. G., de Bont, A., van de Klundert, J., & Reed, M. E. (2015). The organizational dynamics enabling patient portal impacts upon organizational performance and patient health: A qualitative study of Kaiser Permanente. *BMC Health Services Research, 15*, 559. doi:10.1186/s12913-015-1208-2

Patient engagement important, but definitions vary. (2012). *Journal Of AHIMA, 83*(9), 80.

PatientsLikeMe. (2017). About us. Retreived from www.patientslikeme.com/about

Pehora, C., Gajaria, N., Stoute, M., Fracassa, S., Serebale-O'Sullivan, R., & Matava, C. T. (2015). Are parents getting it right? A survey of parents' internet use for children's health care information. *Interactive Journal of Medical Research, 4*(2), e12. doi:10.2196/ijmr.3790

Perez, S. L., Kravitz, R. L., Bell, R. A., Man Shan, C., Paterniti, D. A., & Chan, M. S. (2016). Characterizing internet health information seeking strategies by socioeconomic status: A mixed methods approach. *BMC Medical Informatics & Decision Making, 16*, 1–9. doi:10.1186/s12911-016-0344-x

Perez, S. L., Paterniti, D. A., Wilson, M., Bell, R. A., Chan, M. S., Villareal, C. C., et al. (2015). Characterizing the processes for navigating internet health information using real-time observations: A mixed-methods approach. *Journal of Medical Internet Research, 17*(7), e173. doi:10.2196/jmir.3945

Perret, J. L., Bonevski, B., McDonald, C. F., & Abramson, M. J. (2016). Smoking cessation strategies for patients with asthma: Improving patient outcomes. *Journal of Asthma and Allergy, 9*, 117–128. doi:10.2147/JAA.S85615

Perri-Moore, S., Kapsandoy, S., Doyon, K., Hill, B., Archer, M., Shane-McWhorter, L., et al. (2016). Automated alerts and reminders targeting patients: A review of the literature. *Patient Education and Counseling, 99*(6), 953–959. doi:10.1016/j.pec.2015.12.010

Pinciroli, F., & Pagliari, C. (2015). Understanding the evolving role of the personal health record. *Computers in Biology and Medicine, 59*, 160–163. doi:10.1016/j.compbiomed.2015.02.008

Piwek, L., Ellis, D. A., Andrews, S., & Joinson, A. (2016). The rise of consumer health wearables: Promises and barriers. *Plos Medicine, 13*(2), e1001953. doi:10.1371/journal.pmed.1001953

Poushter, J. (2016). Smartphone ownership and internet usage continues to climb in emerging economies. But advanced economies still have higher rates of technology use. Pew Research Center. Retrieved from www.pewglobal.org/files/2016/02/pew_research_center_global_technology_report_final_february_22__2016.pdf

PR Newswire, (2013, June 13). NSU center designated as WHO collaborating center in consumer health informatics. *PR Newswire US.*

Prybutok, G. L., Koh, C., & Prybutok, V. R. (2014). A content relevance model for social media health information. *CIN: Computers, Informatics, Nursing, 32*(4), 189–200. doi:10.1097/CIN.0000000000000041

Qing, Z., Gibson, B., Hill, B., Butler, J., Christensen, C., Redd, D., et al. (2016). The effect of simulated narratives that leverage EMR data on shared decision-making: A pilot study. *BMC Research Notes, 9*, 1–9. doi:10.1186/s13104-016-2152-x

Rai, A., Chen, L. Pye, J., & Baird, A., (2013). Understanding determinants of consumer mobile health usage intentions, assimilation, and channel preferences. *Journal of Medical Internet Research, 15*(8), e149. doi: 10.2196/jmir.2635

Romano, M., Sardella, M., Alboni, F., Russo, L., Mariotti, R., Nicastro, I., et al. (2015). Is the digital divide an obstacle to ehealth? An analysis of the situation in Europe and in Italy. *Telemedicine and EHealth, 21*(1), 24–35.

Rideout, V., & Katz, V. S. (2016). *Opportunity for all? Technology and learning in lower-income families.* The Joan Ganz Cooney Center at Sesame Workshop. Retrieved from www .joanganzcooneycenter.org/wp-content/uploads/2016/01/jgcc_opportunityforall.pdf

Sands, D. Z., & Wald, J. S. (2014). Transforming health care delivery through consumer engagement, health data transparency, and patient-generated health information. *Yearbook of Medical Informatics, 9,* 170–176. doi:10.15265/IY-2014-0017

Saranto, K., & Hovenga, E. J. (2004). Information literacy—What it is about? Literature review of the concept and the context. *International Journal of Medical Informatics, 73,* 503–13.

Sayakhot, P., & Carolan-Olah, M. (2016). Internet use by pregnant women seeking pregnancy-related information: A systematic review. *BMC Pregnancy & Childbirth, 16,* 1–10. doi:10.1186/s12884-016-0856-5

Schroeder, E. B., Desai, J., Schmittdiel, J. A., Paolino, A. R., Schneider, J. L., Goodrich, G. K., et al. (2015). An innovative approach to informing research: Gathering perspectives on diabetes care challenges from an online patient community. *Interactive Journal of Medical Research, 4*(2), e13. doi:10.2196/ijmr.3856

Shneyderman, Y., Rutten, L. F., Arheart, K. L., Byrne, M. M., Kornfeld, J., & Schwartz, S. J. (2016). Health information seeking and cancer screening adherence rates. *Journal of Cancer Education: The Official Journal of the American Association for Cancer Education, 31*(1), 75–83. doi:10.1007/s13187-015-0791-6

Singh, K., Drouin, K., Newmark, L. P., Rozenblum, R., Lee, J., Landman, A., et al. (2016). Developing a framework for evaluating the patient engagement, quality, and safety of mobile health applications. *Issue Brief (Commonwealth Fund), 5,* 1–11.

Smith, A., & Page, D. (2015). U.S. smartphone use in 2015. Published by Pew Research Center © 2015. Retrieved from www.pewinternet.org/2015/04/01/us-smartphone-use-in-2015/

Smith, T. R. (2016). Developmental surveillance and screening in the electronic health record. *Pediatric Clinics of North America, 63*(5), 933–943. doi:10.1016/j.pcl.2016.06.014

Sonya, L. (2014). The importance of knowing how to get things: Information literacy and the healthcare professional. *Journal of Mental Health, 23*(3), 113–114. doi:10.3109/0963823 7.2014.912748

Sudbury-Riley, L., FitzPatrick, M., & Schulz, P. J. (2017). Exploring the measurement properties of the ehealth literacy scale (eHEALS) among baby boomers: A multinational test of measurement invariance. *Journal of Medical Internet Research, 19*(2), e53. doi:10.2196/jmir.5998

Tan, S. S., & Goonawardene, N. (2017). Internet health information seeking and the patient-physician relationship: A systematic review. *Journal of Medical Internet Research, 19*(1), e9. doi:10.2196/jmir.5729

US Digital Literacy. (2016). Digital literacy and media literacy for today's learners. Retrieved from http://digitalliteracy.us/

US Food and Drug Administration (FDA). (2017). FDA allows marketing of first direct-to-consumer tests that provide genetic risk information for certain conditions. Retrieved from www.fda.gov/newsevents/newsroom/pressannouncements/ucm551185.htm

Usher, W., Gudes, O., & Parekh, S. (2016). Exploring the use of technology pathways to access health information by Australian university students: A multi-dimensional approach. *Health Information Management Journal, 45*(1), 5–15. doi:10.1177/1833358316639450

Vâjâean, C. C., & Băban, A. (2015). Emotional and behavioral consequences of online health information-seeking: The role of ehealth literacy. *Cognitie, Creier, Comportament/Cognition, Brain, Behavior, 19*(4), 327–345.

Valdez, R. S., Holden, R. J., Novak, L. L., & Veinot, T. C. (2015). Transforming consumer health informatics through a patient work framework: Connecting patients to context. *Journal of The American Medical Informatics Association, 22*(1), 2–10. doi:10.1136/amiajnl-2014-002826

van Deursen, A. M., & van Dijk, J. M. (2015). Toward a multifaceted model of internet access for understanding digital divides: An empirical investigation. *Information Society, 31*(5), 379–391. doi:10.1080/01972243.2015.1069770

Vydra, T. P., Cuaresma, E., Kretovics, M., & Bose-Brill, S. (2015). Diffusion and use of tethered personal health records in primary care. *Perspectives in Health Information Management*, 1–16.

Walsh, A. M., Hamilton, K., White, K. M., & Hyde, M. K. (2015). Use of online health information to manage children's health care: A prospective study investigating parental decisions. *BMC Health Services Research, 15*(1), 1–10. doi:10.1186/s12913-015-0793-4

Warner, J. L., Jain, S. K., & Levy, M. A. (2016). Integrating cancer genomic data into electronic health records. Genome Medicine, 81–13. doi:10.1186/s13073-016-0371-3

Watters, A., Bergstrom, A., & Sandefer, R. (2016). Patient engagement and meaningful use: Assessing the impact of the EHR incentive program on cultural competence in healthcare. *Journal of Cultural Diversity, 23*(3), 114–120.

Wiesner, M., Griebel, L., Becker, K., & Pobiruchin, M. (2016). Consumer health informatics in the context of engaged citizens and ehealth services - a new chi meta model. *Studies In Health Technology And Informatics, 225*, 582–586. doi:10.3233/978-1-61499-658-3-58

Yan, M. (2015). Constructing and reading visual information: Visual literacy for library and information science education. *Journal of Visual Literacy, 34*(2), 1–22. doi:10.1080/23796529.2015.11674727

Ye, J., Stevenson, G., & Dobson, S. (2016), Detecting abnormal events on binary sensors in smart home environments. *Pervasive and Mobile Computing, 33*, 32–49. doi:10.1016/j.pmcj.2016.06.012

Zeng, Q. T., & Tse, T. (2006). Exploring and developing consumer health vocabularies. *Journal of the American Medical Informatics Association, 13*(1), 24–29. doi:10.1197/jamia.M1761

Zuzelo, P. R. (2016). Health literacy and its influence on self-care potential. *Holistic Nursing Practice, 30*(5), 305–307. doi:10.1097/HNP.0000000000000168

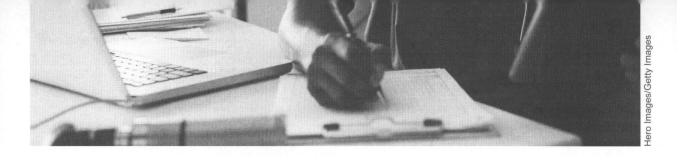

Chapter 19

Connected Healthcare (Telehealth and Technology-Enabled Healthcare)

Lisa Eisele, MSN, RN

 Learning Objectives

After completing this chapter, you should be able to:

- Define common terminology associated with connected health and the delivery of telehealth.

- Identify the historical milestones and driving forces of technology-enabled healthcare.

- Distinguish the delivery modalities and associated technology for telehealth.

- Determine key safety, legal, and ethical considerations for practitioners engaged in delivery of care via telehealth.

- Identify critical patient-safety factors and quality indicators for healthcare delivered via telehealth.

- Determine standards for privacy and information security in connected health.

- Identify the role of the informatics nurse specialist in the evidence-based practice and delivery of technology-enabled healthcare.

- Identify elements of the telehealth network infrastructure, technology selection, bandwidth requirements and utilization.

- Define key considerations for future applications of connected health.

Introduction

Simply stated, connected health is the fusion of healthcare with technology. It is the child of necessity in a family of technology that includes remote monitoring, analytics, virtual access, consumer kiosks and portals, Internet connectivity, smartphones, and other promising solutions to the challenges of providing access to healthcare. These solutions are a win-win for patients, providers, and healthcare administrators who are challenged to improve the environment, access, and quality of care while reducing costs and maximizing existing human and physical resources. In this chapter, you will find the history of telemedicine advancements documented in important literature and research that traces technology-enabled healthcare from its inception to its current state and beyond.

History of Connected Health

Distance communication, traceable to ancient times, is the precursor to modern connected-health (CH) technology. The use of sounds or visible signals corresponding to a prearranged code have allowed distance communication of historic events since the Greek tragedies and the Civil War. Beacon fires through a series of line-of-site relay points carried the news of the fall of Troy over 500 miles across the Aegean Sea, and American military use of the telegraph shared the news of Civil War casualties. Considering the military use of the telegraph to order medical supplies, it is probable that other early applications involved medical consultations (Field, 1996).

Alexander Graham Bell's patent of the telephone, in 1876, advanced technology toward multiplex telegraphy and the development of commercial applications including long-distance telephone connectivity to circuits capable of carrying both still and video signals, audio signals, and data (Field, 1996). In 1906, the first electrocardiographic transmission was accomplished by Willem Einthoven (1860 to 1927), who sent the transmission from the University of Leiden in the Netherlands to the Academic Hospital one mile away. Einthoven went on to develop a system of global electrographic standardization, and received the 1924 Nobel Prize in physiology and medicine (Barold, 2003). The first description of telemedicine in American medical literature was published in 1950, describing the 24-mile transmission of radiologic images between West Chester and Philadelphia, Pennsylvania (Field, 1996).

Connected health advances in the United States and Canada were documented in a series of accomplishments throughout the 1950s, including the transmission of neurological examinations by University of Nebraska faculty to medical students, and later, the development of a link to the Norfolk State Hospital (Madison County, Nebraska) for examinations, diagnostic consultations, and case management. Other early adopters include the City of Miami (Florida) Fire Department's use of voice radio channels to relay electrocardiographic data to physicians at the University of Miami School of Medicine in 1967, and various projects through Massachusetts General Hospital (MGH) dating back to the mid-1960s. One of the principal telemedicine relationships MGH shared was with the Veteran's Administration Hospital in Bedford, Massachusetts—a technology-driven relationship that for over 20 years supported TelePsychiatry from MGH to veterans at Bedford.

The global use of connected health technology has grown exponentially, in part due to the advances associated with early human spaceflight. Prior to the April 1961 Earth orbit of Russian Soviet pilot and cosmonaut, Yuri Gagarin, the United States and Soviets had both performed remote-monitoring experiments to answer the dominant medical questions related to human spaceflight. The National Aeronautics and Space Administration (NASA) played a significant role in the advancement of telemedicine with its use of animals, outfitted with medical-monitoring devices, transmitting biometric data to scientists on Earth via a telemetric link. The data was used to make critical determinations related to human survivability in the absence of gravity by concluding that spaceflight posed little risk to circulatory or respiratory health in nonhuman animals. Early in the 1970s, political influence through the White House Domestic Policy Council explored ways to stimulate the economy by using government programs already in development. As a result, NASA partnered with the Indian Health Service and the Papago (now Tohono O'odham) people of southern Arizona in the deployment of mobile support units that linked rural patients with physicians. Modern day connected health is a spinoff of the beneficial Space Technology Applied to Rural Papago Advanced Health Care (STARPAHC). NASA contributed again when earthquakes in Mexico City (1985) and Soviet Armenia (1988) led to an international telemedicine network for consultations between the disaster locations and medical centers in the United States (National Aeronautics and Space Administration, 2013).

The more recent history of connected health is characterized by three major eras—telecommunications, digital, and Internet. Telecommunications drove the development of connected health, but lacked the technological capability or signal capacity to advance the platform. It was not until the digitalization of telecommunications through the 1990s that significant advances in connected health were possible. Digital telecommunication, through a series of protocols and platforms, provided connectivity to support integrated transmission of voice, video, and data at high speed. For historic context, the digital era quickly morphed into "the era of a more complex and ubiquitous communications network of networks, the Internet" (Bashshur, Reardon, & Shannon, 2000, p. 620).

Current State

It is estimated that the global connected-health market revenues will grow from $23.8 billion in 2016 to roughly $55.1 billion by 2021, with a compound annual growth rate (CAGR) of 18.3% for the five-year period (Research and Markets, 2016). This reflects growing rates of reimbursement and increasing numbers of healthcare providers and patients participating in connected-health options. It is estimated that the number of patients worldwide using telehealth services will rise to roughly seven million by 2018 (Perficient, 2015). This equates to 22-million households using virtual-care solutions, averaging six encounters per year, which include preventive, follow-up, or acute-care services in a variety of care settings (Wang, 2014).

Driving Forces

Over the past 50 years, increasing demand for routine, specialty, and critical-care resources; an aging population; and challenges associated with healthcare staff recruitment and retention, payment, and reimbursement have collided at the intersection of patient safety and healthcare access. *To Err Is Human: Building a Safer Health System* (Kohn, Corrigan, & Donaldson, 2000) is a significant historical patient safety document that has served as a benchmark for advancements since its publication. The document highlights several deficiencies of the American healthcare system, including such systemic issues as fragmentation of care, escalating costs, significant waste of resources, incoherent incentives, an aging and discontented workforce, inequalities in access, lack of investment capital, and a general lack of preparedness for the future. Without being a focus of the study, connected health offers solutions to correct or improve each of the deficiencies cited in this seminal and often-referenced report.

Healthcare technology and the implementation of remote monitoring, analytics, and video teleconferencing technology have all been proven to improve quality and access to healthcare, especially to those patients who are receiving care in rural or underserved communities.

Connected-health options also increase productivity among providers in a variety of ways, leading to their ability to see more patients in a given time period. Benefits include decreased time spent driving for those working in remote locations, less time between patients for those utilizing technology in their office, the ability to assess and intervene without a face-to-face encounter, and the opportunity for improved relationships between providers and patients. The use of connected-health technology allows creative management solutions to address global challenges, such as physician coverage and scope of practice, licensure, regulatory and accreditation considerations, the potential systems impact of deficient services, training and education, and performance measurement. Additionally, connected-health solutions improve infrastructure upon which traditional technology issues such as networking, **bandwidth**, and continuity of operations are addressed. Enterprise and consumer benefits are measured in improved access to healthcare, patient satisfaction, improved clinical outcomes, employee satisfaction, staff retention, and new revenue streams associated with the addition of teleconsultation and remote monitoring.

Underserved Populations: Rural and Remote

In the most recent census of 2010, the Department of Commerce, through the US Census Bureau, reported that 21% of the 311.5 million people in America live in a rural setting. For the purposes of reporting, "rural" is defined as anything that did not meet the urban area (UA) criteria of 50,000 or more people, or the urban cluster (UC) criteria of at least 2,500 and less than 50,000 population-density requirements (US Census Bureau, 2010). With an increase in rural population since the last census, the National Rural Health Association (NRHA) now estimates that approximately 25% of the population lives in rural areas, and are served by only 10% of America's practicing physicians. For rural residents, the distance to main metropolitan centers often places restrictions on their access to essential services, including healthcare specialties. Rural Americans are challenged by other factors that contribute to their risks associated with health. These factors include higher rates of poverty, increasing alcohol and smokeless tobacco use among rural youth, higher rates of hypertension, significant shortages of mental-health resources, higher suicide rates among rural males, and Medicare patients with acute myocardial infarction (AMI) treated in rural hospitals who were less likely to receive recommended treatments (National Rural Health Association, 2016).

Connected health helps to bridge the disparate urban-rural gap by providing a mechanism of care for those who are restricted by distance or mobility, but still prefer a face-to-face option. The Office for the Advancement of Telehealth (OAT) in the Federal Office of Rural Health Policy (FORHP) promotes the use of connected-health technologies for delivery of healthcare, health education, and health-information services. Funding through the Department of Health and Human Services (DHHS) has enabled the OAT to support the development of twelve regional telehealth-resource centers across the country to support the growth of connected health. Their work also supports two national centers focusing on policy and technology. Other notable OAT programs are the *Rural Veterans Health Access Program*, which provides crisis intervention and diagnostic assessments; and the *Rural Child Poverty Telehealth Network Grant Program*, which supports establishing telehealth networks in the delivery of social services, such as early childhood development counseling, and food and nutrition support to rural areas (Department of Health and Human Services, Federal Office of Rural Health Policy 2015a).

Access to Care

The Office of Disease Prevention and Health Promotion (ODPHP) (2018) has identified four synergestic components of access to care: insurance/healthcare coverage, availability of healthcare services, timeliness of care, and workforce. Connected health serves a vital role in this synergy by directly enhancing three of the four critical components, and by indirectly maximizing insurance coverage reimbursement by utilizing services that typically cost less than traditional bricks-and-mortar resources. Barriers to access are significantly reduced when connected health is an option for care delivery.

INSURANCE AND HEALTHCARE COVERAGE By early 2015, an already strained healthcare system felt the net gain of 12 million newly insured Americans as a result of the healthcare exchanges and the Medicaid expansion, resulting from the Affordable Care Act (Congressional Budget Office, Congress of the United States, 2014). Although there are distinct components to the access synergy, it could be argued that, without health insurance or coverage, an individual may not be permitted entry into the system at certain portals. The ODPHP has determined that uninsured people are less likely to receive medical care, more likely to die early, and more likely to have poor-health status.

AVAILABILITY OF HEALTHCARE SERVICES Connected health provides an additional access portal to individuals seeking healthcare services. ODPHP reporting shows that improving the quality of healthcare services is contingent upon having a usual and ongoing source of care. In general, people with usual or established sources have better health outcomes, fewer disparities, and lower healthcare costs. It is felt that the relationship with a primary care provider is especially important as evidenced by greater trust in the provider, good patient-provider communication, and increased likelihood that patients will receive appropriate care.

TIMELINESS OF CARE Timeliness is the system's ability to provide healthcare as soon as the need is recognized. ODPHP measures of timeliness include time spent waiting in doctors' offices and emergency departments, and time between identifying the need for diagnostics, tests or treatments, and actually receiving those services. Connected health significantly reduces wait times for just-in-time care through 24/7 websites such as *Teledoc, Amwell, HealthTap,* and *Doctor On Demand.* These access portals offer interactive video and voice sessions with physicians, therapists, nutritionists, and other specialty providers.

WORKFORCE For the past several years, the number of medical students expressing interest in pursuing a career in primary medicine has decreased. This, combined with unpredictable income, bureaucracy, and healthcare-policy uncertainty, contributes to the lack of desire to enter this field. The ODPHP has identified the need to track the number of practicing primary-care providers, but does not offer solutions to attract and retain them to the field. The growing use of physician extenders (nurse practitioners, advanced-practice nurses, and physician assistants) will help, but connected health provides the greatest opportunity for maximization of existing provider resources.

Cost Savings and Increased Revenue

Tangible benefits of connected health are realized by remote monitoring reimbursement opportunities, the creation of revenue streams through expansion of services to reach patients in remote locations or for consultation services, and by cost savings associated with improved productivity and efficiencies in office space and time utilization. In January 2015, the Centers for Medicare & Medicaid Services (CMS) (n.d.). established a current procedural terminology (CPT) code that allowed providers to bill a monthly fee for monitoring patients with chronic illnesses. Current reimbursement for CPT code 99490 is approximately 50 dollars per month as long as the following criteria are met: (1) The patient has two or more chronic conditions expected to last at least 12 months, or until the death of the patient, (2) the chronic conditions place the patient at significant risk of death, acute exacerbation/decompensation, or functional decline and, (3) a comprehensive care plan is established, implemented, revised or monitored.

Connected Health Modalities

Connected health is the comprehensive term for technology-enabled delivery of distance healthcare. According to the Center for Connected Health Policy, there are four distinct domains of applications: live videoconferencing (synchronous connected health), asynchronous connected health (includes store-and-forward), remote patient monitoring (RPM), and mobile health (mHealth). Connected health leverages the use of technology to deliver healthcare by creating new options outside of traditional settings, which include virtual health kiosks and portals, teleconferencing, videoconferencing, peripheral devices, digital camera imagery, and store-and-forward image transfer.

Rapid growth of this healthcare subset has contributed to the emergence of inconsistent usage of terminology and lack of standardized nomenclature to describe activities and roles associated with connected-healthcare delivery. These inconsistencies contribute to confusion among healthcare providers and consumers, and can blur definitions as they relate to legislation, healthcare policy, and reimbursement. Additional confusion arises when forces within the industry begin to use new terminology in order to distinguish their products and services. For example, virtual health, distance health, interactive health, technology-enabled health, and remote healthcare delivery are not distinct subsets, but are part of the connected-health composite. Use of the "tele" prefix in association with clinical specialties or functions is widely used to distinguish connected-health services.

These inconsistencies were described early during the technology-enabled healthcare surge by Schlachta-Fairchild, Elfrink, and Deickman (2008); even though telemedicine, telehealth, and telenursing were terms with distinct scopes and competencies associated with connected health, they were commonly used interchangeably. In order to promote quality and patient safety in technology-assisted care, and to clarify usage within this text, it is important to distinguish differences in common terms used to describe the delivery of connected health—telemedicine, telehealth, and telenursing.

- **Telemedicine**—Telemedicine is the use of medical information exchanged from one site to another via electronic communications to improve patients' health status. These communications include: videoconferencing, transmission of still images, ehealth including patient portals, remote monitoring, and continuing medical education (American Telemedicine Association, 2016).

- **Telehealth**—Telehealth is the general term used to describe healthcare services delivered utilizing electronic media and is often used to encompass a broader definition of remote healthcare that does not always involve clinical services (American Telemedicine Association, 2016).

- **Telenursing**—Although penned in 2008, the following definition of telenursing by Schlachta-Fairchild, Elfrink, and Deickman remains accurate and comprehensive. "Nurses engaged in telenursing practice continue to assess, plan, intervene, and evaluate the outcomes of nursing care, but they do so using technologies such as the Internet, computers, telephones, digital assessment tools, and telemonitoring equipment" (2008, p.135). Telenursing occurs within the scope and competencies associated with the nursing process. The use of technology requires expertise related to its use in order to render nursing care although neither the nursing process nor scope of practice differ with telenursing.

Based on the growth trajectory of connected health, and the emergence of new technology and innovative solutions to healthcare access, it is likely that the nomenclature will grow increasingly blurred until standardization becomes a priority within the industry. For an example from a historical perspective, a 2007 study found 104 peer-reviewed definitions of the word telemedicine (Sood, 2007). If less is more, the World Health Organization (WHO) continues to say it best: "healing at a distance" (World Health Organization, 2011).

Synchronous Applications

Synchronous connected health applications facilitate interactive, real-time, video and voice interaction and bidirectional communication between patients and healthcare providers. Leveraging synchronous options allows immediate access to services or specialists that might otherwise be inaccessible. The uses are varied, but the result is the delivery of timely care to those in need. Synchronous applications are used widely in hospitals, private practice, school-based healthcare, emergency medical response units, corrections (federal, state, and county jails), federal government (Veterans Health Administration, Department of Defense, and Indian Health Service), offshore, and in the space program. Figure 19-1 depicts an example of synchronous videoconferencing.

VIDEOCONFERENCING Videoconferencing, also known as clinical video telehealth, is the cornerstone of synchronous-connected health technology. It is the platform by which thousands of providers deliver care to millions of patients each year. Early healthcare Videoconferencing sessions were performed over video telephones, often resulting in poor imagery and call quality. Today, advanced technology allows transmission of real-time, high-definition imagery that delivers superior visualization, facilitating rapid diagnosis, especially for dermatology and otolaryngology conditions. Connected-health videoconferencing occurs via private and enterprise conferencing networks, regional networks, state-sponsored networks and Intranet connectivity. Peripheral devices connected to the videoconferencing unit aid the practitioner in assessment and diagnosis at a distance. Common medical peripherals include high-resolution examination cameras, ultrasound probes, electronic stethoscopes, spirometers, 12-lead electrocardiography

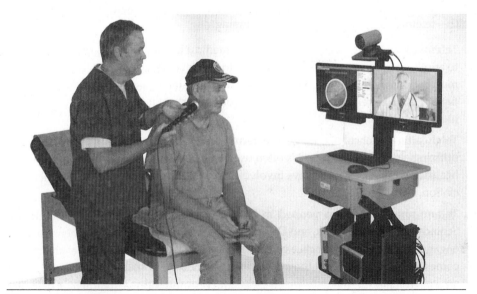

Figure 19-1 • The GlobalMed i8500 Telemedicine Station is deployed around the world as a highly configurable platform to accommodate a wide array of examinations.

SOURCE: Courtesy of GlobalMed.

(EKG), and electroencephalography (EEG). Many of the peripheral devices link to the primary video transmission unit by USB port, or are supported by Bluetooth connected wireless micro technology and cloud-based connectivity.

There is also strong linkage between the use of connected health technology and successful treatment outcomes in adult and pediatric behavioral health populations. Attention-deficit hyperactivity disorder (ADHD) has been studied extensively with consistent data to support the use of telepsychiatry to treat children with ADHD. The Children's Attention-Deficit/Hyperactivity Disorder Telemental Health Treatment Study (CATTS) reported interventions that achieved 46% of the treat-to-target goals compared with 13.6% for augmented primary-care conditions. They found that telepsychiatrists were more likely to adjust medications for patients presenting with higher baseline ADHD severity and comorbid disorders. They concluded that the telepsychiatrists involved in the study showed high-fidelity to evidence-based treatment with care delivered in an effective service model (Rockhill, Fesinmeyer, Garcia, & Myers, 2016).

REMOTE INTENSIVE CARE UNITS AND ASSOCIATED MONITORING Connected health presents an opportunity to improve care to patients in all healthcare settings, especially those who do not have access to specialty services or hospital intensivists. The development of remote or tele-intensive care units was an aggressive system redesign focusing on solutions to the business problem of access to optimal healthcare and specialty services in distant intensive care units. The concept is to use a centralized command center consisting of sophisticated monitoring technology, staffed by highly trained intensivists and critical-care nurses. These centers incorporate decision support systems to track and trend the status of each patient, providing alerts and early detection of trends or patterns requiring intervention. Tele-intensive care units are evolving and focus on four areas of responsibility: performing virtual rounds, managing patient alerts, providing intensive care units (ICU) support, and coaching or providing teaching moments (Goran, 2012). The proliferation of Tele-ICUs coincided with a collaborative study from the New England Health Institute (NEHI) that confirmed the positive contributions made by this technological advancement. The NEHI study found that with Tele-ICU programs in place, ICU mortality rates decreased by more than 20%; ICU length-of-stay decreased 20% hospitals gained significant volumes in ICU; best-practice compliance improved; case margin improved 33% to 80%; total margin increased 136%, considering volume growth; payers realized significant savings; and hospitals achieved payback within the first year (New England Healthcare Institute, 2007). Other literature suggests mortality reduction of 15% by expanding access to trained intensivists, although other studies show little or no impact (Kahn, 2015).

TELESTROKE Telestroke is the use of connected-health technology as a means to overcome limitations of access to stroke care. According to Akbik et al. (2016a) acute ischemic stroke (AIS) is uniquely suited to telemedicine for the following reasons:

- Wide geographic and population distribution of the disease
- Clearly visible clinical findings, often readily identifiable on video
- A narrow therapeutic window
- An existing, proven therapy than can be administered in any facility with basic infrastructure
- Limited specialist availability.

Telestroke services are typically provided from centers staffed with stroke specialists to locations where specialty services are not available, or to remote locations where travel to a higher level of care is prohibitive. Telestroke outcomes and results are compelling, with studies finding that remote consultation led to higher rates of diagnostic and therapeutic interventions, with at least 75% of the consultations leading to meaningful changes in medical management of AIS (Akbik et al., 2016b).

TELEEMERGENCY As technology advances, so do the applications for connected health, especially in the emergency department settings. This technology is especially useful in rural emergency departments who lack the specialists and intensivists to make rapid treatment decisions about patients in critical compromise. Seizures, altered levels of consciousness, and coma can be evaluated immediately through the transmission of EEG data. Ultrasound peripherals for acute appendicitis and other diagnostic applications, spirometers for quickly evaluating pulmonary function in obstruction or restriction, and EKG transmission for rapid diagnosis of myocardial infarction are some of the more frequently used connected-health applications in the emergency setting.

TeleEmergency allows for the immediate treatment of life-threatening symptoms, the stabilization of patients as they prepare for transfer to a higher level of care, and sometimes allows the avoidance of an unnecessary transfer as patients receive emergent care more quickly with less complications.

ROBOTICS The robotic health market holds promise for technological advances targeted to treat the aging American population. Nichol (2016) described three focused areas in medical robotics: direct patient care robots, indirect patient care robots, and home healthcare robots. direct care robots include surgical robots that perform clinical procedures, or provide exoskeletons, and prosthetics to replace lost limbs. Direct care robots, such as those used to perform remote surgery, consist of three major components: the robotic tower is a patient-side cart to which the instruments are connected and mechanically manipulated within the patient; the surgeon's console (where the surgeon sits) controls the actual movement and manipulation of the robotic instruments; and the ancillary vision cart supports a viewing monitor, insufflator, light source, and camera operations (Schwartz, Rais-Bahrami, & Kavoussi, 2015). These systems are commonly used in cardiac, colorectal, general, gynecological, thoracic, urologic, and head/neck surgeries. Figure 19-2 depicts a robotic surgery system.

Indirect care robots streamline automation and reduce labor costs in healthcare by performing courier activities such as transport of medications and specimens in secure-delivery robots, and disinfection-tasking in high-risk spaces. "Germ zapping" robots are deployed as a fast, safe, and cost-effective method of disinfecting patient rooms, operating suites, and intensive care units. Disinfection is achieved through pulsed xenon ultraviolet-emissions, which quickly

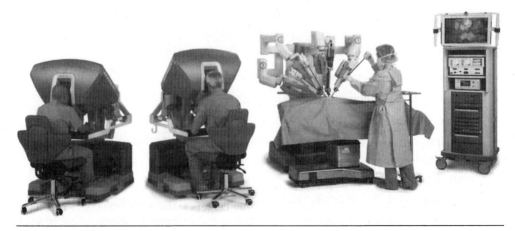

Figure 19-2 • The da Vinci robotic surgical system, Intuitive Surgical Company.

SOURCE: ©[2017] Intuitive Surgical, Inc. Used with permission.

destroy microorganisms that cause healthcare-associated infections such as Clostridium difficile (C. diff), Methicillin-resistant Staphylococcus aureus (MRSA), and the Ebola virus (Xenex, 2015).

Home healthcare robots provide telepresence solutions by providing the aging population with robotic assistance. Their usage ranges from feeding assistance (robotics equipped with feeding utensils) to socially assistive robots (SAR) with advanced communication capabilities, helping the elderly stay connected and safe in their home. SAR capabilities include remote and continuous health monitoring, coaching to facilitate healthy behavior, social applications, fall sensors, and support of cognitive and functional abilities, such as task reminders. SAR acceptance was highest among users who opted to utilize the technology to help compensate for cognitive impairment, increase social engagement, help facilitate risk prevention, and support everyday tasks (Pino, Boulay, Jouen, & Rigaud, 2015).

Asynchronous Applications

REMOTE PATIENT MONITORING AND RISK-STRATIFIED CASE MANAGEMENT
Remote patient monitoring (RPM) is a patient-centric, emerging technology that allows consumers to participate in their own care by using a designated health technology to share health metrics and data with their healthcare provider or monitoring professional. Traditional users of this technology report daily on a device that is either Intranet, smartphone, or POTS-based and answers six to ten questions based on a specific disease-management protocol that has been programmed to the device or application. These protocols ask predetermined questions based on evidence-based disease management, and, depending on the vendor, the questions appear linear or in a decision-tree pattern. Registered nurses and physician extenders are often involved in enhanced case management by utilizing the risk stratification capabilities of RPM technology leading to better management of at-risk populations, including those with chronic diseases and who are high utilizers of healthcare resources. Significant benefits of this platform include enhanced communication between providers and patients, early detection of symptoms, identification of knowledge gaps, identification of risky lifestyle or behavioral choices, medication management and compliance. Figure 19-3 depicts an example of remote patient monitoring.

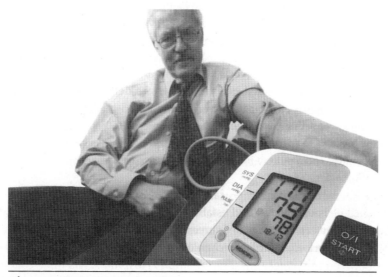

Figure 19-3 • Risk-stratified telemonitoring improves patient outcomes with early intervention.

SOURCE: Brian Maudsley/Shutterstock.

STORE-AND-FORWARD APPLICATIONS Store-and-forward (SF) technology consists of asynchronous connected-health applications that can transmit recorded health information (radiographic images, photos, and videos) through a secure communication network to a provider. The provider evaluates the information, to render a consultation service outside of a real-time patient interaction. SF applications are commonly used where specialty or high-resolution imagery is required. Three of the most common uses are teleradiology, teledermatology, and teleretinal imaging. SF also enables the transmission of electrocardiograms, and data associated with sleep studies (home or clinic-based). Most SF uses rely on established infrastructure enhanced by data transfer.

Smart Homes

Smart homes are dwellings integrated with sensors and actuators intended to monitor the resident and improve their home experience. This technology enables older adults to live independently at home longer, reduces reliance on caregivers or external resources, and provides a cost-efficient approach to safer living. A systematic review of studies of smart home occupants appeared to suggest advantages to clinical outcomes when compared to no intervention or other types of interventions. Smart homes can provide a variety of services, from simple tasking (e.g., room-temperature control) to capabilities including monitoring and transmission of health and wellness data (Liu, Stroulia, Nikolaidis, Miguel-Cruz, & Rincom, 2016). Technology-readiness and technology-acceptance are challenges associated with greater implementation of smart homes.

Implications for Practitioners

The entry into, or development of, connected health within an existing practice requires business planning and establishment of critical components of infrastructure in order to provide safe, effective, high-quality healthcare. Depending on where the provider will be conducting connected-health sessions, the planning may require the establishment of memorandums of understanding (MOU) with landlords or information-technology providers in order to assure that adequate technical support is available to facilitate the delivery of connected healthcare. Important aspects of these MOUs include minimum bandwidth requirements, contingency operations, responsibilities and obligations related to the purchasing and maintenance of connected-health technologies, network-security requirements, contingency plans, and support services required to assure continuity of operations. MOUs usually exist between two physical locations where connected-health services are delivered. For example, an MOU should be in place when a provider is delivering connected-health services from their office to patients who are reporting to another location (clinic, school, or remote location) in order to complete the healthcare encounter. MOUs are required when services are delivered directly between the provider and a patient in their home. These considerations will be discussed later in the practitioner safety section.

Another document of vital importance is the connected-health service agreement (CHSA). The CHSA is negotiated and established between the provider and all locations where patients receive care. This type of agreement is necessary even when all locations are within the same enterprise, as staffing, technology, emergency contacts, and local procedures may differ between the patient sites. For example, Hospital A has three community clinics where patients travel to receive connected-health services from the main hospital. Each clinic provides unique services, has different staffing ratios, and are serviced by different local ambulance services, police, and fire departments. Although all locations are considered

Hospital A service locations, the response to connected health needs and planning for those sessions differs in each location. The CHSA is usually a templated form that specifies provider preferences and requirements for the session. It is the document that addresses issues equating to the provision of safe and effective patient care. The CHSA document establishes standards for each type of connected-health specialty ranging from the ordering of pre-session lab or imaging studies, contingencies for technological failures, points of contact for emergencies on both sides of the encounter, qualifications of the telepresenter (patient side of the encounter), and provision of patient care in the event that an emergency or complication should arise during the course of the connected-health session. The CHSA is a provider and enterprise specific document that should consider local policies, procedures, accreditation, and regulatory standards.

Identifying Telehealth Patient Populations

Would you consider connected health a disruptive innovation? It is certainly worth a pause for consideration as the platform falls within the definition of a disruptive innovation. It has taken a traditional or existing technology and replaced it with an innovation that has resulted in the development of a new industry. Practitioners should approach connected health with that insight, and use it when evaluating patient-provider relationships and determining which patient populations are appropriate for virtual encounters. Disruptive or not, many years of evidence support connected health use in patients with chronic disease, multiple comorbidities, recent hospitalizations, and high-utilizers of healthcare resources, including those who frequent their primary-care provider, urgent-care clinic, or emergency room.

Chronic obstructive pulmonary disease (COPD), congestive heart failure (CHF), and diabetes mellitus (DM) are among the top chronic disease conditions monitored by home telehealth (HT) case managers. Over the past four decades, studies have shown that the HT data allows prediction and preemptive interventions that prevent significant health deterioration, leading to reduction in hospitalizations. In a 7-month study, which included monitoring and follow-up, COPD patients showed significant reduction in ER visits, hospitalizations, length-of- stay, and need for noninvasive mechanical ventilation when compared to conventional care (CC). The cohort of 30 HT patients had 20 ER visits compared to 57 ER visits for the 30 patients receiving conventional care. HT patients had 12 hospitalizations, CC patients had 33 hospitalizations; and length of stay for HR patients was 105 versus 276 for the CC patients. Also, none of the HT patients required noninvasive mechanical ventilation versus eight patients in the CC cohort (Segrelles Calbo et al., 2014).

Patient Safety

ESTABLISHING INCLUSION AND EXCLUSION CRITERIA Perhaps the single most important consideration for patient safety in connected health is establishing criteria for patients to receive care within the virtual environment. Commonly known as inclusion and exclusion criteria, the provider of services must predetermine the cohort of patients who can safely be assessed and treated in the virtual environment. These criteria, in conjunction with patient preferences and individualized assessments of the condition, will allow the provider to make strong decisions regarding the safety and efficacy of connected health in a particular episode of care. For example, stable depression patients are commonly treated through telemental health services, where a patient that is at high risk for suicide might not be a safe candidate for connected health. All patients should be evaluated on a case-by-case basis with the knowledge that connected health will not be an appropriate option for all patients. Other common examples of inclusion criteria are stable patients across the spectrum of medical specialties. Common exclusion criteria may include new onset seizure disorder, active substance abuse, or those with cognitive, functional, or physical limitations that do not allow for optimal assessment in the connected health environment.

ESTABLISHING A SAFETY AND EMERGENCY PLAN FOR TELEHEALTH ENCOUNTERS
Connected-health sessions must exist within a framework that provides for patient safety, emergency plans for crisis, and contingencies for technology failure. Safety plans are unique to the provider-patient encounter, and often involve permission for the provider to notify a patient's emergency contact when an urgent situation arises during the course of the connected-health session. It is also common for providers to have immediate access to emergency-response information (police, fire, and emergency medical) for the patient's geographic location throughout the encounter. Safety planning should consider physical needs/disabilities, emotional needs and interventions, environmental and structural safety, and contingencies for technology-failure.

Practitioner Guidance and Safety Considerations

ESTABLISHING PRIVACY, SESSION CRITERIA, AND INFORMED CONSENT Prior to the start of the telemedicine encounter, and after determining that the patient is appropriate for the scheduled service, the provider shall assure that the privacy of the patient is protected by physically surveying his/her environment and assuring conversations occur in a tone and volume that protect the shared information of the session. The workspaces should be secure, private, reasonably soundproof, and have a lockable door to prevent unexpected entry. Testing should be done to assure that the patient can clearly see the provider, that lighting is sufficient and that there are no visual distractions or glare on the provider field that would be distracting to the patient. Discuss with the patient any concerns they have related to privacy on their end of the encounter, and work toward a solution. For example, some patients may not wish to conduct a session in the presence of a family member or child. If this is the case, provide options to the patient for alternate locations or reschedule the session. Patients should not proceed with a session if they feel privacy will be compromised at their point of care. Establish and discuss criteria for maintaining confidentiality of the connected-health exchanges. Some enterprises have incorporated agreements requesting that patients not record or distribute sessions intended to be confidential patient-provider sessions. If other people are in either the patient or the professional's room, both will be made aware of the other person and must agree to their presence. Discuss the structure and timing of services, scheduling, documentation, potential risks, mitigation of risks, mandatory reporting (such as abuse or neglect), billing, and other nuances of videoconferencing (American Telemedicine Association, 2014).

Care will be conducted within the applicable jurisdictional considerations for the provider's profession at both the site where the provider is practicing and the site where the patient is receiving care. Providers will be cognizant of the provider-patient relationship that exists within the context of connected health and will proceed accordingly with evidence-based care. Healthcare professionals should have the necessary education, training, knowledge, and technical competency to provide safe, quality healthcare within their specialty, and while utilizing devices and software necessary to provide connected-health sessions.

DOCUMENTING THE ENCOUNTER The organization and healthcare professional will document the episode of care in the enterprise system of documentation (electronic health record) and include the documentation elements that are required for appropriate payment of services. This may include the clinical association, town, state, and patient location. However, it is not necessary for the healthcare providers to reveal their specific location to the patient, especially if a provider is located at home at the time of service. However, a mechanism to verify location is critical for compliance with licensing laws where the provider is physically located when providing care, as well at the patient's location when receiving care. This information is also vital to emergency management. Providers should document that the patient consents to the delivery of care via the connected-healthcare technology, and that the patient may schedule in-person care appointments in the event they wish to discontinue their connected-health services.

Legal and Ethical Issues

The legal and regulatory infrastructure for telemedicine has yet to catch up with daily changes in technology, explosive industry growth, and increased utilization of connected-health services. It has created multiple barriers to informal, distance-based care through regulatory challenges such as liability, licensure, and credentialing (Kahn, 2015). While legal challenges are universal, as outlined in Figure 19-4, ethical challenges are considerably more diverse.

Consider these ethical questions:

- Does connected health truly constitute the establishment of a patient-provider relationship?
- What are the implications of significant variability in connected-health research as it relates to healthcare outcomes?
- What are the unintended consequences of connected health?
- Does connected health compromise the traditional concepts and structure of face-to-face, hands-on delivery of healthcare?

The answer to all of these questions is a resounding "we simply don't know." Most providers and patients involved in connected-health encounters would attest that a true relationship exists. Beyond that, the remaining questions remain unanswered. It is prudent to consider

---

1. Credentialing and privileging: Connected-health technologies have created challenges to healthcare organizations that wish to access medical specialties via the platform. Advances have been made through the Centers for Medicare and Medicaid Services (CMS), through the establishment of a new process to credential and privilege providers. Unfortunately, the process conflicts with established policy in many states.
2. Online prescribing: Online prescribing policies vary across the states. Concerns have arisen over the determination of established patient-provider relationships, accuracy of the patient's history given the self-reporting aspect of connected health, and not meeting state medical-board licensing requirements.
3. Malpractice liability: Questions of medical liability increase amid a lack of information on existing malpractice liability within connected health.
4. Licensing of physicians and other healthcare providers: Consultations occurring over great distances require consideration of varied policies governing connected health and physician licensure. Cross-border delivery of healthcare is banned entirely in some states.
5. Informed consent: Medicare does not require informed consent before the delivery of connected-health services, but several states do have Medicaid policies requiring consent. Many connected-health practitioners include a narrative in their encounter notes indicating the patient consents to receive health services using connected health, thus preventing the need to document differently for different reimbursements, and always assuring the patient is informed and consenting to the service.

Figure 19-4 • Five Legal Challenges of Connected Health

these and other ethical considerations as connected-health programs are developed, implemented, and monitored. The traditional ethical principles of in-person healthcare delivery apply equally to connected-health patients, including nonmaleficence, beneficence, fidelity, justice, and patient autonomy (Zubrow, Witzke, & Reynolds, 2015).

LICENSURE PORTABILITY AND CARE ACROSS STATE LINES Licensure portability is one of the critical elements in the strategies required to improve access to quality healthcare through utilization of connected-health services. Because of challenges associated with licensure portability, the Licensure Portability Grant Program awards grants to state professional licensing boards to assist in the development and implementation of state policies that reduce statutory and regulatory barriers to telemedicine (Department of Health and Human Services, Federal Office of Rural Health Policy, 2015b).

PRACTICE STANDARDS The American Telemedicine Association (ATA) has established *Core Operational Guidelines for Telehealth Services Involving Provider-Patient Interactions*. The guidelines consist of scope, associated definitions, administrative, clinical, and technical guidance. The *scope* applies to individual practitioners, group and specialty practices, hospital and healthcare systems, and other providers of health services where connected-health interactions occur between patients and service providers within the United States. The ATA advises that other guidelines and standards addressing specific specialties may exist, and that all documents, as appropriate, should be incorporated into practice. The administrative guidelines state that organizations should:

- Follow the policies and procedures of the governing institution
- Have a systematic quality improvement and performance-management process
- Ensure compliance with relevant legislation and regulations
- Have a mechanism to inform patients and health professionals of their rights and responsibilities with respect to accessing and providing healthcare via connected-health technologies
- Respect patients' requests for in-person care whenever feasible
- Inform and educate the patient in real-time of all pertinent information prior to the start of the connected-health session (as discussed in *Practitioner Guidance and Safety Considerations*)

INFRASTRUCTURE, NETWORK, AND EQUIPMENT CONSIDERATIONS Technical and infrastructure requirements are determined by the type of services and equipment to be utilized in the delivery of connected health. Basic requirements include access to broadband Internet with sufficient bandwidth to transmit the connected health data, connect imaging technology or peripheral devices, access technical support, and train staff (HealthIT.gov, 2016). Equipment should be vetted through the providers who will be utilizing it for delivery of health services. It should be accompanied by vendor training, a comprehensive user manual, access to troubleshooting and ongoing technical support.

The Role of the INS in Connected Health
Development of Clinical Pathways

Clinical pathways are the identification and plotting of healthcare delivery in order to prevent variability that may lead to undesired results. These pathways are the route by which care is delivered in a standardized, consistent, and evidence-based environment. The connected-health clinical pathways differ in regard to the technological versus physical delivery of care. The informatics nurse specialist will help develop clinical pathways that provide for technology-enhanced care. When technology is inserted into a clinical pathway, it must be done in a thoughtful, patient-centric, safe way that is conducive to provider-productivity and satisfaction.

Establishing Criteria for Selection of Equipment and Technology

A common enterprise mistake is the purchase of connected-health equipment without input of providers who will be utilizing the technology for delivery of care, and without consideration of infrastructure requirements to support the session requirements. This approach can lead to the purchase of very expensive paperweights and closets full of dusty, inoperable resources. The best approach is to research a variety of vendors that are specific to the needs of the medical specialty. Although there are some basic, utilitarian connected-health delivery options, most specialties benefit from peripheral devices that are specific to the assessment needs of the medical specialty.

Development of Quality Indicators for Connected Healthcare

The true indicators of quality in connected health are parallel to quality indicators for traditional environments of care. Quality indicators allow organizations to compare their delivery of care at other points within their continuum and to other similar organizations. These indicators and composites focus on outcomes, prevention of complications, patient safety, prevention activities, early interventions, hospitalizations, and utilization of other healthcare resources. The WHO (World Health Organization, 2011) identified four elements considered germane to telemedicine. These remain relevant as a historical marker, but also provide a clear vision for the current and future states of technology-enabled healthcare. It is within these elements that the indicators of connected health quality are rooted.

- Its purpose is to provide clinical support.
- It is intended to overcome geographical barriers, connecting users who are not in the same physical location.
- It involves the use of various types of information and communication technologies.
- Its goal is to improve health outcomes.

Based on the WHO elements, additional quality indicators should include measures of access to care based on wait times for service, expansion of service areas, successful implementation and support of connected-health technologies, and general improvement of health outcomes.

Future Directions

The American Telemedicine Association and the National Consortium of Telehealth Resource Centers are among the nation's leading sources of information and education related to connected-health technologies and programs. The industry predicts explosive growth of connected-health programs over the next five years. This growth is fueled by the refinement of current technology; the advancement of innovations such as biosensors, wearable devices, and new digital platforms; and important changes in healthcare legislation and reimbursement.

Summary

- Connected health is an encompassing term for the delivery of technology-assisted care that occurs outside the traditional face-to-face setting.
- Patient safety is the key driver in all connected-healthcare decisions.
- Establish and share rights and responsibilities for patients and providers engaged in connected health.
- Establish inclusion and exclusion criteria for all connected-health services.
- Develop service agreements, sharing agreements, or memorandums of understanding between all service locations.
- Choose appropriate technology to accomplish optimal results for patient and provider.
- Assure technological and network infrastructure are adequate to meet connected-health demands.
- Each enterprise should establish a connected-health support team to address planning, development, deployment, and sustainability of programs.
- Establish platforms and engagement algorithms that promote patient self management.
- Establish tangible and non tangible data points to track value to the enterprise, the provider, and the patient.
- Track clinical outcomes (hospitalizations, hospital bed days-of-care, readmissions, utilization of healthcare resources, ER visits, PCP visits, reduction in HgbA1c, and blood pressures).
- Track patient and provider satisfaction.
- Develop or consult experts to support connected-health programs in business, administrative, ethical, and legal decisions.

Case Study

Telemedicine in Corrections: The Texas Department of Criminal Justice

The Texas Department of Criminal Justice (TDCJ) is home to the largest prison population in the United States. With more than 150,000 inmates, the TDCJ uses connected health as a way to provide healthcare to inmates in its 31 state prison facilities. Through the establishment of the Correctional Managed Health Care Committee (CMHCC), a collaborative program between the TDCJ, Texas Tech University Health Sciences Center (TTUHSC), and the University of Texas Medical Branch (UTMB), a partnership now exists to ensure that inmates have access to cost-effective, quality healthcare.

Estimates show that over a 14-year period, the use of connected-health technology saved the TDCJ more than $780 million. Other significant findings as a result of the use of connected-health resources were the prevention of approximately 85% of Texan inmates leaving the corrections facility for healthcare, and weeding out offenders who fake illnesses or injuries. A Pew Charitable Trusts report indicates that in some measures the health of inmates has improved.

The collaborative leaves the choice of utilizing telemedicine to the inmate. Most inmates prefer the connected-health option as this usually allows them to return immediately to their housing unit within the system. When inmates leave the prison for a medical appointment, they sometimes are not allowed to return to the cell unit right away. Providers also have a choice in determining if the encounter is appropriate for connected health, or if a face-to-face assessment is needed.

Additional factors that will contribute to the sustainability of this program include the advancing age of the prison population, the limited number of infirmary beds for older inmates, the shortage of healthcare providers, and the rurality of a significant portion of Texas. The risks to correctional officers and hospital personnel are minimized by increased utilization of connected options within prison healthcare and avoidance of transfer outside the system.

Connected-correctional healthcare continues to advance in Texas with plans for medical studies such as CT scans and MRIs, the development of additional treatment protocols, and the expanded use of connected-health peripheral devices such as digital stethoscopes, video otoscope, ultrasound, spirometry, and ECK/EKG monitoring (GlobalMed, 2015).

About the Author

Lisa Eisele, MSN, RN is an informatics nurse specialist who led one of the most robust telemedicine programs in the Veterans Health Administration (VHA), building a strong and sustained community of practice for all modalities of telehealth. Ms. Eisele oversaw the largest deployment of telemedicine technology in the history of the South Central Veterans Healthcare Network, leading to the addition of hundreds of portals to improve access to care for veterans in rural and remote locations. Ms. Eisele continues her work with the VHA in New England as a Chief of Quality, Organizational Performance, and Risk Management.

References

Akbik, F., Hirsch, J. A., Chandra, R. V., Frei, D., Patel, A. B., Rabinov, J. D., et al. (2016a). Telestroke—The promise and the challenge. Part one: Growth and current practice. *Journal of Neurointerventional Surgery, 9*(4), 357–360. doi:10.1136/neurintsurg-2016-012291.

Akbik, F., Hirsch, J. A., Chandra, R. V., Frei, D., Patel, A. B., Rabinov, J. D., et al. (2016b). Telestroke—The promise and the challenge. Part two: Expansion and horizons. *Journal of Neurointerventional Surgery, 9*(4), 361–365. doi:10.1136/neurintsurg-2016-012340

American Telemedicine Association. (2016). Telemedicine nomenclature. Retrieved from www.americantelemed.org/resources/nomenclature#.V1oYzSDD_IU

American Telemedicine Association. (2014). *Core operational guidelines for telehealth services involving provider-patient interactions* Available at Americantelemed.org.

Barold, S. (2003). Willem Einthoven and the birth of clinical electrocardiography a hundred years ago. *Cardiac Electrophysiology Review, 7*(1), 99–104.

Bashshur, R. L., Reardon, T. G., & Shannon, G. W. (2000). Telemedicine: A new health care delivery system. *Annual Review of Public Health, 21*(1), 613–637.

Centers for Medicare & Medicaid Services (CMS). (n.d.). Chronic Care Management Services. Retrieved from www.cms.gov/Outreach-and-Education/Medicare-Learning-Network-MLN/MLNProducts/Downloads/ChronicCareManagement.pdf

Congressional Budget Office, Congress of the United States. (2014). Updated estimates of the effects of the insurance coverage provisions of the affordable care act, April 2014. Retrieved from www.cbo.gov/sites/default/files/cbofiles/attachments/45231-ACA_Estimates.pdf

Department of Health and Human Services, Federal Office of Policy. (2015a). Federal Office of Rural Health Policy. Retrieved from www.hrsa.gov/rural-health/index.html

Department of Health and Human Services, Federal Office of Rural Health Policy. (2015b). Telehealth programs. Retrieved from www.hrsa.gov/rural-health/telehealth/index.html

Field, M. J. (1996). Telemedicine: A guide to assessing telecommunications in health care. Retrieved from www.ncbi.nlm.nih.gov/books/NBK45445/

GlobalMed Group. (2015). Telemedicine in corrections. Retrieved from www.globalmed.com/wp-content/uploads/internal/corrections-whitepaper.pdf

Goran, S. (2012). Making the move: From bedside to camera-side. *Critical Care Nurse, 32*(1), e20–e29.

HealthIT.gov. (2016). What are the technical infrastructure requirements of telehealth? Retrieved from www.healthit.gov/providers-professionals/faqs/what-are-technical-infrastructure-requirements-telehealth

Kahn, J. M. (2015). Virtual visits confronting the challenges of telemedicine. *New England Journal of Medicine, 372*(18), 1684–1685.

Kohn, L. T., Corrigan, J., & Donaldson, M. S. (2000). *To err is human: Building a safer health system.* Washington, DC: National Academy Press.

Liu, L., Stroulia, E., Nikolaidis, I., Miguel-Cruz, A., & Rincom, A. R. (2016). Smart homes and home health monitoring technologies for older adults: A systematic review. *International Journal of Medical Informatics, 91*, 44–59.

National Aeronautics and Space Administration. (2013). A brief history of NASA's contributions to telemedicine. Retrieved from www.nasa.gov/content/a-brief-history-of-nasa-s-contributions-to-telemedicine/#.V1thjCDD_IU

National Rural Health Association. (2016). What's different about rural health care? Retrieved from www.ruralhealthweb.org/go/left/about-rural-health/what-s-different-about-rural-health-care

New England Healthcare Institute. (2007). *Tele-ICUs: Remote management in intensive care units.* Retrieved from www.nehi.net/writable/publication_files/file/tele_icu_final.pdf

Nichol, P. B. (2016). *CIO.* Retrieved from How medical robots will change healthcare. Retrieved from www.cio.com/article/3043172/innovation/how-medical-robots-willchange-healthcarerhealth-get-familiar-with-it.htm

Office of Disease Prevention and Health Promotion (2018). Access to health services. Retrieved from www.healthypeople.gov/2020/topics-objectives/topic/Access-to-Health-Services

Perficient. (2015). Top 10 connected health trends. Retrieved from http://s3.amazonaws.com/rdcms-himss/files/production/public/FileDownloads/2015%20-%2008-%2020%20Perficient%20healthcare-industry-trends-snapshot.pdf

Pino, M., Boulay, M., Jouen, F., & Rigaud, A. S. (2015). Are we ready for robots that care for us? Attitudes and opinions of older adults toward socially assistive robots. *Frontiers in Aging Neuroscience.* Retrieved from http://journal.frontiersin.org/article/10.3389/fnagi.2015.00141/full

Research and Markets. (2016). Global markets for telemedicine technologist. Retrieved from www.researchandmarkets.com/reports/3745706/

Rockhill, C. M., Fesinmeyer, M. D., Garcia, J., & Myers, K. (2016). Telepsychiatrists' medication treatment strategies in the children's attention-deficit/hyperactivity disorder telemental health treatment study. *Journal of Child and Adolescent Psychopharmacology.* 26(8), 662–671.

Schlachta-Fairchild, L., Elfrink, V., & Deickman, A. (2008). Patient safety, telenursing, and telehealth. In Hughes, R. G. *Patient safety and quality: An evidence-based handbook for nurses.* Agency for Healthcare Research and Quality, 3, 135–174. Published by Agency for Healthcare Research and Quality.

Schwartz, M., Rais-Bahrami, S., & Kavoussi, L. (2015). Laparoscopic and robotic surgery of the kidney. In Kavoussi, L. R., Partin, A. W., Peters, C. A., & Wein, A. J. (Ed.). *Campbell-Walsh urology* (11th ed.). (pp. 1446–1483). Philadelphia: Elsevier.

Soriano, J. B., Segrelles Calvo, G., Zamora, E., Ancochea, J., Soriano, J. B., Gonzatez-Gamarra, A., & . . . Fernandez, G. (2014). A home telehealth program for patients with severe COPD: The PROMETE study. *Respiratory Medicine, 108*(3), 453–62.

Sood, S. E. (2007). Differences in public and private sector adoption of telemedicine: Indian case study for sectoral adoption. *Studies in Health Technology and Informatics, 130,* 257–268.

US Census Bureau. (2010). Urban and Rural. Retrieved from www.census.gov/geo/reference/urban-rural.html

Wang, H. (2014). Virtual health care will revolutionize the industry, if we let it. Retrieved from www.forbes.com/sites/ciocentral/2014/04/03/virtual-health-care-visits-will-revolutionize-the-industry-if-we-let-it/#1301a6af5ab5

World Health Organization. (2011). Telemedicine: Opportunities and developments in member states. Retrieved from www.who.int/goe/publications/goe_telemedicine_2010.pdf

Xenex. (2015). Germ zapping robot deployed to destroy germs at william beaumont army medical center. *Hospital & Nursing Home Week.* Retrieved from http://search.proquest.com/docview/1660685163?accountid=30091

Zubrow, M., Witzke, A., & Reynolds, N. (2015). Legal, regulatory, and ethical issues in the use of telemedicine. In Cross, R., & Watson, A. (Eds.). *Telemanagement of inflammatory bowel disease* (pp. 153–177.). New York: Springer.

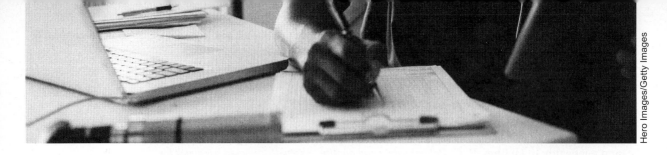

Chapter 20
Public Health Informatics

Marisa L. Wilson, DNSc, MHSc, RN-BC CPHIMS FAAN

 Learning Objectives

After completing this chapter, you should be able to:

- Describe the domain and function of public health.

- Discuss the data and information flows that are key to supporting public health functions.

- Identify critical public health applications used to manage chronic and infectious diseases.

- Examine efforts to facilitate exchange between clinical and public health information systems.

- Describe systems currently in use to manage the public health mandate.

Introduction

Informatics is the science of information management. It is about the collection, processing, representation, and communication of information by computers, humans, and organizations (American Medical Informatics Association, 2017). Informatics draws upon the theories of computer science, information science, and other sciences. Informatics solutions seek to support processes that address a gap or concern along with the people and programs working to meet and eliminate this gap. Informatics processes require three components: (1) knowledge of the domain into which a system is being applied; (2) knowledge of how the information system is to be designed and developed to manage the data and information of the domain; and (3) knowledge of how the organizations and people interact with or use the information system to achieve goals (Haque, Dixon, & Grannis, 2016). The domain focus of this chapter is public and population health.

In the past, public health was largely focused on disease surveillance and protecting specific populations from communicable diseases. In recent years, there has been an increased focus on consumer engagement for self-improvement, the data generated from these activities, and the rapid communication of public health issues and trends to the public (Institute of Medicine (IOM), 2011, 2015). The call for better national security and integration of information and resources after the September 11, 2001 terror attacks is another area of focus (Foldy, Grannis, Ross, & Smith, 2014; Kukafka & Yasnoff, 2007). Public health informatics (PHI) plays a major role in these initiatives. The purpose of this chapter is to increase awareness and sensitivity to selected major issues related to PHI and systems to provide public health information to individuals and populations. The chapter begins by looking at the domain of public health before addressing the informatics challenges.

Exploring Public Heath

This chapter provides a review of the public health domain prior to delving into the specifics of the informatics and information systems needed to support the domain. Understanding public health can be a challenging task when so much focus in healthcare is on the individual experience in the acute setting. Public health transcends the individual to focus on the community and the population. Public health moves beyond the confines of an individual interaction within a hospital, emergency room, or provider office to the activities of people in a local community, state, or nation. In order to understand the requirements of an information system and the necessary informatics processes needed to support the domain, as Haque et al. (2016) directed, one must explore the mission, functions, and tasks that comprise public health.

Providing a succinct definition of public health can be a daunting task. In 1920, C. E. A. Winslow defined public health as "the science and art of preventing disease, prolonging life, and promoting health through organized efforts and informed choices of society, organizations, public and private, communities and individuals" (p. 32). The current definition has changed very little. In 2016, the American Public Health Association (APHA) described public health as the promotion and protection of the health of people and communities "where they live, learn, work, and play" (p. 1). Public health practitioners work to prevent people from getting sick or injured, and they develop programs to promote wellness and encourage healthy behaviors (APHA, 2016). This broad nature of the public health mandate is what makes the domain a challenge to informatics solutions.

The discipline of public health is diverse, encompassing surveillance, case reporting, and prevention activities; consequently, its scope is difficult to fully grasp. On a practical basis, many individuals have had some limited interaction with the public health system, perhaps in the form of filing or obtaining vital records such as birth or death certificates or when reading about an inspection and grading of a favorite restaurant, so their idea of what constitutes public health is limited to those experiences. This provides a very restricted view of the work of public health professionals. If one reflects on the definition of public health, it is apparent that the domain transcends merely bureaucratic functions, also encompassing activities supporting health and wellness in communities, populations, and settings outside of the typical care site or even the health department offices.

Public Health Mandate

In the previous century, vast declines in morbidity and mortality rates were gained through a focus on preventing the spread of communicable diseases. Immunizations, disease screening (especially tuberculosis screening), clean water, hand washing, and other sanitation techniques we now take for granted reduced the spread of communicable diseases and were important factors in increasing life expectancy and improving the health of the population. Today, public health practitioners face new challenges. Emerging epidemics, bioterrorism, antibiotic-resistant microorganisms, and the current struggles with diabetes, obesity, smoking-related illnesses, chronic disease, and health threats from disasters and climate change are just some of the priorities of the public health system that challenge people, processes, and information needs.

There is much more to public health than what may be experienced during brief interactions with local and state level agencies. Public health encompasses more than just checking on the safety of restaurants, collecting vaccination records, and mandating the reporting of the diagnoses of communicable diseases by providers. Public health agencies provide care for indigent populations, oversee the health and safety of food and water supplies, manage the proper disposal of liquid and solid waste, and provide ongoing disease surveillance (Centers for Disease Control and Prevention, 2016). Residents of the United States have been protected and kept healthy by the public health system for over 100 years, but even today most have not had direct contact with the methods in which public health is practiced; Koo, O'Carroll, and LaVenture had noted this trend back in 2001. Thus, to achieve the public health mandate, a unifying approach is needed.

The public health approach to combat these diverse challenges has been well established, and is represented by four general steps as listed below and depicted in Figure 20-1:

1. Identification of the problem, using surveillance to monitor health events and behaviors.
2. Identification of the cause or identification of the risk factors.
3. Identification of what works to address the problem.
4. Identification of implementation and evaluation strategies.

The public health infrastructure responsible for the tasks in this approach is vast, comprising nearly 3,000 county and city health departments and local boards of health; 59 state, territorial, and island nation health departments; tribal health agencies coordinated by the Indian Health Service; over 160,000 laboratories; hospitals and other private providers; and volunteer organizations such as the American Red Cross (Lister, 2005; Salinsky, 2010). This network of agencies requires data and information sharing using informatics techniques and information technology.

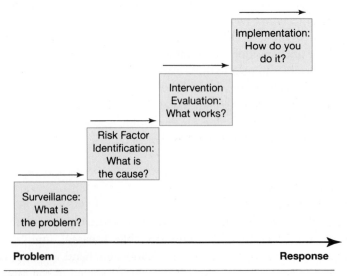

Figure 20-1 • Public health approach.

Reproduced from materials used by the National Center for Injury Prevention and Control, Centers for Disease Control and Prevention, Atlanta, Georgia.

To better understand the methods used in public health, one must understand the unwavering principles. As Koo, O'Carroll, and LaVenture (2001) stated, these principles can be useful as a guide to those attempting to better understand public health. The basic mission of public health is:

- To promote the health of populations and not the health of specific individuals.
- To alter the conditions of the environment that put populations at risk.
- To explore the potential for prevention for all vulnerable populations by exploring the causal chains leading to disease, injury, or disability.
- To reflect the specific governmental context in which public health is practiced.

Based on this mission, one can better understand the activities that comprise the core functions of effective public health systems as named in the landmark report, *The Future of the Public's Health in the 21st Century*, which are: assessment, policy development, and assurance (Institute of Medicine (IOM), 2002). These functions remain relevant today (Centers for Disease Control and Prevention (2017a, 2017b, 2017c). Assessment includes the collection and analysis of information about health problems, which encompass identifying needs, collecting data, and interpreting the data. The Centers for Disease Control and Prevention (2011) lists other tasks essential to support the core functions:

1. Assessment:
   a. Monitor health status to identify community health problems.
   b. Diagnose and investigate health problems and health hazards in the community.
2. Policy Development:
   a. Inform, educate, and empower people about health issues.
   b. Mobilize community partnerships to identify and solve health problems.
   c. Develop policies and plans that support individual and community health efforts.
3. Assurance:
   a. Enforce laws and regulations that protect health and ensure safety.
   b. Link people to needed personal health services and assure the provision of healthcare when otherwise unavailable.
   c. Assure a competent public health and personal healthcare workforce.
   d. Evaluate effectiveness, accessibility, and quality of personal and population-based health services.
   e. Research for new insights and innovative solutions to health problems.

In order to successfully carry out the mission, core functions, and tasks essential to public health, the larger public health services need organizational capacity at the local, state, and national levels; a developed workforce capable of carrying out the tasks; and an integrated and sophisticated information system that can provide real-time (or near real-time) data and information. The nature of public health guides a special set of informatics challenges that are necessary to support the core sciences of surveillance, epidemiology, laboratory results, and prevention effectiveness—all resting on an information system and informatics tools that are needed to assess the risk and health status of a population. Figure 20-2 depicts this foundational relationship.

Data supporting the public health domain must be obtained from multiple, disparate sources such as hospitals, ambulatory centers, laboratories, social service agencies, occupational health sites, pharmacies, and now the Internet using standardized terms and transmission protocols. Patient-specific data then must be aggregated into population-specific information that can be used both to create compelling arguments for policy or program development, and to evaluate outcomes.

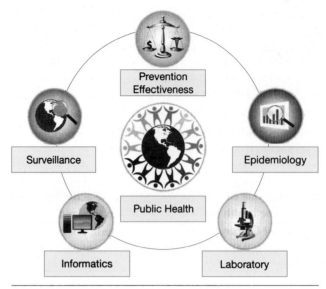

Figure 20-2 • Public health core sciences supported by informatics tools.

Reproduced from Public Health 101 Series. Published by Centers for Disease Control and Prevention.

In 2001, Koo, O'Carroll, and LaVenture identified four grand challenges that continue to face public health practitioners and that influence strategy today:

- Development of a coherent, integrated national public health information system.
- Development of closer integration of public health and clinical care data.
- Addressing the pervasive concerns for patient confidentiality and privacy.
- Application of information technology in unanticipated ways to reengineer public health and create new avenues to protect and promote health and wellbeing.

Public Health Informatics

Data and information are the lifeblood of public health. Public health informatics provides the tools to manage data and information today. Public health informatics (PHI) is defined in several ways, but a widely accepted definition of PHI that remains in use today is "the systematic application of information and computer science and technology to public health practice, research and learning" (Yasnoff, O'Carroll, Koo, Linkins, & Kilbourne, 2000, p. 67). PHI emerged as a specialty when health officials began to investigate how to leverage information technology in systematic ways. In 1995, Friede, Blum, and McDonald wrote: "The combination of the burgeoning interest in health, healthcare reform, and the advent of the Information Age represents a challenge and an opportunity for public health. If public health's effectiveness and profile are to grow, practitioners and researchers will need reliable, timely information with which to make *information-driven decisions*, better ways to communicate, and improved tools to analyze and present new knowledge" (p. 239). Population-level data has to be collected, analyzed, transformed into information, and disseminated efficiently in order to support preventive, as opposed to, curative interventions for groups of individuals, an observation later corroborated by Savel and Foldy (2012).

This began an earnest PHI movement that gained momentum in the late 1990s and early 2000s as technology and systems matured and spread. It is not that public health agencies did not utilize information before the late 1990s and early 2000s. Public health has always been data and information rich. Indeed, the agencies used multiple, disparate reporting systems that ran independently of one another. Early information systems used in public health settings were (and many still are) fundamentally paper-intense with manually entered data, which was then processed in large mainframe systems. Public health has long had mostly paper-driven systems, whereby reports are sent to a central location (a local or state agency) where the data is extracted and developed into information. As an example, birth and death certificates completed by practitioners in multiple settings are often filled out on paper forms that are sent to local or state health departments. The data from these certificates are extracted, reviewed, coded, and developed into information that we use as geographically bound birth and death rates. Moreover, public health has also utilized multiple sources of data for syndromic surveillance, which collects nonspecific information on syndromes before diagnosis, and has great advantages in promoting the early detection of epidemics and reducing the necessities of disease confirmation (Abat, Chaudet, Rolain, Colson, & Raoult, 2016; Yan et al., 2012). Data sources for syndromic surveillance have included data from emergency department visits for certain patient complaints, absentee data collected from schools and work sites, patient chief complaints expressed at provider office visits, calls to nurse hotlines, and prescription requests.

Today, with the proliferation of electronic health records (EHRs) in acute and ambulatory settings, along with mandated health data standards and integration, the reliance on paper-intensive transactions is lessening. The proliferation of systems, however, creates a need for a unifying vision, information systems planning, and systems design, implementation, and data analytics within the public health system in order to use the information to support the health of communities and populations.

Public health has always been about disease surveillance and management, particularly the identification of major disease outbreaks as previously described. However, public health practitioners also work to identify disease causation, distribution of disease, and frequency of disease occurrence or transmission (Macha & McDonough, 2012). Current PHI systems and processes need to support all of these key activities by harnessing the availability of data within EHRs and other systems that store and transfer key data.

PHI is distinguished from other information systems and technology by its emphasis on prevention of illness in populations ((Yu et al., 2015). The focus on population health is linked to prevention as opposed to diagnosis and treatment of an individual patient. Public health has a governmental context, because public health nearly always involves linkages to government agencies at the local, regional, national, or global levels. To make informed public health practice decisions, to develop appropriate policy, and to evaluate the outcomes of programs, timely and accurate data, sourced extensively from disparate systems, must be transformed efficiently into information. To achieve this, effective databases and sources of information for public health systems require application and knowledge from a variety of systems and professions.

The historic 1997 World Health Report cited the need to widely share health information inclusive of epidemiological and statistical data, reports, guidelines, training materials, and periodicals. Today, there are many varied sources of data that can support the public health domain, but the sources often lack standardization in data organization, nomenclature, and electronic transmission (Institute of Medicine, 2015). EHRs, health information exchanges (HIEs), and personal health records (PHRs), all of which are now prevalent in the health-care landscape due to federal requirements and support, are sources of some of the key data that support public health activity. What this means is that the data entered during a patient encounter into an EHR may wind up in a database for public health purposes. Consider documentation of the administration of a vaccine to a pediatric patient. This data will become part of a population-based immunization registry database used for consideration of community-based immunization coverage. Moreover, one has to consider the importance of nontraditional sources of data such as social media entries, mobile applications, wearable devices, nanotechnology, and genomics. Each of these sources supply data and information to describe the health and welfare of populations and communities, which provide a richer portrait of the health of populations. Consider the ability to compare community activity levels and its impact on body mass index by potentially monitoring cumulative steps taken by individuals and captured by wearable devices.

With so many potential sources of data, new and innovative methods are required to collect, store, transmit, organize, exchange, and disseminate all of this data that are gathered and generated during the course of public health work. The solution lies in reconceptualizing and reconfiguring information technology and informatics processes within this domain. Information technology implementations within acute, subacute, and long-term care areas are having a direct impact on public health informatics possibilities. Patient-facing technologies, such as web-based applications, mobile health tools, and personal health records, also provide new possibilities to understand a consumer's contribution to public health.

As described, public health providers have multiple information needs in relationship to healthcare informatics and technology infrastructure. Having the essential components of a health information infrastructure are vital and fundamental to increasing awareness and sensitivity to the types of data sets needed to provide support and improve outcomes used to make data-driven public health decisions. The ability to improve health outcomes and make data-driven decisions within a new or existing health information infrastructure is critical. For example, there is a clear need for valid and reliable databases. It is essential to consider each of these elements as more systems develop to foster and promote collaboration and communication between new and existing health information systems to promote the public's health. Table 20-1 lists 10 essential elements that need to be considered to have a comprehensive, robust health information system that promotes public health informatics.

These essential elements are currently supported by the mandates of federal policy falling within the program, known today as meaningful use, that outlines the foundations for accomplishing the mandate of most of the elements.

Table 20-1   Ten Essential Elements for Health Information Systems Infrastructure

1. Data definitions
2. Coding classification systems
3. Data transmission capability
4. Health information exchange (HIE)
5. Data storage
6. Data analysis
7. Disease staging
8. Electronic health records (EHR)
9. Computerized order entry
10. Decision-support systems

Public Policy Driving Informatics Change

From a policy perspective, the responsibility for public health lies at all governmental levels—local, state, and federal. The reality is that much of the authority for public health is found at the state level. The federal government will influence public health practice through funding decisions, setting national priorities, and by focusing attention on specific problems. The states enforce safety and sanitary codes, conduct inspections, mandate the reporting of certain diseases to state authorities, mandate quarantines, and license healthcare workers. This places responsibility for development of public health information systems in the control of state and local agencies, with national support given by the federal government. Limited resources and a limited informatics workforce challenge the ability to build a strong public health information system.

There has been a new emphasis on the need for a broader information system infrastructure for public health in the last decade. Events and current policies are driving new demand for efficient and effective information systems for public health purposes, beginning at the local level and then moving to the national level. The events of September 11, 2001, and the subsequent anthrax, Ebola, and Zika virus epidemics have crystallized the urgent need for key public health data that is not so localized, as well as informatics applications and skills that could be applied to public health to create a more robust infrastructure in order to respond to these events. Despite this apparent need, federal funding for public health information systems has lagged behind the support given for information systems used in acute-care settings and practitioners' offices. The Health Information Technology for Economic and Clinical Health (HITECH) legislation of 2009 provided billions of dollars for providers and facilities to implement EHR systems, but equivalent funds to strengthen the public health information infrastructure needed to receive, process, and analyze the data from the proliferation of EHRs have not been provided (Edmunds, Thorpe, Sepulveda, & Bezold, 2015).

The proliferation of clinical care information systems in the form of EHRs, PHRs, electronic medication prescribing, and social networking create opportunities to blur the distinction between what is collected on an individual patient, and what may be known about a population. The 2004 provision of the Health Insurance Portability and Accountability Act (HIPAA) generally prohibits disclosure of personal health information without expressed authorization of the individual. However, for public health purposes the law provides for the disclosure of patient information for the purposes of preventing or controlling disease, injury, or disability, and for the purpose of conducting public health surveillance, public health investigations, and public health interventions (HIPAA, 2002). The 2010 Patient Protection and Affordable Care Act (PPACA) establishes policies and mandates for interoperability, standards, and protocols that will facilitate the enrollment of individuals into federal and state health and human services programs through which data must be shared (Congress. gov, n.d.). The HITECH Act, enacted as part of the American Recovery and Reinvestment Act of 2009, promotes the adoption and meaningful use of health information technology (HealthIT.gov, 2015). This has spurred an unprecedented uptake of information technology in primary, secondary, and tertiary care areas. The HITECH Act within DHHS specifically impacts public health by creating opportunities to improve collaboration between clinical and public healthcare at the local and state levels through:

- Implementation of electronic reporting to public health agencies (specifically immunization data, laboratory results, and syndromic surveillance data).

- Improvement of patient-centric preventive care utilizing quality care measures.

- Emphasis on bidirectional communication with clinical providers.
- Mandated standardized data elements and messaging protocols for public health measures.

The drive toward technology-supported and mediated primary, acute, subacute, and long-term healthcare will have major impacts on the way public health data is collected. Public health informaticians are creating opportunities through standardization, nomenclature development, interoperability, and exchange to expand their infrastructure through the work that is underway at the state and national levels. It is hoped that public health will benefit from the advances in information systems and technologies, and will be able to create an efficient and effective information network to support its mission.

Current Public Health Informatics Systems

Public health practice uses a wide variety of data types, data sources, and data management techniques to manage the nation's health. Data to support public health processes can be generated from routine clinical care; however, needed extraction techniques are often missing. In addition, public health processes need data not only from clinical interactions, but also from nonclinical data sources to accurately identify public health trends. Consider the need to integrate birth-defect data with environmental chemical exposure data. Nonclinical information can include data on a patient's geospatial location, socioeconomic status, education levels, environmental factors, crime, or transportation (Haque et al., 2016). Currently, most public health data comes from a patchwork of surveys, surveillance systems, and mandated reporting structures stretched across healthcare systems and local and state health agencies.

Electronic Lab Reporting

Electronic Lab Reporting (ELR) refers to a process of electronically transmitting laboratory results that identify reportable conditions from laboratories across the nation to public health agencies (Haque et al., 2016). Most state public health agencies have the capacity to receive the electronic reports that come from the increased implementation of EHRs. However, there are limitations for public health practitioners in that there is a need to know more than a result. To fully understand the implications of the result, there is a need to know patient demographics, provider information, disease onset, and medication and treatment history.

The National Center for Health Statistics Surveys

The National Center for Health Statistics (NCHS) is a principal source of information related to the health of the nation. The NCHS is the main health statistics agency responsible for compiling national data and information that comes up from local and state agencies to guide actions and policies to improve the health of the nation. The NCHS conducts surveys and collects data through assessments such as:

- The National Health Care Survey, which is designed to answer key questions about healthcare settings and providers.
- The National Health Interview Survey, which collects data on a wide range of health topics through in-person household interviews.
- The National Health and Nutrition Examination Survey, which assesses the health and nutritional status of adults and children through interviews and physical assessments.

- The National Immunization Survey, which is a telephone survey followed by mail to gather information on childhood immunization activity.

- The National Vital Statistics System, which is the oldest and most successful intergovernmental data sharing process in public health, gathering birth, death, marriage, and divorce data through mandated reporting (Centers for Disease Control and Prevention, 2015).

The NCHS oversees, collects, extracts, and disseminates, data standards, interchange processes, and vital statistics information by utilizing contractual and regulatory relationships at the local and state level, as well as procedures for generating birth, death, marriage, divorce, and fetal-death rates (Centers for Disease Control and Prevention, 2016). The NCHS disseminates cause of death, birth rates by maternal age, infant mortality, and fertility data at the national and state level. State health departments also have access to and distribute this data on a county-wide basis. All of the de-identified data sets collected through the various survey mechanisms are available for data analysis through the Center for Disease Control and Prevention, National Center for Health Statistics website at www.cdc.gov/nchs/surveys.htm.

The Behavioral Risk Factor Surveillance System

The Behavioral Risk Factor Surveillance System (BRFSS) is a unique, state-based surveillance system currently active in all 50 states, the District of Columbia, and three territories of the United States. Since 1984, the US Centers for Disease Control and Prevention (CDC), in collaboration with state health departments, has conducted telephone surveys of the civilian, noninstitutionalized adult population (persons aged 18 years or older) as a part of the BRFSS to estimate the prevalence of behaviors linked to specific health problems. States use the BRFSS data to identify emerging health problems, establish and track health objectives, and develop and evaluate public health policies and programs. Many states also use BRFSS data to support health-related legislative efforts. BRFSS prevalence and trend data may be obtained and reviewed at http://apps.nccd.cdc.gov/BRFSS.

Surveillance Systems

Syndromic surveillance refers to a variety of processes that focus on near real-time use of early disease indicators that come from prediagnostic data, such as symptoms and assessment data, used to detect and characterize events that may need public health investigation before a diagnosis is definitively made (Ziemann, Fouillet, Brand, & Krafft, 2016). Public health surveillance is the ongoing systematic collection, analysis, and interpretation of data, closely integrated with the timely dissemination of these data to those responsible for preventing and controlling disease and injury (World Health Organization, 2017). Surveillance can be based on indicator factors, such as the number of new cases of diarrhea reported to healthcare providers; active systems, whereby staff go out and seek information; passive systems, which rely on reports submitted to local or state agencies that are mandated based on certain conditions (e.g., sexually transmitted diseases); or syndromes that rely on both active and passive reporting, but are based on clinical features as opposed to actual diagnoses (Abat et al., 2016).

The Stage 1 Meaningful Use criteria, established by the Office of the National Coordinator and the Centers for Medicaid and Medicare Services (CMS) through the 2009 ARRA, contain provisions that create standards for the submission of electronic data to public health agencies. These standards specifically include immunizations, certain reportable laboratory results, and syndromic surveillance consisting of prediagnostic reporting of data that detain and characterize unusual activity for public health field investigation (Public Health Information Network [PHIN], 2012).

Population Health Disease Registries

Population-based disease registries contain records for individuals who reside in certain defined geographic areas, and who meet certain criteria for a specific disease. Public health agencies have traditionally maintained these disease-specific registries to support epidemiological analyses and emergency public health activity coordinated with clinical stakeholders. These include the following.

1. Chronic disease registries—capturing case data on conditions, such as cardiovascular disease, tobacco and alcohol use, physical activity, and nutrition. This data is gathered from clinical records and survey activity.
2. Immunization registries—often called immunization information systems (IIS), these are the result of a mandated transmission of immunization data from providers to an IIS in a public health agency. IIS assist with the determination of immunization coverage and, if bidirectional data exchange occurs, can reduce duplication of immunization (Curran et al., 2014).
3. Cancer registries—cancer registries capture details for each cancer episode of care in the United States. These registries include data on patient history, diagnosis, treatment, and status. Data are first collected at the local registry level, and are then merged to form population-based cancer data. This data are used to calculate incidence, survival rates, efficacy, treatment, and quality of life.

New Technological Sources of Public Health Information

The Meaningful Use mandate of the 2009 ARRA undergirds many new opportunities to redevelop the public health information systems' infrastructure. The proliferation of web-based applications and information sources are creating new informatics tools for the development of public health information.

Electronic Health Records

Implementation of certified EHRs in ambulatory and acute settings (and somewhat to a lesser extent in long-term care settings) provides an opportunity to harness the interoperability standards imposed in order to access data in near real time. EHRs may provide laboratory results reporting, syndromic surveillance, immunization, and behavioral risk-factor data as part of the regular course of healthcare business instead of as a separate reporting process.

Personal Heath Records

PHRs are not a new concept. Many patients have managed a paper-based PHR for years. Patients keep track of doctors' names, appointments, medications, allergies, and lab results, often in a notebook or on a calendar. Only recently has the electronic form garnered increased attention. The electronic PHR can take multiple forms, ranging from stand-alone software for one's computer that utilizes a USB drive to secure websites tethered to a specific practice, health insurance company, or healthcare enterprise. Each of these approaches supports different health needs such as tracking visits, enabling secure email with providers, scheduling appointments, refilling medications, and integrating clinical data generated by the provider with that provided by the patient. For example, a diabetic patient may have access to a PHR that not only displays laboratory results and medications prescribed, but may also allow the patient to enter blood glucose results, insulin coverage, diet information, exercise, weight, and mental status.

PHRs hold the potential to improve health monitoring, and may even foster entirely new approaches to this public health function. Through PHRs, individuals could easily share their health data anonymously with public health agencies. Such reporting networks could be both passive, where population data are anonymously analyzed in order to assess the prevalence of health issues, and active, where citizens elect to share targeted health information of interest to public health agencies. These approaches could enhance information gathering and reduce the resources necessary to support current health monitoring systems. They could also further engage individuals as sentinels in protecting their own health and the health of their family, their community, and, ultimately, the nation (Weitzman, Kelemen, Kaci, & Mandl, 2012; Institute of Medicine, 2016).

Health Information Exchange

Health information exchange (HIE) refers to the process of reliable, standard, and interoperable electronic health information sharing. This may encompass laboratory results, radiology findings, diagnoses, medications prescribed, and allergies. Specifically, an HIE is an electronic mobilization of healthcare information across organizations within a region, a community, or healthcare system.

HIE provides the capability to electronically move clinical information among disparate healthcare information systems while maintaining the meaning of the information being exchanged. The goal of HIE is to facilitate access to and retrieval of clinical data to provide safer and more timely, efficient, effective, and equitable patient-centered care, regardless of the source of the care.

Essential to HIE is the capability to utilize nationally recognized standards to enable interoperability, security, and confidentiality of the information. Moreover, statewide and local policies will dictate the authorization of those who access the information. HIE will support the sharing of health-related information to facilitate coordinated care through the health trajectory with the use of EHRs, because they are the source of the HIE data. HIE will also provide key information to public health agencies.

Geographic Information Systems

A geographic information system (GIS) integrates hardware, software, and data for capturing, managing, analyzing, and displaying all forms of geographically referenced information. A GIS allows public health practitioners to view, understand, question, interpret, and visualize data in many ways that may reveal relationships, patterns, and trends in the form of maps, globes, reports, and charts.

GISs are being used in public health to model where people live and the environments to which they are exposed throughout their lives. A GIS allows one to pinpoint service area needs with much more accuracy. It also allows a visual representation of geographical distribution, which is one of the most frequently considered factors in public health and epidemiologic research (Ostad et al., 2016). Additionally, a GIS can be used to identify and monitor the health status of communities, target diagnoses and investigations of health problems, inform and educate communities about hazards and health concerns, link resources within communities, and advocate for local policy. So important is geographic specificity to public health that the World Health Organization has created a program of support for GISs solely at www.esri.com/what-is-gis/overview.html.

Infodemiology

Infodemiology was named and defined by Eysenbach (2009), as "the science of distribution and determinants of information in an electronic medium, specifically the Internet, or in a population, with the ultimate aim to inform public health and public policy" (e11). The placement of this information in social media and the Internet enables collection and analysis in a frame very close to real time. Among other things, infodemiology may be used to analyze Internet queries about a particular disease to identify pending outbreaks (e.g., influenza); to conduct syndromic surveillance by following personal status updates on Twitter; and to assess the availability of health information (Eysenbach, 2009). Chew and Eysenbach (2010) archived and analyzed over two-million Twitter posts containing the keywords "swine flu" and "H1N1." They randomly selected a subset of the tweets for analysis, and found that with the rise of participatory web and social media tools, the user-generated content had the potential to serve as a near real-time source of data sufficient to trigger a public health response, and also as a vehicle for knowledge dissemination to the public. Another, more recent example of the technique in South Korea used search engine inquiries and social media data to estimate flu outbreaks (Hyekyung et al., 2016).

Future Directions

PHI is a fairly new specialty, and, as in all specialties requiring the use of data, information, and information systems, work has been done to identify core informatics competencies needed by all persons working in the public health field, as well as for informaticists working in the field. Basic competencies address the use of information for public health practice, the use of IT to support personal effectiveness, and the management of IT projects to improve the effectiveness of the public health system (O'Carroll, 2002). This work was significant because it established a baseline for skill sets that must be addressed in the preparation of the workforce. However, the fact that the public health workforce is drawn from a number of different disciplines makes it difficult to ensure that everyone enters the field with the prerequisite skill sets. O'Carroll was also careful to note that these competencies will continue to evolve over time and are not necessarily mutually exclusive of basic competencies identified in other disciplines. The competencies identified for the informaticist in public health (Centers for Disease Control and Prevention and University of Washington's Center for Public Health Informatics, 2009) are similar to those identified by the American Nurses Association (2015) in *Nursing Informatics: Scope & Standards of Practice*, and are shown here in Table 20-2.

Support for public health informatics in the general informatics community is present. The American Medical Informatics Association (AMIA) has a workgroup devoted to PHI. There are also two open access journals devoted to the field: the *Online Journal of Public Health Informatics* and *International Journal of Public Health Informatics* (IJPHI). Table 20-3 provides a few exemplars of resources available for public health and public health informatics.

Table 20-2   Core Competencies for Public Health Informaticians

Public Health Informatician	Senior Public Health Informatician
Supports development of strategic direction for public health informatics within the enterprise.	Leads creation of strategic direction for public health informatics.
Participates in development of knowledge management tools for the enterprise.	Leads knowledge management for the enterprise.
Uses informatics standards.	Ensures use of informatics standards.
Ensures that knowledge, information, and data needs of project or program users and stakeholders are met.	Ensures that knowledge, information, and data needs of users and stakeholders are met.
Supports information system development, procurement, and implementation that meet public health program needs.	Ensures that information system development, procurement, and implementation meet public health program needs.
Manages IT operations related to project or program (for public health agencies with internal IT operations).	Ensures IT operations are managed effectively to support public health programs (for public health agencies with internal IT operations).
Monitors IT operations managed by external organizations.	Ensures adequacy of IT operations managed by external organizations.
Communicates with cross-disciplinary leaders and team members.	Communicates with elected officials, policymakers, agency staff, and the public.
Evaluates information systems and applications.	Ensures evaluation of information systems and applications.
Participates in applied public health informatics research for new insights and innovative solutions to health problems.	Conducts applied public health informatics research for new insights and innovative solutions to health problems.
Contributes to development of public health information systems that are interoperable with other relevant information systems.	Ensures that public health information systems are interoperable with other relevant information systems.
Supports use of informatics to integrate clinical health, environmental risk, and population health.	Uses informatics to integrate clinical health, environmental risk, and population health.
Implements solutions that ensure confidentiality, security, and integrity while maximizing availability of information for public health.	Develops solutions that ensure confidentiality, security, and integrity while maximizing availability of information for public health.
Conducts education and training in public health informatics.	Contributes to progress in the field of public health informatics.

SOURCE: Core Competencies for Public Health Informaticians from Competencies for Public Health Informaticians. Published by U.S. Department of Health and Human Services.

Table 20-3   Public Health Informatics Web Resources

American Public Health Association	www.apha.org/what-is-public-health
AMIA—Public Health Informatics	www.amia.org/applications-informatics/public-health-informatics
CDC Public Health Information Network	www.cdc.gov/phin/
Cochrane Public Health Group	http://ph.cochrane.org
HIMSS—Public Health Informatics	www.himss.org/public-health-informatics
National Association of County and City Health Officials	www.naccho.org/programs/public-health-infrastructure/health-it
National Center for Health Statistics	www.cdc.gov/nchs/
National Health Interview Survey	www.cdc.gov/nchs/nhis.htm
National Indian Health Board	www.nihb.org/public_health/phrc.php
National Vital Statistics System	www.cdc.gov/nchs/nvss.htm
Public Health Informatics Institute	www.phii.org/resources/

Summary

- Public health informatics is defined as the systematic application of information science, computer science, and information technology to public health practice, research, and learning.
- Informatics and information technology play a major role in supporting public health functions of disease surveillance, protection of population health, disaster management, and improved consumer health.
- Initiatives to connect data from EHRs with public health databases will improve tracking for immunizations, and serve as an early alert of threats to public health.
- Improved access to public health data and information will better inform public policy.
- Work is needed to ensure a public health workforce that is prepared with the skills to develop a public health informatics infrastructure.

Case Study

You are about to present a lecture to your senior nursing students enrolled in their community health class on public health and informatics. The topic under discussion is Zika virus transmission in a community. Discuss the data collection and workflow processes that would be engaged in the collection of data used to notify public health officials of a possible outbreak.

About the Author

Marisa L. Wilson, DNSc, MHSc, RN-BC, CPHIMS FAAN is an Associate Professor and Specialty Track coordinator for the MSN Nursing Informatics program at the University of Alabama at Birmingham School of Nursing. Dr. Wilson has over 30 years of experience in public health and clinical informatics, and she has been engaged in academia for over a decade leading graduate students to push for better infusion of technology at the points of care.

References

Abat, C., Chaudet, H., Rolain, J., Colson, P., & Raoult, D. (2016). Traditional and syndromic surveillance of infectious diseases and pathogens. *International Journal of Infectious Diseases: Official Publication of the International Society for Infectious Diseases, 48*, 22–28. doi:10.1016/j.ijid.2016.04.021

American Medical Informatics Association. (2017). The Science of Informatics. Retrieved from www.amia.org/about-amia/science-informatics

American Nurses Association. (2015). *Nursing informatics: Scope & standards of practice* (2nd ed.). Silver Spring, MD: Nursesbooks.org.

American Public Health Association (APHA). (2016). What is public health? Retrieved from www.apha.org/what-is-public-health

Centers for Disease Control and Prevention (CDC) and University of Washington's Center for Public Health Informatics. (2009). *Competencies for public health informaticians.* Atlanta, GA: Department of Health and Human Services, Centers for Disease Control and Prevention. Retrieved from www.cdc.gov/InformaticsCompetencies/downloads/PHI_Competencies.pdf

Centers for Disease Control and Prevention (2011). The Public Health Workforce an Agenda For The 21st Century : A Report of the Public Health Functions Project. Published by U.S. Department of Health and Human Services.

Centers for Disease Control and Prevention. (2015). Surveys and data collection systems. Retrieved from www.cdc.gov/nchs/surveys.htm

Centers for Disease Control and Prevention. (2016). NCHS overview. Retrieved from www.cdc.gov/nchs/data/factsheets/factsheet_overview.htm

Centers for Disease Control and Prevention. (2017a). National public health performance standards. Retrieved from www.cdc.gov/stltpublichealth/nphps/index.html

Centers for Disease Control and Prevention. (2017b). The public health system and the 10 essential public health services. Retrieved from www.cdc.gov/stltpublichealth/publichealthservices/essentialhealthservices.html

Centers for Disease Control and Prevention. (2017c). State, tribal, local & territorial Public Health Professionals Gateway: The Public Health system & the 10 Essential Public Health services. Retrieved from www.cdc.gov/stltpublichealth/publichealthservices/essentialhealthservices.html

Chew, C., & Eysenbach, G. (2010). Pandemics in the age of Twitter: Content analysis of tweets during the 2009 H1N1 outbreak. *PLOS ONE, 5*(11).

Congress.gov. (n.d.). H.R.3590—Patient protection and affordable care act. Retrieved from www.congress.gov/bill/111th-congress/house-bill/3590

Curran, E. A., Seib, K. G., Wells, K., Hannan, C., Bednarczyk, R. A., Hinman, A. R., & Omer, S. B. (2014). A national survey of immunization programs regarding immunization information systems data sharing and use. *Journal of Public Health Management and Practice, 20*(6), 591–597.

Edmunds, M., Thorpe, L., Sepulveda, M., & Bezold, C. (2015). The future of public health informatics: Alternative scenarios and recommended strategies. *Frontiers in Public Health Services & Systems Research, 4*(2), 1–13. doi:10.13063/2327-9214.1156

Eysenbach, G. (2009). Infodemiology and infoveillance: Framework for an emerging set of public health informatics methods to analyze search, communication and publication behavior on the Internet. *Journal of Medical Internet Research, 11*(1), e11.

Foldy, S., Grannis, S., Ross, D., & Smith, T. (2014). A ride in the time machine: Information management capabilities health departments will need. *American Journal of Public Health, 104*(9), 1592–1600. doi:10.2105/AJPH.2014.301956

Friede, A., Blum, H. L., & McDonald, M. (1995). Public health informatics: How information age technology can strengthen public health. *Annual Review of Public Health, 16*, 239–252. Published by Annual Review of Public Health, © 1995. doi: 10.1146/annurev.pu.16.050195.001323.

Haque, S. N., Dixon, B. E., & Grannis, S. J. (2016). *Clinical informatics study guide: Text and review.* Cham, Switzerland: Springer International.

Health Insurance Portability and Accountability Act (HIPAA) Privacy Rule. (2002). US government publishing office, *45*, CFR Parts 164, Retrieved from www.access.gpo.gov/nara/cfr/waisidx_02/45cfr164_02.html

HealthIT.gov. (2015). Meaningful Use definition and objectives. Retrieved from www.healthit.gov/providers-professionals/meaningful-use-definition-objectives

Hyekyung, W., Youngtae, C., Eunyoung, S., Jong-Koo, L., Chang-Gun, L., & Seong Hwan, K. (2016). Estimating influenza outbreaks using both search engine query data and social media data in South Korea. *Journal of Medical Internet Research, 18*(7), e177. doi:10.2196/jmir.4955

Institute of Medicine (IOM). (2002). *The future of the public's health in the 21st century.* Washington, DC: National Academies Press.

Institute of Medicine (IOM). (2011). *Innovation in health literacy research: Workshop summary.* Washington, DC: National Academies Press.

Institute of Medicine (IOM). (2015). *Vital signs.* Washington, DC: National Academies Press.

Institute of Medicine (IOM). (2016). Metrics that matter for population health action: Workshop summary. Washington, DC: National Academies Press.

Koo, D., O'Carroll, P., & LaVenture, M. (2001). Public health 101 for informaticians. *Journal of the American Medical Informatics Association, 8*(6), 585–597.

Kukafka, R., & Yasnoff, W. A. (2007). Public health informatics. *Journal of Biomedical Informatics, 40*(4), 365–369.

Lister, S. A. (2005). An overview of the US public health system in the context of emergency preparedness. Retrieved from www.fas.org/sgp/crs/homesec/RL31719.pdf

Macha, K., & McDonough, J. P. (2012). *Epidemiology for advanced nursing practice.* Sudbury, MA: Jones & Bartlett Learning LLC.

O'Carroll, P. W. (2002). *Public health informatics competency working group: Informatics competencies for public health professionals.* Seattle, WA: Northwest Center for Public Health Practice.

Ostad, M., Shirian, S., Pishro, F., Abbasi, T., Ai, A., & Azimi, F. (2016). Control of cutaneous leishmaniasis using geographic information systems from 2010 to 2014 in Khuzestan Province, Iran. *PLOS ONE, 11*(7), e0159546. doi:10.1371/journal.pone.0159546

Public Health Information Network. (2012). Meaningful use fact sheet. Retrieved from www.cdc.gov/phin/library/PHIN_Fact_Sheets/FS_MU_SS_120511a.pdf

Salinsky, E. (2010). *Governmental public health: An overview of state and local public health agencies.* Background Paper No. 77, National Health Policy Forum, George Washington University. Retrieved from www.nhpf.org/library/background-papers/BP77_GovPublicHealth_08-18-2010.pdf

Savel T. G., & Foldy, S. (2012). The role of public health informatics in enhancing public health surveillance. *Morbidity & Mortality Weekly Report, 61*20–24.

Weitzman, E., Kelemen, S., Kaci, L., & Mandl, K. (2012). Willingness to share personal health record data for care improvement and public health: A survey of experienced personal health record users. *BMC Medical Informatics and Decision Making, 12,* 39. Retrieved from https://doi.org/10.1186/1472-6947–12-39

Winslow, C. E. A. (1920). The untilled fields of public health. *Science, 51*(1306), 23–33. Published by The American Association for the Advancement of Science.

World Health Organization (WHO). (1997). The World Health Report 1996—fighting disease, fostering development. © 1996. Retrieved from www.who.int/whr/1996/en/index.html.

World Health Organization (WHO). (2017). Public health surveillance. Retrieved from www.who.int/topics/public_health_surveillance/en/

Yan, W., Nie, S., Xu, B., Dong, H., Palm, L., & Diwan, V. (2012). Establishing a web-based, integrated surveillance system for early detection of disease epidemic in rural China: A field experimental study. *Medical Informatics & Decision Making, 12,* 4.

Yasnoff, W. A., O'Carroll, P. W., Koo, D., Linkins, R. W., & Kilbourne, E. M. (2000). Public health informatics: Improving and transforming public health in the information age. Journal of *Public Health Management Practice, 6*(6), 67–75.

Yu, X., Xie, Y., Pan, X., Mayfield-Johnson, S., Whipple, J., & Azadbakht, E. (2015). Developing an evidence-based public health informatics course. *Journal of the Medical Library Association, 103*(4), 194–197. doi:10.3163/1536-5050.103.4.007

Ziemann, A., Fouillet, A., Brand, H., & Krafft, T. (2016). Success factors of European syndromic surveillance systems: A worked example of applying qualitative comparative analysis. *PLOS ONE, 11*(5), e0155535.

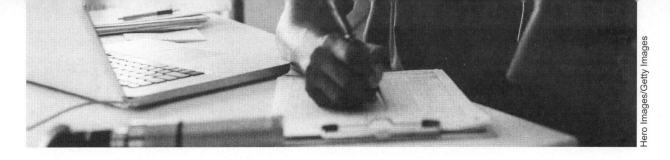

Appendix A
Hardware and Software

Athena Fernandes, DNP, MSN, RN-BC

A computer is an electronic device used to capture, store, process, and retrieve data. A computer is made up of hardware and software. Hardware refers to the physical components of the computer, such as:

- Input devices: These are devices used to enter or capture data electronically. Examples are: keyboard, mouse, stylus, touch screen, barcode scanner.

- Storage devices: These devices are used to store data. An example of a storage device within a computer is its hard drive.

- Central processing unit (CPU): This piece of hardware is the "brain" of the computer. It processes and manipulates data.

- Output devices: These devices are used to present or display data to the user via monitors, terminals, printers, speakers, and so on.

Software refers to the programs and instructions used by the computer to operate and process information. Examples of software applications commonly used by informaticists include: Microsoft Office (Excel, Word, Outlook, PowerPoint, and Access), Visio, Microsoft Project, and Adobe Acrobat. Examples of some electronic health record software applications include: Epic, Allscripts, Cerner Millennium, NextGen, and Centricity.

Peripheral Hardware

Peripheral hardware refers to equipment or devices that can be externally connected to a computer. Connections can be through wires or cables, or can be wireless (radio wave connection). Some examples of peripherals are: monitors, keyboards, mice, printers, secondary storage devices, backup systems, scanners, and webcams.

- Monitors are devices with screens that display input and output data to the user.

- Keyboards are devices, similar to a typewriter, that contain keys to send commands and/or data to a computer.

- A mouse (plural = mice) is a device used to move an on-screen pointer or cursor to a specific location on a monitor screen. Other examples of pointing devices include joysticks, trackballs, and touch pads.

- Printers are devices that convert data stored in electronic format into human-readable output on paper or other surfaces.

- Modems are electronic devices that allow for transmission of data along telephone, cable, or fiber-optic lines.

- Scanners are electronic devices that capture data from documents and images and convert to electronic format for digital storage.

- Webcams are cameras that are built into the computer or connected externally to the computer, to capture live images and transmit the live feed over the Internet.

Secondary storage devices are devices used to store data outside of the computer's main data storage, its internal hard drive. These devices are typically used to: (a) store backup information in the event of data loss; (b) place data into a portable format; (c) store archived or historical information for data retention; and (d) allow for additional data storage capacity that the computer may not have. For secondary storage, devices such as USB flash drives, DVD drives, external hard drives, web drives, or cloud backup may be used.

Backup systems are devices that create and store copies of data files from the primary computer system where the original data are stored. The backup files are stored on a different device and in a different location from the original files. In the event of data loss or primary computer system outage, these backup systems (depending on how the system is configured) can be accessed for data retrieval. When working with electronic health records (EHRs), it is important to establish a robust backup system to ensure that clinicians have access to patient data during planned EHR downtimes or unplanned system outages so that patient care is not compromised.

Types of Computers

Many types of computers exist, based on their size, processing power, purpose, and use. These include supercomputers, mainframes, personal computers, laptops, and mobile devices.

- Supercomputers: These computers process at heightened operational capacity. They are the fastest and the most powerful of computers. They are used in various industries for complex calculations and scientific computations such as those needed for weather forecasting, molecular modeling, quantum mechanics, and so on.

- Mainframes: Also known as "big iron," these oversized computers are capable of processing large amounts of data. They have traditionally been used by large corporations to centrally process information and then distribute it.

- Personal computers: These computers are built to be used by one individual at a time, and therefore are smaller in size, are not as powerful as supercomputers or mainframes, and are much less expensive. These computers are typically used in a business or personal setting to conduct day-to-day operations such as sending and receiving emails, writing documents, and shopping online.

- Laptops: Laptops are lightweight personal computers that are easily portable and can fit on a person's lap. They have the capacity to run on a battery that can be recharged via an AC adapter. These computers are ideal for traveling, for business presentations, and for working remotely. They can be connected to a docking station to allow them to be recharged and to connect them to peripherals such as bigger speakers, monitors, keyboards, and so on.

- Mobile devices: These devices are much smaller in size than a laptop and run on a mobile-device operating system. The two predominant mobile device operating systems on the market are iOS and Android mobile. These devices have a touch screen with a built in keyboard, and users can use a stylus (similar to a pen with a scratch-resistant tip) or a finger for data input. Like laptops, mobile devices can operate on a rechargeable battery. However, these devices are not as powerful as laptops and are not ideal for conducting day-to-day business operations such as writing documents, working with spreadsheets, and so on. Examples of mobile devices include tablets and smartphones.

- Tablets: These are mobile personal computers that are flat and much smaller in size than a laptop (7 to 11 inches). They are typically used to engage in social media, play computer games, shop online, take pictures and videos, and access email.

- Smartphones: These devices are similar to tablets, but even smaller. Unlike tablets, these devices can also be used as a phone. They can fit in a purse or a pocket, which makes them a convenient handheld personal assistant to be used for reminders, alarms, access to one's calendar, stay connected on social media, listen to music, obtain navigation information, connect to the internet, and so on.

Basic Networks

A network consists of two or more electronic devices that are interconnected with hardware and software, for information exchange or resource sharing. For example, a network printer in an office may connect several computers to one printer in order to share the printer resource.

Virtual private networks (VPNs) are networks that are extended across the Internet such that a point-to-point connection can be made from the registered user's remote computer to the private network. A VPN connection allows the user to remotely connect to a private network (such as a school or a business) and access its resources just as if the user were locally connected to the private network.

Types of Computer Networks

Local area networks (LANs) are computer networks comprised of computers and/or other devices, which are interconnected within a confined geographical area. The simplest form of a LAN is a household network where all the electronic devices within the household are connected. A more complex LAN would be a network of computers connected within an office building or small business. A LAN allows for resource sharing, such as sharing files or a network printer.

Wireless local area networks (WLANs) are local area networks connected together wirelessly. Wi-Fi is an example of wireless technology for enabling WLANs.

Wide area networks (WANs) are computer networks comprising of LANs and cover a larger geographical area, such as an enterprise. The Internet, also known as the Net, is comprised of several networks that are interconnected and is an example of a WAN. Intranets are networks that are private and confined to within organizations, while extranets are public networks.

Networking Architecture

Peer-to-peer (P2P) is a type of networking architecture where all the computers on the network function as equals or peers, without a hierarchy. This type of networking system is ideal for file-sharing, as each computer can share files that are downloadable by the other computers.

Client–Server is a type of networking architecture whereby many computers (clients) are connected to one server. In this configuration, the client is called a "fat client" because the software application is installed and processed on the local client. The clients rely on the server to host, manage, and provide resources to the clients when needed.

Server-based computing or thin client technology is a type of networking architecture whereby the software application is installed and processed on the server. The client in this configuration is referred to as a "thin client" or a "dumb terminal," and is simply involved in data capture, data transmission to the server, and data display to the end user. The processing of the information is done by the server.

About the Author

Athena Fernandes, DNP, MSN, RN-BC is a Senior Physician Systems Analyst at Penn Medicine Chester County Hospital. She is a board certified nurse informaticist, with a master's degree in nursing informatics. Dr. Fernandes is actively involved on professional committees at the American Nursing Informatics Association (ANIA) and the Greater Delaware Valley ANIA Chapter.

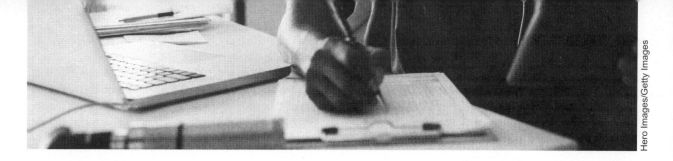

Appendix B
The Internet and the World Wide Web

Athena Fernandes, DNP, MSN, RN-BC

The Internet is a network of networks that was initiated in the 1960s by the US Department of Defense to collaborate and share information among governmental, research and academic organizations. Today, the Internet, or the Net as it is commonly known, is the largest electronic network of networks, connecting individuals and private and public organizations to data and information on the Net. The Internet can be accessed via several types of electronic devices including personal computers, laptops, mobile devices, and smart devices referred to as the Internet of things (smartwatches, smart refrigerators, smart cars, and so on).

A connection to the Internet is made possible via a fee-based subscription to an Internet service provider (ISP) or by connecting through free Wi-Fi. Many businesses that cater to the public, such as the hospitality industry, offer their customers free Wi-Fi service. Access to the Internet is made available via telephone lines, cable lines, digital-subscriber lines (DSLs), fiber optic lines, wirelessly through Wi-Fi, or via satellite. The Internet makes it possible to send and receive electronic messages via email; transfer files electronically from one location to another; conduct database searches; remotely access resources; find journals, articles, and other published information; network with colleagues; work collaboratively in a virtual environment on projects; and so on.

The ease with which the Internet connects computers and other electronic devices to one another exposes it to certain vulnerabilities. These include: (a) data security and unauthorized access to information; (b) data validity and integrity issues related to the quality and reliability of the information presented on websites; (c) concerns that a user's personal information may be captured by websites and used for purposes that the user did not authorize; (d) the risk of introducing computer viruses and malware that could destroy or compromise data and devices; and (e) the lack of Internet protocols and governing regulations.

The World Wide Web

The World Wide Web (WWW), also known as the web, comprises a collection of websites that are connected to the Internet. The content on the web may consist of text, graphics, videos, and images. The web uses hyperlinks to jump to content residing on other web pages and websites. Hyperlinks are web addresses that point to the location where the content resides on the web. Hyperlinks are embedded within a phrase, a word, an image, or other content on a web page.

Another way to access websites is via uniform resource locators (URLs), which are similar to a postal address in that a URL provides the location of the content on the web and the server on which it resides. The beginning portion of a web address contains the words "http" or "https" ("s" means secure). Hyper text transfer protocol (http) is a protocol used to define how messages are formatted and sent across the web. The web is accessed via a web browser.

Web Browsers

A browser or web browser is an application that is used to access the Internet. The browser uses a URL to locate and access Internet content. Examples of web browsers include Internet Explorer, Mozilla Firefox, Google Chrome, and Safari.

Internet Search Tools

Search tools are used to make it easier to find information on the Internet. The most commonly used Internet search tool is a search engine. Search engines take keywords entered by the user, search Internet content, and return material that matches the keywords. Examples of popular search engines include Google, Yahoo!, Ask.com, Bing, and AOL.com. Search engines vary in how they search the Internet and return matches. Therefore, results returned via one search engine may differ from another.

Meta search engines, also known as aggregators, are search tools that simultaneously search several search engines to return results that match the user's search criteria. Examples of meta search engines include Dogpile, Sputtr, Clusty, and Search.com. OmniMedicalSearch is a meta search engine used to search for medical information.

Portals

A portal or web portal is a site that serves as a gateway or starting point to access varied types of information such as email, discussion boards, current events, search tools, online shopping, and so on. The information is organized and presented in a manner that is user-friendly. By capturing user information, content presented to the user via a portal may be tailored to the user's interests. Patient portals are becoming increasingly popular today both in outpatient and inpatient settings. These portals allow patients to login to the portal via a user ID and password, and access their medical records electronically. Patients are able to view their laboratory test results, see past appointments, make future appointments, and communicate with their healthcare provider via email.

About the Author

Athena Fernandes, DNP, MSN, RN-BC is a Senior Physician Systems Analyst at Penn Medicine Chester County Hospital. She is a board certified nurse informaticist, with a master's degree in nursing informatics. Dr. Fernandes is actively involved on professional committees at the American Nursing Informatics Association (ANIA) and the Greater Delaware Valley ANIA Chapter.

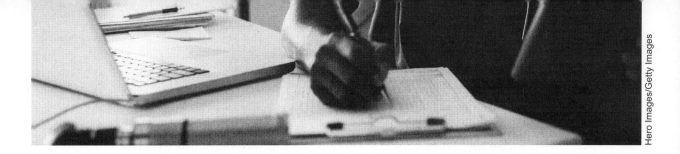

Appendix C

An Overview of Tools for the Informatics Nurse

Carolyn Sipes, PhD, CNS, APN, PMP, RN-BC

A nurse informaticist, or essentially any nurse—be it in a practice or leadership role—can always benefit from tools that help organize a variety of tasks and activities or identify quality issues.

Tools for Processes

Examples of four different types of tools frequently used when defining or monitoring a process include workflows, cause-and-effect diagrams, checklists, and scatter diagrams. This is a category of diagramming techniques to use when identifying risks and quality management concerns. Examples are included below.

Workflows

How tasks move from one to the next and the order in which they flow is known as a workflow. Drawing out and using a workflow can be useful when organizing assignments or any work that needs to be completed within a certain timeframe. Within a workflow are the activities, decision points, and other attributes related to the process to be defined. Using this process, define what needs to be completed first, working through an entire sequence of activities step by step. Sketching out a visual diagram of the task or activity can help make sure nothing is omitted.

The workflow example below moves through three steps, then identifies a decision that needs to be made before continuing to step four, with continuation through the entire process until completed.

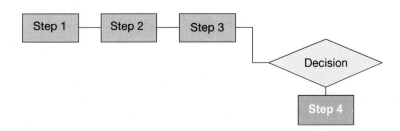

Cause-and-Effect or Fishbone Diagramming

Another useful tool, a cause-and-effect diagram, also known as a fishbone diagram, is used to identify and trace problems and then track the cause back to the root. This is also called root-cause analysis. The first step in the process is to state what the problem is, then ask "why" any number of times until the source or cause has been identified. Examples of items on the arrows or causes might be people, technology, a process, or different environments.

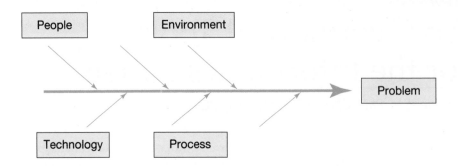

Checklists

Checklists are another simple way of gathering data in order to organize facts in an easy way so an issue or problem can be reviewed in more detail. Some of the most common examples are checklists for frequencies of an event or consequences of using a particular process.

Category of Issue	Frequency/Date of Occurrence	Consequence if Not Resolved
1		
2		
3		

Scatter or Correlation Charts

A scatter or correlation chart provides a quick, visual way of looking at how one variable or item relates to another, either in a positive, negative way or no (zero) correlation. Variables are plotted out on a regression line, x- and y-axis. If the line goes up to the right, it represents a positive correlation; if it goes down to the left, it represents a negative correlation.

The x-axis could represent something as simple as temperature, and the y-axis something like time. In this example, temperature goes up over time.

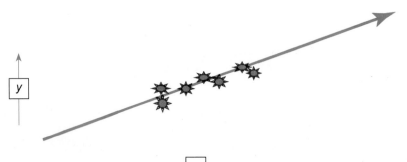

More Checklists

Another type of tracking chart is known as the responsible, accountable, consulted, and informed (RACI) checklist. When a group is assigned different levels of responsibilities where each member has a different task, it is important to track who is doing what; for example, who is responsible and who might just be consulted or just kept informed about the task.

Tasks/Activities	Owner/Responsible	Accountable	Consulted	Informed
Task 1				
Task 2				

Gantt Chart

A Gantt chart is another way to track different tasks and provide a quick visual representation of due dates, including duration times and start and end dates as well as tasks, subtasks, and who is responsible for making sure the task is completed.

Task Number	Task Name	Task Duration	Owner	3/13	3/20	3/27
Task 1						
Task 2						
Task 3						

There are other commercial tools available to use depending on the specific activity. These include many from the Microsoft Office suite, such as Access to develop databases, Excel to develop and track spreadsheets, and Project to help track projects in more detail. These tools typically are used by organizations for specific projects or purposes.

Testing and Testing Types

There are many different types of tests run before an application is made available to the end users. Testing is done to make sure the system is functioning as designed; in other words, it works the way the end users require it to work in order to accomplish daily tasks such as clinical documentation in a patient record. Tests are completed in phases as the system is built and prior to end users actually using the system, again to make sure everything is working properly. Some of the different types of tests include functional, load testing, regression, stress testing, acceptance, and security testing.

The written examples of how a certain task or process flows, what might happen in that particular situation or case, what a workflow might be, and/or tools used in the specific instances are called use cases. Use cases are very common in the testing process prior to implementation of electronic health record systems (EHRS). Many of the types of testing described below include an example of a use case.

Acceptance Testing

This occurs when the end users are asked to test the functionality of a system or module to make sure it works as it is supposed to. This is based on the workflow to a particular department. End users are given access to the functionality; they login and go through a number of test scripts, entering patient data in the different modules to make sure everything is working properly and accurately.

An example or use case of a clinical documentation test script might include entering patient information such as physical assessment, vital signs, and medication and procedures orders, then making sure the information populates each of the correct areas of the echart.

Functional Testing

This is another type of testing that occurs before the system goes "live." Functional testing is done to make sure information entered into a patient record goes to the correct place; for example, x-ray orders go to the correct place and departments.

Interface Testing

In interface testing, data is tracked to make sure it flows across an interface—a place where two systems interact or communicate—to the correct target.

A use case might examine an order for a radiology procedure written in an order-entry program. The order is expected to move across an interface to the radiology information system. The radiology department acknowledges receipt of the order, which is communicated back to the order-entry program.

Regression Testing

Regression testing involves using repeated episodes of testing with the same test scripts/ functions. Using the same test scripts provides a standard for this kind of iterative testing. This type of testing is especially important after there has been an upgrade or fix to the system. This is a standardized process used to make sure that the fix or upgrade did not cause some issue, break something else, or impact the remaining system in any way.

System Testing

System testing occurs when all of the different tests have been completed and all problems addressed. The entire system is turned on for what is called a dry run. The main test includes the question, "Do *all* of the different functions work together as designed?"

Graphical User Interface Testing

Graphical user interface (GUI) testing includes testing of software to make sure it meets expectations and requirements defined in the legal documents, scope, and charter developed during project design and planning phases. There are many functions tested during this phase, such as all data entry meets design requirements, moving from tab to tab works flawlessly, all information entered into the system populates each area and module appropriately, the minimum number of tabs/tab functions is needed to reach a specific tab (e.g., when inputting medication or procedure orders for a patient, what is the number of places or screens required to complete entry of a medication order?), and the category lists/drop-downs are correct.

Load Testing

Load testing is designed to test the system at the highest use times. This test is conducted during peak activity times to test system response rates. Response rates can be assessed by the speed with which different key areas can be populated with information and data, and by the number of users that can be using the system at the same time before performance degrades.

Time tests are run when the system is at peak capacity with both information and number of users. The outcome of testing may indicate a need for more RAM and computing power.

Security Testing

The process designed to test a variety of internal and external challenges to security—such as hacking the system—is called security testing. Security testing also monitors password challenges, confidentially of patient data, and backup plans in event of breaches such as those from outside threats including human and nonhuman (e.g., weather issues). This area requires expertise in security tools and knowledge in application and malicious programs, as well as in new web applications and how they can impact overall system security.

Usability Testing

Usability testing is a process where end users have full access to the software/system in an environment where there is no impact on real patients. Users are observed on how well they react and move through difference tasks. End users are observed and debriefed for factors such as ease of use, whether it is too difficult to tab through a workflow, the number of clicks it takes to get to the right screen, and if the screens are pleasing and easy to work with. Many times, surveys are conducted at the end of the test to obtain additional feedback. This information is prioritized based on critical need and impact on workflow.

Summary

In summary, this has been an overview of the key tools that may be used in your organization for a variety of reasons, such as quality management, risk assessment, project management in varying levels of detail, or assessment of a workflow/process. The second part defined a few of the testing models and methodologies used with EHRS implementations that may be more familiar. This is only a partial list of many, many tools and testing methods available to be used in a variety of settings. It is only meant to provide an introduction, with a recommendation that there is much more to explore.

About the Author

Carolyn Sipes teaches nursing informatics at Chamberlain College of Nursing. She has more than 30 years' experience in management, consulting, and teaching that includes national and international implementation of electronic health records (EHRs). She holds project management professional (PMP) certification through the Project Management Institute (PMI), eight Epic clinical systems certifications, is board certified by the American Nurses Credentialing Center in Nursing Informatics (RN-BC), and is an ANCC Nursing Informatics Content expert. Dr. Sipes has published and presented extensively and authored the book, *Project Management for the Advanced Practice Nurse*.

Glossary

Administrative information systems   Systems that support patient care by managing financial and demographic information and providing reporting capabilities.

Admission/Discharge/Transfer system   Tracks patient activities and location from admission through all transfers within a facility through discharge.

Affordable Care Act   US legislation intended to improve healthcare quality through using information technology, ensuring affordable care, and increasing the number of insured persons.

Agency for Healthcare Research and Quality   Agency within the Department of Health and Human Services devoted to improving healthcare quality and safety.

Alert/Alarm fatigue   Phenomenon that occurs when the volume of alerts, alarms, or warning messages acts contrary to intention through desensitizing the clinician to the indicators and/or the purpose.

American Nurses Association   Professional organization for nurses.

Analytics   Discovery, interpretation, and communication of meaningful patterns from data to offer solutions and drive decisions.

Anesthesia information management system   Supports real-time anesthetic management of the patient in the operating suite.

Antivirus software   Set of computer programs capable of finding and eliminating viruses and other malicious programs from scanned disks, computers, and networks.

Association for Perioperative Registered Nurses   Professional organization representing perioperative registered nurses.

Asynchronous connected health   Healthcare services in a setting other than face-to-face that involves asynchronous exchange between a patient and provider.

Audiovisual monitor   Electronic device for displaying video and audio output from an information source.

Audit trail   Electronic tool that can track system access by individual user, by user class, or by all persons who viewed a specific client record.

Authentication   Action that verifies the authority of users to receive specified data.

Authorization   Process that sets level-of-access privileges and provides training for healthcare workers to locate and obtain correct patient-level information during their daily workflow, based upon their need to know.

Automatic sign-off   Mechanism that logs a user off the computer after a specific period of inactivity.

Back loaded   Information that is preloaded into the system before the go-live date.

Bandwidth   Measure of the information carrying capacity of a communications channel.

Barcode scanning   Optical-scanning technology used for positive patient identification, administration of correct medications, and inventory control.

Best of breed   Refers to the best available technology solution for a given purpose.

Big data   Very large data sets that are beyond human capability to analyze or manage without the aid of information technology.

Bioinformatics   Applying informatics skills to understand and organize information associated with life at the molecular and genetic levels, inclusive of research, taxonomies, and standard terminologies.

Biometrics   A unique, measurable characteristic or trait of a human being for automatically recognizing or verifying identity.

Business-continuity management   Process to ensure that organizations can withstand any disruption to normal functioning.

Business-continuity planning   Combines information technology and disaster recovery planning with business functions recovery planning.

Business impact assessment or analysis   Process of determining the critical functions of the organization and the information vital to maintain operations, as well as the applications, databases, hardware, and communications facilities that use, house, or support this information.

Business intelligence   Integration of business data from different sources to optimize its use and understanding in business decisions; data are comprised of strategies and processes, as well as a tool set.

Certificate authority   Trusted third party that issues digital certificates that certify ownership of a public key.

Change control board   An organizational entity that handles requests for changes or issues in order to keep project scope manageable as plans to implement HIT move forward.

Chief nursing informatics officer   An executive leadership role that represents nursing interests with informatics-related practices, policies, and issues.

Classification system   Approach that uses mutually exclusive categories for specific purposes such as describing the details of a patient encounter for clinical, administrative, or reimbursement issues.

Clinical Care Classification System   Nursing classification designed to document the six steps of the nursing process across the care continuum. Consists of two interconnected terminologies—the CCC of Nursing Diagnosis and Outcomes and the CCC of Nursing Interventions.

Clinical-data networks   Entities developed to support research on patient outcomes rather than the care delivered; typically comprised of several types of healthcare systems that partner to conduct research.

Clinical decision support system   Supports healthcare practitioners in making patient-care decisions by integrating patient data with current clinical knowledge.

Clinical information systems   Large computerized database management systems used to access the patient data that are needed to plan, implement, and evaluate care. May also be known as *patient care information systems.*

Clinical nurse specialist   Advanced-practice nurse prepared at the graduate level to practice in a specialty area who often engages in research, supports direct-care nurses, and helps drive practice changes.

Clinical-research informatics   Application of informatics to methods supporting clinical and translational research, particularly knowledge discovery and secondary use of data.

Clinical terminology   Concepts that support clinical constructs, such as diagnostic studies, history and physical examinations, visit notes, ancillary department information, nursing notes, assessments, flow sheets, vital signs, and outcome measures. This can be mapped to a broader classification system for administrative, regulatory, and fiscal reporting requirements.

Closed source   Software owned by a vendor and for which a customer pays a fee to use but does not own.

Cloud computing   Internet-based, on-demand model of computing that relies upon shared resources; this model provides higher-level service than may be available locally with less investment of resources.

Codes   Letters, numbers, or a combination thereof, that represent concepts in a computer system.

Codified   Concept with an assigned code.

Cognitive walkthrough   This usability assessment method is a detailed review of a sequence of real or proposed actions to complete a task in a system.

Communication plan   Tool used in phase two of project management (planning) that shows how each upper-leadership shareholder and team member will receive communication and updates on the project status and issues.

Computer forensics   Collection of electronic evidence for purposes of litigation and internal investigations.

Computerized provider (or practitioner) order system   An application that supports direct electronic entry of patient-care-related orders by authorized practitioners and direct transmission of those orders to designated entities.

Computer literacy   Familiarity with the use of computers, including software tools such as word processing, spreadsheets, databases, presentation graphics, and email.

Confidentiality   Tacit understanding that private information shared in a situation in which a relationship has been established for the purpose of treatment or delivery of services will remain protected.

Concept   Expression with a single unambiguous meaning, although it may have one or more representations called *synonyms* or *terms.* Used to document ideas and express orders,

assessments, and outcomes within an EHR; they are uniquely identified by codes.

Configurability   Refers to the extent that a given software product can be adapted or changed to meet a user's preferences.

Connected health   Model or platform by which technology-assisted healthcare is delivered between at least two points, involving either synchronous assessment or asynchronous exchange.

Consultants   Outside experts brought in to support/educate project team members and/or end users.

Consumer health informatics   Use of electronic information and communication to improve medical outcomes and healthcare decision making from the patient/consumer perspective.

Contextual inquiry   When an informaticist interviews and observes users at their actual sites, one person at a time, focusing on users' points of view.

Continuity of care record   Technical informatics standard that provides a snapshot of a person's current health and healthcare to a provider who does not have access to that person's electronic health record.

Continuity planning   Essential component of strategic planning designed to maintain business operations.

Continuous-quality-improvement system   Provides continuous monitoring and evaluation of performance and supports audit capability; also known as *quality-assurance system.*

Criteria-based standards   Technical specifications that include *defining* characteristics, content, formats, and workflows for use of the health information exchange.

Critical-care information system   Integrates captured physiological data with practitioner documentation and clinical data management functions, as well as access and communication with remote experts.

C suite   Term used to refer to a corporation's senior executives, such as the chief executive officer (CEO).

Current Procedural Terminology   Classification system that lists medical services and procedures performed by physicians, and is used for physician billing and payer reimbursement.

Current state   What is occurring now and might not be working.

Cybercrime   Commonly refers to the theft of personal information stored on computers, such as Social Security numbers.

Data   Collection of numbers, characters, or facts that are gathered according to some perceived need for analysis and, possibly, action at a later point in time.

Database   File structure that supports the storage of data in an organized fashion and allows data retrieval as meaningful information.

Database administrator   Person responsible for overseeing all activities related to maintaining a database and optimizing its use.

Data cleansing   Use of software to improve the quality of data to ensure that it is accurate enough for use in data mining and warehousing.

Data governance   Collection of policies, standards, processes, and controls applied to an organization's data to ensure that it is available to appropriate persons when, where, and in the format needed while maintaining security.

Data integrity Ability to collect; store; and retrieve correct, complete, and current data so that the data are available to authorized users when needed.

Data management Process of controlling the storage, retrieval, and use of data to optimize accuracy and utility while safeguarding integrity.

Data mining Technique that looks for hidden patterns and relationships in large groups of data using software.

Data modeling Identification of data requirements to support processes for an information system; this is a key step in the design of a database or HER.

Data science Systematic study of digital data.

Data scrubbing See *data cleansing*.

Data warehouse Provides a powerful method of managing and analyzing data.

Decision-support software Computer programs that organize information to aid choices related to patient care or administrative issues.

Dental informatics Sub-discipline of clinical informatics dedicated to the improvement of dental health.

Device integration Ability of systems to "talk" to each other, for example, cardiac monitors that automatically download data into the electronic health record system.

Digital camera imagery Stores images digitally for ease of transmission and storage.

Digital curation The long-term preservation and maintenance of digital data for later access and use.

Digital literacy Use of computer technology and smartphones to read and interpret media, reproduce data and images, and evaluate and apply knowledge gained through exploration of the digital world; it may be used interchangeably with computer literacy.

Digitization Conversion of data and information into an electronic format.

Disaster Manmade or natural event with the potential to cause considerable damage and possibly loss of life.

Disaster recovery Processes that help organizations deal with disruptive events.

Discovery informatics Scientific models and theories used to create computer-based discovery of new learning in big data, reducing reliance on human cognition.

Disease registries Collections of secondary data related to patients with a specific diagnosis, condition, or procedure, used for tracking clinical care and outcomes.

Disruptive innovation A new product, service, or process that begins in a small market (small number of consumers) and rapidly attracts a larger market until it replaces existing dominant products, services, or processes.

Dissemination Process of widely transmitting or circulating data and information, including research knowledge.

Doctorate of Nursing Practice Terminal degree with emphasis on evidence-based practice, quality improvement, and systems leadership.

Downtime Period of time when an information system is not operational or available for use.

Educational-needs assessment Process to obtain data on educational opportunities.

eHealth Wide range of healthcare activities involving the electronic transfer of health-related information on the Internet.

eHealth literacy Ability to use electronic sources to search for, find, comprehend, and evaluate information and images found online, and apply acquired knowledge to address or solve a health issue.

Electronic documentation Digital capture of assessments and interventions that permit simultaneous use of electronic health records from multiple sites by multiple users; formats may vary but structured data is commonly used, which may support standard terminologies.

Electronic health record system Database-management software enabling the many functions needed to create and maintain an electronic health record.

Electronic intensive-care unit Remote care option that allows critically-ill patients to remain in rural hospitals with support from intensivists and ICU nurses at another location.

Electronic lab reporting Process of electronically transmitting laboratory results that identify reportable conditions from laboratories across the nation to public health agencies.

Electronic medical record Legal record created in hospitals and ambulatory settings of a single encounter or visit that is the source of data for the electronic health record.

Emotional intelligence Structured approach to being aware of emotions—modifying emotional reactions.

Enterprise system Information system that improves the functions of a business entity or organization through integration and coordination of its processes.

Ergonomics Scientific study of work and space, including details that impact productivity and health.

Expanding search criteria Strategies to improve database search results, such as adding Boolean operators "and", "or", "not," or text phrases.

External environment Includes those interested parties and competitors who are outside the healthcare institution.

Feature creep Uncontrolled addition of features or functions without regard to timelines or budget.

Federal Register Daily publication for rules, proposed rules, and notices of the US Government.

File deletion software Overwrites files with meaningless information so that sensitive information cannot be accessed.

Filtered resources Materials that have been pre-appraised for quality and content.

Financial system Uses patient demographic data and insurance information to charge for services and receive reimbursement; this is integrated with the registration system.

Firewall Type of gateway designed to protect private network resources from outside hackers, network damage, and theft or misuse of information.

Five phases of the project management life cycle Design or initiation, planning, implementation, monitoring and control, and closure with lessons learned.

Function Task that may be automated or performed manually.

Functional test Final process in project management phase two (planning) that ensures the innovation works as designed.

Future state What is desired and planned for in the project.

Gantt chart Graphic presentation that shows a project schedule with start and finish dates of selected component tasks and the person responsible for each task or sub-task; it is used for at-a-glance management.

Gap analysis Comparison of actual performance with potential or desired performance.

Garbage can model A model of organizational decision making, including policy making processes.

Geographic information system Hardware, software, and data for capturing, managing, analyzing, and displaying all forms of geographically referenced information.

Goal alignment Linking individual goal outcomes with organization goal outcomes.

Goals and objectives In the context of project management, goals identify the high-level context for the project in alignment with the organization's mission; project objectives delineate specific, measureable, achievable, relevant, and time-specific activities to achieve the goal(s).

Go-live Date when an information system is first used, or the process of starting to use an information system.

Grief model Refers to work by theorist Kubler-Ross on the stages of grief, which are also seen with major changes generated by a HIT implementation.

Hardware Physical components of a computer.

Healthcare Information Exchange Electronic sharing of patient information such as demographic data, allergies, presenting complaint, diagnostic test values, and other relevant data between providers such as primary physicians, specialists, hospitals, and ambulatory care settings according to nationally recognized standards.

Healthcare information system Computer hardware and software dedicated to the collection, storage, processing, retrieval, and communication of patient care information in a healthcare organization.

Healthcare terminology standards Strategy to enable and support widespread interoperability among healthcare software applications for the purpose of sharing information.

Health games (gamification) A means to educate consumers on health issues.

Health-information networks Entities that enable the exchange of patient-level information within a multi-site healthcare organization, within a collection of such organizations in one state, or within a collection of such organizations across states.

Health Insurance Portability and Accountability Act Also known as the Kennedy–Kassebaum Bill, it is the first federal legislation to protect automatic client records and to mandate that all electronic transactions include only HIPAA compliant codes.

Health information technology Information systems and other information technology used to record, monitor, and deliver patient care as well as perform managerial and organizational functions.

Health literacy Degree to which individuals can obtain, process, and understand the basic health information and services needed to make appropriate health decisions.

Help desk First line of user support within an organization. It is a support service, rather than a specific location, for computer users that is often available 24 hours a day by calling a special telephone number. Help desk staff have an information system or computer background and are familiar with all of the software applications and hardware in use.

Heuristic evaluations Assessments of a product according to accepted guidelines or published usability principles.

Hospital information system Group of information systems used within a hospital or enterprise that support and enhance patient care, and consists of two major types of information systems: clinical and administrative.

Human-computer interaction The study of how people design, implement, evaluate, and use interactive computer systems.

Human factors The scientific study of the interaction between people, machines, and their work environments.

Human-resources information system Provides tracking for payroll purposes, such as attendance and paid-time-off; health benefits, including insurance information; and career development.

ID management Administrative area that deals with identifying individuals in a system and controlling their access to resources.

Implantable medical device A surgically implanted item used to treat or monitor a medical condition or improve the function of a particular body part; pacemakers and defibrillators are a common example.

Implementation science Studies how change takes place.

Infodemiology Science of distribution and determinants of information in an electronic format with the ultimate aim to inform public health and public policy; it may also be called *information epidemiology*.

Informatics Science and art of turning data into information.

Informatics competencies Ability to perform the tasks associated with informatics.

Information Collection of data that have been interpreted and examined for patterns and structure.

Information-and-data privacy Right to choose the conditions and extent to which information and beliefs are shared.

Information consent Occurs when an individual authorizes healthcare personnel to use and share personal information based on an informed understanding of how this information will be used for treatment purposes.

Information literacy Ability to recognize when information is needed as well as the skills to find, evaluate, and use needed information effectively.

Information networks Set of standards, specifications, hardware, software, and policies that enable information exchange.

Information security Protection of confidential information against inadvertent disclosure or threats to its integrity.

Information system A computer system that uses hardware and software to process data into information in order to solve a problem.

Information-system security Protection of information systems and the information housed on them from unauthorized use or threats to integrity.

Interface terminology   Also known as *point of care terminology*, it consists of terms familiar to clinicians.

International Classification of Diseases   An international standard diagnostic classification for health-management purposes and clinical use; it is used to classify mortality and morbidity data from patient records.

International Classification of Nursing Practice   A system that serves to unify various approved nursing languages and classification systems to ensure the acceptance of common meanings across different settings.

International standards   Technical informatics standards allowing worldwide communication of patient information.

Internet of things   Devices with embedded microchips, sensors, and actuators that use Internet Protocol (IP) to share data with other machines or software over communications networks, examples include thermostats, appliances, and more.

Interoperability   The ability of two entities, human or machine, to exchange and predictably use data or information while retaining the original meaning of that data.

Keyword   Significant term or concept used to index resources and, later, to search for resources containing the same word.

Kiosks   Specially housed computer systems designed for public use in unattended areas for access to health programs or search sites.

Knowledge databases   Collections of literature and research evidence that are indexed to support organized search and retrieval.

Knowledge   Synthesis of information derived from several sources to produce a single concept or idea.

Knowledge discovery in databases   Extraction of implicit, unknown, and potentially useful information from data.

Knowledge management   Structured process for the generation, storage, distribution, and application of both tacit knowledge (personal experience) and explicit knowledge (evidence).

Knowledge management systems   Sets of information systems that enable organizations to tap the expertise of their human resources to improve performance.

Knowledge translation   Applying research to practice.

Kotter's change management theory   One of several foundational theories of leading others through planned change; it delineates an eight-step process indicating buy-in from administration as important for success.

Kubler-Ross   Theorist who identified stages of grief, which are also seen with major changes generated by a HIT implementation; also referred to as *the grief model*.

Lab-on-a-chip   Emerging informatics technology that provides point of care complex biochemical analyses via small-volume samples for the purpose of early diagnosis, preventing debilitating illness, and containing costs.

Laboratory information systems   Computer system for use by laboratories that provides many benefits as a result of automated order entry.

Learning curve   Time required for end users to adapt to and efficiently, effectively, and competently use an information technology system or subsystem.

Lewin's change model   One of several foundational theories for leading others through planned change; identifies three steps: unfreezing, changing, and refreezing.

Literacy   Ability to process and critique meaning using reading, writing, and oral language within a specific context.

Lobbyists   Experts at encouraging others to act in a predetermined way.

Logical Observation Identifiers, Names, and Codes   Terminology that includes laboratory and clinical observations.

Maintenance   An information system life cycle phase that includes evaluation; the period in which new behaviors, such as work flows and processes, are solidified.

Malicious software   Programs written for the purpose of stealing information, causing annoyance, or performing covert actions.

Master person index   Enterprise-wide database containing a unique identifier for every person (patient) registered at the organization.

Meaningful use   Use of health information technology (HIT) legislated by the American Recovery and Reinvestment Act of 2009 to collect specific data with the intent to improve care and population health, engage patients, and ensure privacy and security.

Measurable   Refers to an observable, quantifiable entity that can support a decision; in project management, measureable entities track progress and determine completion.

Measures of success   Benchmarks by which a project may be deemed as having met its intended purpose(s), such as user acceptance or fulfilling business objectives.

Medical informatics   Application of informatics to all of the healthcare disciplines as well as the practice of medicine.

Membership fee   Health information exchange model that calls for stakeholders to pay to support shared services for all.

Metadata   Set of data that provides information about how, when, and by whom data are collected, formatted, and stored.

Metrics   Quantifiable indicators that determine the progress or conclusion of work toward a specific goal.

mHealth   Use of wireless devices and sensor networks to access healthcare information or services from the community, or to transmit information to providers.

Mission   Purpose or reason for an organization's existence, representing the fundamental and unique aspirations that differentiate it from others.

Must-haves   Components deemed critical for inclusion in an information system.

National Health Information Network   The Office of the National Coordinator (ONC) for Health Information Technology (HIT) initiative to provide the standards, services, and policies that enable secure health information exchange (HIE) over the Internet.

Network   Combination of hardware and software that allows the communication and electronic transfer of information between computers.

Nice-to-haves   Desired components considered non-critical for inclusion in an information system; these are features that can wait until system optimization.

North American Nursing Diagnosis International Terminology to identify human responses to health promotion, risk, and disease that is recognized by the American Nurses Association.

Nursing Interventions Classification A standardized classification of interventions that describes the activities that nurses perform.

Nurse practitioners Advanced-practice nurses prepared at the graduate level and qualified to assume some of the duties and responsibilities associated with physicians—help to drive practice changes.

Omaha system American Nurses Association recognized research-based taxonomy that provides a framework for integrating and sharing clinical data. It is widely used in settings such as home care, hospice, public health, school health, and prisons.

One vendor Refers to a suite of related, interoperable software applications that collectively make data more accessible, even though some individual applications may not provide the most highly rated solution for a given purpose.

Ontology System that organizes concepts by meaning, describing their definitional structure/relationship as well as organizing the concepts for storage and retrieval of semantically accurate data.

Open source Software available for use and modification by the public at no cost.

Operating room information system Provides software functions to manage real-time patient care in the perioperative period, to monitor and manage surgical resources, to support documentation, and to enable operational analyses; also known as *surgical information systems* or *perioperative information systems*.

Operational and business models Prototypes for the management of health information networks for the health information exchange.

Password Alphanumeric code required for access and use of some computers or information systems as a security measure against unauthorized use. The password does not appear on the monitor display when it is keyed in.

Perioperative information system See *Operating room information system*

Perioperative Nursing Data Set Standardized perioperative nursing vocabulary provides nurses with a clear, precise, and universal language for clinical problems and surgical treatments.

Peripheral devices Any device attached externally to a computer (e.g., scanners, mouse pointers, printers, keyboards, and clinical monitors such as pulse oximeters and weight scales).

Personal Health Record Lifelong tool for managing health information, such as disease conditions, allergies, medications, past surgeries, and other relevant information.

Pharmacy information systems Support the management and distribution of pharmacological products and related devices including inventory control, alerts, and reporting capability.

Phishing A ruse to get consumers to divulge personal information through social engineering and technical subterfuge via the use of electronic communication.

Physiological monitoring systems Obtain and electronically store real-time patient data, collected intermittently or continuously, related to a variety of physiological parameters; data may be integrated with electronic health records.

Picture archiving and communication system Supports electronic storage, retrieval, presentation, and sharing of digital images from x-rays, magnetic resonance imaging (MRI), computerized tomography, ultrasound, and other imaging technologies.

Playground Software environment where people can use a new system or application within a facility without fear of causing damage.

Point of care Computer access at the actual worksite, which, in the delivery of healthcare, is at the patient's bedside.

Policies Written documents articulating sets of ideas or plans for making decisions; they may be generated by governments, organizations, groups, or individuals.

Policy entrepreneur Person who commits interest, time, and money to moving a proposed policy forward.

Politics Process of persuading someone to accept your perspective to act on bills, policies, and programs.

Portal Websites that collect information from the user and offer personalized features for individual users that may require registration.

Portal for access An electronic access point for authorized users to sign on to a system or health information exchange to view, record, retrieve, download information, or contact a provider.

Predictive analytics Uses past and current data to forecast the likelihood that an event will occur; also known as *predictive modeling*.

Predictive modeling See *Predictive analytics*.

Privacy Freedom from intrusion as well as control over the exposure of personal information.

Production environment Point at which a planned information system is actually used to process and retrieve information and support the delivery of services.

Program and service fee Health information exchange model that charges stakeholders for participation in services.

Project Management Institute Private organization that defines standards and methodologies for organizing projects into structured processes and formats, provides educational resources on project management, and manages the certification of project managers.

Project management life cycle Sequence of activities or phases conducted to design or initiate, plan, implement, monitor, control, and conclude any endeavor, including deployment of information technology.

Project planning Early phase in project management life cycle.

Project scope Defines the size and details of an effort.

Public health Promotion and protection of the health of people and the communities where they work and live.

Public health informatics Application of information and computer science and technology to public health practice, research, and learning.

Public key infrastructure Provides a unique code for each user.

Push or pull function Two communication methods that can be built into communication software as optional functions. The push method distributes data and information without a request from a receiver. The pull method requires a user to actively access desired data and information.

Quality-assurance system See *continuous-quality-improvement system*.

Radio frequency Wireless technology that creates detectable electromagnetic waves; common examples include anti-theft tags on store inventory and identification badges.

Radiology information system Provides scheduling of diagnostic tests, communication of patient information, generation of patient instructions and preparation procedures, and file room management.

Real-time analytics Examines current data to foster learning and prediction; in clinical settings, it uses point of care data from multiple sources to present immediate, actionable information to clinicians.

Record-locator service Computer service to access and find health records registered to a single individual.

Reference terminology Set of concepts with definitional relationships that is frequently an ontology and, therefore, can be used to support data aggregation, disaggregation, retrieval, and analysis.

Registration and scheduling system Collects and electronically stores client identification and demographic data, which is verified and updated at each visit; it provides a framework for managing patients' identities and appointments across clinical information systems, as well as information for billing and other administrative purposes.

Remote access The ability to use the resources contained on a network, or an information system, from a location outside of the facility where they are physically located.

Remote patient monitoring Personal health and medical data collected from an individual at one site via electronic communication technologies and transmitted to a provider at a different site for use in care and related support.

Repository Central storage location for data.

Request for Information A document sent to vendors that explains the institution's plans for purchasing and installing an information system with the goal of determining which vendors can meet the organization's basic requirements.

Request for Proposal Document sent to vendors detailing the requirements of a potential information system with the purpose of soliciting proposals from vendors that describe their capabilities to meet these requirements.

Resource availability Extent to which planned-for resources are capable or ready to be used when needed in a project.

Results reporting An application that enables direct electronic sharing of an individual's laboratory and other diagnostic test results within that person's electronic health record.

Risk assessment and management plan Project management phase two (planning) tool that documents, ranks, and tracks risks and determines how risks will be handled.

Risk-management system Identifies and documents potential risks and develops strategies to deal with them.

Roll-out Staggered, or rolling, system implementation, sometimes refers to the preceding marketing campaign as well.

Sabotage Intentional destruction of computer equipment or records to disrupt services.

Scope creep Unexpected and uncontrolled growth of user expectations as a project progresses.

Scope document Written description of a project's goal(s) and what must be done to achieve the goal(s).

Shared electronic health record A type of electronic health record (EHR) supported by an electronic health record system (EHRS) that allows clinicians to access an individual patient's EHR data and information located at different facilities.

Site visit A scheduled information-gathering trip to another organization using the information system under consideration for adoption.

Smart pumps Infusion devices with software that sets parameters for fluid and medication infusion and communicates with pharmacy or medication administration systems.

Smart technology Integrated technology that saves time and physical burdens, and improves patient outcomes.

SNOMED Clinical Terms Globally recognized, controlled-healthcare vocabulary that provides a common language for electronic health records.

Software Computer programs or stored sequences of instructions to the computer.

Spam Unwanted or "junk" mail.

Sponsor For each project, this is an individual with overall accountability for the successful achievement of the project meeting the business goals agreed to by the organization.

Spyware Data collection mechanism that installs itself without the user's permission during web browsing or when downloading software.

Stakeholders Persons with a vested interest in a project because it will impact them in some way.

Standardized terminologies Structured, controlled languages developed according to terminology development guidelines and approved by an authoritative body.

Strategic plan A process that creates an entity's vision of the future, develops broad goals for reaching that future, and specifies high-level steps for achieving these goals.

Strategic planning Development of a comprehensive, long-range plan for guiding the activities and operations of an organization.

Strategic thinking Vision or process that an organization uses to determine what its future should look like.

Structural (imaging) informatics Research and practice applications representing, managing, and using information about the physical organization of the body.

Subject-matter experts People who have an advanced level of knowledge about a particular field or topic.

Surgical information system See *operating room information system* or *perioperative information system*.

Survivability Capability of a system, as a whole, to fulfill its mission in a timely manner, in the presence of attacks, failures, or accidents.

Sustainable models   Refers to business models that enable health information networks to function in the present environment and adapt to future environments.

SWOT analysis   A process that examines the strengths, weaknesses, opportunities, and threats of a given situation.

Syndromic surveillance   Near real-time use of early disease indicators from pre-diagnostic data, such as symptoms and assessment data, to detect and characterize events that may need public health investigation before diagnosis occurs.

System check   A mechanism provided by a computer system to assist users by prompting them to complete a task, verify information, or prevent entry of inappropriate information.

System development life cycle   A sequence of activities in the planning, designing, testing, implementation, and evaluation of an information system or sub-system.

Task analysis   One of the most well-known collections of usability techniques, involving systematic methods of determining what users are required to do with systems by accounting for behavioral actions between users and computers. It is used to determine the goals of a new system and the role of information technology in user activities.

Team selection   An activity that needs to occur in the first phase of project management.

Teleconferencing   Use of computers, audio and video equipment, and communication links to provide interaction between two or more persons at two or more sites.

Telehealth   Provision of information to healthcare providers and consumers and the delivery of services to clients at remote sites through the use of telecommunication and computer technology.

Telemedicine   Use of telecommunication technologies and computers to provide medical information and services to clients at another site.

Telenursing   Use of telecommunications and computer technology for the delivery of nursing care to clients at another location.

Telepresenter   A clinically and technically trained facilitator on the "patient end" of a connected health encounter that assists in assuring high quality clinical care and patient safety.

Test environment   A separate software program similar to the one used for the actual application or information system that allows programming changes to be tested prior to their implementation in the actual system, thereby protecting the "real" system from unwanted alterations.

Think aloud protocol   Usability method where users talk about what they are doing as they interact with an application. Interactions are observed or recorded and analyzed.

Threat source   Intent or method that targets a vulnerability or triggers a vulnerability.

Tracking board   A data display to provide situational awareness.

Training environment   A separate software application that mirrors the actual information system but permits learners to practice skills without harm to the system or data contained in it. Makes use of fictitious clients and scenarios for instruction and practice.

Transaction fee   Health information exchange model that charges fees for services or products on the basis of benefit to the participants.

Translational bioinformatics   Integration of bioinformatics, structural informatics, statistics, clinical informatics, and data mining to provide a foundation for personalized medicine.

Trusted third party or certificate authority   Term used to refer to an entity that issues digital certificates that certify ownership of a public key.

Unfiltered resources   Materials without limits of quality or specific criteria.

Unified medical language system   Attempt to standardize terms used in healthcare delivery. It is a metathesaurus that contains more than a hundred source vocabularies.

Usability   Specific issues of human performance in achieving specific goals during computer interactions within a particular context.

Usefulness   How well an informatics application meets the needs of the user, within a specific context.

User acceptance   Point at which users think that a new informatics application makes work easier and more effective and efficient.

User experience   Concept addressing all aspects of a user's interaction with a service, system, or HIT product.

Vendor Evaluation Matrix Tool   A tool that facilitates selection of health information technology, consisting of a method for prioritizing vendors and assessment questions that address functionality and usability; it is available through HealthIT.gov.

Videoconferencing   Face-to-face meeting of persons at separate locations through the use of telecommunications and computer technology.

Virus   A malicious program that can disrupt or destroy data.

Vision   Future-oriented, high-level view of what an organization would like to become that provides direction for planning purposes.

Vulnerability   Flaw or weakness in system procedures, design, implementation, or internal controls that could accidentally or intentionally be used to breach security or violate the system's security policy.

Wearable technologies   Fitness tracking and monitoring devices that collect and transmit specific patient data.

Wireless body area network   Specialized communication network that uses sensors in or on the body to monitor and convey data to healthcare providers via the Internet.

Wisdom   Application of knowledge to manage and solve problems.

Work breakdown structure   A plan to develop project timelines or schedule a hierarchical arrangement of all specific tasks by using project-planning software.

Workforce plan   Systematic, written plan addressing informatics training for healthcare staff.

Worm   A malicious program named for the type of damage left behind. It often uses network communication practices to spread itself.

Wrist wearable unit   A smartwatch with the capability to monitor and transmit wearers' activity.

Index